NEUROPHYSIOLOGIE UND PSYCHOPHYSIK DES VISUELLEN SYSTEMS

THE VISUAL SYSTEM: NEUROPHYSIOLOGY AND PSYCHOPHYSICS

SYMPOSION FREIBURG/BR., 28.8.–3.9.1960

HERAUSGEGEBEN VON / EDITED BY

RICHARD JUNG   HANS KORNHUBER

FREIBURG / BR.

MIT 217 ABBILDUNGEN / WITH 217 FIGURES

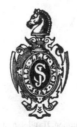

Springer-Verlag
Berlin Heidelberg GmbH
1961

ISBN 978-3-662-22222-5   ISBN 978-3-662-22221-8 (eBook)
DOI 10.1007/978-3-662-22221-8

© by Springer-Verlag Berlin Heidelberg 1961
Ursprünglich erschienen bei Springer-Verlag oHG. Berlin · Göttingen · Heidelberg 1961.
Softcover reprint of the hardcover 1st edition 1961

Inhaltsverzeichnis

Teilnehmerverzeichnis

*Akimoto, H., Neuropsychiatrische Klinik der Universität Tokyo (Japan)

Arduini, A., Istituto di Fisiologia della Università di Pisa (Italien)

Barlow, H., Physiological Laboratory, University of Cambridge (England)

*Bartley, S. H., Michigan State University, Dept. of Psychology, East Lansing (USA)

Baumgardt, E., Laboratoire de Physiologie générale, Université de Paris (Frankreich)

Baumgartner, G., Abteilung für klinische Neurophysiologie der Universität Freiburg/Br.

Beresford, W. A., University Laboratory of Physiology, Oxford (England)

Best, W., Universitäts-Augenklinik, Bonn/Rh.

*Bishop, G. H., School of Medicine, Dept. of Psychiatry and Neurology, Laboratory of Neurophysiology, Washington University, St. Louis (USA)

Bornschein, H., Physiologisches Institut der Universität Wien (Österreich)

Bremer, F., Laboratoire de Pathologie Générale, Université de Bruxelles (Belgien)

Creutzfeldt, O., Dt. Forschungsanstalt für Psychiatrie, Max Planck-Institut, München

DeValois, R. L., Department of Psychology, Indiana University, Bloomington (USA)

Dodt, E., William Kerckhoff-Institut der Max-Planck-Gesellschaft, Bad Nauheim

Donner, K. O., Zoologisches Laboratorium der Universität Helsingfors (Finnland)

Doty, R. W., Center for Brain Research, University of Rochester (USA)

Fillenz, M., University Laboratory of Physiology, Oxford (England)

Galifret, Y., Section de Psychologie experimentale, Collège de France, Paris (Frankreich)

Glees, P., Institut für Histologie und Experimentelle Neuroanatomie, Göttingen

Grüsser, O.-J., und U. Grüsser-Cornehls, Universitäts-Klinik für psychische und Nervenkrankheiten, Göttingen

Hurvich, L. M., und D. Hurvich-Jameson, New York University, Washington Square College of Arts and Science, Dept. of Psychology, New York (USA)

Jaeger, W., Universitäts-Augenklinik, Heidelberg

Jung, R., Abteilung für klinische Neurophysiologie der Universität Freiburg/Br.

Kornhuber, H., Abteilung für klinische Neurophysiologie der Universität Freiburg/Br.

*Lennox-Buchthal, M. A., Universitetets Neurofysiologiske Institut, Kopenhagen (Dänemark)

MacNichol, E. F. jr., The Thomas C. Jenkins Department of Biophysics, The Johns Hopkins University, Baltimore (USA)

Metzger, W., Psychologisches Institut der Universität Münster/Westf.

Monjé, W., Institut für angewandte Physiologie der Universität Kiel

*Motokawa, K., Department of Physiology, Tohoku-University, Sendai (Japan)

Schober, H., Institut für Physiologische Optik, München

Sickel, W., Physiologisches Institut der Karl-Marx-Universität, Leipzig

*Sjöstrand, F. S., Department of Zoology, University of California, Los Angeles (USA)

Söderberg, U., Nobel Institute of Neurophysiology, Karolinska Institutet, Stockholm (Schweden)

Svaetichin, G., Instituto Venezolano de Investigaciones Cientificas, Caracas (Venezuela)

Teuber, H.-L., Department of Psychiatry and Neurology, New York University, Bellevue Medical Center, New York University College of Medicine, New York (USA)

---

* Schriftliche Mitteilung und Diskussion.

*Tomita, T., Department of Physiology, School of Medicine, Keio University, Shinanomachi, Tokyo (Japan)

Vallecalle, E., Instituto de Medicina Experimental, Universidad Central de Venezuela, Caracas (Venezuela)

Verzeano, M., University of California, Medical Center, School of Medicine, Department of Biophysics and Nuclear Medicine Los Angeles (USA)

*Villegas, G.M., Laboratorio de Ultraestructura, Instituto Venezolano de Investigaciones Cientificas, Caracas (Venezuela)

*Villegas, J., Instituto Venezolano de Investigaciones Cientificas, Caracas (Venezuela)

Whitteridge, D., Department of Physiology, University New Building, Edinburgh (Schottland)

Widén, L., Department of Clinical Neurophysiology, Serafimerlasarettet, Stockholm (Schweden)

Wolbarsht, M. L., Physiciology Division, Naval Medical Research Institute, National Naval Medical Center, Bethesda (USA)

_____

* Schriftliche Mitteilung und Diskussion.

Einleitung

Dieses Symposion ist ein Versuch, die subjektive und objektive Sinnesphysiologie des Sehens in Verbindung zu bringen. Die Neurophysiologen, die Einzelmechanismen des peripheren und zentralen Sehsystems untersuchen, sollen mit den Psychologen und Sinnesphysiologen diskutieren, die über die Psychophysik der Sehwahrnehmung beim Menschen arbeiten. Unsere gemeinsame Diskussion ist zunächst ein Experiment. Ob es gelingt, muß sich erst zeigen.

Zwei methodisch völlig verschiedene wissenschaftliche Richtungen zu vereinigen, hat seine Gefahren: Äquivokationen und kritiklose Übernahmen der mit anderen Methoden gewonnenen Ergebnisse können entstehen. Nicht nur die verschiedene Methodik, auch die Verschiedenheit der Untersuchungsobjekte — Katzen und Affen oder sogar Fische auf der einen, Menschen und ihre Wahrnehmungsleistungen auf der anderen Seite — erschweren die Verbindung. Dazu kommen die Unterschiede einer alten und jungen Wissenschaft. Die subjektive Physiologie des Sehens ist ein Werk des 19. Jahrhunderts: FECHNERs „Psychophysik" erschien 1860, vor genau 100 Jahren, HELMHOLTZ' Handbuch in seinen ersten Teilen ebenfalls 1858 und 1860, HERINGs erstes Buch 1861, nachdem PURKINJE bereits 1819 und 1825 die Sehphysiologie eingeleitet hatte. Zwar beschrieb HOLMGREN das Elektroretinogramm schon 1865, doch stammt die Elektrophysiologie des zentralen Sehsystems vorwiegend aus den letzten drei Jahrzehnten, seitdem BISHOP und BARTLEY sowie FISCHER, KORNMÜLLER und TÖNNIES 1932 Belichtungseffekte an der Sehrinde registrierten. Die Neuronenphysiologie des visuellen Systems hat sich vorwiegend in den letzten 20 Jahren entwickelt. HARTLINEs erste Mitteilung über das Limulusauge 1932 blieb zunächst ohne Resonanz, aber seine Einzelfaserregistrierungen am Froschauge 1938 zeigten die receptiven Felder mit Erregungs- und Hemmungs-Konvergenz und begründeten alle späteren Untersuchungen. GRANITs Buch erschien 1947 und die Neuronenableitungen vom visuellen Cortex begannen erst vor 9 Jahren.

Dennoch führen die Wege beider Forschungszweige in dieselbe Richtung und beide haben im Grunde ein gleiches Ziel: Das visuelle System in seinen Funktionen und Leistungen zu erklären und zu verstehen, indem Lichtreize und ihre neuronalen oder psychophysiologischen Effekte messend verglichen werden. Unsere neurophysiologische Arbeit der letzten Jahre ergab so zahlreiche Parallelen mit psychophysischen Ergebnissen, daß es lohnend erschien, auf diesem Symposion gemeinsame Wege zu suchen und die gegenseitige Beziehung und Verständigung zwischen Neurophysiologie und Psychophysik zu fördern.

In einem Symposion ist die Teilnehmerzahl notwendig beschränkt, und auch die Themen müssen begrenzt werden, wenn die Diskussion fruchtbar sein soll. Das Hauptgewicht liegt bei der *Elektrophysiologie*, doch war es notwendig, die Elektronenmikroskopie mit aufzunehmen, da sie viele entscheidende physiologische Anregungen gegeben hat. Auf andere wichtige Forschungsrichtungen, deren Aufnahme anfangs geplant war, mußten wir verzichten. Die Optokinetik und ihre Beziehung zum Sehen hätte ein eigenes Symposion erfordert. Die Photochemie fiel aus, nachdem WALD und RUSHTON absagen mußten. Auch in der Neurophysiologie vermissen wir viele Forscher, die Wichtiges hätten beitragen können: HARTLINE, der Begründer der Neuronenphysiologie des visuellen Systems, war leider verhindert, ebenso FUORTES, so daß wir auf das Limulus-Auge verzichteten. GRANIT, KUFFLER und seine Schüler HUBEL und WIESEL, die für die Diskussion der rezeptiven Felder und Kontrasterscheinungen eingeladen waren, vermissen wir besonders, ebenso wie SMIRNOW, BYZOW und CHANG aus Rußland und China. Bedauerliche Absagen kamen ferner von P. O. BISHOP (Sidney), BURNS (Montreal), BRINDLEY (Cambridge), ENROTH (Stockholm), EVARTS (Bethesda), FERNÁNDEZ-MORÁN (Boston), INGVAR (Lund), KLÜVER (Chikago), KOHLER (Innsbruck) LETTVIN (Boston), LINDSLEY (Los Angeles), MACKAY (London), MÜLLER-LIMMROTH (Münster), O'LEARY (St. Louis) und RATLIFF (New York).

Um so mehr hat uns gefreut, daß andere Kollegen ihre Beiträge schriftlich übersandt haben, nachdem sie persönlich verhindert waren: BARTLEY und G. BISHOP, die Pioniere der Elektrophysiologie des visuellen Systems, die japanischen Kollegen AKIMOTO, MOTOKAWA und TOMITA, sowie VILLEGAS, LENNOX-BUCHTHAL und SJÖSTRAND. So können sie wenigstens indirekt an der Diskussion teilnehmen und zum Gelingen unseres Experiments beitragen.

Ein gutes Experiment muß auch exakt geplant und technisch gut vorbereitet werden. Diese technischen Vorbereitungen hat Dr. KORNHUBER übernommen und mit dem ihm eigenen Impetus durchgeführt. Wir danken ihm und den anderen Mitarbeitern, die bei diesem Symposion geholfen haben, besonders herzlich. Ferner danken wir für finanzielle Unterstützung der Medizinischen Fakultät der Universität Freiburg mit ihrer Hoffmann-La Roche-Stiftung, den Firmen Schwarzer (München-Pasing), Ciba-A.G. (Wehr) und Boehringer (Mannheim) der National Science Foundation (Washington, D.C.) für Reiseunterstützung der amerikanischen Teilnehmer, sowie vor allem dem Springer-Verlag für die Ermöglichung einer raschen Publikation.

Auf die ursprüngliche Form des Symposions bei den Griechen, Gespräch und Diskussion mit einem Weingelage zu verbinden, müssen wir zwar verzichten. Doch soll statt simultaner Verbindung von Rede und Weintrinken, die der Wissenschaft nicht förderlich ist, geistige und leibliche Nahrung mit badischem Wein *sukzessiv* verabreicht werden. So hoffen wir, daß Vorträge und Diskussionen als Tischgespräche beim Wein fortgesetzt werden.

Wenn es gelingt, Neurophysiologen und Psychologen zu fruchtbarem Gedankenaustausch zu bringen, neue Anregungen zu geben und Verbindungen zwischen der klassischen Psychophysik und der modernen Neurophysiologie zu schaffen, so wird das Experiment dieses Symposions nicht vergeblich sein und vielleicht zu ähnlichen Tagungen in späteren Jahren anregen.

R. JUNG

A. Retina

I. Ultramikroskopische Grundlagen der Retina-Physiologie

Comparative Ultrastructure of the Retina in Fish, Monkey and Man*

With 5 Figures

Comparative studies of the fine structure of the retina have been carried out by the author in several species of the vertebrate series ranging from the fish to the monkey (*19, 20, 21*). In those studies, the ultrastructure and organization of the elements present in all the retinal layers have been analyzed, and the findings of other authors (*2, 3—6, 7, 8, 12—17*) in the receptor layer have been confirmed.

A new method of fixation for electron microscopy has recently been developed in our Laboratory. This method consists of a modification of the classical silver impregnation method of Golgi and was applied to the fish and human retina.

The present work is intended to present a comparative study of the fine structure of the retina of the fish, monkey and man.

Material and Method. Two types of fixatives were used: 1) buffered 2 per cent osmium tetroxide (*10*) and 2) a buffered mixture of 2 per cent potassium dichromate plus 1 per cent osmium tetroxide followed by a silver impregnation with 0.5 per cent silver nitrate (*21*). Retinae of fish (Centropomidae Sp.) and man were fixed in both types of fixatives, while the retina of monkey (Macaca Irus and Mulatta) was fixed only with the osmium tetroxide solution. After fixing and dehydrating, the retinae were embedded in a prepolymerized mixture of n-butyl and methyl-metacrylate (*1*) or in araldite (Nysem method).

Results. For morphological studies one can consider the vertebrate retina as a five-layered structure taking into consideration three main types of cells and the connections between them (Fig. 1). The five layers are, considering the most externally situated first, the following: 1 — the receptor layer; 2 — the external neuropile; 3 — the bipolar cell layer; 4 — the inner plexiform layer or internal neuropile; 5 — the ganglion cell layer. An additional layer, the pigment epithelium, covers the outer surface of the retina.

The total thickness of the fish retina is about 240 μ, while the monkey and the human retinae are 100—110 μ thick. The individual thickness of each of the five retinal layers for each type of retina can be seen in Table 1.

---

* From the Laboratorio de Ultraestructura, Instituto Venezolano de Investigaciones Cientificas (IVIC), Caracas, Venezuela.

1*

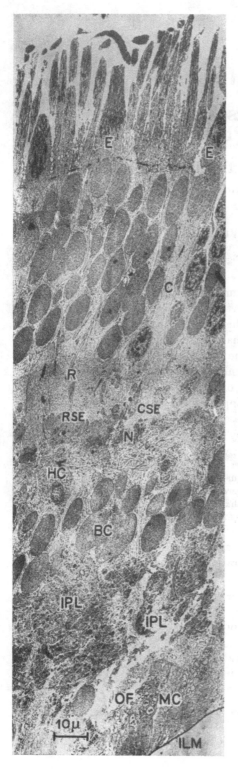

Receptor layer. The receptor layer consists of rods and cones. They are elongated cells with the same structural pattern already described by others (*2, 3—6, 7, 8, 12—17*). Both types of receptors exist in the fish, monkey and human retinae, the rods being always smaller than the cones (Fig. 1). Double cones appear only in the fish retina and they show a symmetrical arrangement around the single cones (*19—21, 22*). The receptor layer is divided into two zones by the external limiting membrane which embraces the receptor bodies just below the inner segment. The relationship existing between the receptors and the external limiting membrane has already been described (*20, 21*). From the external limiting membrane to the synaptic ending, the receptor cell appears as a slim cytoplasmic portion with an enlargement occupied by the nucleus (Fig. 1). The cytoplasm contains filaments ~ 200 Å thick. Due to the difference in caliber of both types of receptors of the monkey and human retina, the filaments are relatively more abundant in the rods than in the cones. In the fish retina, it has not been possible to follow the receptor bodies in their whole length (*21*); this might be due to the abundancy of receptors and the thinness and tortuous shape of their bodies.

In the three types of retinae studied here, the receptor synaptic endings are pyramidal and large in the cones and ovoid and smaller in the rods (Fig. 1). Synaptic microvesicles completely fill the cytoplasm of this portion of the recep-

Fig. 1. *Human retina.* Composite electron micrograph showing a longitudinal section through the five retinal layers. One cone (*C*) is observed in its whole length from the ellipsoidal region (*E*) to the synaptic ending (*CSE*). Segments of the rod bodies (*R*) appear at several places. The rod synaptic endings (*RSE*) present ovoidal shapes and are seen grouped around the cones synaptic endings. The external neuropile (*N*) intermingled with the plexus formed by the horizontal cells (*HC*) appears between the synaptic endings and the bipolar cells (*BC*). The zone situated between the inner plexiform layer (*IPL*) and the fifth layer is not well preserved. Bundles of optic fibers (*OF*) are observed separated by MÜLLER cytoplasmic columns (*MC*). These columns arise from the internal limiting membrane (*ILM*)

tor cell. The microvesicles are ~ 500 Å in diameter in the fish receptors and its approximate concentration is about the same for rods and cones ($200-220$ per μ^2). In the monkey and human retina, the diameter of the microvesicles is $300-400$ Å, the approximate concentration of them being greater in the rod than in the cone synaptic endings. There are ~ 170 microvesicles per μ^2 in the cones of both retinae; ~ 190 microvesicles per μ^2 in the rods of the monkey retina and ~ 250 microvesicles per μ^2 in the same type of receptor of the human retina.

External neuropile. The connection between the receptor and the bipolar cells is a complicated structure, $1\ \mu$ thick, which we have named external neuropile (*19—21*). It is formed by the intertwining of the dendrites of the bipolar cells before they penetrate the base of the receptor synaptic endings (Figs. 2, 5). The dendritic processes are cytoplasmic portions which range in size from $0.1-0.4\ \mu$ (man and monkey) to $0.5-1.2\ \mu$ (fish) and contain filaments and numerous rounded mitochondria.

In the vertebrate series the neuropile is constant and it is always situated between the receptor synaptic endings and the external horizontal cells. In the fish,

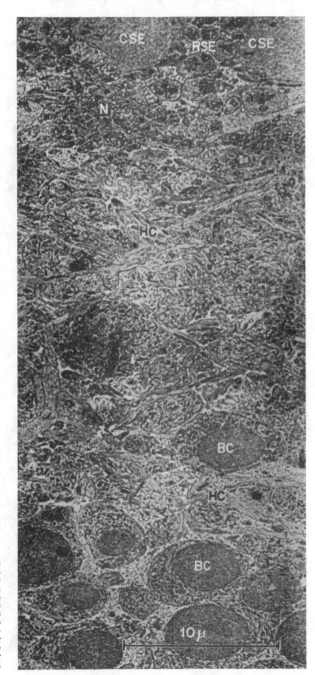

Fig. 2. Composite electron micrograph showing an oblique section through the second retinal layer and the outermost regions of the third layer. Rod (*RSE*) and cone synaptic endings (*CSE*) are observed at one side, while the bipolar cells (*BC*) are seen at the opposite side. The external neuropile (*N*) and the plexus formed by the horizontal cells (*HC*) occupy the center position. Among the bipolars and the receptor endings portions of Müller cytoplasm can be distinctly observed

the internal limiting structures of this layer are readily distinguished due to the greater size of the horizontal cells and their linear arrangement. In the primate retina the horizontal cells are small and thin and their processes form a plexus in the horizontal plane. This plexus is intermingled with the neuropile, the limit of both structures being vague (Fig. 2).

Third retinal layer. Three types of cells form this layer. The horizontal, the bipolar and the amacrine cells. In the primate retina, the last mentioned type has not yet been identified with the electron microscope.

Horizontal cells: In the fish (*19—21*), the horizontal cells are large structures which occupy almost all of the third retinal layer. They are of two different types, the external and the internal horizontal cells. The external horizontal cells lie in the outermost part of the third layer. They are grouped in a single row which delimits the external neuropile at its inner side (*21*).

The internal horizontal cells are grouped in two rows and are larger than the external hori-

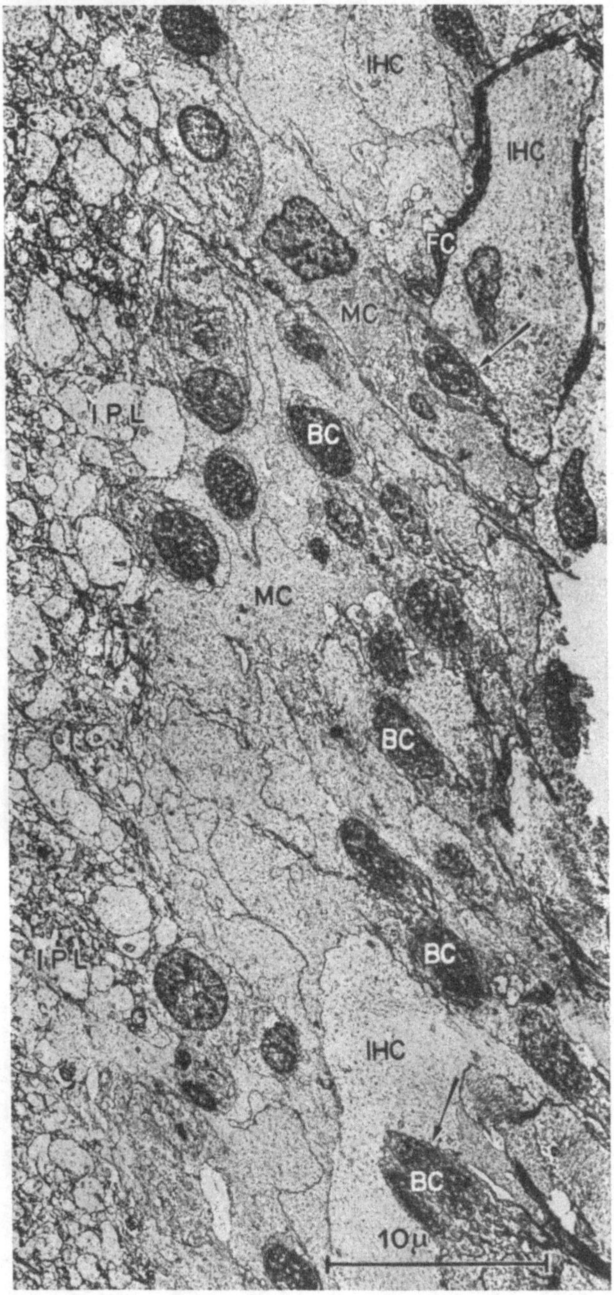

Fig. 3. Longitudinal section through the innermost region of the third layer of the *fish retina* fixed by the Golgi method. The inner plexiform layer (*IPL*) can be seen at the inner side. The composite electron micrograph shows a gap between the rows of internal horizontal cells (*IHC*). This gap is occupied by the bipolar (*BC*) and the Müller cells (*MC*) which present their maximal extension at this region. The lower situated bipolar cells are observed surrounded by the Müller cytoplasm, while some other bipolars are seen in close contact with the horizontal cells (arrow). Notice how the cells forming the first row of internal horizontal cells are lined by the strips of dense cytoplasm (*FC*)

zontal cells (40—80 μ in diameter, *19—21*) (Fig. 3). The cytoplasm of the internal horizontal cells contains closely packed filaments, 70 Å thick, and few mitochondria, while the cytoplasm of the external horizontal cells does not

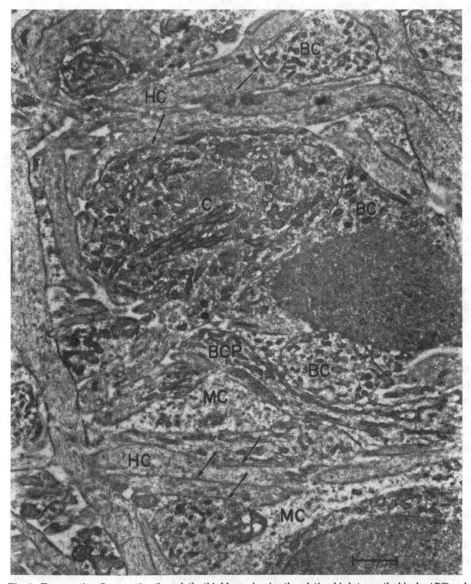

Fig. 4. *Human retina*. Cross section through the third layer showing the relationship between the bipolar (*BC*) and the horizontal cells (*HC*). Part of a cell with the same cytoplasmic features of the bipolars and containing a peculiarly "ciliary structure" (*C*) can be observed at the center. Portions of Müller cytoplasm (*MC*) occupy the free spaces among the other cells. Notice the different cytoplasmic characteristics of the Müller, the bipolar (*BCP*) and the horizontal (*HC*) cell processes. Arrows show the membrane-to-membrane contacts between the horizontal and the bipolar cells

present filaments and contains numerous mitochondria. The cells are connected to each other by processes which are short in the external horizontal cells and long (up to 10 μ in length) in the internal cells. In a three dimensional view each row appears as a net, the meshes of which are occupied by the bipolar cells and their processes and by the processes of the Müller cells. In cross sections of the fish retina, the internal horizontal cells appear star-shaped due to the greater length of their processes (19—21).

Strips of fibrous and dense cytoplasm which line the internal horizontal cells forming the first row have been observed (21) (Fig. 3). These strips separate the two rows of internal horizontal cells and also separate the first row from the external horizontal cells. The density of the cytoplasm of these strips is due to the presence of closely packed membranous microtubuli (21). In the monkey and human retina, the horizontal cells do not form a net, but a plexus which lies between the bipolar cells and the external neuropile, both limits being imprecise (Fig. 2). In these types of retinae, the horizontal cells are reduced to delicate and fibrous cytoplasmic portions which contain few elongated mitochondria. The most internally situated processes of the plexus make membrane-to-membrane contact with the bipolar cells (~ 60 Å intercellular spaces) (Fig. 4).

In the fish, the outermost situated bipolar cells and their processes have the same membrane-to-membrane relationship with the external and internal horizontal cells. No horizontal cells have been observed between the external neuropile and the bipolar cells in the foveal region of the monkey (Fig. 5).

Bipolar cells: The bipolar cells are small rounded cells with a relatively large nucleus, 4—5 μ in diameter, surrounded by a cytoplasmic rim which contains granules, small and numerous mitochondria, endoplasmic reticulum and a Golgi complex. The two processes arising from the cell body present the same cytoplasmic characteristics and besides contain filaments.

The bipolar cells are abundant in the primate retina and they almost fill the third retinal layer (Fig. 1). Small cytoplasmic portions belonging to the Müller cells separate the bipolar cells from each other, but in some cases the bipolar cells make direct contact.

A particular structure like a bundle of cilia is present in the cytoplasm in several of the bipolars situated near the receptor endings (Fig. 4). The general characteristics of the cells bearing the "ciliary structure" are the same as those of the other bipolar cells. The question is if these cells are really bipolars or if they are as the receptors cells derived from the ependymal epithelium.

In the fish retina, the bipolar cells are predominantly situated towards the internal region of the third layer. Other bipolar cells are found at the level of the internal horizontal cells and a few can be seen among the external horizontal cells. The internally situated bipolars are surrounded by the Müller cells (Fig. 3) while the other bipolars situated among the horizontal cells have a close relationship with these cells without any interposed Müller cytoplasm (Fig. 3). The nuclei of the Müller cells are situated in the innermost region of the third retinal layer of the fish. These cells are also of maximum size in this position (Fig. 3).

In the same region, amacrine cells have been observed (21), limited in number, with a 10 μ diameter and cytoplasmic characteristics similar to those of the astrocytes of the central nervous system (11). The scanty processes of the amacrine cells have been observed penetrating the inner plexiform layer. These processes are 1—3 μ thick and run horizontally in the outermost part of the fourth retinal layer.

Inner plexiform layer. Morphologically the fourth retinal layer is a feltwork

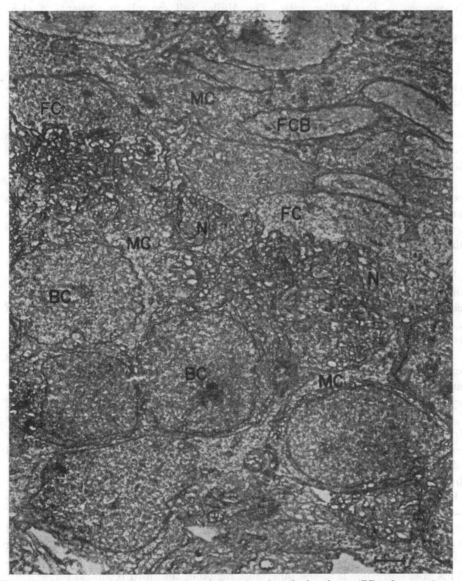

Fig. 5. *Monkey retina.* Longitudinal section through the region where the foveal cones (*FC*) make synaptic connections with the bipolar cells (*BC*). Due to the length and direction of their traject, the bodies of the foveal cones (*FCB*) appear obliquely sectioned. Notice that no horizontal cells are observed between the external neuropile (*N*) and the bipolar cells. Portions of Müller cytoplasm (*MC*) separate the cells from each other

of different types of processes which separate the ganglion cells from the cells forming the third retinal layer. In this feltwork lie the synaptic connections between the bipolar and the ganglion cells.

In the primate retina, this layer appears formed by two types of fine processes; one type with small mitochondria and filaments and the other type which contains microvesicles and larger mitochondria. The uniformity of the feltwork is interrupted by the presence of large irregularly shaped cytoplasmic portions belonging to the Müller cells. The Müller cell cytoplasm presents a clear matrix and contains numerous small dense granules and a few small mitochondria (Figs. 1, 2,3).

In the inner plexiform layer of the fish retina, there appear the same processes described for the primate retina and also two more types which predominate in the outermost part of the layer. These two types are the amacrine cell processes and some myelinated nerve fibers which run in a perpendicular plane (21).

Ganglion cell layer. This layer is formed by the ganglion cells and the optic nerve fibers. The internal limiting membrane separates the layer from the vitreous body. Pyramidal columns belonging to the Müller cells arise from this membrane to penetrate all the retinal layers and end in the external limiting membrane.

In the fish, the ganglion cells are small neurons, ~ 5 μ in diameter with a rounded nucleus and a cytoplasm rich in granules, endoplasmic reticulum, mitochondria and small vacuoles. The ganglion cells are not numerous and can be observed in groups of 2 or 3 cells near the inner plexiform layer. The optic nerve fibers, all myelinated in this fish, occupy the rest of the fifth layer.

In the monkey and human retina, the ganglion cells have the same structural characteristics as those of the fish, the size being greater (~ 20 μ). The dendrites of the ganglion cells contain filaments and less granules and organelles than the cell body. These dendrites penetrate the inner plexiform layer. Another type of ganglion cell can also be observed in the primate retina; it presents the same pattern as the other type but its size can be as small as 5 μ in diameter.

The optic nerve fibers are unmyelinated fibers grouped in bundles which run in the same direction and are situated near the ganglion cell bodies. The bundles and the ganglion cells are surrounded by the Müller cells which appear as clear cytoplasmic portions with numerous small granules and few mitochondria (Fig. 1).

Müller cells. The Müller cells are the supporting tissue of the retina. They arise from the internal limiting membrane and penetrate the retinal layers to end in the external limiting membrane. The limiting membranes can be considered as part of the plasma membrane of the Müller cells (20, 21). The external limiting membrane appears thickened and desmosome-like structures have been observed where the plasma membranes of adjacent Müller cells come in contact (20). Spaces ~ 60 Å wide separate these cells from all other retinal structures.

In man and monkey retina, the Müller fibers present two areas of maximal extension, the fifth layer and the zone of the receptor synaptic endings, the former area being greater. In the fish, only one area of maximal extension is observed. This area corresponds to the innermost region of the third retinal layer.

No blood vessels have been seen in the retina of the fish, while in the primate retina, the blood vessels, some of them of great size, are observed from the inner border to the vicinity of the receptor synaptic endings. Blood vessels have not been observed in the receptor layer.

In the fifth layer, the blood vessels are seen near the ganglion cells. They are separated from these cells by portions of Müller cytoplasm. Some horizontal cell processes are observed in the vicinity of the blood vessels which are situated in the external region of the third layer.

Table 1. *Thickness of the retinal layers expressed in micra (μ)*

	fish	monkey	man
Receptor layer	~ 140	50—60	60—70
External neuropile	~ 1	~ 1	~ 1
Bipolar layer	~ 40	~ 16	~ 18
Inner plexiform layer	~ 40	~ 15	~ 16
Ganglion cell layer	~ 20	~ 13	~ 15
Total retinal thickness	~ 240	~ 100	~ 115

Comments. In the vertebrate series, the retina is organized following the same structural pattern. From fish to man, the main types of cells present the same general characteristics, the differences being the size and the number of the cells. There is a striking resemblance between the monkey and the human retina, while the presence of double cones, giant horizontal cells and myelinated optic fibers, among other characteristics, make the fish retina appear different. Of particular importance in the fish is the relationship existing between the bipolars and the Müller and horizontal cells. The majority of the bipolar cells are situated in the inner region of the third layer and are surrounded by the Müller cells which present their maximal extension in the same region. Other bipolars lie among the horizontal cells and have close relationship with them without any interposed cytoplasm. The color response recorded from the same fish was localized at the level at which the bipolars are in greater number, while the response to the luminosity was recorded from the zone of the horizontal cells (*9, 18*).

The bipolars connected to the foveal cones of the monkey are also surrounded by Müller cytoplasm. No horizontal cells have been observed in the same region. The general structural characteristics of the horizontal cells do not resemble those of the neurons, and in the fish their relationship to the luminosity response (*18*) leads us to think of the possibility that the horizontal cells are satellite glial cells of the bipolars.

The Müller cells would play the same role as the horizontal cells for the bipolars related to the color response. In the monkey, both types of cells, the Müller and the horizontal cells, have been seen in close relationship with the blood vessels of the zone.

The disposition of the limiting membranes in relation to the Müller cells have been considered previously and an analogy between the Müller cell and the Schwann cell and the oligodendroglia has also been suggested (*21*).

Other types of glial cells present in the retina might be the amacrine cells and the strips of dense cytoplasm which surround the internal horizontal cells of the fish. In a previous work (*21*) the resemblance between the astrocytes and the amacrine cells has been analyzed.

Summary

Comparative studies of the fine structure of the retina have been carried out in the fish (Centropomidae), monkey (Macaca) and man. There is a similarity between the retinae of monkey and man, while the presence of double cones, giant horizontal cells and myelinated optic fibers make the fish retina appear different. In the fish, the horizontal cells are of two different types, the external horizontal cells and the internal horizontal cells. They are grouped in rows and each row, in a three-dimensional view, appears as a net. The meshes of these nets are occupied by the bipolars and the Müller cell processes. The bipolar cells are grouped mainly towards the inner region of the third layer and they are surrounded by the Müller cell processes. Other bipolars are situated among the horizontal cells and establish close relationship with these cells without any interposed Müller cytoplasm.

In the primate retina, the horizontal cells are delicate and fibrous cytoplasmic portions which form a plexus intermingled with the external neuropile. There are membrane-to-membrane connections between the horizontal cells and the bipolar-like cells situated in the outer region of the third layer. Spaces ~ 60 Å wide separate the retinal structures from each other. The possibility of the horizontal and the Müller cells being the glial cell of the retina is discussed.

Acknowledgement

The author wishes to express her thanks to Mr. JOSEPH SUTER and Mr. G. GEISLER for their technical assistance. The help of Miss ELUSKA BARUCH in the preparation of the manuscript is gratefully acknowledged.

References

1. BORISKO, E.: Recent Developments in Methacrylate Embedding. 1. A Study of the Polymerization Damage Phenomenon by Phase Contrast Microscope. J. biophys. biochem. Cytol. 2 (Suppl.), 3 (1956).
2. CARASSO, N.: Etude au microscope electronique des synapses des cellules visuelles chez le tetard de l'Alytes Obstetricans. C. R. Acad. Sci. (Paris) 245, 216 (1957).
3. DE ROBERTIS, E.: Electron Microscope Observations on the Submicroscopic Organization of the Retinal Rods. J. biophys. biochem. Cytol. 2, 319 (1956).
4. — Morphogenesis of the Retinal Rods. An Electron Miscroscope Study. J. biophys. biochem. Cytol. 2 (Suppl.), 209 (1956).
5. — and C. M. FRANCHI: Electron Miscroscope Observations on Synaptic Vesicles in Synapses of the Retinal Rods and Cones. J. biophys. biochem. Cytol. 2, 307 (1956).
6. — and A. LASANSKY: Submicroscopic Organization of Retinal Cones of the Rabbit. J. biophys. biochem. Cytol. 4, 743 (1958).
7. LADMAN, A. J.: The Fine Structure of the Rod-Bipolar Cell Synapse in the Retina of the Albino Rat. J. biophys. biochem. Cytol. 4, 459 (1958).
8. LASANSKY, A., and E. DE ROBERTIS: Electron Microscopy of Retinal Photoreceptors. The Use of Chromation Following Formaldehyde Fixation as a Complementary Technique to Osmium Tetroxide Fixation. J. biophys. biochem. Cytol. 7, 493 (1960).
9. MACNICHOL, jr., E. F., L. MACPHERSON and G. SVAETICHIN: Studies on Spectral Response Curves from the Fish Retina. Symp. on Visual Problems of Colour, Teddington, England, 531, 1957.
10. PALADE, G. E.: A Study of Fixation for Electron Microscopy. J. exp. Med. 95, 285 (1952).
11. SCHULTZ, R. L., E. A. MAYNARD and D. C. PEASE: Electron Microscopy of Neurons and Neuroglia of Cerebral Cortex and Corpus Callosum. Amer. J. Anat. 100, 369 (1957).
12. SJÖSTRAND, F. S.: An Electron Microscope Study of the Retinal Rods of the Guinea Pig Eye. J. cell comp. Physiol. 33, 383 (1949).
13. — The Ultrastructure of the Outer Segments of Rods and Cones of the Eye as Revealed by the Electron Microscope. J. cell. comp. Physiol. 42, 15 (1953).
14. — The Ultrastructure of the Inner segments of the Retinal Rods of the Guinea Pig Eye as Revealed by Electron Microscopy. J. cell. comp. Physiol. 42, 45 (1953).

15. SJÖSTRAND, F. S.: and G. ELFVIN: Some Observations on the Structure of the Retinal Receptors of the Toad Eye as Revealed by the Electron Microscope. Electron Microscopy Proceedings of the Stockholm Conference, September. 194 S. Stockholm: Almqvist & Wiksell 1956.
16. — Ultrastructure of Retinal Rod Synapses of the Guinea Pig Eye as Revealed by Three-Dimensional Reconstructions from Serial Sections. J. Ultrastr. Res. 2, 122 (1958).
17. — Fine Structure of Cytoplasm: the Organization of Membranous Layers. Rev. Mod. Phys. 31, 301 (1959).
18. SVAETICHIN, G., and W. KRATTENMACHER: Photostimulation of Single Cones. Proceedings of the XXI International Congress of Physiological Sciences, Buenos Aires, 267 (1959).
19. VILLEGAS, G. M., and J. SUTER: Functional Organization and Ultrastructure of the Vertebrate Retina. Proceedings of the XXI International Congress of Physiological Sciences, Buenos Aires, 289 (1959).
20. — Electron Microscopic Study of the Vertebrate Retina. J. gen. Physiol. 43 (Suppl. II), 15 (1960).
21. — and J. SUTER: The Fine Structure of the Fish Retina. The Use of the Method of Golgi for Electron Microscopy. Sent to publication.
22. WALLS, G. L.: The Vertebrate Eye and its Adaptative Radiation. 587 S. Bloomfield Hills, Michigan: Cranbook Press 1942.

Discussion see p. 22

Topographic Relationship between Neurons, Synapses and Glia Cells*

By

FRITIOF S. SJÖSTRAND

With 6 Figures

According to the neuron doctrine the junctions between neurons, the synapses, are special regions where the activity in the nervous system can be regulated to a certain extent as, for instance, through a one-way transmission of impulses, through facilitation, and through inhibition.

From a physiological point of view the possibility has been discussed that the individual neurons might be capable of a rather high degree of integrative activity. This would mean that the firing of the neuron would be modulated by a more complex interaction of all incoming signals than can be accounted for by the simple concept of an all or none signal transmission over its synaptic contacts with more or less fixed inhibitory or facilitating connections. To explain how the neuron may integrate the varied patterns of incoming signals to a corresponding spectrum of responses it has been proposed that the surface of the neuron is differentiated into a number of functionally different regions. The type of response of the neuron to an incoming signal would then depend on the functional characteristics of the regions over which the signal is transmitted as well as on the effect of other incoming signals on other parts of the neuronal surface.

From a morphological point of view there are no indications of any structural differentiation of the neuronal surface as far as the plasma membrane is concerned that would support this hypothesis. However, this paper will discuss the possibility

* From the Department of Zoology, University of California, Los Angeles, USA.

that the assumed functional differentiation of the neuronal surface might be ascribed to the topographical relationship between the neurons and the various types of satellite cells as for instance the neuroglia in the brain and the Müller's cells in the retina. A hypothesis has been proposed (SJÖSTRAND 1960) according to which the satellite cells in fact represent what is characterized as the extracellular space of nervous tissue. This hypothesis was first proposed for the retina (SJÖSTRAND 1958), but the same arguments apply to brain tissue as well as to peripheral nerves. This hypothesis gives a new role to the satellite cells and would give a logically satisfactory explanation to the fact that conducting elements in nervous tissue are associated with satellite cells. The functional significance that this hypothesis ascribes to the satellite cells would make the topographical relationships between the neurons and these cells appear important, since the conductivity of the neuronal surface would be limited to those areas of the surface which were covered by satellite cells.

From a morphological point of view it seems reasonable to assume that the topographical relations between the neuron surface and the neuroglia or corresponding elements in, for instance, the retina, the Müller's cells, might be of paramount importance in determining the functional properties of the neuronal surface.

Let us now discuss the basis for this hypothesis. The neurophysiologists consider the central nervous system as consisting of neurons bathing in an extracellular fluid. Determination of the sodium or chloride space has encouraged such a concept by giving values as high as twenty to thirty percent for the volume of what is considered the extracellular space. Light microscopy has not presented any conclusive evidence against or in favor of the existence of any such space because the silver impregnation methods used to demonstrate neuronal morphology are effective only when the impregnation is confined to a limited number of cells and does not involve all the cellular elements. Furthermore, light microscopists have accepted preservation of the tissue so poor as to be unacceptable for modern electron microscopy.

Several studies of the retina (SJÖSTRAND 1956, 1958) and the brain (DEMPSEY and WISLOCKI 1955, FARQUHAR and HARTMANN 1957, MAYNARD and PEASE 1955, SCHULTZ, MAYNARD and PEASE 1957, WYCKOFF and YOUNG 1954) by means of electron microscopy have demonstrated a striking close-packing of the cellular elements in nervous tissue. The neurons are embedded in satellite elements, which in the retina are represented by the Müller's cells, in the central nervous system by the neuroglia, and in peripheral nerves by the Schwann cells. In the first two cases the satellite elements cover the surfaces of the neurons in an incomplete way, leaving certain areas of the neurons free for synaptic contact areas as well as for areas where adjacent ganglion cells are in direct contact without any interposed glia.

Let us now examine the boundaries between the neurons and the satellite cells. We can choose either a neuron in the brain tissue, a neuron or a receptor in the retina or an unmyelinated nerve fiber to demonstrate the structural features of these cell boundaries. If we choose the synaptic region of the retinal receptors of the guinea pig eye as a model for this demonstration we will base our description on a case where the structural relationships have been studied by means of three-dimensional reconstructions from uninterrupted series of sections (SJÖSTRAND

1958). This has made it possible to identify the various parts of the satellite cells in spite of the very complex mixing of satellite cell processes with receptor cell parts and neuronal dendrites.

The cell boundary appears in the sections of tissue fixed in osmium tetroxide solution as consisting of two about 50 Å-thick opaque lines separated by a ca. 100 Å wide less opaque interspace (Fig. 1, 2). The opaque lines represent layers

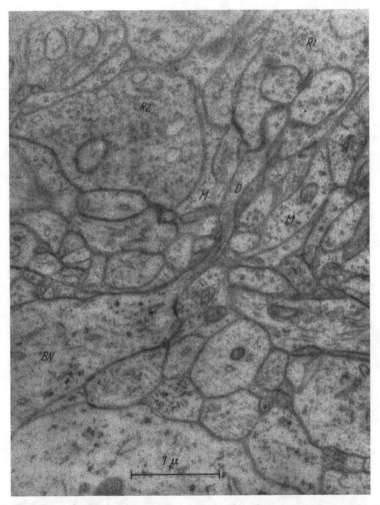

Fig. 1. Section through the outer plexiform layer of a guinea pig retina showing two synaptic bodies *R1* and *R2* of two receptor cells, *R1* of the α type, *R2* of the β type. In the lower left corner part of a bipolar nerve cell with a dendrite extending to and making synaptic contact with receptor *R1*. The end of the dendrite is located in an invagination of the plasma membrane of the receptor at its vitreal pole. Some parts of Müller's cells are indicated by *M*.

This picture is from section number 20 in a series of 40 sections used for three dimensional reconstruction of the synaptic structures of the receptor cells as well as of their synaptic relations. The model made in connection with the reconstruction is shown in Figs. 3—4. × 35,000. (From F. S. SJÖSTRAND, 1958)

consisting of material that interacts with osmium tetroxide, which is an efficient electron stain due to the heavy osmium atoms. Each opaque line represents an osmiophilic component of the plasma membranes of the two adjacent cells.

The striking feature of the cell boundary is the constancy of the dimensions of the osmiophilic layer of the plasma membranes as well as of the less opaque interspace separating the osmiophilic layers of adjacent plasma membranes. The situation is identical to that observed in other tissues consisting of closely packed cells. It is furthermore striking that the two opaque layers do not fuse but are always separated by this light interspace. This appearance of the cell boundaries as

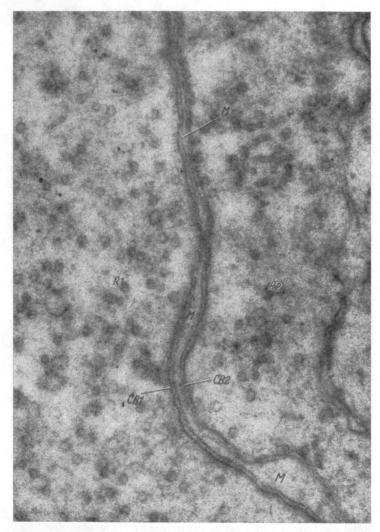

Fig. 2. Parts of two synaptic bodies of two receptor cells *R1* and *R2* in the guinea pig retina with a thin layer of Müller's cell cytoplasm interposed, *M*. Each plasma membrane appears as an osmiophilic layer. Two cell boundaries *CB1* and *CB2* separate the two receptor cells, each appearing as two osmiophilic layers separated by a light interspace. Of the two osmiophilic layers in each cell boundary one belongs to the plasma membrane of the receptor cell and one to the plasma membrane of the Müller's cell. × 90,000. (From F. S. SJÖSTRAND, 1957)

represented by the tubular epithelium of the mouse kidney was interpreted in terms of molecular architecture by SJÖSTRAND and RHODIN (1953) and SJÖSTRAND (1956). The constancy of the dimension of the light interspace was assumed to depend on the existence of some cementing material filling the space between the osmiophilic layers. Deductions and analogies made from observations of certain layered lipo-protein structures like the myelin sheath (SJÖSTRAND 1953, 1956) and the outer segments of retinal rods and cones (SJÖSTRAND 1949, 1953, 1959) had led to the assumption that the light interspace separating osmiophilic layers contains the double layers of oriented lipid molecules which, on indirect evidence, have been assumed to represent one basic component of the plasma membrane (DANIELLI and DAVSON 1934).

Observations made on material fixed in potassium permanganate seem to support this interpretation. In this material the plasma membrane appears as a triple-layered structure with a total thickness of 75 Å (ROBERTSON 1957). When two Schwann cells are closely packed the two triple-layered components of adjacent plasma membranes fuse to form a five-layered structure with a thicker middle opaque layer (SJÖSTRAND 1960).

When examining the relationship between the plasma membrane and the myelin sheath structural pattern it seems justifiable to conclude that the triple-layered component observed in potassium permanganate-fixed material contains a double layer of lipid molecules, presumably sandwiched between two very thin layers of protein or one layer of protein and one constisting of polysaccharides (ROBERTSON 1959, SJÖSTRAND 1960). The relationship between these patterns is easy to determine due to the fact that the myelin sheath pattern is continuous with the Schwann cell plasma membrane. The interpretation of the myelin sheath pattern as observed in the electron microscope, with respect to the localization of the lipid and the protein layers, seems rather well established and corresponds to that originally proposed by SJÖSTRAND (1953).

It also becomes obvious that the triple-layered component is mainly located in what appears as a light interspace between densely stained layers in osmium-fixed material. This relationship suggests itself when comparing osmium-fixed and potassium permanganate-fixed myelin sheaths where the plasma membrane of the Schwann cell can in both cases be traced through the invagination all the way to the myelin sheath pattern. The potassium permanganate seems to stain a component of the plasma membrane which remains unstained in osmium-fixed material. This component is located in the middle of the invagination and is continuous with the intraperiod layer of the myelin sheath pattern which appears weakly stained in osmium-fixed material (SJÖSTRAND 1953) and intensely stained in potassium permanganate-fixed material (ROBERTSON 1957). At the outer surface of the Schwann cell this middle layer splits up in two thinner layers which now appear as a component of the Schwann cell plasma membrane.

Since the triple-layered components of the two plasma membranes at a cell boundary fuse to form a five-layered boundary pattern like the pattern observed at the Schwann cell invagination it has been concluded (SJÖSTRAND 1960) that this triple-layered component is mainly located in the ca. 100 Å wide interspace which is observed separating the osmiophilic layers at cell boundaries in osmium-fixed material. The potassium permanganate thus would indicate the location of the lipid double layers in the light interspace which is observed in osmium-fixed material (SJÖSTRAND 1960). This would be in accordance with the interpretation of this osmium pattern which was proposed by SJÖSTRAND and RHODIN (1953) and by SJÖSTRAND (1956).

It has furthermore been proposed (SJÖSTRAND 1960) that the plasma membrane consists of an additional layer of presumably protein nature located on the cytoplasmic side of the triple-layered component observed in potassium permanganate-fixed material, and that this additional layer accounts for a greater part of the osmium stained layer in osmium-fixed material.

The consequences of these observations are that we have no direct evidence for the existence of any extracellular space between the cells in nervous tissue. There might be a possibility that a highly hydrated layer of protein or mucopolysaccharides is present in the middle of the ca. 100 Å wide interspace between cells observed in osmium-fixed tissue, but the width of this space can not exceed a few tenths Ångström units.

The physiologist, who frequently is much aware of the artifacts involved in morphological studies, will point to the fact that fixation and embedding of tissue is associated with shrinkage. Modern techniques of preservation and embedding which have been worked out in connection with electron microscopy of tissues make it possible, however, to preserve tissue with considerably less distortion than did earlier techniques. Shrinkage involves a reduction of the volume of the cells. The cells are the osmotic units, which retain a limiting membrane during the whole fixation and embedding procedure. The shrinkage of the cells results in an increase of the distances between the cells, that is, in an *increase* of the extracellular space in tissues where such an extracellular space is obviously present. Therefore, shrinkage is unlikely to cause an *obliteration* of any extracellular space in nervous tissue.

The report of ROBERTSON (1958) on the effect of exposure of nervous tissue to hypo-, iso- or hypertonic media before fixation has not been confirmed by our own studies. According to ROBERTSON the cell boundaries would swell in hypotonic media, a result which seems somewhat strange in the light of the discussion presented above according to which an increase in width of the extracellular space would be associated with a shrinkage of the cells. This would be expected to occur primarily in connection with exposure to a hypertonic medium.

Experiments have been made in which nervous tissue has been exposed to distilled water or strongly hypertonic media for two hours before fixation without introducing any appreciable change in the width of the space separating the osmiophilic layers of adjacent plasma membranes at cell boundaries (ELFVIN, unpublished). The tendency was toward an *increase* of this width after treatment in *hypertonic* media.

These observations make it justifiable to question the existence in the nervous tissue of an extracellular space of the dimensions generally assumed by neurophysiologists.

The logical consequence will then be to look for any space to take over the functional properties of the "extracellular space". I have proposed that the satellite elements of the nervous system such as the Müller's cells in the retina or the neuroglia would be most likely to represent this "extracellular space" (SJÖSTRAND 1958, 1960). Such an assumption would give a satisfactory explanation for the fact that neurons are associated with satellite cells. It would mean that the "outside" of the excitable membrane would be controlled with the precision by which a cell can control the composition of its cytoplasm. It would also mean that possibly the excitable membrane is a composite membrane to which both the neuronal and the glial plasma membranes contribute.

This hypothesis has some obvious implications. It would mean that the ionic composition of the cytoplasm of the glia cells with respect to K^+ and Na^+ would be drastically different from what is conventionally accepted for cellular cytoplasm. The permeability of the plasma membrane to ions would be different, with Na^+ passing freely through and the K^+ diffusion being restricted, perhaps through a

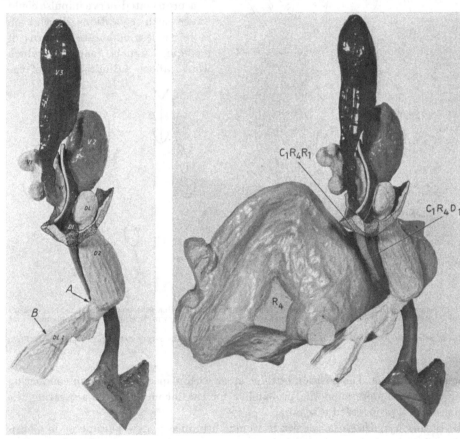

Fig. 3   Fig. 4

Fig. 3. Plastic model of receptor synapse from the guinea pig retina (after removal of the plasma membrane). This is a true three-dimensional reconstruction from a series of 40 sections, which are represented in Fig. 1. $D1$ and $D2$ are dendrites entering into synaptic contact with the receptor (Receptor $R1$ in Fig. 1.) (From F. S. SJÖSTRAND 1958)

Fig. 4. The synaptic bodies of receptor $R1$ and $R4$ have been assembled to show contact relations. (From F. S. SJÖSTRAND, 1958)

K^+ pump similar to the Na^+ pump of the axon. Preliminary experiments seem to point to striking differences in the permeability properties of the plasma membranes of neurons as compared to those of satellite cells.

If we assume that the glia elements represent the outside milieu of the neurons it will be of great importance to analyze the topographical relations between the glia cells and the ganglion cells. Only certain parts of the surface of the latter cells are covered by glia cells. These parts would represent the conducting paths or "streets" along the surface. The width of these streets and the arrangement of these streets would then introduce factors which would affect the response of the neuron and would allow integration of reactions initiated at various spots along the different streets.

The final response of the neuron eventually resulting in a firing off of a propagated nerve impulse could under such conditions depend on more or less elaborate patterns of incoming signals, each of which would affect a limited area of the

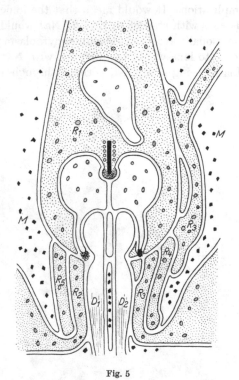

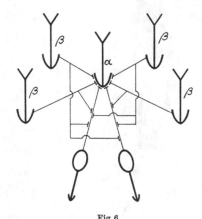

Fig. 5   Fig 6

Fig. 5. Schematic drawing of receptor synaptic body in the guinea pig retina with dendritic terminal branches *D 1* and *D 2* and branches from adjacent receptor synaptic bodies *R2—R5* shown. *M* Müller's cell cytoplasm. (From F. S. SJÖSTRAND, 1958)

Fig. 6. Schematic presentation of contact relations of one receptor of the α-type in the guinea pig retina. (From F. S. SJÖSTRAND, 1958)

neuronal surface. The position of these areas with respect to the main conducting streets would determine the probability for the incoming signal activating the neuron in a propagated discharge.

If this hypothesis is correct it would introduce a new parameter in neurophysiology, and the analysis of the street maps of the neurons would become an important problem in neuroanatomy.

Speculation can push us to imagine that in the process of learning the street maps of neurons are being changed by changes in the topographical relations between neurons and glial elements.

The three-dimensional reconstruction of the synaptic contacts of the retinal receptors in the guinea pig eye (Fig. 3—5) that was mentioned above can serve as a model for the kind of structural analysis which has to be performed in order to reveal the topographical relationships between the neurons and the neuroglia. Such studies would allow a complete mapping of the neuron surface with quantitative data for various synaptic contact relationships. In the retina this study allowed the demonstration of rather extensive interreceptor contacts of presumably synaptic character (Fig. 5—6). These contacts were assumed to exert inhibitory influences on the receptors, an assumption that would allow a simple explanation of certain features of the simultaneous contrast phenomenon (SJÖSTRAND 1958). Electron microscopy is today technically well enough developed to attack this kind of problem in a systematic way.

Summary

1. Detailed analysis of the structural relationship between the plasma membranes of receptor cells, neurons and satellite cells in the retina, and peripheral nerve fibers, as well as in the central nervous system, exclude the existence of any appreciable extracellular space. The satellite elements are proposed to represent what is referred to as the "extracellular space".

2. Only part of the surface of the neurons is covered by satellite cells and is assumed to be able to conduct an impulse. The arrangement of these areas over the cell body and the dendrites of the neuron is proposed to play an important role for an integrative action at the level of the single neuron.

3. Contact relations between receptor cells and bipolars in the guinea pig retina make it reasonable to assume extensive interreceptor synaptic contacts in addition to the receptor-bipolar synapses.

References

DANIELLI, J. F., and H. DAVSON: A contribution to the theory of permeability of thin films. J. cell. comp. Physiol. 5, 495 (1934).

DEMPSEY, E. W., and G. B. WISLOCKI: An electron microscopic study of the blood-brain barrier in the rat, employing silver nitrate as a vital stain. J. biophys. biochem. Cytol. 1, 245 (1955).

FARQUHAR, M. G., and J. F. HARTMANN: Neuroglial structure and relationship as revealed by electron microscopy. J. Neuropath. exp. Neurol. 16, 18 (1957).

MAYNARD, E. A., and D. C. PEASE: New observations on the ultrastructure of the membranes of frog peripheral nerve fibers. Anat. Rec. 121, 440 (1955).

ROBERTSON, J. D.: New observations on the ultrastructure of the membranes of frog peripheral nerve fibers. J. biophys. biochem. Cytol. 3, 1043 (1957).

— Structural alterations in nerve fibers produced by hypotonic and hypertonic solutions. J. biophys. biochem. Cytol. 4, 349 (1958).

— The ultrastructure of cell membranes and their derivatives. Biochem. Soc. Symposia Cambridge (England) 16, 3 (1959).

SCHULTZ, R. L., E. A. MAYNARD and D. C. PEASE: Electron microscopy of neurons and neuroglia of cerebral cortex and corpus callosum. Amer. J. Anat. 100, 369 (1957).

SJÖSTRAND, F. S.: An electron microscope study of the retinal rods of the guinea pig eye. J. cell. comp. Physiol. 33, 383 (1949).

— The ultrastructure of the outer segments of rods and cones of the eye as revealed by the electron microscope. J. cell. comp. Physiol. 42, 15 (1953).

— The lamellated structure of the nerve myelin sheath as revealed by high resolution electron microscopy. Experientia (Basel) 9, 68 (1953).

— The ultrastructure of cells as revealed by the electron microscope. Int. Rev. Cytol. 5, 455 (1956).

— Die Elektronenmikroskopie als morphologische Untersuchungstechnik. Verh. anat. Ges. 53. Versamml. Stockholm, 1956. Jena: Fischer Verlag 1957.

— Ultrastructure of retinal rod synapses of the guinea pig eye as revealed by three-dimensional reconstructions from serial sections. J. Ultrastr. Res. 2, 122 (1958).

SJÖSTRAND, F. S.: The ultrastructure of the retinal receptors of the vertebrate eye. Ergebn. Biol. **21**, 128 (1959).
— Electron microscopy of myelin and nerve cells and tissue, *in* CUMINGS, J. N. (Ed.). Modern Scientific Aspects of Neurology. London: Edward Arnold Publishers Ltd. 1960.
— — and J. RHODIN: The ultrastructure of the proximal convoluted tubules of the mouse kidney as revealed by high resolution electron microscopy. Exp. Cell. Res. **4**. 426 (1953).
WYCKOFF, R. W. G., and J. Z. YOUNG: The organization within neurons. The nerve cell surface. J. Anat. Lond. **88**, 568 (1954).

Discussion to VILLEGAS and SJÖSTRAND

P. GLEES: 1. Light microscopy of the monkey's retina shows in the nuclear layer of the receptors two types of nuclei, large pale staining and small darkly staining nuclei. Which are the nuclei of rod or cones and which are neuroglia nuclei? Can electron microscopy shed any "light" on these?

2. How far do capillaries reach in the receptor layer?

W. SICKEL: 1. Lassen sich an den elektronenmikroskopischen Aufnahmen der Netzhaut "compartments" mit den nach TOMITAs Doppelmikroelektroden-Befunden zu fordernden Dimensionen erweisen?

2. Welche Unterschiede bestehen bei Stäbchen und Zapfen hinsichtlich Zahl und Anordnung von Mitochondrien?

H.-L. TEUBER: Is there a species difference in the concentration of Müller fibers, especially as regards fish and monkey retinae? I am also wondering about the distribution of Müller fibers in the retina of the cat. WEISKRANTZ[1] found that these elements seemed to undergo a rather selective atrophy in kittens reared with partial visual deprivation. These results are particularly intriguing because RIESEN[2] had shown earlier that such kittens failed to show normal pattern perception when brought into a normal visual environment.

These kittens were reared in a dark room until they were 17 weeks old. From the 14th week on, they were given daily exposures to light for $^1/_2$ hour, with diffuse light to one eye, and normal stimulation to the other. Apparently this form of rearing produces atrophy of Müller fibers and an associated agnosia-like syndrome, with peculiar difficulties in the interocular transfer of visually-guided habits.

R. JUNG: Wenn die elektronenmikroskopischen Ergebnisse eines praktisch fehlenden Extracellularraumes im ZNS den Verhältnissen in vivo entsprechen, so ist es logisch und notwendig, auch unsere physiologischen Vorstellungen über intra- und extracelluläre Vorgänge der Membranerregung zu verändern. Dr. SVAETICHIN hat schon einige Konsequenzen dieser Art angedeutet und wir werden nach seinem Vortrag noch über die Rolle der Glia diskutieren.

Die schönen Bilder von Dr. VILLEGAS zeigen klar die Ultrastruktur der menschlichen Retina. Physiologisch bedeutungsvoll und neu ist der Hinweis, daß die Horizontalzellen zur Glia gehören, während sie bisher als neuronale Strukturen angesehen wurden. Wie soll man sich nun die Verbindungsfunktion dieser Gliazellen zwischen den Zapfen vorstellen, als echte Erregungskoordination oder nur als trophische Speicherfunktion für Natrium oder photochemische Vorgänge? Gibt es histochemische Hinweise für die Sonderstellung der gliösen Horizontal- und Müllerzellen?

SJÖSTRANDs Befunde über die enge Anlagerung der Glia-Zellen an die Neurone und sein Hinweis, daß auch der schmale intercelluläre Spalt mit Lipoidmolekülen auszementiert ist, läßt dem Neurophysiologen keinen Extracellularraum mehr, aus dem die Neuronenmembran ihre Na-Ionen gewinnen könnte. Glia- und Schwannzellen müssen ihn ersetzen. Statt von „intercellulärem" und „extracellulärem" Raum würden wir daher in der Elektrophysiologie

[1] WEISKRANTZ, L.: Sensory deprivation and the cat's optic system. Nature (Lond.) **181**, 1047—1050 (1958).
[2] RIESEN, A. H., M. I. KURKE and J. C. MELLINGER: Interocular transfer of habits learned monocularly in visually naive and visually experienced cats. J. comp. physiol. Psychol. **46**, 166—172 (1953).

besser von *intraneuronalem* und *extraneuronalem* Raum sprechen. Dann kann vorläufig offen bleiben, ob und wie der extraneuronale Raum in seiner Elektrolytstruktur von der Glia, von Satelliten- und Schwannzellen gebildet und modifiziert wird. Bevor wir genauere Vorstellungen entwickeln, würden wir als Neurophysiologen gerne mehr über den *Natrium- und Kalium-Gehalt der Gliazellen und über ihre Membranpermeabilität* wissen. Wenn Eccles Doppelmikroelektrodenmethode mit Elektrophorese verschiedener Ionen für große Gliazellen anwendbar ist, könnte man so ihre Membraneigenschaften bestimmen und Ionenverhältnisse aufklären. Vielleicht können auch Elektrolytbestimmungen von Gliomen Hinweise auf den elektrophysiologisch zu postulierenden Na-Speicher der Gliazellen geben.

G. Villegas (to Glees): 1. We have not observed any neuroglia nuclei in the receptor layer of the monkey retina, but we have seen two types of nuclei corresponding to the rods and cones. The cone nuclei are rectangularly shaped and are situated closer to the external limiting membrane than the rod nuclei.

2. In monkey and man retinae, capillaries stop at the bipolar zone and they do not penetrate the receptor layer. In the fish retina no capillaries have been observed in the retinal layers.

(to Sickel): In the fish there is a clear difference between cones and rods in relation to the number and order of the mitochondria. The rods have 5 to 7 mitochondria arranged as a semilunar structure around the connecting cilium and the cones have many rounded closely packed mitochondria which fill completely the ellipsoid. In monkey and man, the mitochondria are elongated in both receptors, but they are more numerous in the cones due to the greater size of this type of receptor.

I leave the other question to Dr. Svaetichin since it is closely related to electrophysiology.

(to Teuber): There might be a difference in the concentration of the Müller fibers in fish and monkey retinae, but as far as I know it has not been studied. Generally speaking, the Müller cells in the fish and monkey retinae are similar structures, the difference being mainly in the size and the place of the retina where they present their maximal extension. In the fish the Müller cell shows its larger expansion at the level of the inner third of the bipolar layer. At this level the Müller cell contains its nucleus. In the monkey, due to the abundancy of bipolars, the Müller cells are reduced to thin strands among the bipolars. However, between the synaptic endings of the receptors and at the level of the internal limiting membrane the Müller cytoplasm occupies quite a large space. We have not made any electronmicroscopic study of the cat retina, but presumably the Müller cell occupies also a large space between the receptors of that retina.

Closing Remarks: Comparative electronmicroscopic study of the vertebrate retina has shown the same general pattern from fish to man. The retina is a structure consisting of three cellular layers and two synaptic layers. The cellular layers are formed by three types of nerve cells, which are the receptors, the bipolars and the ganglion cells. Crossing the retina from the internal limiting membrane to the external limiting membrane the Müller cells fill all the spaces existing between the different cells. Since the Müller cytoplasm adjusts its shape to the spaces left between the cells, there exist only intermembranous spaces about 100 Å wide in the whole retina.

Another type of cell described in the retina is the horizontal cell, which is quite large in the fish retina. The ultrastructural pattern of such a cell does not resemble that described for the neurons. This fact, together with the lack of an axon, which we have not been able to see with the electron microscope so far, leads us to consider the horizontal cell as a glial cell. A close relationship between the horizontal cells and some bipolars has been shown in the fish and human retinae. It has also been shown in the fish retina that the Müller cells occupy quite a large space in the bipolar zone, while in the monkey and man retinae the places of more extension of the Müller cells are the zone of the synaptic endings of the receptors and the zone close to the internal limiting membrane.

F. S. Sjöstrand: The hypothesis that the satellite elements represent what has generally been designated as an extracellular space will be tested in our laboratory by using radioactive tracer techniques for the analysis of, for instance, the Na concentration in satellite cells.

The nuclei of the cone cells are located immediately vitreal of the outer limiting membrane and appear larger than the rod nuclei. There are no Müller's cell nuclei in the nuclear layer of the receptors.

There exist large spaces, several microns in width, occupied by Müller's cells separating groups of bipolar nerve cells and receptor synapses in the guinea pig retina. The three dimensional shape of these wide spaces observed in sections has not yet been analyzed. Their distribution in different parts of the retina and precise dimensions have not been analyzed.

There seem to be more mitochondria in the cone cells than in the rod cells corresponding to the larger volume of the former cells.

II. Receptoren, Gliazellen und Retinaneurone

Electrical Activity of Single Neurons in the Frog's Retina[1,2]

By

T. Tomita, M. Murakami, Y. Hashimoto and Y. Sasaki

With 6 Figures

After a long lasting controversy concerning the origin of the ERG, opinions of investigators now appear to be approaching the general agreement that the major source of the fast components of ERG, or PII and PIII of Granit, is not in the receptors themselves but anterior to them. However, the allocation of the ERG in the retina is still very incomplete, since no one has succeeded yet in identifying the cell type that is responsible for the generation of ERG, nor in clarifying the mechanism of its generation. As a step to enter into these problems, we have been working during the last one year on the frog's retina, trying to obtain intracellularly some responses that could reasonably be correlated with the ERG. A preliminary report has been submitted for publication by Naka, Inoma, Kosugi and Tong (1960). For this kind of experiment, one needs pipettes much more slender than the ordinary superfine micropipettes, as the cells to be impaled are small.

Our pipettes now in use for this purpose are made, after the method of Naka, by pulling borosilicate glass tubings after heated in a U-shaped iridium-platinum ribbon of 50 μ in thickness and 7 mm in width. The pipettes thus made are characterized by shallow tapering and small diameter (less than 0.1 μ). After filling them with 3 M-KCl by boiling, their tip is checked under a high power microscope. The tip looks blurred, of course, as the size is far below the resolving power of any light microscope, but in well made pipettes the blurred image becomes fainter and fainter towards the tip until finally it just dissolves into the background. This kind of microscopic examination also serves for discarding pipettes which contain air bubbles. The pipettes thus selected are further checked with a megohmmeter. Those ready for use show resistances around 200 MΩ when measured with their tips immersed in 3 M-KCl solution.

The excised frog's eye is cut along its equator and the vitreous humor is drained off by means of small pieces of "Kleenex" tissue arranged radially with their one end in the vitreous a short distance across the cut edge of the eye, and the other end in contact with a piece of filter paper on which the eye is mounted. The eye together with the filter paper underneath is then mounted on an Ag-AgCl plate which serves as the indifferent electrode.

For the illumination of the eye, the two-channel photostimulator described by Tomita, Murakami and Hashimoto (1960) was used. Most experiments were carried out at room temperatures between 10 and 15° C.

[1] From the Department of Physiology, Keio University School of Medicine, Tokyo, Japan.

[2] This research work was done with the support of Research Grant No. MGl-60-1 (M 26-59-26) (Tsuneo Tomita, Responsible Investigator) from US Army Research and Development Group, Far East (9852).

When a pipette is inserted into the retina from its anterior surface, three types of impulse discharge, on-, on/off- and off-type, are obtained from a most superficial retinal layer. The spike height often exceeds 50 mV. As a feature common to these responses, they comprise impulse spikes accompanied by no discerned slow potential change. In addition, their receptive field is usually some distance from the site of recording, indicating that they are responses of single optic nerve fibers. For convenience sake, they will be called the Group-I responses.

During further advancement of pipette, spontaneous discharges are often observed which are likely due to injury of some small cells, but from a depth some 70 to 80 μ more from the depth for Group-I responses, fairly stable responses such as illustrated in Fig. 1 are obtained. They are characterized by impulse spikes superimposed on slow potential changes resembling an ERG or some components of it. In Fig. 1 A which represents the on/off-type, the membrane shows, when

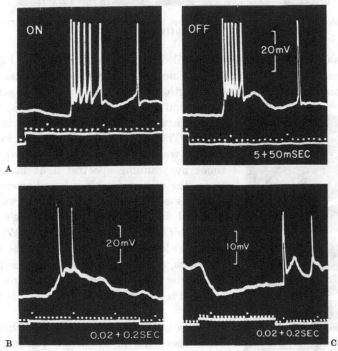

Fig. 1. A—C. Three types of Group-II responses. A on/off-type. Depolarizations at "on" and "off" usually showed irregular fluctuations unreproducible in repetition of illumination. B on-type, elicited by a small light spot on the site of recording. Diffuse illumination did not change the type of response. C off-type, fluctuations before the onset of illumination being subsiding off-effect of the preceding response in repetition of the sweep. Record-A was obtained with compensation of the input capacitance, while B and C without, which resulted in a reduction of the spike height nearly by half

light is on, an initial small hyperpolarization followed by depolarization with impulse spikes on it, and another depolarization, when light is off, with an off-discharge. There are also two other types; on-type (Fig. 1 B) and off-type (Fig. 1 C). In the on-type, depolarization occurs only during illumination, while in the off-type the cell is hyperpolarized during illumination with a rebound at "off". All the above three types, which will be called the Group-II responses, are elicited by a small light spot on the site of recording as well as by diffuse illumination.

Beyond this depth, no impulse spike is detectable, but from a layer some 40 μ deeper, pipettes often pick up a purely slow potential very similar to the S-potential from the fish retina excepting that the area effect is smaller in the frog than in

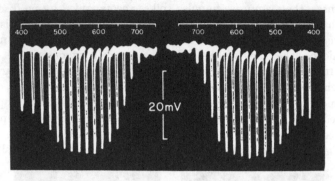

Fig. 2. L-type spectral curve of Group-III response (frog), by a method similar to that of Svaetichin and Mac-NICHOL (1958)

the fish. This type of responses will be called the Group-III responses. Fig. 2 shows a spectral response curve of such. Each negative deflection is response to a flash of monochromatic light whose wave lengths were changing in steps of some 20 mμ throughout the visible spectral range, from blue to red (left) and then in the opposite direction (right). The response was so stable in this case that we were able to repeat the recording several times by scanning spectral light in both directions. The response peak is found around 570 mμ which is a little longer than the wave length maximal in sensitivity of the frog's photopic dominator curve (Granit 1942). While many points are left to be investigated on the Group-III responses, a number of observations suggest that in the frog the luminosity-type response as shown in Fig. 2 is almost the only response, if not exclusively.

There was indication that some other response types also exist in the frog's retina, but those in the above three groups were most common.

Attention will now be directed to the slow potential changes in Group-II and III responses. It is suspected that some of these slow potential

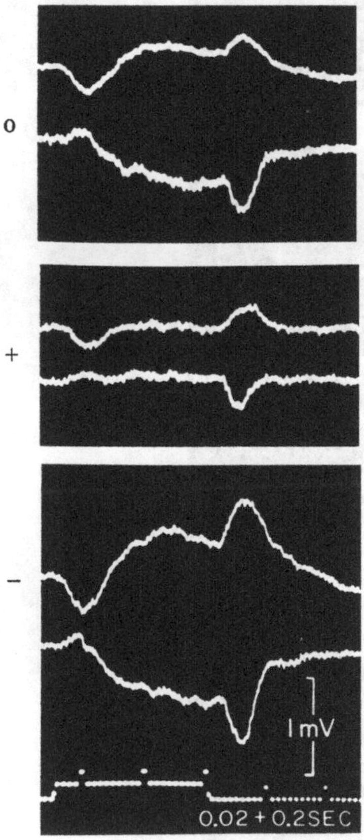

Fig. 3. Effect of polarizing current across the retina on the size of ERG (upper tracings). O control, without polarizing current. + vitreous side positive. — vitreous side negative. In these recordings, a coaxial microelectrode of Tomita was used, its external pipette being on the retinal surface for recording the ERG, and the internal pipette deep in the retina for obtaining intraretinal action potential or EIRG (lower tracings). The same effect on the ERG and EIRG support the view of Tomita et al. (1960) that the two responses are same in nature but reversed in polarity because of leading-off from opposite sides of the ERG generating layer

changes might be a constituent of the ERG. The slow component in Group-II responses resembles the ERG or some components of it, and the Group-III responses the component PIII. In any case, if one of these slow potentials is a constituent of the ERG, any agent that is known to influence the ERG should also influence it in a similar manner. In an attempt to test this point, the effect of polarizing current across the retina on the ERG was compared with that on these slow potential changes. Result on the ERG confirmed the experiment of GRANIT and HELME (1939). As shown in Fig. 3, the ERG is augmented by current applied with the vitreous side as cathode and is suppressed by current in the opposite direction. However, the effect of polarizing current on Group-III responses was various, showing no constant result. Current in one direction augmented some responses but suppressed some others, while giving little effect to the rest. With regard to the Group-II responses, the effect was regularly opposite to that on the ERG. As is illustrated in Fig. 4, the slow response was enhanced by current applied with the vitreous side as anode instead of as cathode, and was suppressed by current in the opposite direction.

This result on the slow component in Group-II responses may suggest one of two alternatives: The slow component has nothing to do with the ERG, or it does constitute the ERG but appearing differently owing to the difference in recording conditions. The latter possibility is based on the following assumptions: First, the ERG is a field effect of current produced in certain cell types arranged longitudinally. A limited region of the membrane near one end of such a cell acts as a miniature source of the ERG, giving rise to a current which flows, for instance, into the cell at this region and flows out of the cell across the remaining part of the membrane to the extracellular· space to make a closed circuit. Second, the conductance of this remaining part of the membrane, which then acts as a current barrier, is increased by an extrinsic polarizing current in one direction, while decreased by current in the opposite direction. On the above two assumptions, the density of current of the ERG is increased with an increase in the membrane conductance, resulting in a bigger field effect or a bigger ERG. Intracellularly, on the other hand, the potential becomes smaller because the current barrier is removed partially due to the membrane conductance increase. While the first assumption appears not to be unlogical, there is no material at hand to

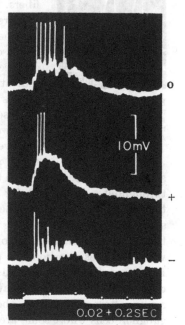

Fig. 4. Effect of polarizing current across the retina on Group-II response of on-type. Symbols on the right indicate the same as in Fig. 3

prove or disprove the second. Any conclusion, therefore, is left open to the future.

Turning the subject, the problem of localization of the Group-II responses will be discussed. BROWN and WIESEL (1959) report an experiment similar to ours but using the cat's unopened eye. Inspite of the difference in material, their result is amazingly similar to ours excepting one point that they could not reveal the slow component in our Group-II responses, probably because of their extracellular recording. The Group-II responses appear to correspond to the impulse activities that they believe arise from the bipolar cell layer. It is peculiar, however, that the neurons that give rise to the Group-II responses are readily invaded by antidromic impulses which are elicited in the optic nerve fibers by means of a coaxial stimulating needle electrode placed on the optic disc. Three antidromic impulses from an on-type neuron whose response to light was shown in Fig. 1 B are illustrated in Fig. 5. As is seen, each impulse spike is followed by a second elevation, occasionally with another spike on top of it (C). The nature of the second elevation is unknown, but it appears to be related to deterioration of the neuron. It was often observed that the second elevation manifests itself only after a neuron has been impaled for a while.

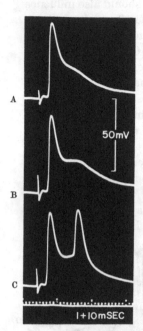

Fig. 5. Three antidromic impulses from within Group-II neuron whose response to light is shown in Fig. 1 A. No compensation of input capacitance

This physiological evidence appears to show that the Group-II responses originate not from the bipolar cells but from ganglion cells connected directly with optic nerve fibers. Questions may arise to this view.

First, the depth at which the Group-II responses are obtained does not agree with the ganglion cell layer. A result of our histological measurement of the thickness of each retinal layer is shown schematically in Fig. 6, arrows indicating approximate depths for the three major response groups as judged from readings of the micrometer gauge. As is seen, the depth for Group-II responses is a little too far away from the ganglion cell layer. It is necessary, however, to take into account a possible dislocation of cells when pushed by the tip of a pipette. During lowering a pipette, we often hear from loudspeaker an impulse activity of one single neuron throughout a distance as far as 50 μ or more before the pipette actually impales the cell, and after having once impaled the pipette can be pulled back about the same distance without losing intracellular recording. The difficulty of identifying the cell types from readings of the micrometer gauge may also be well understood when one tries insertion of a pipette from the receptor side of the isolated retina. It is very common in this case that all the three response groups are detectable only after the pipette is located much closer to the internal limiting membrane. As an alternative to the above, the Group-II responses might originate from ganglion cells whose soma are displaced into the inner nuclear layer. Existence of such ganglion cells is found histologically (cf. Polyak, 1957, Figs. 146 and 147). There is also a possibility that the recording was from ganglion cell dendrites in the inner plexiform layer.

Second, the latency of antidromic impulses which usually amounts to 2—3 msec. (see Fig. 5) is extremely long compared with the distance between the sites of stimulation and recording (2—3 mm). This fact has made us suspect that the impulses obtained by stimulation to the optic disc might not be antidromic but orthodromic, being transmitted via synapses from some cells which are sensitive enough to be excited by current spreading from the site of stimulation. This agrees also with our knowledge that the retina is very sensitive to electrical stimulation. However, there now appears to be little possibility for this: 1. Impulses elicited in single optic nerve fibers by stimulation to the optic disc show about the same latency as those from within Group-II neurons. This is true of fibers whose receptive field is at a very peripheral retinal region and, therefore, of little chance to be excited by spreading current. 2. If the long latency were the result of spreading current as suspected, a sudden shortening of the latency should occur when the intensity of stimulation is increased further until the fiber under observation is excited at the optic disc. However, this never happened. 3. When the region of the optic disc is inactivated locally (this could be done easily by passing d.c. current through the stimulating coaxial metal electrode, i.e. by products of electrolysis), stimulation fails to elicit impulses in Group-II neurons as well as in optic nerve fibers. Thus, the long latency must be attributed to an excitation delay of some unknown reason at the site of stimulation. It may be worthy of note that this observation on the frog's retina makes a good contrast with that on the fish in which the latency is found to be constantly less than 1 msec.

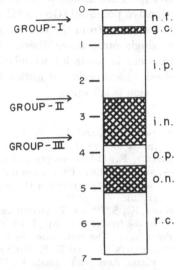

Fig. 6. Schematic diagram showing the retina thickness (frog) and approximate depths for Group-I, II and III responses. Numerals show distances in steps of 35 μ. *n.f.* nerve fiber layer, *g.c.* ganglion cell layer, *i.p.* inner plexiform layer, *i.n.* inner nuclear layer, *o.p.* outer plexiform layer, *o.n.* outer nuclear layer, *r.c.* rod and cone layer

Third, the response of Group-II neurons to stimulation of the optic disc might be a result of activation of some efferent fibers in the optic nerve, the potential described by the name of second elevation (cf. Fig. 5) constituting an EPSP. However, in an experiment using stimulation of gradually increasing intensity, the second elevation, if existed, could never be dissociated from the spike potential.

In conclusion, we have actually no conclusion. We only described some of our recent observations on the frog's retina using very fine micropipettes. For determining the cell types responsible for the different responses mentioned, development of a method is keenly awaited of visualizing under a microscope the retinal cells to be probed, or of labelling the cells that have been probed for later histological identification.

Summary

A minute pipette electrode (less than 0.1 μ in tip diameter) inserted into the frog's retina from its anterior surface records well isolated response whose configuration is different according to the depth of recording. The most frequently observed response patterns are classified into three groups. The Group-I response obtained from the most superficial retinal layer comprises impulses, of either on-, off- or on/off-type, which often exceed 50 mV in spike height but not accompanying any discerned slow potential change. The Group-II response obtained from a layer lying some $70-80\,\mu$ deeper also shows a discharge of impulses similar to the Group-I but is featured by their being superimposed on a conspicuous slow potential change resembling the ERG or some components of it. Beyond the depth for Group-II no impulses are detectable, but there is a layer yielding a sustained negative potential (Group-III response) that resembles the potential recorded by Svaetichin from the fish retina. The origin of the Group-I response is identified as single optic nerve fibers. Attempt to identify the cell type for the Group-II response is made by stimulating the whole bundle of the optic nerve fibers to check the invasion of antidromic impulses upon the Group-II neuron, but the question is left open.

References

Brown, K. T., and T. N. Wiesel: Intraretinal recording with micropipette electrodes in the intact cat eye. J. Physiol. 149, 537—562 (1959).
Granit, R.: Colour receptors of the frog's retina. Acta physiol. scand. 3, 137—151 (1942).
—, and T. Helme: Changes in retinal excitability due to polarization and some observations on the relation between the processes in retina and nerve. J. Neurophysiol. 2, 556—565 (1939).
Naka, K., S. Inoma, Y. Kosugi and C. Tong: Recording of action potentials from single cells in the frog retina. Jap. J. Physiol. 10, 436—442 (1960).
Polyak, S.: The vertebrate visual system. The University of Chicago Press (1957).
Svaetichin, G., and E. F. MacNichol: Retinal mechanisms for chromatic and achromatic vision. Ann. N. Y. Acad. Sci. 74, 385—404 (1958).
Tomita, T., M. Murakami and Y. Hashimoto: On the R membrane in the frog's eye: Its localization, and relation to the retinal action potential. J. gen. Physiol. 43, No. 6, Suppl., 81—94 (1960).

Discussion

E. F. MacNichol: First, I should like to congratulate Dr. Tomita for having accomplished what we have tried repeatedly and failed to do; that is to record the internal potentials of small ganglion cells and to show the relationship between the membrane potential and impulse discharge.

Although Dr. Tomita's results were not unexpected in the light of what we know about other neurons, it is gratifying to find that the ganglion cells behave in the same way as they do. In addition, Dr. Tomita's paper furnishes an excellent illustration of a fact which is not always appreciated: namely that very small micropipettes having resistances greater than 50 megohms will record from structures not accessible to ordinary micropipettes having resistances less than 20 megohms.

Although very large electrodes can be used for internal recording from spinal motoneurons and giant axons, according to Hunt very fine ones are required to penetrate internuncials without injuring them. Similarly, Fuortes obtained slow responses in the ommatidia of Limulus of over 60 mv. in amplitude. We had never seen more than 40 mv. of response in the course of literally thousands of punctures. We decided that the smaller electrodes used by Fuortes must have penetrated very small structures without injury. This conjecture was verified when Yeandle and Benolken, in our laboratory, pulled much finer microelectrodes than we had been using and regularly obtained the large potentials described by Fuortes. Similarly I believe that our failure to obtain in the goldfish retina long lasting chromatic responses of the type described by Svaetichin was due to our using electrodes which were so large that they caused injury. We hope that if we do the experiment with very small pipettes we will get responses which last for a long enough time to permit quantitative studies that can be correlated with the ganglion cell discharges in the same animal.

R. Jung: Wenn Dr. Tomita selbst auf Konklusionen seiner schönen intracellulären Ableitungen mit ultrafeinen Mikroelektroden verzichtet, so ist es für uns schwer, solche zu diskutieren. Die Lokalisation der langsamen Potentiale der Gruppe-III entspricht etwa derjenigen von GRÜSSER bei der Katze in der äußeren plexiformen Schicht. Besonders wichtig sind TOMITAs Abb. 1A und C. Sie zeigen eine deutliche Hyperpolarisation als direkten Nachweis der Lichthemmung in on/off- und off-Neuronen.

Die Latenzzeitunterschiede antidromer Reizung bei Fisch und Frosch sind wohl am besten durch verschiedene Leitungsgeschwindigkeiten myelinisierter und unmyelinisierter Opticusfasern zu erklären. Die antidrome Reizung der Group-II-responses von TOMITA spricht zwar nicht sicher gegen Spikes von Bipolarzellen, weil antidrom auch andere Neurone über rückläufige Kollateralen synaptisch erregt werden können, ähnlich PHILLIPS' Befunden an Betz-Zellen des motorischen Cortex. Doch scheinen nach TOMITAs Bildern echte antidrome Spikes von dislozierten Ganglionzellen oder ihren Dendriten wahrscheinlich.

P. GLEES: The slow antidromic propagation of impulses by intraretinal optic fibres could partially be accounted for by the extreme thinness of these fibres and by the absence of myelin in the mammalian intraretinal optic nerve fibres. What is the histology of the optic fibres in TOMITA's frogs?

E. DODT: Die antidromen Effekte könnten auch durch efferente Opticusfasern kompliziert sein, insbesondere die Doppelentladung.

W. SICKEL: Eine den Reiz besonders bei Dunkeladaptation beträchtlich überdauernde Nachwirkung kann ebenfalls den von SVAETICHIN gezeigten Experimenten MITARAIs entnommen werden. Das gleiche ergibt sich aus Spike-Ableitungen der mit geeigneter Lösung umspülten isolierten Froschretina, bei der off-bursts wachsender Latenz mit steigender Reizintensität auftreten (vgl. Abb. 2 meines Vortrags).

T. TOMITA: Thank you for your valuable criticisms. Drs. JUNG and GLEES are probably right in interpretation of the long latency of antidromic impulses in the frog retina. We have not examined our material histologically, but in the frog, when its opened eye is viewed through a dissection microscope under strong falling light, the intraretinal optic fibers are hardly discernible, while in the fish the fibers are clearly seen as white threads running radially from the optic disc. The difference may be attributed to nonmyelinated and myelinated fibers.

With regard to the cell type of Group-II neurons. After submission of this paper, we noticed a paper of BYZOV[1] dealing with observations very similar to ours but using extracellular micropipette electrodes. He mentions that some neurons in the bipolar cell layer respond with impulses to illumination and also to antidromic stimulation of the optic nerve. He considers them as Dogiel's cells or the ganglion cells displaced in the bipolar cell layer. While these neurons are very likely to correspond to our Group-II, there is at least one problem to be solved before one can conclude that the Group-II neurons are a kind of ganglion cells. In the Group-II neurons of on/off-type which outnumber the other two types, response to "on" of light regularly starts with a hyperpolarization that closely resembles in shape the a-wave of the ERG (cf. Fig. 1 A) though it is far larger in amplitude, showing sometimes 5 mV or more, than the a-wave obtained in the standard manner. If this type of response were from ganglion cells, the initial hyperpolarization should conduct electrotonically along the optic nerve. However, the absence of any trace of such has been shown by BERNHARD[2]. Consequently, the possibility is still preserved that the impulses elicited in Group-II neurons by stimulation of the optic nerve may not be direct but of postsynaptic nature, being produced in such a way as was suggested by Dr. JUNG or by Dr. DODT. The situations are confusing like this, but our effort to identify the cell type of Group-II neurons will continue, as I believe this is very important for furthering the understanding of intraretinal mechanisms.

---

[1] BYZOV, A. L.: Source of the impulses recorded from the inner layers of the frog retina (in Russian). Biofizika 4, 414—421 (1959).

[2] BERNHARD, C. G.: Temporal sequence of component potentials in the frog's retina and the electrotonic potential in the optic nerve. Acta Physiol. scand. 3, 301—310 (1942).

The Physiological Basis of Simultaneous Contrast in the Retina*

By

Koiti Motokawa, Eizo Yamashita and Tetsuro Ogawa

With 4 Figures

The loci of contrast effects in the visual system have been a subject of controversies in the literature of vision. Among others, Helmholtz (9) was firm in his opinion that simultaneous contrast depends on "judgment". Hering (10) assigned the phenomena of contrast to a physiological rather than to a psychological mechanism. Sherrington's classical experiments (26, 27) made with rotating discs may be interpreted as indicating that the physiological processes for contrast occur at a lower level of the nervous system than that required for binocular fusion. Brückner (4) found that in clinical cases with injury above the level of the lateral geniculate, color contrast could be induced into the injured half of the visual system by stimulation of the other half. In his studies on 'retinal induction' measured with electrical phosphenes as an index, Motokawa (14) suggested the peripheral nature of this phenomenon on the basis of the findings obtained from cases of homonymous hemianopsia. Kohata (12) showed that 'retinal induction' was abolished by a mechanical pressure as small as 50 g applied to the eyeball, while the photosensitivity of the eye was almost unaffected by such a slight pressure. All these phenomena suggest the retinal origin of 'retinal induction'. It was, however, demonstrated by Motokawa, Komatsu and Watanabe (16) that 'retinal induction' could be induced from the contralateral eye. This phenomenon together with the well-known phenomena of binocular contrast necessitates some central mechanisms.

In what follows some purely physiological data to be correlated with simultaneous contrast will be presented.

The carp's retina was isolated following the technique of Ottoson and Svaetichin (22) and mounted with the receptor side upwards on a small patch of Ringer-soaked black cloth covering a small silver plate which served as an indifferent electrode.

Unitary discharge of a ganglion cell was recorded with a 3 M KCl-filled microelectrode inserted into a depth of about 200 μ from the receptor side. Slow potentials were recorded with a microelectrode from the superficial layer. For recording these potentials A.C. amplifiers with a cathode follower input stage were used, the overall time constant of which was 100 msec. for slow potentials and 1.0 msec. for spike activity.

Slow potentials and spike activity of the fish retina

A slow potential in response to a light stimulus of small size is generally simple in form; it consists of a positive deflection which declines slowly during illumination to reach a steady level. At cessation of illumination a slight overswing towards the negative direction is usually seen. In the surrounding non-illuminated area there appears a slow potential which is similarly simple in form, but in polarity opposite to that obtained at the illuminated locus. The distribution of the negative slow potentials relative to the positive ones at the site of illumination is characteristic and of great importance for the physiology of pattern vision. The distribution was

---

* From the Department of Physiology, Tohoku University, Sendai, Japan.

mapped in such a way that a test spot 0.2×0.2 mm. in size was moved step by step along a straight line across the fixed recording electrode to take a record for each position of the test spot. An example is illustrated by a broken curve in Fig. 1, in which the magnitudes of responses are plotted as ordinates against distances from the electrode tip to the center of the illuminated area. The position and

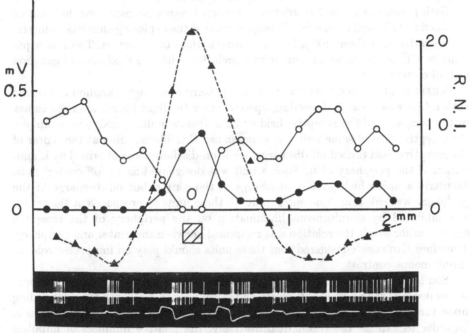

Fig. 1. Simultaneous recordings of slow electric responses (lower beam in inset) and unitary discharge of retinal ganglion cell (upper beam in inset). Magnitudes of slow responses and relative numbers of impulses *(R. N. I.)* are plotted as a function of distances between electrode tip and center of light spot. Open and filled circles connected with solid line represent 'on' and 'off' discharges respectively, and filled triangles connected with broken line represent slow responses. Size and position of stimulus are shown by shaded square. Intensity and duration of stimulus were 1250 lux and 0.4 sec. respectively

size of the illuminated area are shown by shaded square under the distribution curve. As can be seen in this figure, the positive potential falls off from the center towards the periphery of the illuminated area and changes its polarity at a short distance from 0.4 to 0.6 mm. from the margin of the light spot. The negative potential reaches a maximum at the distance from 0.8 to 1.2 mm. and extends as far as from 2 to 3 mm.

In other series of experiments the light spot was fixed at a certain point, and the recording electrode was moved step by step along a straight line passing through the illuminated part. The results obtained were essentially the same as above.

With a microelectrode inserted into various depths it was found that the positive potential was maximal at the surface and in its vicinity, and decreased very steeply around an apparent depth of about 100 μ from the receptor side. According to the histological investigation by OIKAWA, OGAWA and MOTOKAWA (21), receptor cells are included in a range of apparent depths from 0 to 100 μ. Therefore, the receptor layer may be responsible for the production of positive potentials, although contribution by other kinds of tissue is not excluded.

Similar experiments were done at a certain horizontal distance away from the margin of the illuminated part, but at various depths to get information of the laminar distribution of negative slow potentials, and it was found that the magnitude of the negative response was maximal around a depth of 100 μ from the receptor side. From these experiments it is apparent that the positive and negative slow potentials originate in different layers of the retina.

Both potentials are not restricted to inverted retina preparations, but can be obtained equally well from eyebulb preparations, if the exploring electrode is inserted into a depth of about 200 μ from the inner surface of the retina. These slow potentials will be shown to have definite correlation with the discharge of ganglion cells of certain type.

KUFFLER (13) found that the discharge pattern of a single ganglion cell of the cat's retina was variable depending upon whether the light illuminated the center or the periphery of the receptive field or both areas simultaneously; for example, the receptive field of some unit was so organized that illumination at the center of the receptive field caused off-discharge, while on-discharge was obtained by illumination of the periphery of it. Such a unit was designated as an 'off-center' unit. Similarly a unit which gave on-discharge at the center, but off-discharge at the periphery was called an 'on-center' unit. In these units the response at the center was inhibited by simultaneous illumination on the periphery of the receptive field; in other words the relation was reciprocal between the center and periphery. Therefore KUFFLER considered that these units should play an important role for simultaneous contrast.

Similar units with contrast organization have been found in the carp's retina. An example is shown in Fig. 1, which shows changes in discharge type depending upon the distance between the locus of illumination and the recording electrode. In order to express the result quantitatively, the relative numbers of impulses (R.N.I.) which refer to the numbers for 0.3 sec. after the onset and termination of the light stimulus respectively were plotted as a function of distances from the center of the illuminated area. The curve connecting open circles refers to the on-discharge, and the one connecting solid circles to the off-discharge. The distribution curve of slow potentials (the broken curve) may be compared with the data concerning the impulse discharges, because they were obtained from one and the same preparation by simultaneous recording. As can be seen in this figure, the positive slow potentials correspond to the off-discharge, while the negative ones correspond to the on-discharge. Thus the slow potentials are connected closely with the contrast organization of the receptive field of a unit of this type.

It is to be noted that the extent of the receptive field is of the same order as that of the field of slow potentials. BARLOW, FITZHUGH and KUFFLER (1) showed that the receptive field became narrower with increasing light adaptation of the retina. The field of negative potentials around a retinal image shrinks also with increasing intensities of background illumination. From these similarities it is likely that the effects of slow potentials are reflected in the impulse discharge of ganglion cells, or that the effects of slow potentials are transmitted to the central nervous system. It must, however, be noted that we have encountered a number of ganglion cells which had no contrast organization, for example, units of 'pure on' or 'pure off' type; in these units the type of discharge remained the same throughout the whole extent of the receptive field and no inhibitory interaction could be observed between the center and periphery of the receptive field. Therefore they do not seem to contribute to the physiological mechanism for simultaneous contrast.

Color contrast and the functional organization of the receptive field

In some units the type of discharge depended not only upon the locus of illumination within the receptive field, but also upon the wave-length of the illuminating

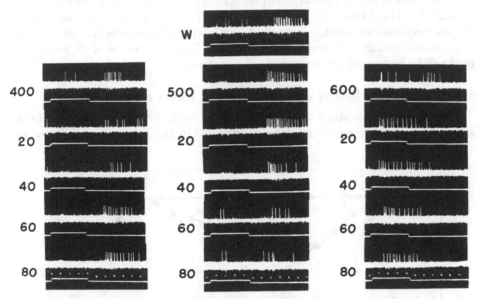

Fig. 2. Dependence of discharge pattern upon wave-lengths of stimulus lights. Numerals indicate wave-lengths (mμ). W stands for white light. Stimulating light spot (0.4 × 0.4 mm. in size) was centered upon tip of microelectrode. Height of spike was about 200 μV. Time mark 0.1 sec

light used. An example is shown in Fig. 2. The unit illustrated in this figure was an 'off-center' unit as examined by a test spot of white light.

The colored lights used were obtained by a set of interference filters whose width of the transmission band was each less than 20 mμ. The energy of these lights was made equal by suitable neutral tint filters. The test light was centered on the tip of the microelectrode placed at the center of the receptive field. Within a range between 400 and 540 mμ this unit showed a burst of spikes at 'off'. To the lights of 560—600 mμ it responded both at the onset and cessation of illumination. But the lights of wave-lengths longer than 620 mμ elicited only 'on' responses which lasted longer than the period of illumination. This change in discharge type was not due to the differences in brightness, because changes in intensity alone caused no alteration in discharge type.

When the functional organization of this unit was examined with the blue-green light of 500 mμ it proved to be an 'off-center' unit just as when searched with the white light, but it was found to be an 'on-center' unit, when tested with the light of 640 mμ complementary to the blue-green light used above. Complementarity is the known characteristic of color contrast. The unit under consideration responded most actively to both preferential portions of the spectrum, that is

3*

640 mμ and 500 mμ, and these wave-lengths are complementary to each other. The reciprocal relation with respect to the effects of wave-lengths is obvious in such a manner that the response type at the center of the receptive field was 'off' to the blue-green light, but 'on' to the red light.

WAGNER, MACNICHOL and WOLBARSHT (28) investigated the receptive fields of certain ganglion cells in the goldfish retina and obtained results very similar to ours. The most interesting finding by these authors seems to be that the 'on' and 'off' responses could be light-adapted separately: Adaptation to a steady background of red light raised the threshold of the 'off' responses, but the threshold of the 'on' responses was slightly lowered. A blue adapting light made the 'on' process less sensitive and the 'off' process more sensitive. These properties of the receptive field will be important for successive color contrast.

The field of slow potentials and border contrast

When the stimulus size is larger than a certain limit, the form of response at the site of illumination is not so simple as is illustrated in Fig. 1, but as complicated as

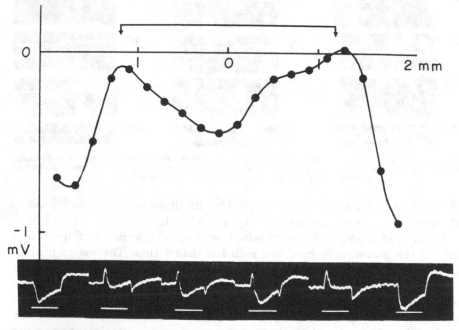

Fig. 3. Potential field within and without retinal image 2.5 × 2.5 mm in size. Magnitude of response was measured from base line to steady level of response, and plotted as ordinate against distance between electrode tip and center of illumination as abscissa. Horizontal line with arrows at ends shows extent of illumination. Insets are some examples of real records. Horizontal bars in insets indicate duration of stimulus of 0.6 sec. Intensity 25 lux

the form of an electroretinogram of the frog. Examples are shown in the inset of Fig. 3. The response of the carp's retina obtained within the illuminated area consists of a biphasic 'on' response, initially positive, then negative, and a negative 'off' response. Judging from their polarity the initial positive deflection would correspond to the a-wave, and the later negative one to the b-wave of the usual ERG. The response obtained around the illuminated area is usually a pure negative potential, but can be preceded by a small positive deflection, when stray light is effective. The carp's retina is a favorite material for obtaining a pure negative potential, although such is obtainable under special conditions also from other vertebrate retinas (3). The negative potential represents a physiological process conducting laterally through some nervous tissue, because it was shown in a previous paper (18) that the negative potential in the dark area around an illuminated part was abolished by a mechanical cut along the boundary between both bright and dark areas. This process is considered to be induced from the photoreceptors into a proximal layer probably consisting of horizontal cells and conducted laterally. The conduction velocity was measured in such a way that the latencies of negative potentials recorded at various distances from the margin of an illuminated part were expressed as a function of distance (17). The relation was linear, and from this relation a value of 110 mm. per sec. was obtained on an average. This value is of the same order as that of the conduction velocity of 'retinal induction' determined in the light-adapted human retina (15).

Strong summation can be seen among negative potentials produced simultaneously in the retina, because they are propagating graded responses. On the contrary, the positive potential shows no sign of lateral conduction, and its tendency to spatial summation is only slight; some apparent summation of positive potentials which can be seen in the dark-adapted retina is greatly reduced by light adaptation, because the effect of stray light which obviously summates is reduced by background illumination.

The biphasic 'on' response to a large stimulus mentioned above may be regarded as an interference product of positive and negative potentials. The positive component is a direct effect of illumination at the illuminated locus, but the negative one is a summation product of potentials conducted from a wide region, so that the initial positive, later negative deflections of the 'on' response will be produced. The attempts to analyze the ERG into components of different polarities have been made by different authors such as PIPER (23), GRANIT (6) and others. The present investigation is in line with the classical analyses in that the two components of different polarities are assumed, but it is a new concept to regard one component as a local process and the other as a propagating, diffuse process. It should be recollected that there were controversies concerning the question whether the ERG is a local process or a diffuse one (2, 5, 7). The origin of the ERG will be discussed in detail elsewhere, and only some aspects important for simultaneous contrast will be mentioned here.

When the slow potentials of the central and peripheral parts of the illuminated area are compared with each other, it will be found that the positivity is more prominent (negativity is less prominent) in the peripheral part than in the central part. In Fig. 3 the magnitudes of negative deflections are plotted as a function of distances from the center of the illuminated area. The curve so obtained is M-shaped showing that there is a distribution of slow potentials characteristic for simultaneous contrast at the margin of the illuminated area; the positivity of response is maximal at the margin and falls off very steeply towards the outside of the illuminated area and reaches a minimum at a short distance from the boundary. Such a distribution of visual excitation at the boundary has ever been imagined, but experimental evidence has been lacking.

Such a characteristic distribution of slow potentials can be accounted for in terms of the properties of both potentials mentioned above. The positive potential at a point within the illuminated area is a local process and will be depressed by the negative potentials induced from neighboring excited points. The depression will be less marked at the margin of the illuminated area, because no depressant effect comes from the neighboring non-illuminated area. In consequence, a maximum of positivity or minimum of negativity will be established at the margin of the illuminated area. The negative process induced from the illuminated part into the surrounding area will decline with increasing distances away from the boundary because of either decremental conduction of the process or increasing reduction in the number of elements involved. On the other hand, stray light whose amount shows an exponential decrement with lateral distance causes a gradient of positive potential from the boundary towards the surrounding area. The observed maximum of negativity located at a short distance from the boundary has been produced by interaction of these two opposing processes.

The question now arises as to the site of interaction between positive and negative potentials. As has been stated above, the positive potential is produced in the receptor layer or tissue closely connected with receptors, while the negative potential is maximally recorded at a depth of about 100 μ from the receptor side. If the interaction were a physical process occurring somewhere in the volume conductor represented by these layers, the result of interaction would be an algebraic sum of both potentials. In reality, however, the positive potential is so predominant that the interaction between positive and negative potentials of equal magnitude will result in a positive potential of reduced amplitude. The interaction must, therefore, be a physiological one occurring at some special seats such as synapses. The seat of interaction is not located in the synapses between ganglion cells and bipolar cells, because the interaction can be recorded most clearly with a microelectrode inserted into a depth less than 100 μ from the receptor side; no remarkable slow potential can be recorded from the ganglion cell layer from which isolated spikes of considerable amplitude may be obtained.

In one of the schemata proposed by POLYAK (24) it is shown that a horizontal cell makes a synapse with a receptor cell. Such a synapse will be an adequate one as the seat of interaction under consideration. For this schema to be adopted it must be taken for granted that the positive potential is produced in the receptor cells while the negative one represents the activity of the laterally connecting nervous pathways including horizontal cells. It is to be noted that a negative slow potential can be elicited by electrical stimulation with a microelectrode inserted into a depth of about 100 μ from the receptor side (19). The negative potential elicited by electrical stimulation propagates laterally at the same velocity as the negative potential induced by a light stimulus (20). But we have not yet succeeded in eliciting a positive potential by electrical stimulation, and this situation makes it likely that the positive potential originates in the receptor cells; it must be produced by some photochemical products, and electrical stimulation will not be effective to cause photochemical reactions.

As has been stated above, the positive potential is a direct effect of a light stimulus, but cannot be a generator potential which fires the second neurons. It may be a positive potential picked up from the source of the current caused by some generator potential, but all attempts to prove a phase reversal of potential with a microelectrode advanced from the receptor side into deeper layers have failed. Therefore the question as to the origin and mode of action of the positive potential awaits further studies. At any rate, it should be assumed that there is a nervous mechanism responsible for simultaneous contrast at a retinal level located closely to the receptor layer. This is, however, not the only mechanism for simultaneous contrast in the vertebrate retinas, for the ganglion cell level may be regarded as another seat of interaction having possible relation to contrast effects. In the vertebrate retinas a great number of receptors converge onto a common ganglion cell which represents a seat of interaction and integration.

It has been shown above that the receptive field of some ganglion cells is so organized that the excitation at the central part is inhibited by simultaneous excitation of the peripheral part, and vice versa. This is obviously an organization essential to contrast, as was pointed out by KUFFLER, and is not a mere replica of the contrast mechanism postulated at a more distal level. There are some grounds to assume that the organization of such a unit depends on the synaptic organization of the ganglion cell or the arrangement of excitatory and inhibitory synapses at that level. One of the grounds is that a neighboring ganglion cell can be of entirely different discharge type; units of 'pure on' or 'pure off' type are scattered among units with contrast organization. This fact would be difficult to understand if the contrast organization were predetermined by a more distal mechanism. If this interpretation is correct, there are in the vertebrate retina at least two levels at which lateral inhibition takes place so as to cause contrast effects.

In the following example it will be seen how the mechanisms at the two levels cooperate. We determined precisely the receptive field of a ganglion cell. The central part of the receptive field responded with an off-discharge to a test spot, and the peripheral part with an on-discharge, the intermediary zone responding with an on-off-discharge. Illumination of an area outside the receptive field caused no response whatsoever. The off-discharge was reduced in comparison with that caused by a test spot restricted to the central part, when the whole area of the receptive field was illuminated. This effect may be due to the contrast organization at the ganglion cell level or lateral inhibition at the slow potential level or more probably due to both factors.

When the area of illumination was further increased so as to involve the area beyond the limits of the receptive field, the off-discharge was increased above the response to the stimulus just covering the receptive field. From this finding it is apparent that the area whose illumination had no direct influence upon the discharge of the ganglion cell can have indirect influence upon it. This indirect effect cannot be ascribed to the synaptic action at the ganglion cell level, because the ganglion cell makes synapses with the neurons connected with the receptive field, but receives no direct influence from any area outside the receptive field. The indirect effect must, therefore, be due to the lateral inhibition occurring at the more distal level. The curious fact stated above may be accounted for in terms of 'disinhibition': The activity of the peripheral zone of the receptive field will be inhibited by the activation of the surrounding area. In consequence, the inhibitory effect of the peripheral zone upon the central part will be lessened so that the off-discharge will be enhanced above that caused by illumination of the whole receptive field. It seems that the lateral effect of negative slow potentials is broader and diffuser than the one to be ascribed to the ganglion cell level. The contrast effect seems to be somewhat restricted in space but more accentuated in pattern by the organization at the ganglion cell level.

Comments

Physiological evidence for border contrast was provided by Ratliff and Hartline (25) at the optic nerve level and by Jung (11) at the cortical level.

In the experiments of Hartline, Wagner and Ratliff (8) the discharge of impulses in the single optic nerve fiber originating from an ommatidium of the lateral eye of Limulus was shown to be inhibited by activation of neighboring ommatidia. The depression of the frequency of discharge (inhibition) increased approximately linearly with the logarithm of the intensity of illumination on receptors in its vicinity. Inhibition was greater the larger the area of the eye illuminated in its vicinity. The degree of inhibition diminished with increasing distance, but might extend for several millimeters. All these properties apply well to the negative slow potentials of the fish retina, but we do not know whether a similar slow potential can be found also in the Limulus eye.

In the experiments of Ratliff and Hartline (25) it was found that a maximum and minimum of the discharge rate appeared on either side of the boundary between brightly and dimly illuminated areas, and this fact was interpreted by these authors as representing a physiological basis of border contrast. It was emphasized that lateral inhibition alone will do to account for this fact. The interpretation proposed by these authors is as follows: "A unit which is within the dimly illuminated region, but which is near this boundary, will be inhibited not only by dimly illuminated neighbors but also by brightly illuminated ones. The total inhibitions exerted on it will therefore be greater than that exerted upon other dimly illuminated elements that are farther from the boundary; consequently its frequency of response will be less than theirs. Similarly, a unit within but near the boundary of the brightly illuminated field will have a higher frequency of discharge than other equally illuminated units which are located well within the bright field but which are subject to stronger inhibition since all their immediate neighbors are also brightly illuminated. Thus differences in the activity of elements on either side of the boundary will be exaggerated and the discontinuity in this pattern of illumination will be accentuated in the pattern of neural response."

We have interpreted our similar pattern of slow potentials on the same principle as Ratliff and Hartline. The lateral inhibition in the Limulus eye is mediated by the nervous interconnections in the plexus of fibers just behind the layer of ommatidia. Similarly, the lateral spread of the negative slow potentials in the fish retina was located in the lateral nervous connections including horizontal cells. In the Limulus eye the inhibition is exerted directly upon the sensitive structure within the ommatidium, because it was observed when the impulses were recorded by a microelectrode thrust into an ommatidium as well as when they were recorded more proximally in single fibers dissected from the optic nerve. In the fish eye the synapse between a receptor cell and a horizontal cell was regarded as the seat of interaction between positive and negative potentials. Thus similarity is very close between the mechanism for contrast in the Limulus eye and the first order mechanism for contrast in the fish eye.

In the Limulus eye there is no nerve cell intercalated between an ommatidium and its optic nerve fiber, nerve impulses traversing the fiber pathway from ommatidia to optic nerve in either direction. Therefore the second order mechanism for contrast such as that observed in the fish retina is lacking in the Limulus eye. The synaptic organization at the ganglion cells in the vertebrate retina must be a device for elaborating the neural pattern predetermined by a more distally located crude mechanism. The differences between both sorts of eyes are schematized in Fig. 4. The most conspicuous difference consists in the convergence from the receptors (R) within its receptive field (P C P) onto a ganglion cell (G) via bipolar cells (B). The synapses marked by minus signs corresponding to the central part (C) of the receptive field will be, say — inhibitory — and yield off-discharge, while those marked by plus signs corresponding to the peripheral part (P) will be facilitatory and yield on-discharge. In the Limulus eye in

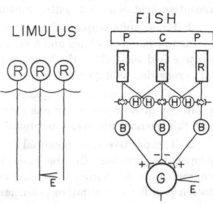

Fig. 4. Schematic representation of nervous connections in Limulus and fish eyes. R receptor; H horizontal cell; B bipolar cell; G ganglion cell; E recording electrode; P and C periphery and center of receptive field. Further explanation in text

which there is no such synaptic system the response is only of 'on' type, and no phenomenon to be called a 'post-inhibitory rebound' can be seen.

The first order mechanism for contrast is represented by a nervous connection including horizontal cells (H) in this diagram. Whether or not the action of this system is completely similar to that of the system for lateral inhibition in the Limulus eye will have to be clarified in further studies.

In the experiments of BAUMGARTNER and HAKAS, reported by JUNG (11) a large contrasting stimulus of white and black was arranged in various positions relative to the receptive field for a cortical neuron of certain type, B-neuron, to investigate how the discharge of this neuron depended upon the stimulus pattern. When the receptive field corresponded to white at the border to the dark field, the strongest on-discharge appeared. A reverse discharge type, showing an off-discharge, similar to a D-neuron reaction, was seen when the receptive field projected to the dark region. This sort of approach is of great value, because it will provide a clue to the phenomena of binocular contrast which cannot be accounted for in terms of the contrast mechanisms in the retina.

Summary

With 3 M KCl-filled microelectrodes slow potentials and spike activity of ganglion cells were recorded simultaneously in the isolated retina of the carp. The slow potentials were well recorded in the layer within 100 μ from the receptor side, while the spike activity was recorded in depths of about 200 μ.

1. The slow potentials recorded within an illuminated area were positive in polarity relative to an indifferent electrode placed beneath the inverted retina.

In the surrounding area there appeared negative potentials which had the maximal amplitude at a short distance from the margin of the illuminated area and extended as far as a few millimeters.

2. Units of various discharge types were found, for example, 'on-center' units, 'off-center' units, 'pure on' units, 'pure off' units, etc. It was shown that the distribution of slow potentials had certain relation to the discharge pattern within the receptive field of an 'off-center' unit or an 'on-center' unit.

3. Some units responded most actively to both preferential portions of the spectrum, that is, 640 mμ and 500 mμ. The response type at the center of the receptive field was 'off' to the blue-green light, but 'on' to the red light. These units were regarded as important for color contrast.

4. When the retina was exposed to a stimulus larger than a certain limit, the positivity of slow potentials was maximal at the margin of the illuminated area, and this phenomenon was interpreted as physiological evidence of border contrast.

5. The positive slow potential is a local process, while the negative one is a propagating process. On the basis of these properties the spatial distribution characteristic for border contrast was accounted for in terms of interaction between positive and negative potentials.

6. Two retinal mechanisms for simultaneous contrast were postulated at the slow potential level and the ganglion cell level.

References

1. BARLOW, H. B., R. FITZHUGH and S. W. KUFFLER: Change of organization in the receptive fields of the cat's retina during dark adaptation. J. Physiol. 137, 338—354 (1957).
2. BOYNTON, R. M., and L. A. RIGGS: The effect of stimulus area and intensity upon the human retinal response. J. exp. Psychol. 42, 217—226 (1951).
3. BRINDLEY, G. S.: Responses to illumination recorded by microelectrodes from the frog's retina. J. Physiol. 134, 360—384 (1956).
4. BRÜCKNER, A.: Über Anpassung des Sehorgans. Schweiz. med. Wschr. 6, 245—252 (1925).
5. FRY, G. A., and S. H. BARTLEY: The relation of stray light in the eye to the retinal action potential. Amer. J. Physiol. 111, 335—340 (1935).
6. GRANIT, R.: The components of the retinal action potential in mammals and their relation to the discharge in the optic nerve. J. Physiol. 77, 207—240 (1933).
7. — B. RUBINSTEIN and P. O. THERMAN: A new type of interaction experiment with the retinal action potential. J. Physiol. 85, 34 P. (1935).
8. HARTLINE, H. K., H. G. WAGNER and F. RATLIFF: Inhibition in the eye of Limulus. J. gen. Physiol. 39, 651—673 (1956).
9. HELMHOLTZ, H.: Handbuch der physiologischen Optik. Hamburg und Leipzig 1886.
10. HERING, E.: Grundzüge der Lehre vom Lichtsinn. Berlin: Springer 1920.
11. JUNG, R.: Microphysiology of cortical neurons and its significance for psychophysiology. An. Fac. Med. Montevideo 44, 323—332 (1959).
12. KOHATA, T.: Suppression of color contrast and retinal induction by mechanical pressure applied to the eyeball. Tôhoku J. exp. Med. 66, 239—250 (1957).
13. KUFFLER, S. W.: Discharge patterns and functional organization of mammalian retina. J. Neurophysiol. 16, 37—68 (1953).
14. MOTOKAWA, K.: Physiological induction in human retina as basis of color and brightness contrast. J. Neurophysiol. 12, 475—488 (1949).
15. — and M. KOMATSU: Propagation velocity and total reflection of spreading induction induced in the light-adapted human retina. Tôhoku J. exp. Med. 67, 149—158 (1958).
16. — — and K. WATANABE: Binocular contrast and physiological induction. Tôhoku J. exp. Med. 70, 39—48 (1959).

17. Мотокаwa, K., T. Oikawa and T. Ogawa: Slow potentials induced from the illuminated part into the surrounding area of the retina. Jap. J. Physiol. 9, 218—227 (1959).
18. — — K. Tasaki and T. Ogawa: The spatial distribution of electric responses to focal illumination of the carp's retina. Tôhoku J. exp. Med. 70, 151—164 (1959).
19. — E. Yamashita and T. Ogawa: Responses of retinal network to electrical stimulation. Tôhoku J. exp. Med. 71, 41—53 (1959).
20. — — — Interaction of slow potentials of the retina evoked by photic and electric stimuli. Tôhoku J. exp. Med. 71, 67—77 (1959).
21. Oikawa, T., T. Ogawa and K. Motokawa: Origin of so-called cone action potential. J. Neurophysiol. 22, 102—111 (1959).
22. Ottoson, D., and G. Svaetichin: Electrophysiological investigations of the frog retina. Cold Spr. Harb. Symp. quant. Biol. 17, 165—177 (1952).
23. Piper, H.: Über die Netzhautströme. Arch. Anat. Physiol. 85—132 (1911).
24. Polyak, S. L.: The retina. VII, 607 pp. Chicago: Chicago Univ. Press. 1941.
25. Ratliff, F., and H. K. Hartline: The responses of Limulus optic nerve fibers to patterns of illumination on the receptor mosaic. J. gen. Physiol. 42, 1241—1255 (1959).
26. Sherrington, C. S.: On reciprocal action in the retina as studied by means of some rotating discs. J. Physiol. 21, 33—54 (1897).
27. — On binocular flicker and the correlation of activity of "corresponding" retinal points. Brit. J. Psychol. 1, 26—60 (1904).
28. Wagner, H. G., E. F. MacNichol and M. L. Wolbarsht: Opponent color responses in retinal ganglion cells. Science 131, 1314 (1960).

Discussion

M. L. Wolbarsht: The diagram showing "off" center field with "off" receptors in the center of the field and "on" receptors on the periphery is probably incorrect, as both "on" and "off" responses can be recorded by properly stimulating the receptors located in the center of the receptive field.

G. Baumgartner: Man könnte sich auch vorstellen, daß die langsamen Potentiale mit Vorgängen zu tun haben, die der Organisation des rezeptiven Feldes zugrundeliegen. In diesem Falle sollte man aber erwarten, daß mit zunehmender Lichtadaptation das Gebiet, in dem die negativen Potentiale registriert werden können, größer wird. Prof. Motokawa berichtet aber gerade das Gegenteil, Verkleinerung des Feldes mit zunehmender Lichtadaptation. Sind bei voll lichtadaptierter Retina noch negative Potentiale zu registrieren? — Ist dies nicht der Fall, so ist es möglich, daß es sich bei den langsamen Potentialen nur um Sekundärphänomene ohne direkte Kontrastwirksamkeit handelt, da der Kontrast mit der Helladaptation positiv korreliert.

M. Monjé: Als Vertreter der subjektiven Sinnesphysiologie möchte ich ein Wort zum Simultankontrast sagen: Wir haben unseren Vpn eine kreisförmige Marke (Durchmesser 10′) dargeboten und haben die Empfindlichkeit (sensitivity) in der Nachbarschaft dieser Marke mit Hilfe von kleinen Prüfreizen (Durchmesser 1,5′) untersucht. Wir fanden dabei die Empfindlichkeit im Bereiche des Randkontrastes herabgesetzt (Diapositiv). Der Anstieg der Empfindlichkeit war nicht in allen Richtungen gleich steil; er ist u. a. von individuellen Faktoren abhängig.

R. Jung: Monjés Ergebnisse entsprechen den Befunden von Harms und Aulhorn über veränderte subjektive Schwellen in der Region des Simultankontrasts beim Menschen. Dies paßt wiederum zu Baumgartners neuronalen Befunden im Kontrastfeld der Katze, die im Randbezirk die massivste Aktivierung der Einzelneurone ergaben. In diesem Gebiet wächst die Signal-Noise-Ratio und dadurch wird auch die Schwelle erhöht.

M. Monjé: Ja, der Einfluß der hellen Scheibe ist von ihrer Leuchtdichte abhängig, er ist um so größer und reicht um so weiter, je höher die Leuchtdichte ist (Diapositiv). — Wir haben weiter die Empfindlichkeit im Bereich des Binnenkontrastes bestimmt, indem wir die Empfindlichkeit im Innern der Scheibe gemessen haben. Wir haben ein Absinken der Empfindlichkeit in der Mitte gefunden. Die Kurven sind denen von Motokawa ganz ähnlich. Es freut mich, daß wir hier objektiv bestätigt finden, was wir auch subjektiv schon nachgewiesen haben.

W. Metzger: Ich möchte in diesem Zusammenhang auf alte Versuche von St. Blachowski[1] hinweisen. Blachowski hat anscheinend mit größerem Reizfeld gearbeitet. Dabei war das Ergebnis für die Umgebung des Reizfeldes genau dasselbe wie bei Monjé. Im Innern des Feldes aber umgekehrt, wenn ich mich recht erinnere.

M. Monjé: Die Unterschiede zwischen den Befunden von Blachowski und mir lassen sich tatsächlich weitgehend auf die verschiedenen Versuchsbedingungen zurückführen. Sie sind von mir in meiner Arbeit „Über die Lichtempfindlichkeit im Bereich des Rand- und Binnenkontrastes"[2] ausführlich diskutiert worden.

L. M. Hurvich: In connection with Prof. Monjé's remarks, a large number of psychophysical experiments on humans show interactive effects on visual threshold measurements. We should, moreover, not overlook an extensive related literature motivated by more practical interests, namely the study of visibility under glare conditions. In the presence of bright sources marked threshold increases have been demonstrated and the dependence of these increases on a wide variety of parameters has been rather exhaustively explored.

R. Jung: Die wichtigste Frage, die von mehreren Teilnehmern geäußert wurde und die uns Prof. Motokawa vielleicht schriftlich beantworten kann, ist folgende: *Sind die langsamen Potentiale, die im Kontrast eine Umkehr zeigen, intracellulär abgeleitete* (wie Svaetichins Ableitungen beim Fisch und Grüssers bei der Katze) *oder sind sie diffuse intraretinale Potentiale?* Die starke Summation spricht vielleicht gegen intracelluläre und mehr für intraretinale Potentiale, und Svaetichin hat auch diese Meinung geäußert. Ist ein Dipoleffekt durch die seitlichen Durchschneidungsversuche ausgeschlossen?

Wenn es sich um intracelluläre Potentiale handelt, würden sie gut zu Grüssers Vorstellungen über die synaptische Auslösung der nächsten neuronalen Spikes in reziproken Neuronensystemen durch positiv und negativ gerichtete Receptorpotentiale passen und damit auch zu Baumgartners Befunden über on- und off-Umkehr im Grenzkontrast.

Wenn Motokawa die positive Komponente als lokalen, die negative als fortgeleiteten Prozeß ansieht, entstehen dann positive und negative Komponenten in verschiedenen Strukturen? Welche Zellstrukturen kommen in Frage, wenn die Horizontalzellen nach Svaetichin und Villegas Gliazellen sind?

K. Motokawa: Psychophysical experiments of Prof. Monjé and others seem to receive physiological grounds from our experiments. The effect of light adaptation upon the field of negative potentials also seems to be in line with the well-known experiment by Hess and Pretori who showed that the apparent brightness of an inner field depends on the ratio of the illuminances at the inner and outer fields. Since the ratio was reduced on raising the level of light adaptation in our experiment, the apparent brightness or contrast would be reduced under such conditions. This situation would correspond to the observed reduction of the outer field of negative potentials under light adaptation. It is, therefore, difficult for me to understand the interpretation offered by Dr. Baumgartner.

Next, I should like to reply to Prof. Jung. The positive and negative slow potentials mentioned above were recorded extracellularly, and only the latter shows a diffuse character and strong summation. The negative potential cannot spread across a mechanical cut which is made between the illuminated and surrounding areas. This fact together with its low conduction velocity suggests that the spread of the negative potential is a physiological spread. The maximum of the localized positive potential is found at the receptor layer or its neighborhood, while that of the diffuse negative potential is located in the layer containing horizontal cells and

---

[1] Z. Sinnesphysiol. **47**, 291 (1913).
[2] Pflügers Arch. ges. Physiol. **262**, 92 (1955).

bipolar cells. The positive potential is reduced markedly by a shunt-effect when the isolated retina is immersed into the Ringer's solution, but the negative potential is affected only slightly by this procedure. It seems that the horizontal cells are the most probable seat of lateral conduction, although the nature of the horizontal cells is not clear at present, as pointed out by SVAETICHIN and VILLEGAS.

I agree with Dr. WOLBARSHT in that the discharge type of a unit is not fixed, but can be different depending upon the intensity, duration, wavelength and size of the illumination.

Kontrastlichteffekte an retinalen Ganglienzellen: Ableitungen vom Tractus opticus der Katze*

Von

GÜNTER BAUMGARTNER

Mit 5 Abbildungen

Durch KUFFLERs Untersuchungen (1952 und 1953) mit Lichtpunktreizen ist die antagonistische Organisation der rezeptiven Felder einzelner retinaler Ganglienzellen der Katze bekannt geworden, nachdem HARTLINE schon 1949 auf ähnliche Mechanismen lateraler Hemmung am Limulus-Auge hingewiesen hatte. Die Ganglienzellen der Retina reagieren danach bei isolierter Belichtung ihres rezeptiven Feldzentrums umgekehrt wie bei Belichtung der Peripherie. On-Zentrum-Neurone werden also durch isolierte Belichtung der Feldperipherie gehemmt, off-Zentrum-Neurone aktiviert. Dies gilt allerdings nur für die helladaptierte Retina. Bei zunehmender Dunkeladaptation wird die antagonistische Randzone des rezeptiven Feldes kleiner. Wie BARLOW, FITZHUGH u. KUFFLER (1957) gezeigt haben, ist in der voll dunkeladaptierten Retina kein Randzonenantagonismus mehr nachweisbar.

Um zu erfahren, wie sich diese Feldorganisation bei einfachen Kontrastreizen auswirkt, welche Information on- und off-Zentrum-Neurone auch bei Reaktionsumkehr übertragen, und in welcher Weise die verschiedenen visuellen Zentren an der Kontrastbildung beteiligt sind, haben wir die Reaktionen der visuellen Neurone bei einfachen Hell-Dunkel-Reizen im *Tractus opticus, Corpus geniculatum laterale* und *Cortex* (Area 17) registriert (BAUMGARTNER u. HAKAS 1959, 1960). In dieser Mitteilung wird nur auf Neurone des Tractus opticus eingegangen.

Methodik. Zur Ableitung wurde der Tract. opt. durch Resektion der darüberliegenden Großhirngebiete freigelegt und die Mikroelektrode (mit 3 mol KCl gefüllte Glascapillaren) unter Sichtkontrolle eingeführt. Als Kontrastreiz wurde ein Gitter aus senkrechten Metallstreifen und freien Zwischenräumen verwandt, welches vor einer gleichmäßig ausgeleuchteten Milchglasscheibe (30° × 50°) in Intervallen von 42,5′ verschiebbar war. Die Hellfeldbreite war zwischen 5° 41′ und 0° variabel. Nach 8 Gitterverschiebungen war bei gleichgroßen Hell- und Dunkelfeldern (5° 41′) der anfänglich aufgehellte Gesichtsfeldbereich dunkel, der zunächst beschattete hell. Das Gesichtsfeld der Katze war so abgedunkelt, daß über zwei getrennt verschließbare Oculare nur die Milchglasscheibe gesehen werden konnte. Die Augen der Katze waren durch Durchtrennung der äußeren Augenmuskel oder Curare immobilisiert und durch eine Hintergrundsbeleuchtung von 30 Lux leicht helladaptiert. Die Cornea wurde durch einen Dauertropf feucht gehalten. Die operative Vorbereitung erfolgte in Äthernarkose. Zur Ableitung selbst wurde die Katze durch einen hohen Querschnitt (encéphale isolé, BREMER 1938) ruhiggestellt.

---

* Aus der Abteilung für Klinische Neurophysiologie der Universität Freiburg i. Br.

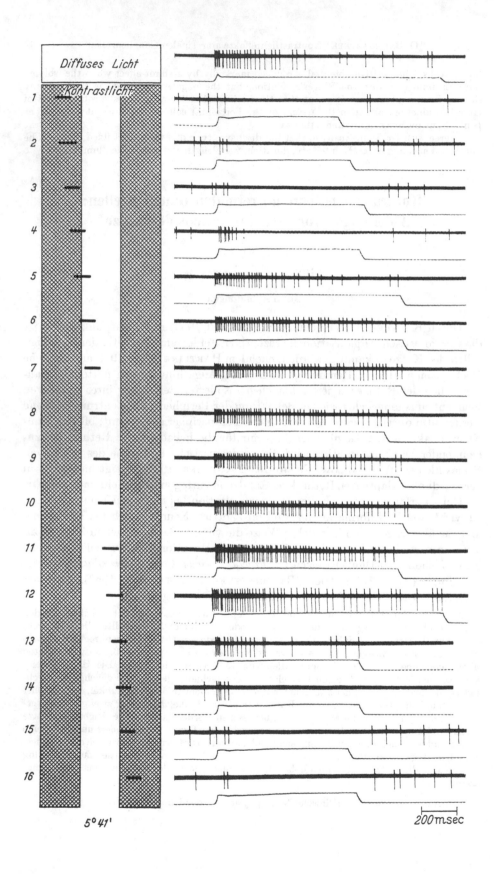

Diffuses Licht

Kontrastlicht

5° 41'

200 msec

Zunächst wurde ein auf diffuse Belichtung (300 Lux, weißes Licht einer breitbandigen Niedervoltlampe) der Milchglasscheibe reagierendes Neuron gesucht. Zeigte das Neuron bei Vorbeibewegen des Gitters bei eingeschaltetem Licht durch sakkadierende Impulsstöße, daß es das Gitter „sah" und nicht nur durch Streulicht aktiviert war, so wurde es weiter getestet. Dazu wurden in jeder Gitterposition die Reaktionen auf Belichtung registriert und in einer Belichtungspause das Gitter in die nächste Position gebracht. Blieb das Neuron an der Elektrode, so wurde es mit verschiedenen Hellfeldbreiten untersucht.

Ergebnisse. Abbildung 1 a u. b zeigt das Beispiel eines on-Zentrum-Neurons bei Kontrastreizung. Zum Vergleich ist die Reaktion auf diffuse Belichtung

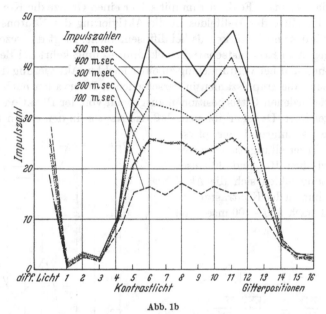

Abb. 1b

Abb. 1 a u. b. On-Zentrum-Faser des Tractus opticus bei diffusem Lichtreiz und Kontrastbelichtung. a Links: Schema der retinalen Projektion *des Kontrastfeldes* auf das rezeptive Feldzentrum bei verschiedener Gitterposition. Der horizontale Durchmesser des Feldzentrums (schwarzer Balken) und seine Ausleuchtung durch den Kontrastreiz in den verschiedenen Gitterpositionen ist größen- und lagerichtig angegeben. *Rechts: Neuronale Reaktionen* bei den entsprechenden Gitterpositionen. Die Dauer des Lichtreizes wird durch eine Photozelle markiert, die unter jeder neuronalen Reaktion abgebildet ist. Hell (weiß)- und Dunkelfelder (schraffiert) sind in diesem Beispiel von gleicher Breite (5° 41'). b Abhängigkeit des Kontrasteffektes von der Zeit: Impulszahlen des Neurons in den verschiedenen Gitterpositionen. Die Kurven zeigen die Impulszahl in den ersten 100, 200, 300, 400 und 500 msc nach Belichtung

vorangestellt. Vor der Abbildung des Neurons ist schematisch die Kontrastsituation gezeichnet. In das Kontrastfeld ist größen- und lagerichtig der horizontale Durchmesser des rezeptiven Feldzentrums in den verschiedenen Gitterpositionen eingetragen. Die dahinter befindlichen neuronalen Reaktionen entsprechen der davor angegebenen Ausleuchtung des rezeptiven Feldes.

Der horizontale Durchmesser des Feldzentrums selbst wurde unter der Annahme bestimmt, daß es bei Belichtung auch nur eines Teiles des Feldzentrums zur Aktivierung des Neurons kommt. Mißt man unter dieser Voraussetzung die Größe der Feldverschiebung (F_v) vom Beginn bis zum Ende der Aktivierung und kennt man die Hellfeldbreite (F_b), so ergibt die Feldverschiebung (F_v) weniger der Hellfeldbreite (F_b) die Größe der Verschiebung (D) zwischen den beiden gegenüberliegenden Grenzen des Feldzentrums (s. Abb. 2). Bei Kenntnis des Abstandes des Gitters vom Auge (d) ergibt sich daraus der Sehwinkel $\left(\dfrac{D}{d} = \text{tg}\,\varepsilon\right)$, woraus sich der horizontale Durchmesser einfach errechnen läßt. Dabei sind wir im Anschluß an Barlow et al. (1957) davon ausgegangen, daß einem Sehwinkel von 4°30′ 1 mm auf der Retina der Katze entspricht. Der auf diese Weise gemessene Horizontaldurchmesser der rezeptiven Feldzentren von 5 on-Zentrum-Neuronen des Tr. opt. lag zwischen 0,52 und 0,85 mm. Die einzelnen Neuronen wurden jeweils mehrfach mit verschiedenen Hellfeldbreiten gemessen.

Aus Abb. 1a ist ersichtlich, daß das on-Zentrum-Neuron maximal aktiviert wird, wenn das rezeptive Feldzentrum mit seiner einen Grenze die Kontrastgrenze berührt. In der Mitte des Hellfeldes ist die Aktivierung des Neurons etwas verringert, aber immer noch stärker als bei diffusem Licht. Liegt das rezeptive Feldzentrum dagegen im Kontrastschatten, so kommt es umgekehrt bei Belichtung zu einer Hemmung und bei Verdunkelung zu einer leichten Aktivierung des Neurons. In Abb. 1b sind die Impulszahlen in verschiedenen Intervallen nach Belichtung über den verschiedenen Gitterpositionen ausgehend von der Reaktion auf diffuses Licht aufgezeichnet. Dabei ergibt sich, daß das Neuron in den ersten 100 msec so reagiert, wie es aufgrund der physikalischen Lichtverteilung zu erwarten ist. Erst zwischen 100 und 300 msec nach Belichtung bilden sich die Aktivierungsmaxima an der Kontrastgrenze aus. Sie sind nach 300—400 msec voll ausgeprägt.

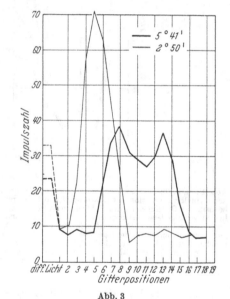

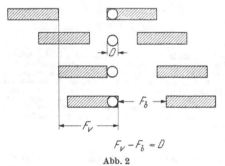

$$F_v - F_b = 0$$

Abb. 2   Abb. 3

Abb. 2. Schematische Darstellung der Messung des horizontalen Durchmessers eines on-Feldzentrums mit dem Kontrastgitter (//// Dunkelfeld, F_b Hellfeldbreite, F_v Feldverschiebung, D Verschiebung zwischen den Grenzen des Feldzentrums), s. Text, S. 47

Abb. 3. *Impulszahlen einer on-Zentrum-Faser des Tractus opticus bei Kontrastreizen mit unterschiedlicher Hellfeldbreite (5° 41′, 2° 50′)*. Ausgezählt wurden jeweils die Entladungen in den ersten 500 msec nach Belichtung in verschiedenen Gitterpositionen

Auf Abb. 3 sind 2 Aktivierungsverläufe einer anderen Tractusfaser dargestellt, welche mit verschiedenen Hellfeldbreiten (5°41′ und 2°50′) getestet wurde. Man sieht, daß die Aktivierung bei schmalem Hellfeld wesentlich stärker ist als bei breitem und daß es nur noch zu einem Aktivierungsmaxima kommt. Diese Aktivierungssteigerung ist dabei nicht nur durch die etwas erhöhte Ausgangsaktivität des Neurons bei der Testung mit schmalem Hellfeld zu erklären.

Das Verhalten einer on-off-Faser im Kontrast zeigt Abb. 4a und b. Für die schematische Darstellung des Kontrastes gilt das gleiche wie für Abb. 1a (s. o.). Die Felddurchmesser wurden bei off-Zentrum-Fasern lediglich unter der Voraussetzung bestimmt, daß Belichtung des Zentrums hemmt. Man hat deshalb die Feldverschiebung zwischen zwei on-Maxima zu messen, wie aus Abb. 5 hervorgeht. Aktivierungsmaxima bei Belichtung müssen auftreten, wenn das Feldzentrum gerade völlig beschattet und der größtmögliche Bereich der aktivierenden Randzone belichtet wird. Die Dunkelfeldbreite (Fb) abzüglich der Feldverschiebung (Fv) ergibt dann die Verschiebung (D) zwischen den beiden Grenzen des Feldzentrums, woraus sich bei Kenntnis des Augenabstandes (d) wieder der Sehwinkel und damit auch die horizontale Durchmessergröße des rezeptiven Feldzentrums auf der Retina errechnen läßt.

Auf Abb. 4a sieht man, daß die bei diffuser Belichtung nach einer präexcitatorischen Hemmung auftretende on-Reaktion im Kontrast verschwindet. Die Lichthemmung wird also unter Kontrastbedingungen vollständig, und zwar dann, wenn das rezeptive Feldzentrum an der Kontrastgrenze im Hellfeld liegt. Wird das rezeptive Feldzentrum in den Kontrastschatten gebracht, so zeigt das Neuron auf Belichtung dagegen eine verstärkte on-Aktivierung und eine Verminderung des off-Effektes. Bei Auszählung der Impulse in den ersten 500 msec nach Belichtung ergibt sich wiederum, daß die on-Aktivierung eine Tendenz zu einem Doppelgipfel mit Maxima an den Kontrastgrenzen zeigt. Im Gegensatz zu dem on-Zentrum-Neuron liegt die Aktivierungskurve aber im Dunkelfeld des Kontrastbereiches. Der horizontale Durchmesser des rezeptiven Feldzentrums dieses Neurons betrug 0,85 mm.

Besprechung. Das Verhalten der Neurone des Tract. opt. unter Kontrastbedingungen ist danach so, wie es aufgrund KUFFLERs Lichtpunkt-Untersuchungen an Ganglienzellen der Retina zu erwarten ist. Durch Beschattung der Feldperipherie im Kontrast wird die bei diffuser Belichtung antagonistische Randzonenhemmung der on-Zentrum-Neurone vermindert. Die on-Zentrum-Neurone werden deshalb an der Kontrastgrenze maximal aktiviert. Inmitten eines breiten Hellfeldes nimmt die Hemmung durch gleichzeitige Belichtung beider Randzonen wieder zu, was das Absinken der Aktivierungskurve und damit deren M-förmigen Verlauf erklärt. Beschattet man die Randzone durch Verschmälerung des Hellfeldes von beiden Seiten, so nimmt erwartungsgemäß bis zu einer von Neuron zu Neuron unterschiedlichen Hellfeldbreite zwischen 2—3° die Aktivierung stark zu. Wird das Feldzentrum selbst in den Kontrastschatten gebracht, so kommt es über die Belichtung der hemmenden Randzone zu einer Hemmung des Neurons bei Belichtung und einer leichten Aktivierung bei Verdunkelung.

Die off-Zentrum-Neurone, zu denen die reinen off- und die präexcitatorisch gehemmten on-off-Neurone gehören, zeigen umgekehrt bei Belichtung im Kontrast dann eine Aktivierung, wenn ihr Feldzentrum im Kontrastschatten liegt. Auch hier ist die maximale Aktivierung an der Kontrastgrenze durch die Belichtung der in diesem Falle antagonistisch aktivierenden Randzone (laterale Aktivierung) einfach zu erklären. Die völlige Lichthemmung der on-off-Neurone mit präexcitatorischer Hemmung bei Annäherung an die Kontrastgrenze zeigt, daß die späte on-Aktivierung über die antagonistische Randzone ausgelöst wird. Bei einseitiger Beschattung der Randzone reicht die von ihr ausgehende Aktivierung nicht mehr aus,

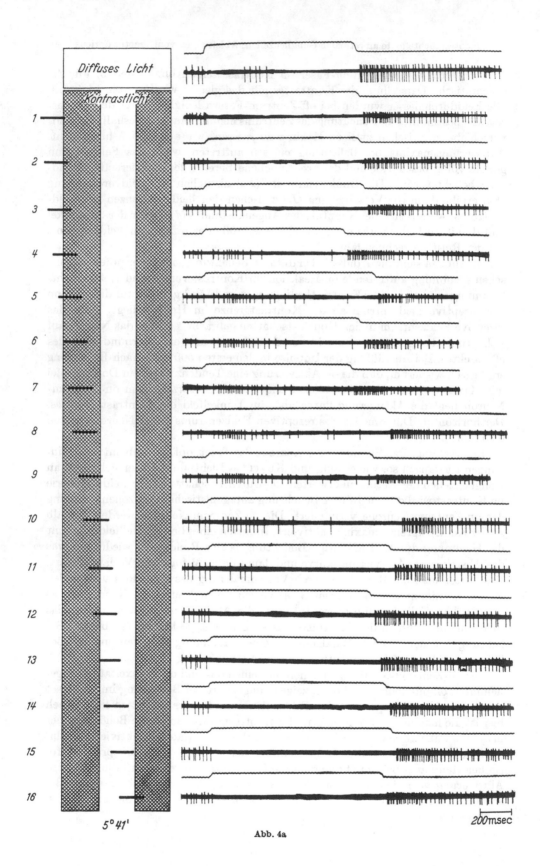

Abb. 4a

die vom Feldzentrum direkt durchgeschaltete und dadurch bei diffuser Belichtung immer primär auftretende Hemmung zu durchbrechen, d. h. die Hemmung bei Belichtung wird vollständig. Das Kontrastverhalten der präexcitatorisch gehemmten on-off-Neurone zeigt also,daß es sich bei ihnen um off-Zentrum-Neurone handelt.Die Äquivalente dieser on-off-Neurone mit off-Zentren sind on-off-Neurone, deren rezeptive Felder eine on-Zentrum-Organisation aufweisen. Diese Neurone reagieren demzufolge ohne präexcitatorische Hemmung auf Belichtung, während dagegen die off-Aktivierung erst nach einer langen Latenz auftritt. Sie sind bei den von uns als Test verwendeten Lichtintensitäten sehr selten ($< 1\%$).

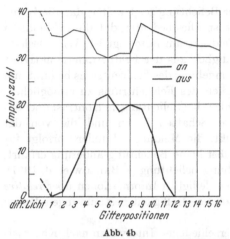

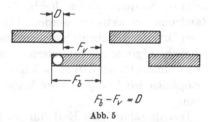

$$F_b - F_v = D$$

Abb. 4b   Abb. 5

Abb. 4 a u. b. *Kontrastreaktionen eines on-off-D-Neurons des Tractus opticus* (off-Zentrum-Faser, die bei diffuser Belichtung eine on-off-Reaktion zeigt). a *Neuronale Reaktionen in verschiedenen Gitterpositionen* (Anordnung entsprechend Abb. 1). Die Photozelle wurde hier über der jeweiligen Neuronreaktion registriert. b. *Impulszahlen des Neurons 500 msec nach Belichtung (——) und Verdunkelung (——)*

Abb. 5. Schematische Darstellung der Messung des horizontalen Durchmessers eines off-Feldzentrums mit dem Kontrastgitter. (//// Dunkelfeld, F_b Dunkelfeldbreite, F_v Feldverschiebung, D Verschiebung zwischen den Grenzen des Feldzentrums) s. Text, S. 49

Die Reaktionen der on- und off-Tractusfasern auf Kontrastlichtreize bestätigen also die früheren Befunde KUFFLERs und BARLOWs et al. erneut (s. a. HUBEL 1960). Gleichzeitig zeigen sie, daß *das neuronale Verhalten weitgehend mit der subjektiven Kontrastwahrnehmung korreliert, sofern man die Helligkeitswahrnehmung mit den on-Zentrum-Neuronen, die Dunkelwahrnehmung mit den off-Zentrum-Neuronen in Verbindung bringt.* Denn die on-Neurone werden im Hellfeld an der Kontrastgrenze, also dort maximal aktiviert, wo subjektiv der größte Helligkeitseindruck (Grenzkontrast) entsteht. Off- und präexcitatorisch on-off-Neurone zeigen dagegen, wenn sie auf Belichtung aktiviert werden im Dunkelfeld an der Kontrastgrenze, also dort eine maximale Aktivierung, wo subjektiv der stärkste Dunkeleindruck eintritt. Denn durch den Kontrast kommt es bei Belichtung zu einer Kontrastverdunkelung des Dunkelfeldes mit Maxima an der Grenze zum Hellfeld. Der leichten subjektiven Aufhellung der Dunkelfelder bei Verdunkelung geht eine Aktivierung der on-Neurone, deren Feldzentren im Kontrastschatten liegen, parallel (s. Abb. 1a).

Die Verbindung neuronaler Reaktionen bei der Katze mit subjektiv sinnesphysiologischen Erfahrungen setzt sich über ein weites, völlig unbekanntes Gebiet hinweg und ist zweifellos gewagt. Die Korrelationen sind jedoch so eindeutig, daß sie kaum zufällig sein können und es wahrscheinlich ist, daß auch beim Menschen ähnliche Mechanismen von Bedeutung sind. Setzt man dies voraus, so läßt das

4*

Verhalten der Opticusfasern im Kontrast schließen, daß die on-Zentrum-Neurone der Katze bei Aktivierung immer „heller", die off-Zentrum-Neurone immer „dunkler" für den Bereich ihres rezeptiven Feldzentrums melden. Dabei ist es gleichgültig, ob die Aktivierung bei Belichtung oder Verdunkelung erfolgt. Wenn es im Kontrast zur Reaktionsumkehr eines Neurons kommt, dann entsteht diese immer nur bei Beschattung des Feldzentrums durch Belichtung der antagonistischen Randzone.

Das Verhalten der Neurone bei diffuser Belichtung zeigt weiter, daß die Lichtreaktion des Feldzentrums stets dominant ist. Dies bedeutet, daß die Information einer retinalen Ganglienzelle durch ihr Feldzentrum festgelegt ist. Wird deshalb im Kontrast eine Opticusganglienzelle lediglich aus der Feldperipherie aktiviert oder gehemmt, so wird das Licht aus der Umgebung des Feldzentrums benutzt, um eine Information über die relative Helligkeit des Feldzentrums zu ermöglichen. So erfolgt beispielsweise die Meldung „dunkler" bei Belichtung im Kontrast über off-Zentrum-Neurone, deren Feldzentren im Schatten liegen und die von der Randzone her aktiviert werden. Das heißt, die Meldung „dunkler" erfolgt für einen Ort der Netzhautoberfläche, der selbst keine Belichtungsänderung erfährt, lediglich aufgrund der veränderten Umgebungsbelichtung (s. BARLOW et al. 1957). Es ist einleuchtend, daß ein solches System lediglich Informationen über *relative Helligkeitsveränderungen*, aber keine absoluten Helligkeitsbestimmungen liefern kann.

Die Auszählung der Entladungen in verschiedenen Intervallen nach Kontrastbelichtung hat ergeben, daß sich der Einfluß der Feldperipherie durch laterale Hemmung (s. Abb. 1b) erst verzögert bemerkbar macht. Dies ist verständlich, da die Erregung des Feldzentrums über weniger Synapsen (minimal bisynaptisch) zur Ganglienzelle gelangt als die Erregung der Feldperipherie. Die Reaktion in den ersten 100 msec nach Kontrastbelichtung zeigt deshalb lediglich die physikalische Lichtverteilung im rezeptiven Feldzentrum für die verschiedenen Gitterpositionen an. Erst danach wird durch die mit längerer Latenz aus der Feldperipherie auf die Ganglienzelle konvergierenden Impulse deren Aktivität modifiziert und kontrastabhängig gemacht.

Summary

1. The responses of retinal ganglion cells recorded from their axons in the optic tract fibers of the cat to contrast patterns of black and white stripes are described. The contrasting stimulus was moved at small intervals across the visual field. In every position of the pattern, the neuronal responses to light-on and off were recorded.

2. By this contrast stimulation, the diameter of the neuronal receptive field center can be measured by correlating the neuronal responses in different positions of the contrasting grid with its lateral shift.

3. The activation of optic tract fibers is always stronger near the contrast borders than at diffuse illumination of the same intensity.

4. The responses of optic tract fibers to stimulation correspond to KUFFLER's antagonistic organization of their receptive fields and can be explained by lateral inhibition or lateral activation of the field center from the surrounding field.

5. On-center neurons show the strongest activation if their receptive field center is made brighter and their surrounding field darker by contrast light stimulation. Conversely, off-center neurons exposed to contrast illumination exhibit the strongest activation if their receptive field centers lie in the dark field of the contrast stimulus and their surrounding field is illuminated.

6. Activation of on-center neurons always occurs where contrast stimulation subjectively would correspond to a perception of increased brightness. Conversely, activation of off-center neurons occurs where contrast stimulation leads to subjective perception of darkening. This correspondance suggests that on-center neurons transmit the information "brighter", off-center neurons the information "darker". It is then irrelevant, whether activation of these neurons occurs at light-on or light-off.

7. The responses of optic tract neurons therefore can be separated in *2 classes: on-center neurons and off-center neurons*. These antagonistic neuronal systems signal relative brightness information and darkness information respectively and thus assure specificity and constancy of brightness vision and correlate well with subjective perceptions in simultaneous brightness contrast.

Literatur

1. BARLOW, H. B., R. FITZHUGH and S. W. KUFFLER: Change of organization in the receptive fields of the cat's retina during dark adaptation. J. Physiol. (Lond.) 137, 338—354 (1957).
2. BAUMGARTNER, G., u. P. HAKAS: Reaktionen einzelner Opticusneurone und corticaler Nervenzellen der Katze im Hell-Dunkel-Grenzfeld (Simultankontrast). Pflügers Arch. ges. Physiol. 270, 29 (1959).
3. — Vergleich der rezeptiven Felder einzelner on-Neurone des Nervus opticus, des Corpus geniculatum laterale und des optischen Cortex der Katze. Zbl. Neurol. Psychiat. 155, 243—244 (1960).
4. BREMER, F.: L'activité électrique de l'écorce cérébrale. Paris: Hermann Cie. 1938.
5. HARTLINE, H. K.: Inhibition of visual receptors by illuminating in the limulus eye. Fed. Proc. 8, 69 (1949).
6. HUBEL, D.: Single unit activity in lateral geniculate body and optic tract of unrestrained cats. J. Physiol. (Lond.) 150, 91—104 (1960).
7. KUFFLER, S. W.: Neurons in the retina: organization, inhibition and excitation problems. Cold Spring Harbor Symposion on quantitative Biology 17, 281—292 (1952).
8. — Discharge patterns and functional organization of mammalian retina. J. Neurophysiol. 16, 37—69 (1953).

Diskussion

L. M. HURVICH: I wonder whether Dr. BAUMGARTNER has had an opportunity to use spectral stimuli in addition to black and white stimuli in this type of situation and if so what sort of differentiating signals are obtained? The dominating note here with respect to the quality or colour signal seems to be of spatial differentiation. SVAETICHIN localises the achromatic and chromatic signals in two different levels and says that he believes these spatially differentiated signals are maintained all the way to the cortex. The MacNICHOL and WOLBARSHT goldfish data show different kinds of responses in the same layer but are interpreted as indicating specificity of different ganglionic cells. DE VALOIS says that this is essentially his view also. Since we have already reached the point where "on" responses from a cell are assumed to have a different color coding from "off" responses in the same cell then I wonder if the assignment of different types of responses to different spatial loci may not be a consequence of the limitations of the electrophysiological techniques of the moment and whether with further refinement of technique we might find that the same tissue can respond differentially to different stimuli.

M. L. WOLBARSHT: The question of the distribution of "on" and "off" receptors in the receptive fields of "on-off" ganglien cells has not been answered yet, e. g. are there "on" receptors in the center of the "off" center field ? The color separation technique which WAGNER, MACNICHOL and I have used in the goldfish does not appear to be applicable to the cat, but some drug such as alcohol may allow experiment in which one process, the inhibition is removed.

M. MONJÉ: Wir haben den Kontrast nach der klassischen Methode untersucht, indem wir in der Umgebung eines hellen Fleckes von 10′ Durchm. die Empfindlichkeit gemessen haben. Im Bereiche des Randkontrastes fanden wir eine Herabsetzung der Empfindlichkeit, die um so größer war, je höher die Leuchtdichte der kontrasterregenden Marke war. Ihre Ausdehnung scheint eine geringere Rolle zu spielen. Die Steilheit des Anstiegs ist in den verschiedenen Meridianen verschieden, die fixierte Stelle allerdings stets dieselbe, denn der Anstieg wurde in verschiedenen Versuchen übereinstimmend gefunden. Wir konnten ferner feststellen, daß die Empfindlichkeit im Inneren der Kontrastmarke, im Bereich des Binnenkontrastes, mit Sicherheit herabgesetzt ist. In größeren geradlinig begrenzten Flächen fehlt diese Empfindlichkeitssenkung; subjektiv können also solche Flächen heller sein als objektiv gleich helle, aber kleinere Scheiben. Versuche am Stabgitter-Kontrast von HERMANN bestätigen die Ergebnisse. Die Senkung der Empfindlichkeit in der Umgebung eines Lichtpunktes ist wahrscheinlich die Voraussetzung dafür, daß das Auge in der Lage ist, den Lichtpunkt zu fixieren (vgl. M. MONJÉ, Über die Lichtempfindlichkeit im Bereiche des Rand- und Binnenkontrastes).[1]

G. BAUMGARTNER (zu HURVICH): Wir haben bisher lediglich Schwarz-Weiß-Kontraste untersucht, weil wir auf Grund der Verhaltensversuche angenommen haben, daß die Katze keine nennenswerte Farbdiskrimination besitzt. Ich kann also keine Angaben über farbspezifische Fasern machen. Bei der Verwandtschaft von Farb- und Helligkeitskontrasten ist aber wahrscheinlich, daß das gleiche Organisationsprinzip, welches wir beim Schwarz-Weiß-Sehen finden, auch für die Farbrezeption gilt. Das würde besagen, daß es Felder gibt, die nach Farbpaaren antagonistisch angeordnet sind, und auf ähnliche Phänomene haben DE VALOIS und WOLBARSHT schon hingewiesen. Die Schwierigkeit der Übertragung des Hell-Dunkel-Mechanismus auf das Farbensehen ist die Tatsache, daß bei Farbpaaren beide Farben Lichtenergie zuführen, während beim Schwarz-Weiß-Sehen nur durch das weiße Licht Energie zugeführt wird. Eine direkte Analogie ist also kaum möglich, obwohl die Farbenkontraste für antagonistische Feldorganisationen wie beim Hell-Dunkel-System sprechen. Vielleicht könnte die Annahme weiterführen, daß die komplementären Gegenfarben für entsprechende Farbreceptoren jeweils „schwarz", d. h. nicht aktivierend sind.

Zu WOLBARSHT: Die neuronalen Reaktionen auf *Helligkeitskontrastreize* lassen sich auch ohne die Annahme von zwei verschiedenen Receptortypen (on- und off-Receptoren) durch die Organisation der rezeptiven Felder verstehen. Man hat nur vorauszusetzen, daß der gleiche Receptorentyp im Zentrum eines on-Feldes mit der zugehörigen Opticusfaser aktivierend, in der Peripherie des Feldes dagegen hemmend verschaltet ist. Umgekehrt ist für ein off-Zentrum-Neuron anzunehmen, daß das Feldzentrum hemmend und die Feldperipherie mit aktivierenden Impulsen auf die zugehörige Opticusganglienzelle konvergiert. Mir ist diese Auffassung sympathischer als die Annahme von getrennten on- und off-Receptoren, da ich mir schlecht vorstellen kann, was ein Receptor aufnehmen soll, wenn keine Lichtenergie mehr auf die Retina trifft.

Unter diesem Gesichtspunkt läuft Dr. WOLBARSHTs Frage darauf hinaus, ob durch alleinige Reizung des off-Zentrums eines on-off-Neurons auch on-Reaktionen auslösbar sind oder nicht. Bei den bisherigen Versuchen war dies nie der Fall. Auszuschließen ist dies jedoch noch nicht, weil bisher nur geringe Helligkeitsvariationen im Kontrast getestet wurden. Bei unterschiedlich verlaufenden Empfindlichkeitskurven für on- und off-Reaktionen sind deshalb Reaktionsumkehrungen denkbar. Auf Grund der neuronalen Reaktionen bei diffusen Lichtreizen verschiedener Intensität ist dies jedoch weniger wahrscheinlich.

Zu MONJÉ: Die Empfindlichkeitsverminderung in der Kontrastumgebung läßt sich neuronal durch die im Bereich des Grenzkontrastes gesteigerte Grundaktivität erklären, sofern man diese als einen erhöhten Störpegel (noise) auffaßt. Die Verminderung der Empfindlichkeit im

---

[1] Pflügers Arch. ges. Physiol. **262**, 92 (1955).

Bereich der Kontrastgrenze verhindert, daß das abgebeugte Licht überschwellig wird. Die Kontrastgrenze wird dadurch verschärft. Das gleiche gilt meines Erachtens für die von Ihnen festgestellte Empfindlichkeitsverminderung im Innern der Helligkeitsmarke. Ich glaube nicht, daß diese Empfindlichkeitsverminderung ein Phänomen des „Binnenkontrastes" ist, zumal Sie ebenfalls wie frühere Untersucher festgestellt haben, daß bei besseren Voraussetzungen zur Ausbildung des „Binnenkontrastes", d. h. in größeren Flächen, diese Verminderung fehlt.

Neuronal sind Binnen- und Randkontrast nicht zu unterscheiden. Die neuronalen Mechanismen, die der Kontrastbildung zugrunde liegen, sind bei diffuser Belichtung genau so vorhanden wie bei Kontrastreizen und verursachen den „Binnenkontrast", der eine Art Kontrast ohne Kontrast ist. Dieser „Binnenkontrast" sollte unter neuronalem Gesichtspunkt zu einer Empfindlichkeitssteigerung führen und dies wurde auch schon mehrfach subjektiv sinnesphysiologisch nachgewiesen (BLACHOWSKI[1] 1913, KRÜGER u. BONAME[1] 1955 und andere). Wenn Sie eine Empfindlichkeitssenkung auch im Zentrum der Lichtmarke festgestellt haben, so ist dies wahrscheinlich durch die relativ kleine Marke von 10' bedingt. Man findet nämlich bei indirekten Feldbestimmungen mittels des Hermannschen Gitters auch im fovealen Sehen Feldzentrumsdurchmesser von ungefähr 4—5' (vgl. S. 309). Das besagt, daß bei einer Lichtmarkengröße von 10' eine Trennung von Rand- und Binnenkontrast noch nicht möglich ist. Die empfindlichkeitssenkende Wirkung des Randkontrastes muß in diesem Falle also bis ins Zentrum reichen.

Glial Control of Neuronal Networks and Receptors[2]

By

GUNNAR SVAETICHIN, MIGUEL LAUFER, GENYO MITARAI, RICHARD FATEHCHAND, EDMUNDO VALLECALLE and JORGE VILLEGAS

pg. 445

The Effect of Temperature, Carbon Dioxide and Ammonia on the Neuron-Glia Unit[2]

By

MIGUEL LAUFER, GUNNAR SVAETICHIN, GENYO MITARAI, RICHARD FATEHCHAND EDMUNDO VALLECALLE and JORGE VILLEGAS

pg. 457

Glia-Neuron Interactions and Adaptational Mechanisms of the Retina[2]

By

GENYO MITARAI, GUNNAR SVAETICHIN, EDMUNDO VALLECALLE, RICHARD FATEHCHAND, JORGE VILLEGAS and MIGUEL LAUFER

pg. 463

[1] ST. BLACHOWSKI: Studien über den Binnenkontrast. Z. Psychol-Physiol. Sinnesorg. II, 47, 291—330 (1913). — L. KRÜGER and J. R. BONAME: A retinal excitation gradient in a uniform area of stimulation. J. exp. Psychol. 49, 220—224 (1955).

[2] From the Instituto Venezolano de Investigaciones Cientificas, Caracas, Venezuela.

Studies on the Retinal Ganglion Cells[1]

By

Jorge Villegas

The Retina as Model for the Functional Organization of the Nervous System[1]

By

Edmundo Vallecalle and Gunnar Svaetichin

Discussion

III. Lokalisation und Bedeutung der retinalen „Receptorpotentiale" ("Cone potentials", "EIRG")

Gruppendiskussion

Receptorabhängige R-Potentiale der Katzenretina[2]

Von

O.-J. Grüsser[3]

Mit 2 Abbildungen

In der Retina der Katze (Cerveau isolé Präparation) lassen sich mit Mikroelektroden, deren Spitzendurchmesser unter $0,5\,\mu$ beträgt, intraretinale DC-Potentiale (*1, 2, 4—7, 8a*) ableiten, die den von Svaetichin (*8, 11*) in der Fischretina entdeckten Potentialen (*13*) ähneln. Diese langsamen R-Potentiale zeigten folgende physiologischen Eigenschaften (*4—7*):

[1] From the Instituto Venezolano de Investigaciones Cientificas (IVIC) Caracas, Venezuela.
[2] Aus der Abteilung für Klinische Neurophysiologie der Universität Freiburg i. Br.
[3] Universitätsnervenklinik Göttingen. Mit Unterstützung der Deutschen Forschungsgemeinschaft.

1. Die absolute Schwelle lag für „weißes Licht" einer Wolframbandlampe zwischen 0,5 und 5 Lux.

2. Das Ruhepotential lag zwischen 15 und 40 mV. Der „wirkliche" Wert ist wahrscheinlich höher, da das Ruhepotential in der Regel um so höher war, je dünner die Mikroelektrodenspitze war.

3. Auf weißes Dauerlicht erfolgte eine Hyperpolarisation (Negativierung) um 3 bis 30 mV. Zwischen 2 und 500 Lux ergab sich näherungsweise eine logarithmische Abhängigkeit zwischen der Amplitude des R-Reaktionspotentials und der Beleuchtungsstärke.

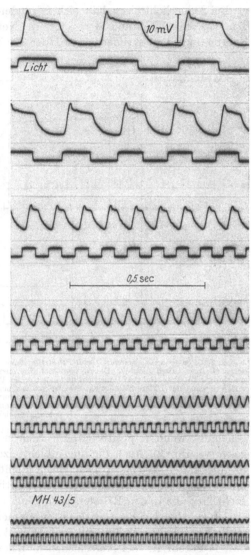

4. Die Flimmerfusionsfrequenz (CFF) bei 200 Lux lag über 70 Lichtreizen pro sec (Hell-Dunkel-Verhältnis 1:1). Sie ist damit deutlich höher als die Flimmerfusionsfrequenz retinaler Neurone unter gleichen Versuchsbedingungen (9) (Abbildung 1).

5. Die Amplitude (A), die Anstiegsteilheit $\frac{(-dA)}{dt}$ und das Flächenintegral des R-Potentials über dem Ruhepotential nahmen mit steigender Flimmerfrequenz bis zur CFF ab.

6. Die Latenzzeit der on-Reaktionen verkürzte sich mit Erhöhung der Beleuchtungsstärke und war um 3—5 msec kürzer als die kürzeste Latenzzeit der on-Neurone in der Retina unter gleichen Lichtreizbedingungen. Die Latenzzeit war unabhängig von der Flimmerfrequenz.

7. Orientierende Untersuchungen mit farbigen Lichtreizen ergaben im gesamten Spektralbereich nur Hyperpolarisation auf Belichtung. Eine Analogie zum L-Typ SVAETICHINs in der Fischretina ist anzunehmen.

Abb. 1. R-Potential MH 43/5 Flimmerlicht 200 Lux. Flimmerfusionsfrequenz über 70 Lichtreizen pro Sekunde (aus 5)

8. Nach Elektrocoagulation der Arteria centralis retinae können unverändert R-Potentiale registriert werden, Neuronentladungen mit spikes dagegen nicht.

9. Messungen der Einstichtiefe von der Membrana limitans interna aus ergaben die äußere plexiforme Schicht als wahrscheinlichen Ableitort der R-Potentiale.

10. Die R-Potentiale sind außerordentlich kleinen Einheiten zuzuordnen. Bewegungen der Mikroelektrode um wenige μ brachten sofort das Ruhepotential zum Verschwinden. Es war sehr viel schwerer, R-Potentiale zu registrieren als spike-Entladungen, wobei sich in der Katzenretina Pulsationen äußerst ungünstig auswirkten.

Bei Dauerlichtreizen läßt sich folgender zeitlicher Zusammenhang zwischen den R-Potentialen und der retinalen Neuronenaktivität herstellen: Die on-Neurone werden aktiviert, wenn der Differentialquotient (dA/dt) negativ ist,

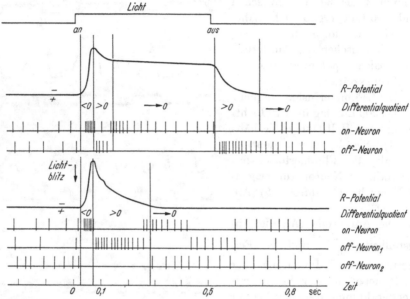

Abb. 2. *Zeitliche Beziehung zwischen dem R-Potential und den retinalen Neuronen (on- und off-System) bei Dauerlicht und einem kurzen Lichtblitz.* Die rhythmischen Neuronentladungen nach dem Lichtblitz haben keine Entsprechung im R-Potential. Auf Dauerlicht und in den ersten Phasen nach einem Lichtblitz werden die on-Neurone aktiviert, wenn der Differentialquotient des R-Potentials negativ, gehemmt, wenn er positiv ist. Die off-Neurone verhalten sich umgekehrt. Hemmung und Erregung sind immer relativ zum vorausgehenden Aktivierungsgrad. Einige off-Neurone (off$_2$) werden nach Lichtblitzen erst dann aktiviert, wenn das R-Potential wieder das Ruhepotential erreicht hat

gehemmt, wenn er positiv ist. Die Neurone des off-Systems verhalten sich umgekehrt (Abb. 2). Auch für kurze Lichtreize gilt dieser zeitliche Zusammenhang für die ersten 200 msec nach einem Lichtblitz. Im retinalen Neuronensystem findet man jedoch rhythmische Nachaktivierungsphasen bis 2 sec nach dem Lichtblitz, die in den R-Potentialen keine Entsprechung haben. (6)

Ob der beschriebene zeitliche Zusammenhang ein Kausalzusammenhang ist, muß offen bleiben. Auffallend ist jedoch, daß auch zwischen der Anstiegsteilheit des R-Potentials bei verschiedenen Beleuchtungsstärken und bei Flimmerbelichtung und der Latenzzeit der retinalen on-Neurone eine konstante zeitliche Beziehung besteht: Die Anstiegsteilheit ($-dA/dt$) nimmt mit Verminderung der Beleuchtungsstärke ab, die Latenzzeit der on-Neurone zu (3,9). Das gleiche gilt für Flimmerlicht: mit steigender Flimmerfrequenz nimmt die Anstiegsteilheit des R-Potentials ab, die Latenzzeit der on-Neurone bis zur CFF zu.

Wir glauben, daß es sich bei den registrierten Potentialen um Ableitungen aus synaptischen Strukturen (Zapfen-Bipolaren) handelt. Die einzelne Receptorzelle wird als Kondensator-Widerstands-System aufgefaßt, in dem durch Zerfalls-produkte der Sehfarbstoffe die Kondensatorkomponente während der Belichtung verändert wird.

Diese Änderung des C-Gliedes kommt möglicherweise durch eine Änderung der Dielektrizitätskonstante zustande. An den synaptischen Strukturen bedingt die Kapazitätsänderung eine Potentialänderung, für die nach der Kondensator-formel keine Ladungsänderung notwendig ist. Die Potentialänderung in den synaptischen Strukturen hat eine Wanderung der "synaptic vesicles" zur Folge, die eine postsynaptische Erregung auslösen.

Das morphologische Substrat für die C-Komponente wird in den geschichteten Lipoproteinstrukturen des Außengliedes gesehen, die mit den Sehfarbstoffschichten abwechseln. Das Substrat der R-Komponente stellen die übrigen Receptor-strukturen (Innenglied usw.) dar, wobei der schmalen Verbindung zwischen Außen- und Innenglied (bei einigen Receptortypen etwa 1 μ) eine besondere Be-deutung zukommen kann.

Die RC-Hypothese der Receptorerregung hat den Vorteil, daß mit ihr auch erklärt werden könnte, warum durch die Absorption weniger Photonen, also durch den Zerfall weniger Sehfarbstoffmoleküle eine weitergeleitete Erregung zustande kommen kann. Der geringfügige Sehfarbstoffzerfall ändert durch ein „Leck" innerhalb des Dielektrikums die Dielektrizitätskonstante und damit die Kapazität bzw. die Spannung im RC-System[1]. Die Wirkung des Zerfalls weniger Moleküle mit Hilfe einer direkten Wirkung auf die Ionenladung der Membran zu erklären, erscheint mir unmöglich.

Gegen die SVAETICHINsche Hypothese der Entstehung der langsamen Potentiale in dem System der Müllerzellen wird kritisch eingewandt:

a) Würden die R-Potentiale ein „negatives Abbild" der retinalen Neuronen-entladungen darstellen, so wäre schwer zu verstehen, warum sie die rhythmischen Entladungen der retinalen Neurone nicht ebenfalls zeigen. Zum anderen müßten dann auch Potentiale zu finden sein, die bei „Licht aus" hyperpolarisieren, da bei intracellulären Ableitungen die off-Neurone während der Dunkelphase de-polarisiert werden.

Es wäre auch schwer zu verstehen, warum sich die Latenzzeiten der retinalen on-Neurone bei Flimmerlicht anders verhalten als die Latenzzeit der R-Potentiale und warum die CFF der Neurone unter gleichen Bedingungen niedriger ist als die CFF der R-Potentiale.

b) Würden die R-Potentiale in den Müllerzellen jedoch das negative Abbild von Potentialänderungen in den Receptoren sein, wobei den Müllerzellen die Funktion des „Extracellulärraumes" der Receptorzellen zukommen würde, so ergeben sich ebenfalls Schwierigkeiten.

So wäre z. B. nach den zur Zeit anerkannten Membrantheorien schwer zu erklären, daß ein negatives Ruhepotential besteht, wenn man den Receptorzellen ebenfalls ein negatives Ruhepotential zuschreibt. Wenn ich Dr. SVAETICHIN richtig verstanden habe, so meint er, daß die Receptorzellen ein höheres Ruhe-potential als die Müllerzellen haben und in der Hyperpolarisation der − in die

---

[1] Anmerk. b. d. Korrektur: WALD hat 1956 [in FORD Symposium on Enzymes: Units of biological structure and function (O. H. GAEBLER, ed.), p. 355] eine ähnliche Auffassung ver-treten.

Müllerzellen lokalisierten — R-Potentiale die Depolarisation der Receptorzellen zum Ausdruck kommt. Würde es sich um einen echten Membranvorgang handeln, so müßte man nach dieser Hypothese annehmen, daß diese hypothetische Receptor-Depolarisation relativ zum Membranpotential der Receptorzellen gering ist. Dies wäre nochmals eine neue Annahme in der Lehre von der Erregung der Membran.

Ein Teil des Ruhepotentials der Nervenzelle läßt sich durch ein Donnan-Potential erklären. Ein gleichzeitiges negatives extra- und intracelluläres Ruhepotential läßt sich schwer mit Donnan-Gleichgewichten in Einklang bringen.

c) Die Zeitkonstante der üblichen Nervenzellmembranen liegt um 4 msec (Eccles u. Mitarb.). Sieht man im Abfall des R-Reaktionspotentials bei „Licht aus" den Ausdruck eines Membranvorganges, so würden sich bei einer Zeitkonstante von etwa 40—70 msec ebenfalls völlig neue Eigenschaften für die gemeinsame Receptor-Müllerzell-Membran ergeben. Die genauen elektrischen Eigenschaften dieser Grenzfläche können allerdings nur durch direkte elektrische Reizung bestimmt werden.

d) Dr. Svaetichin und Dr. Vallecalle (12) haben die Möglichkeit offen gelassen, daß die hypothetische Müllerzell-Erregung nicht als reiner Membranvorgang aufzufassen ist, sondern die Ionenkonzentrationsänderung quantitativ wiedergibt. Gegen diese Erklärung spricht, daß bei der Erregung der Nervenzelle nur kleine Bruchteile der intracellulären Ionen pro Entladung durch die Membran wandern, so daß kaum anzunehmen ist, daß sich nach kurzen Erregungen das extracelluläre Ionenmilieu in Form von quantitativ meßbaren Potentialen ändert.

Vielleicht können diese Einwände durch spätere Berechnungen und experimentelle Messungen widerlegt werden. Dann würden sich allerdings durch die Svaetichinsche Hypothese völlig neue Gesichtspunkte für nervöse Erregungsvorgänge — auch im zentralen Nervensystem — ergeben.

Herrn Dipl. Chem. R. Reich, Max-Planck-Institut für Physikalische Chemie Göttingen, danke ich für kritische Anregungen.

Literatur

1. Brown, K. T., and T. N. Wiesel: Intraretinal recording in the unopened cat eye. Amer. J. Ophthal. **46**, 91—98 (1958).
2. — — Intraretinal recording with micropipettes in the intact eye. J. Physiol. (Lond.) **149**, 537—562 (1959).
3. Enroth, Ch.: The mechanism of flicker and fusion studied on single retinal elements in the dark-adapted eye of the cat. Acta physiol. scand. **27**, Suppl. 100, 1—67 (1952).
4. Grüsser, O.-J.: Receptorpotentiale einzelner retinaler Zapfen der Katze. Naturwissenschaften **44**, 522 (1957).
5. — Receptorabhängige Potentiale der Katzenretina und ihre Reaktionen auf Flimmerlicht. Pflügers Arch. ges. Physiol. **271**, 511—525 (1960).
6. — u. A. Grützner: Neurophysiologische Grundlagen der periodischen Nachbildphasen nach Lichtblitzen. Albrecht v. Graefes Arch. Ophthal. **160**, 65—93 (1958).
7. Jung, R., O. Creutzfeldt u. O.-J. Grüsser: Die Mikrophysiologie corticaler Neurone und ihre Bedeutung für die Sinnes- und Hirnfunktionen. Dtsch. med. Wschr. **82**, 1050 bis 1054 (1957).
8. MacNichol, E. J., and G. Svaetichin: Electric responses from the isolated retinas of fishes. Amer. J. Ophthal **46**, 26—46 (1958).
8a. Motokawa, K., T. Oikawa and K. Tasaki: Receptor potential of vertebrate retina. J. Neurophysiol. **20**, 186—199 (1957).

9. Reidemeister, Ch., u. O.-J. Grüsser: Flimmerlichtuntersuchungen an der Katzenretina. I. On-Neurone und on-off-Neurone. Z. Biol. 111, 241—253 (1959).
10. Sjöstrand, F. S.: The ultrastructure of the retinal receptors of the vertebrate eye. Ergebn. Biol. 21, 128—160 (1959).
11. Svaetichin, G.: Spectral response curves from single cones. Acta physiol. scand. 39, Suppl. 134, 19—46 (1956).
12. — M. Laufer, G. Mitarai, R. Fatehchand, E. Vallecalle, and J. Villegas: Glial control of neuronal networks and receptors. Dieses Symposion.
13. Tomita, T.: A study on the origin of intraretinal action potential of the cyprinid fish by means of pencil-type microelectrode. Jap. J. Physiol. 7, 80—85 (1957).

Origin of the R-Potential in the Mammalian Retina*

By

Gunnar Svaetichin

With 1 Figure

The R-potentials, recorded from the mammalian retina, have characteristics very similar to the L-response recorded from the fish. Dr. Grüsser concludes from his localization experiments that the recording site of the electrode is close to the synaptic endings of the cones. As far as we know, no electron microscope studies exist of the cat retina, but the work of Dr. Gloria Villegas on the monkey retina shows that the Müller fibers have their largest expansion at the level of the synaptic endings of the rods and cones. The cone synapses in the fish retina are the largest of their kind ($10\,\mu$), and are much larger than those of the cat. We do not believe that it has been possible to obtain any intra-synaptic potentials, as post-synaptic potentials are difficult to be obtained in extra-cellular recordings. Therefore, in analogy with the findings obtained in the fish retina, we are inclined to believe that the R-potential of the cat is either recorded from the Müller fiber at the level of the synaptic endings or, possibly from some "horizontal cell of glial nature", located at the level of the bipolars, very close to the outer plexiform layer. We do believe that this kind of potential reflects the post-synaptic activity, as it has been observed in the intra-cellular recordings from the glial extra-neuronal space in the fish retina.

We are perfectly aware of the difficulties arising when presenting the concept of neuro-glia interaction as a working hypothesis for electrophysiological studies of the nervous activity. We do think, however, that our efforts are worth while, since we are trying to find a general interpretation of the recent findings of electrophysiology and ultra-structural neuro-histology in terms of common concepts of membrane physiology.

We refer the discussion to the points raised by Dr. Grüsser, concerning some problems of membrane physiology to our original papers, in order to avoid repeating ourselves.

In this connection I want to mention that we made, together with Dr. Mitarai, some recordings from the isolated mammalian retina, and we were able to obtain responses, very similar to the R-potentials of the cat retina, recorded by Dr. Grüsser. We were working mainly on the isolated retinae of dogs and monkeys.

The isolated retina was kept in a moist chamber in an atmosphere of O_2 and 5% of CO_2. Under these conditions the retina was functioning well for a few hours,

* From Instituto Venezolano de Investigaciones Cientificas, Caracas, Venezuela.

producing spike activity in the ganglion cell layer and slow potentials originating somewhere in the neighborhood of the bipolar cells. However, if the isolated mammalian retina was being kept in a pure O_2 atmosphere without CO_2, it went into a state of hyper-excitability. The ganglion cells were firing spikes continuously at a high frequency, and the surface recording showed oscillations very similar to the so called brain waves. The lack of CO_2 created a kind of an epileptic seizure which was stopped instantaneously when CO_2 was added, for instance by expiring towards the retina. A similar behaviour was observed sometimes on an isolated fish retina; however, it appeared clearly that a mammalian retina is much more sensitive to the lack of CO_2. All these facts will be discussed in more details in a

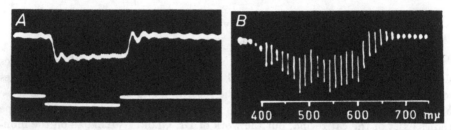

Fig. 1. *Dog retina, isolated. Microelectrode recordings from bipolar layer.* A: Graded response to illumination (300 msec) with hyperpolarization and oscillations of 24 and 80 per sec. B: Corresponding spectral response curve. Due to an error, the energy of the light stimuli in the long wave end of the spectrum was too low, which might be the reason for the absence of responses from 650 mμ onwards

paper by LAUFER et al. in this symposium. Hence, the secret in being able to work on the isolated mammalian retina is the use of CO_2, as otherwise the retina is exhausting itself within a few minutes.

When a superfine glass capillary electrode was introduced into the dog retina from the receptor side, at a depth corresponding to the bipolar layer, there appeared suddenly a negative resting potential and, when the retina was subjected to a light stimulus, a hyperpolarizing response was obtained, like the one shown on the left hand picture of Fig. 1. At "on" and "off" of the recording, as shown in the left hand picture (Fig. 1A) oscillations of the frequencies of 24 and 80 c/sec are seen. Note the phase reversal of the oscillations at "on" and "off". Similar responses were observed in the isolated monkey retina.

The right hand picture (Fig. 1B) shows a spectral response curve, recorded from the dog retina, showing the spectral characteristics of this kind of response, which is very similar to the obtained from the fish retina, and it corresponds most likely to the R-potential registered by Dr. GRÜSSER in the cat retina. The spectral response curve shows four sub-maxima, situated at 410, 481, 542 and 590 mμ. This response is probably recorded from a glial cell in the dog retina, and it looks like a photopic luminosity curve indeed; further, the sub-maxima seem to agree quite well with the submaxima obtained in recordings from the fish and the sub-maxima of the photopic luminosity curve of man.

Discussion

F. BREMER (to SVAETICHIN): To the clinical argument based on the contrasting effects on the ERG of retinal degeneration and of optic nerve atrophy one can add an experimental argument. P. DANIS succeeded in cutting the optic nerve in the rat without interference with the retinal vascularisation. The section resulted ultimately in a considerable loss of ganglion cells as a consequence of retrograde degeneration. Yet the ERG of these rats showed only slight modifications, a fact contrasting with the complete abolition of the ERG of rats suffering from a spontaneous degeneration of the retinal receptors.

(to GRÜSSER): Could Dr. GRÜSSER explain us how, in his mind, the slow unitary potential he picked up, presumably from the receptor-bipolar synaptic complex, exerts by its growing phase an excitatory effect responsible for the *on* discharge, and by its fast decaying phase an inhibitory effect resulting in the cessation of this discharge and followed by the *off*-discharge. Such opposite effects, which should depend, if I understood well, from the direction of the slope of the membrane depolarization, are certainly not familiar electrophysiological processes.

O.-J. GRÜSSER: Die Beziehung zwischen dem Differentialquotienten des R-Potentials und der Aktivierung bzw. Hemmung im retinalen on- bzw. off-Neuronensystem ist zunächst rein deskriptiv. Ich könnte mir vorstellen, daß die Geschwindigkeit, mit der ein elektrisches Feld im Bereich der synaptischen Strukturen aufgebaut wird, eine Rolle spielt für die Geschwindigkeit, mit der die synaptischen Überträgersubstanzen vom prä- ins postsynaptische Substrat wandern. Wenn man eine bestimmte Halbwertszeit für die „Lebensdauer" der postsynaptisch angelangten "vesicles" annimmt, wäre ihre Zahl, die in jedem Augenblick wirksam ist, zunächst bei Erregungsbeginn abhängig von den initialen elektrischen Feldänderungen in der Zeiteinheit, später dagegen nur noch von der Feldstärke.

M. WOLBARSHT: Most of the discussion has been concerned with the correlation of the structures shown by electron microscopy with the structures postulated by the electro-physiologists. Our problem connected with this correlation is that the electron microscopist is usually unable to find many of the postulated membrane and synaptic structures in the excised retina which still appears to have in vivo electrical properties.

W. SICKEL (zu SVAETICHIN): Die Empfehlung, der isolierten Säugernetzhaut, die zweifellos eine Reihe von Vorteilen auch für die hier diskutierten Probleme bietet, eine Atmosphäre von 95% O_2 und 5% CO_2 zu bieten, entspricht dem Vorgehen bei der Untersuchung auch anderer isolierter Organe. Die geschilderten Entartungserscheinungen bei Fortlassung der Kohlensäure — Hypersensibilität und schließlich Erschöpfung — sind auch an der umströmten Froschnetzhaut (S. 80) zu beobachten und entsprechen in vielen Details — Auftreten des switchboard effect (GRANIT), Spontanaktivität — einer extremen Dunkeladaptation. Auch die von GOURAS beschriebene spreading depression tritt an der Netzhaut bevorzugt bei Dunkeladaptation auf. Diese Effekte lassen sich, ebenso wie in Ihren Versuchen durch CO_2, durch Senkung des p_H-Wertes (oder Helladaptation) beseitigen oder vermeiden. Andererseits zeigen auch extreme Helladaptation und Schädigungen verschiedener Art — Druck (WALLER), Temperatur (NIKIFOROWSKI), übrigens auch CO_2 in 10%iger Beimischung — Gemeinsamkeiten, so daß man wohl berechtigt ist, in der Applikation von CO_2 die Justierung eines physiologischen Puffers zu sehen, um so mehr als sich das CO_2/HCO_3'- System in unseren Versuchen durch Phosphatpuffer ersetzbar, d. h. unspezifisch, erwies.

Problematischer dagegen erscheint mir die Anwendung so hoher Sauerstoff-Spannungen. Sie dienen bei der Untersuchung isolierter Organe zur Kompensation für den in Fortfall gekommenen Konvektionstransport. Nun liegt aber die Dicke der Netzhaut — besonders wenn sie von beiden Seiten aus versorgt wird — unterhalb der Warburgschen Grenzschichtdicke und manche Species (pauk-, an-angische) weisen vorwiegend oder ausschließlich Diffusionsversorgung der Netzhaut auf, ohne daß je höhere als der Zimmerluft entsprechende O_2-Partialdrucke auftreten. Reiner Sauerstoff erweist sich bereits im Sinne eines Pasteur-Effektes als toxisch und macht daher durch Senkung des p_H-Wertes — besonders wirksam auf dem Wege über CO_2 — eine Zurückdrängung der Oxydationen (SLATER) erforderlich.

Wir haben es vorgezogen, die Netzhaut in ein flüssiges Medium zu inkubieren, das die hier interessierenden Variablen leicht zu beherrschen erlaubt. In meinem Beitrag sind die einzuhaltenden Bedingungen aufgeführt. Bemerkenswert ist die erforderliche Bewegung des Mediums (HOPPE-SEYLER), besonders dann, wenn dieses nicht in dünner Schicht an Luft grenzt: gewissermaßen das Gegenstück zu Ihrer Beobachtung der Auswaschung von CO_2 in reiner — strömender — O_2-Atmosphäre; hier eine Retention.

Es erscheint danach wichtig, einen bestimmten p_H-Bereich, dessen genaue Einstellung einer Einflußnahme durch die adaptierende Lichtwirkung unterliegt, zu wahren, da andernfalls die energieliefernden Reaktionen des Stoffwechsels in ein Mißverhältnis zu der Belastung — durch Licht — des Systems geraten. Es ist bestechend, diese Beziehungen im Detail unter dem Bild basaler Regulationsmechanismen wie anläßlich des CIBA-Symposions (1959) zu diskutieren, wodurch vielleicht auf einer stofflichen Basis eine Erklärung zu finden wäre für eine bremsende Stabilisierung (R. Jung), d. h. für das Phänomen, daß angesichts reichlichen Substrat- wie Sauerstoff-Angebotes das System nicht in hellen Flammen steht. Es hat den Anschein, als arbeite das biologische Objekt nicht nur mit der Präzision, sondern auch — pulsatorisch — nach den Funktionsprinzipien eines Uhrwerkes.

O.-J. Grüsser (Schlußwort): Die recht unterschiedlichen Meinungen in der Diskussion zeigen, daß die methodische Genauigkeit zur Lokalisation der Mikroelektrodenspitze noch nicht so groß ist, daß mit ihr sichere Resultate festgestellt werden können. Auch Untersucher, die mit sehr ähnlichen Methoden der Mikroelektrophorese von Farbstoffen gearbeitet haben, kamen zu etwas verschiedenen Resultaten über die Lokalisation des R-Potentials (bzw. S-Potentials).

Vielleicht helfen vergleichende neurophysiologische Untersuchungen etwas weiter. Ergänzend möchte ich auf Untersuchungen von Naka und Kuwabara[1,2] hinweisen, die mit Mikroelektroden aus einzelnen Sehzellen der Fliege *Lucilia caesar* registriert und Kurven publiziert haben, die in der Form den R-Potentialen der Katzenretina verblüffend ähnlich sind.

Ähnliche Befunde erhoben kürzlich Burkhardt und Autrum[3] an der Fliege *Calliphora erythrocephala*, wobei nach Ansicht dieser Autoren kein Zweifel bestand, daß intracellulär aus einzelnen Sehzellen registriert wurde. Die von Burkhardt und Autrum publizierten Reaktionspotentiale gleichen zum Teil in der Form zum Verwechseln den gezeigten R-Potentialen aus der Katzenretina, hatten jedoch regelmäßig positive Polarisationsrichtung.

Da bei den genannten Fliegen eine eindeutige Trennung zwischen Sehzellen und weiterleitenden Elementen besteht, kann man nicht daran zweifeln, daß die Sehzellen langsame Generatorpotentiale bei Lichteinfall erzeugen. Dies ist natürlich kein Beweis, aber immerhin ein Hinweis dafür, daß die R-Potentiale der Katzenretina doch in enger Beziehung zu den Receptoren stehen können, da es bisher keinen Anhalt gibt, prinzipiell andersartige Mechanismen des visuellen Primärprozesses bei Vertebraten im Vergleich zu Nichtvertebraten anzunehmen.

IV. Vergleichende Physiologie, Adaptation und Stoffwechsel der Retina

Elektroretinographische Untersuchungen über das adaptive Verhalten tierischer Netzhäute[4,5]

Von

Eberhard Dodt

Mit 5 Abbildungen

Nach den Untersuchungen von Willibald Kühne (1877—1882) über die Bleichung und Regeneration des in den Stäbchen der Wirbeltiere reichlich vor-

[1] Naka, K., and M. Kuwabara: Electrical response from the compound eye of LUCILIA. J. Ins. Physiol. **3**, 41—49 (1959).

[2] Kuwabara, M., and K. Naka: Response of a single retinula cell to polarized light. Nature (Lond.) **184**, 455—456 (1959).

[3] Burkhardt, D., u. H. Autrum: Die Belichtungspotentiale einzelner Sehzellen von Calliphora erythrocephala Meig. Z. Naturforsch. **15 b**, 612—616 (1960).

[4] Aus dem W. G. Kerckhoff-Herzforschungsinstitut der Max Planck-Gesellschaft, Bad Nauheim.

[5] Mit Unterstützung der Deutschen Forschungsgemeinschaft.

handenen Sehpurpurs glaubte man lange Zeit, der Mechanismus der Dunkel- und Helladaptation bestünde im wesentlichen in einer Zunahme und Abnahme der Photopigmentkonzentration in den Sinneszellen der Netzhaut. Zweifel an einer solchen photochemischen Theorie der Helligkeitsanpassung wurden bereits frühzeitig geäußert. FRITJOF HOLMGREN, einer der Entdecker des Elektroretinogramms, beobachtete 1882 beim Kaninchen auch nach vollständiger Bleichung des Sehpurpurs auf Lichteinfall Schwankungen des Retinastromes, woraus er folgerte, daß die Erregung der Netzhaut in keiner wesentlichen Beziehung zu den Bleichungs- und Regenerationserscheinungen des Sehpurpurs stehe. Zu ähnlichen Schlußfolgerungen gelangten GRANIT, MUNSTERHJELM und ZEWI (1939), die bei Fröschen und Katzen während Dunkeladaptation keine direkte Beziehung zwischen der Amplitude der b-Welle im Elektroretinogramm und der gleichzeitig gemessenen Sehpurpurkonzentration feststellen konnten. Weitere experimentelle Einwände gegen die photochemische Theorie der Helligkeitsanpassung wurden von BAUMGARDT (1950) und HAGINS und RUSHTON (1953) vorgebracht, wonach die Reizschwelle eines dunkeladaptierten Auges bis zum 10^6fachen ansteigen kann, ohne daß nennenswerte Bleichung des Sehpurpurs eintritt. Dennoch hält WALD (1957), wohl auf Grund von simultanen Bestimmungen der Reizschwelle und der Sehpurpurkonzentration bei Ratten im Vitamin A-Mangel (DOWLING und WALD 1958), an einer Proportionalität zwischen dem Logarithmus der Reizschwelle und der Sehpurpurkonzentration fest. Außer durch Bleichung der Photopigmente, die erst bei sehr hoher retinaler Beleuchtung beobachtet wird (RUSHTON 1959), kann eine Änderung der Augenempfindlichkeit durch Variation der Pupillenweite und auf Grund nervöser Vorgänge innerhalb der Netzhaut erfolgen. So vergrößert sich beim Übergang von Hell- zu Dunkeladaptation die Ausdehnung des rezeptiven Feldes (KUFFLER 1952), wodurch über räumliche Summation eine stärkere Integration der Erregungen zustandekommt (ARDEN und WEALE 1954).

Der folgende Bericht gibt einen Überblick über die an tierischen Netzhäuten bei elektroretinographischer (Massen-) Ableitung zu beobachtenden Veränderungen der retinalen Reizschwelle während Hell- und Dunkeladaptation. Die Versuche wurden bei maximal weiter, lichtstarrer Pupille und Belichtung von etwa drei Viertel der gesamten Netzhaut durchgeführt. Gemeinsam mit ECHTE wurden an vollständig (12 Std.) dunkeladaptierten, pigmentierten Ratten Messungen und Berechnungen über das Verhältnis zwischen absoluter Schwelle, Unterschiedsschwelle (increment threshold) und Sehpurpurkonzentration angestellt. Zur Bestimmung der Reizschwelle wurde die für eine konstante, schwellennahe Antwort im Elektroretinogramm notwendige Lichtenergie zunächst während Dunkeladaptation, dann bei zunehmender adaptiver Beleuchtung gemessen (Abb. 1, Kreise und Ordinate links). In der gleichen Abbildung (Linie und Ordinate rechts) ist die jeweils vorliegende Sehpurpurkonzentration eingezeichnet, wobei der Berechnung der von DARTNALL, GOODEVE und LYTHGOE (1938) für Halbbleichung des Sehpurpurs in vitro gemessene Wert von 10^{16} Quanta/cm² zu Grunde gelegt wurde.

Bei Annahme einer molekularen Reaktion für die Sehpurpurbleichung (HECHT 1921) wurde die Sehpurpurkonzentration $(1/p)$ nach der Formel $\log p = 3 \times 10^{-5}$ $E \cdot t$ berechnet (E in lumen/m², t in sec). Der Wert für E wurde nach LE GRAND (1957) unter Benutzung folgender Werte berechnet: Maximale Leuchtdichte hinter der zur Adaptation (Xenonlampe) verwandten Mattscheibe = 2620 Nit; Pupillen-

Öffnung $= 0,2$ cm²; Gesamtbrechkraft des Rattenauges $= 275$ Dioptrien (Dodt und Heerd 1960); Durchlässigkeitsfaktor der lichtbrechenden Medien $= 0,8$. Dauer der Helladaptation (t) jeweils 6 min. Regenerative Vorgänge blieben bei der Berechnung unberücksichtigt.

Für die Reizschwelle ergibt sich nach Abb. 1 für eine adaptive Beleuchtung von $2,6 \times 10^{-3}$ bis $2,6 \times 10^{3}$ Nit ein annähernd der Beleuchtung entsprechender Empfindlichkeitsverlust ($\Delta I/I =$ konst. $= 1,0$), während die Sehpurpurkonzentration sich wesentlich anders verhält, und zwar keineswegs proportional mit der

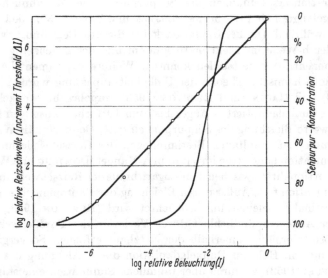

Abb. 1. Absolute Schwelle und Unterschiedsschwelle (increment threshold Δ I) der Ratte (gefüllte und offene Kreise, Ordinate links) und Sehpurpurkonzentration (Linie und Ordinate rechts) bei stufenweise zunehmender adaptiver Beleuchtung (I). Dauer der Helladaptation auf jeder Stufe 6 min. Null-Abszisse $= 5,2 \times 10^4$ Trolands. Reizschwelle $=$ relative Energie für eine konstante Antwort im Elektroretinogramm von 0,06 mV. (Nach Dodt und Echte 1961)

Beleuchtungsstärke abnimmt. Bei Steigerung der adaptiven Beleuchtung bis zu 2,6 Nit, was etwa dem 10000fachen der Dunkelschwelle entspricht, vermindert sich die Sehpurpurkonzentration nur um wenige Prozent, um bei weiterer Steigerung der retinalen Beleuchtung außerordentlich stark abzunehmen (vgl. Rushton 1956). Die in der Abbildung vorgenommene Zuordnung der Ordinaten (Reizschwelle und Sehpurpurkonzentration) ist daher willkürlich.

Betrachtet man nur jenen Beleuchtungsbereich, der dem steilsten Abfall der Sehpurpurkonzentration entspricht (log $-1,5$ bis $-3,0$ der adaptiven Beleuchtung), so läßt sich leicht eine Übereinstimmung zwischen dem Logarithmus der Reizschwelle und der Sehpurpurkonzentration herstellen. Unter experimentellen Bedingungen wäre solche Übereinstimmung bei einer nicht voll dunkeladaptierten Netzhaut denkbar. Nach Mitteilung von Professor Wald betrug die Sehpurpurkonzentration in Dowlings Versuchen am Ende der Helladaptation 5%. Die anschließend gemessene totale Dunkeladaptationszeit von 2 Std. gegenüber mehr als 7 Std. in den mit Echte durchgeführten Versuchen (siehe Tab. 1) läßt vermuten, daß die Ratten in Dowlings Versuchen zu Beginn nicht vollständig dunkeladaptiert waren.

Kommen für die in Abb. 1 beschriebenen Schwellenveränderungen photochemische Faktoren nur bei sehr hoher adaptiver Beleuchtung in Frage, fragt man nach der Art der Prozesse, die für die Empfindlichkeitsabnahme bis zum Eintritt photochemischer Adaptation verantwortlich sind. Da die Versuche bei erweiterter Pupille und bei Belichtung von etwa drei Viertel der gesamten Netzhaut durchgeführt wurden, scheiden einige der obengenannten Möglichkeiten (Pupillenverengung, verminderte räumliche Summation) praktisch aus. Dennoch ist auch hier wohl in erster Linie an nervöse Prozesse zu denken. Hierfür spricht einmal die Verminderung der maximalen b-Wellen-Amplitude schon bei geringer adaptiver Beleuchtung, die durch stärkere Testreize nicht kompensiert werden kann (ELENIUS und DODT, unveröffentliche Beobachtungen). Zum anderen stellt sich die Reizschwelle bei plötzlicher Steigerung der adaptiven Beleuchtung außerordentlich schnell auf einen Wert ein, der sich im weiteren Verlauf der einzelnen Helladaptation kaum noch verändert (während die Sehpurpurkonzentration gleichermaßen mit Stärke und Dauer der retinalen Beleuchtung variiert). Bei der nicht

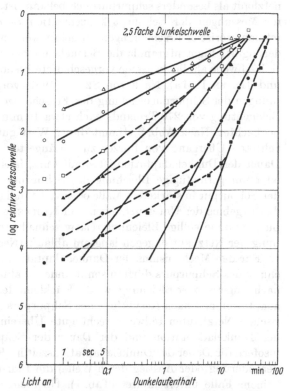

Abb. 2. Dunkeladaptationskurven des Frosches nach verschiedener adaptiver Beleuchtung konstanter Dauer (30 min). Ordinate = relative Energie weißen Lichts für eine konstante Antwort im Elektroretinogramm von 0,02 mV; Null-Ordinate = Energie für eine solche Antwort nach 12 Std. Dunkeladaptation. Retinale Beleuchtung während Helladaptation (Trolands): 0,4 (offene Dreiecke); 1,7 (offene Kreise); 26 (offene Quadrate); 210 (gefüllte Dreiecke); 3300 (gefüllte Kreise); 52400 (gefüllte Quadrate).(Nach DODT und JESSEN 1961 a)

photochemisch bedingten Veränderung der Reizschwelle während Helladaptation handelt es sich offenbar um Prozesse ähnlich der α-Adaptation (SCHOUTEN und ORNSTEIN 1939), für die ein nervöser Hemmungsmechanismus angenommen werden muß.

Eine weitere Versuchsserie behandelt die Veränderungen der Reizschwelle während Dunkeladaptation. Wie MÜLLER (1931) und viele andere nach ihm gezeigt haben, ist die Dauer der Dunkeladaptation von dem Produkt aus Stärke und Dauer der vorhergehenden adaptiven Beleuchtung abhängig (β-Adaptation, SCHOUTEN und ORNSTEIN 1939). Bei Betrachtung von Abb. 2, die die Veränderung der Reizschwelle des Frosches während Dunkeladaptation wiedergibt, sieht man die Dunkeladaptationskurve um so stärker verzögert, je stärker die adaptive Beleuchtung während Helladaptation ist. Betrachtet man jedoch die totale Dauer der Dunkeladaptation (z. B. die Rückkehr der Reizschwelle bis zum 2,5fachen der ursprünglichen Dunkelkontrolle), so ist diese nach einer halbstündigen Beleuchtung bis zu 210 Trolands relativ kurz (15—25 min), während sie nach einer Beleuchtung von 3300 und 52 000 Trolands mehr als das Doppelte beträgt (55—65 min).

Welches ist hier die zugehörige Sehpurpurkonzentration ? Obwohl die Froschnetzhaut als besonders sehpurpurreich bekannt ist, ist der Frosch kein ideales Tier für Messungen der Sehpurpurkonzentration *in vivo*, da durch Helladaptation retinomotorische Erscheinungen ausgelöst werden, wobei insbesondere die Wanderung der Pigmentgranula die Beleuchtung der Sinneszellen modifiziert und die Reizschwelle ähnlich wie eine vorgeschaltete Blende beträchtlich verändert (Dodt und Jessen 1961 a). Nach von Segal (1957) vorgenommenen Schwellenbestimmungen der Sehpurpurbleichung des Frosches *in vivo* werden bei einer retinalen Beleuchtung von 270 Trolands nach etwa 10 min erste Bleichungserscheinungen beobachtet. Nach Abb. 2 stimmt dieser Wert gut mit dem experimentell beobachteten Übergang von kurzer zu verlängerter Adaptationsdauer überein. Die Dauer der Dunkeladaptation ist somit kurz, falls während Helladaptation keine oder nur geringfügige Bleichung des Sehpurpurs eintritt, dagegen lang, sobald der Sehpurpur in stärkerem Maße oder vollständig gebleicht ist. Dies ist praktisch das Ergebnis der Untersuchungen von Kühne, wonach die Resynthese des Sehpurpurs ohne völlige Bleichung relativ schnell (Anagenese), nach völliger Entfärbung der Netzhaut dagegen langsam abläuft (Neogenese).

Für den Mechanismus der Dunkeladaptation nach Helladaptation ohne Bleichung des Sehpurpurs dürften somit andere Faktoren im Vordergrund stehen als nach eingetretener Bleichung, wo die Rückkehr der Reizschwelle während Dunkeladaptation erst nach Resynthese des Sehpurpurs erfolgt. Tatsächlich wird bei tierischen Netzhäuten teilweise recht gute Übereinstimmung zwischen der Dauer der Dunkeladaptation und der Dauer der Sehpurpurregeneration beobachtet, insofern die Dauer der Dunkeladaptationszeit im Elektroretinogramm (Schwellenveränderung oder Anstieg der b-Welle) die Dauer der Sehpurpurregeneration in keinem Falle unterschreitet (Tab. 1). Über ein entsprechendes Verhalten beim Menschen wurde kürzlich von Rushton (1959) berichtet.

Tabelle 1

Tierart	Dauer der Dunkeladaptation im Elektroretinogramm (Stunden)		Dauer der Sehpurpurregeneration in vivo (Stunden)	
Frosch	3 (bei 16,4° C)	(18)	3 (bei 17° C)	(41)
Katze.	>2	(8)	1—2	(33)
Kaninchen . . .	>4	(15)	1—2	(33)
Ratte.	≫7	(7)	7—8	(28)

Andere Versuche beschäftigen sich mit der zeitlichen Änderung der Reizschwellen während Dunkeladaptation, wobei hier besonders die von Aubert (1865) und Kohlrausch (1931) beschriebene Diskontinuität der Dunkeladaptationskurve interessiert. Nach Kohlrausch ist dieser Knick dadurch bedingt, daß jeweils das System mit geringerer Reizschwelle (Zapfen oder Stäbchen) den Kurvenverlauf bestimmt, insofern beim Menschen bis zum Knick die Helligkeitskurve des Tagessehens (Maximum bei 560 mμ), nach dem Knick jene des Dämmerungssehens (Maximum bei 500 mμ) beobachtet wird. Ganz ähnliche Verhältnisse lassen sich elektroretinographisch beim Froschauge nachweisen (Dodt und Jessen

1961a). Ein wesentlich anderes Bild ergibt sich beim Kaninchen. Hier erhält man nach intensiver Helladaptation eine Dunkeladaptationskurve mit einem Knick bei etwa einer Stunde, wobei die relativen Reizschwellen für 462 und 605 mμ vor und nach dem Knick gleich sind und mit den bei vollständiger Dunkeladaptation erhaltenen Werten übereinstimmen (Abb. 3). Bereits frühere Versuche mit WALTHER (1958a) hatten ergeben, daß beim Kaninchen die bei frequenter intermittierender Lichtreizung (40—50 Lichtreize/sec) gemessene Spektralsensitivität im Gegensatz zur Katze mit der Absorptionskurve des Sehpurpurs übereinstimmt.

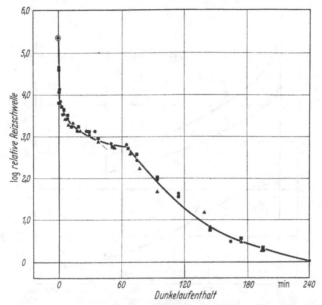

Abb. 3. Dunkeladaptationskurve des Kaninchens für verschiedene Testreize: Weiß (Kreise), 462 mμ (Quadrate), 605 mμ (Dreiecke). Ordinate = relative Lichtenergie für eine konstante Antwort im Elektroretinogramm von 0,025 mV, Null-Ordinate = Energie für eine solche Antwort nach 4 Std. Dunkeladaptation. Retinale Beleuchtung während Helladaptation = 7,5 × 10⁵ Trolands. (Umgezeichnet nach DODT und ELENIUS 1960)

In der Terminologie der Duplizitätslehre würde man ein solches Verhalten in der Weise interpretieren, daß beim Kaninchen neben den Stäbchen auch die Zapfen als visuelles Pigment Sehpurpur und offenbar nur dieses enthalten. Eine solche Schlußfolgerung führt indessen zu Schwierigkeiten. So wurde von RUSHTON u. Mitarb. (1955) beim Kaninchen nach vollständiger Bleichung der Photopigmente in vivo während Dunkeladaptation ein lineares Ansteigen der Sehpurpurkonzentration beobachtet, d. h. in der Regenerationskurve des Sehpurpurs ist ein Knick nicht zu erkennen. Wie hierzu von RUSHTON (persönliche Mitteilung) bemerkt wurde, kann der Knick in der Dunkeladaptationskurve des Kaninchens möglicherweise dadurch entstehen, daß bei Helladaptation nur etwa drei Viertel der Netzhaut direkt gebleicht wurden, während das Elektroretinogramm während Dunkeladaptation durch die Wirkung von Streulicht die Aktivität der gesamten Netzhaut wiedergibt, also auch jenes Teils der Netzhaut, der während Helladaptation nicht direkt dem Licht ausgesetzt war. Eine solche Möglichkeit ist indessen nicht sehr wahrscheinlich, da bei der pigmentierten Ratte ein Knick in der Dunkeladaptationskurve nur für langwelliges Licht nachweisbar ist, das von Sehpurpur in weit

70   E. DODT:

geringerem Maße als weißes oder langwelliges Licht absorbiert wird (Abb. 4 C). Wir möchten vielmehr annehmen, daß die Zahl dieser „Sehpurpur-Zapfen" beim Kaninchen zwar ausreicht, die Reizschwelle im Elektroretinogramm zu bestimmen, doch läßt offenbar ihre räumliche Verteilung innerhalb der Netzhaut oder die in ihnen vorliegende Sehpurpurkonzentration eine densitometrische Messung nicht zu.

Besondere Schwierigkeiten bereitet vorläufig noch die Erklärung des im Vergleich zum totalen Achromaten verzögerten b-Wellen-Anstiegs im Elektroretinogramm des normalen menschlichen Auges während Dunkeladaptation. Hierzu

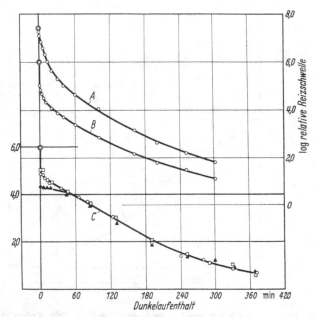

Abb. 4. Dunkeladaptationskurven der pigmentierten Ratte. Ordinaten: relative Lichtenergie für eine konstante Antwort im Elektroretinogramm von 0,06 mV. Null-Ordinate = Energie für eine solche Antwort nach 12 Std. Dunkeladaptation. A und B (Ordinate rechts): Mittelwerte von 10 Tieren (B) und 5 Tieren (A), adaptive Beleuchtung (Dauer 30 min): 7 × 10³ Trolands (B), 5,2 × 10⁴ Trolands (A). C (Ordinate links): Dunkeladaptationskurve (Einzelversuch) nach 30 min Helladaptation mit 7 × 10³ Trolands. Testreize: weiß (Kreise), 462 mμ (Quadrate), 605 mμ (Dreiecke). (Nach DODT und ECHTE 1961)

wurde von ELENIUS und HECK (1958) die suggestive Annahme einer Hemmung der Stäbchenaktivität durch die lichtaktivierten Zapfen entwickelt. Es erscheint jedoch fraglich, ob die Verzögerung der Reizschwellensenkung nach stärkerer Helladaptation generell auf einen solchen Mechanismus zurückgeführt werden kann. So wird beim Frosch eine Verschiebung der Helligkeitswerte im Spektrum, d. h. eine Aktivierung von Zapfen bereits bei einer adaptiven Beleuchtung beobachtet, die während des nachfolgenden Dunkelaufenthaltes noch nicht zu einer verlängerten Adaptationsdauer führt (DODT und JESSEN 1961a). Umgekehrt wird bei der Ratte mit zunehmender Intensität der adaptiven Beleuchtung eine Verzögerung der Dunkeladaptation ohne Knick sichtbar (Abb. 4A und B).

In den bisher beschriebenen Versuchen war häufig von Stäbchen und Zapfen die Rede, um die mutmaßlich beteiligten Arten von Sinneszellen zu kennzeichnen. Frosch, Katze und Kaninchen verfügen, obgleich in verschiedenen Proportionen, sowohl über Stäbchen als auch über Zapfen. Bei sämtlichen dieser Tiere ist ein deutlicher Knick in der Dunkeladaptationskurve zu erkennen, doch zeigt sich bei Katze und Kaninchen bereits vor dem Knick die Tätigkeit von Sehpurpurelementen (vgl. Abb. 3). Somit ist weder die Gegenwart von Zapfen noch das Auftreten eines Knicks generell mit einer Purkinje-Verschiebung verknüpft, während eine Purkinje-Verschiebung ohne Knick in der Dunkeladaptationskurve nicht beobachtet wird (Abb. 4 C).

Tabelle 2 gibt für verschiedene tierische Netzhäute eine Zusammenstellung der jeweils vorliegenden Arten von Sinneszellen sowie den elektroretinographischen Nachweis einer Purkinje-Verschiebung und eines Kohlrausch-Knicks in der Dunkeladaptationskurve. Demnach wird bei gemischten Netzhäuten nach intensiver Helladaptation regelmäßig ein diskontinuierlicher Verlauf der Dunkeladaptationskurve beobachtet, während dieser bei solchen Netzhäuten, die entweder nur Stäbchen oder nur Zapfen besitzen, in der Regel vermißt wird. Eine Ausnahme machen lediglich die nachtaktiven Geckos, deren Netzhäute nach Untersuchungen von TANSLEY (1959) und anderen eine homogene Receptorpopulation zeigen, die entwicklungsgeschichtlich aus Zapfen entstanden sein soll. Obwohl die Netzhäute dieser Tiere Sinneszellen nur einer Art aufweisen, zeigt sich hier nach Versuchen mit JESSEN beim Wechsel von Dunkel- zu Helladaptation ein vollständiger Übergang

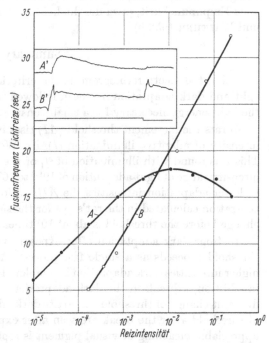

Abb. 5. Tarentola mauritanica. Einzelversuch. Fusionsfrequenz intermittierender Lichtreize (Ordinate) gegen Reizintensität (Abszisse) während Dunkeladaptation (A und gefüllte Kreise) und nach 20 min Helladaptation mit 8 × 10³ Trolands (B und offene Kreise). Maximale Reizintensität (Abszisse 10⁰) = 5,3 × 10⁴ Trolands. Im oberen Teil des Diagramms sind Einzelreiz-Elektroretinogramme während Dunkeladaptation (A') und nach Helladaptation (B') wiedergegeben. Reizdauer 3,7 sec (A'); 2,0 sec (B'). (Nach DODT und JESSEN 1961b)

von skotopischer zu photopischer Netzhautfunktion: Je nach Adaptationszustand werden im Elektroretinogramm skotopische und photopische Potentialformen

Tabelle 2

Tierart	Stäbchen	Zapfen	Purkinje-Verschiebung im Elektroretinogramm während Dunkeladaptation	Kohlrausch-Knick im Elektroretinogramm während Dunkeladaptation
Frosch	+	+ (17)	+ (21)	+ (30)
Katze.....	+	+ (35)	+/− (8)	+ (8)
Kaninchen ..	+	+ (24)	− (8)	+ (8)
Ratte.....	+	+/− (40;6)	+ (7)	für langwellige Lichtreize + (7)
Grauhörnchen .	−	+ (37)	− (37)	− (37)
Gecko	keine Differenzierung (5)		− (11)	+ (11)

beobachtet, und bei intermittierender Belichtung werden mit diesen je nach Adaptationszustand ganz verschiedene Verschmelzungsfrequenz-Intensitätskurven registriert (Abb. 5). Diese Netzhäute verhalten sich somit bei Wechsel des Adaptationszustandes ganz ähnlich wie gemischte Netzhäute, zeigen im übrigen eine zweigeteilte Dunkeladaptationskurve und im dunkeladaptierten Zustand eine sehr hohe Empfindlichkeit, etwa der dunkeladaptierten Katze vergleichbar (vgl. DODT und WALTHER 1958 b).

Summary

Using the electroretinogram as the criterion the change of threshold during light and dark adaptation has been followed in different animals by determining the light energy necessary for a small constant b-wave.

In rats the increment threshold (ΔI) rises in about the same proportion as the intensity of adaptive illumination (I), i. e. Weber's law $\Delta I/I =$ const. is obeyed. This was found with illumination of $^3/_4$ of the total retinal surface and within an intensity range of light adaptation of $10^{1,5}$ to 10^7 times the absolute dark threshold, at lower adaptation intensities the $\Delta I/I$-ratio being smaller. The rhodopsin concentration calculated in the rat's eye for the same adaptive illuminations does not change before the threshold is about 10^4 times the absolute dark threshold.

In frogs dark adaptation after exposure to white light up to 10^4 times dark threshold proceeds as a single fast process. After light adaptation to somewhat higher intensities dark adaptation is completed in about the same time but there is, in addition, a break in the dark adaptation curve separating two phases with a different change of threshold. Bipartite dark adaptation curves with a slow change of threshold after the break are seen after exposure to light intensities for which appreciable bleaching of visual pigment is reported.

In frogs, cats, rabbits and rats the total dark adaptation time for a small constant b-wave after strong light adaptation is of the same order or even longer than the time period reported for full regeneration of visual purple after a total bleach.

After strong light adaptation the change of threshold during dark adaptation in frogs, cats, rabbits and nocturnal geckos consists of two branches, an early cone and a late rod branch with a kink at their intersection. In frogs and cats the visibility curve during the cone branch is different from that of the rod branch while in rabbits and geckos the visibility curve does not change with the state of adaptation.

The retinae of nocturnal geckos which possess sense cells of only one type exhibit electrical responses of the photopic type in the light adapted state and during the cone branch of the dark adaptation curve while after the break the shape of potentials is purely of the scotopic type.

It is concluded 1) that both nervous and photochemical processes contribute to the change of threshold during light and dark adaptation, changes in the concentration of visual pigment being caused only by strong illumination; 2) that the branching of the dark adaptation curve is due to nervous interaction rather than to different types of sense cells; 3) that a shift of the visibility curve during light and dark adaptation cannot be predicted from the duplicity of the sensory epithelium.

Literatur

1. ARDEN, G. B., and R. A. WEALE: Nervous mechanisms and dark adaptation. J. Physiol. (Lond.) **125**, 417—426 (1954).
2. AUBERT, H.: Physiologie der Netzhaut. Breslau 1865.
3. BAUMGARDT, E.: Les théories photochimiques classiques et quantiques de la vision. Rev. opt. **28**, 661—690 (1950).
4. DARTNALL, H. J. A., C. F. GOODEVE and R. J. LYTHGOE: The effect of temperature on the photochemical bleaching of visual purple solutions. Proc. roy. soc. A **164**, 216—230 (1938).
5. DETWILER, S. R.: Studies on the retina. An experimental study of the gecko retina. J. comp. Neurol. **36**, 125—141 (1923).
6. — Vertebrate photoreceptors. New York 1943.
7. DODT, E., and K. ECHTE: Dark and light adaptation in the pigmented and white rat as measured by the electroretinogram threshold. J. Neurophysiol. **24**, No. 5 (1961).
8. — and V. ELENIUS: Change of threshold during dark adaptation measured with orange and blue light in cats and rabbits. Experientia (Basel) **14**, 313 (1960).
9. — and E. HEERD: The light gathering power of some vertebrate eyes. Manuscript (1960).
10. — u. K. H. JESSEN: Das adaptive Verhalten der Froschnetzhaut, untersucht mit der Methode der konstanten elektrischen Antwort. Vision Research (1961 a).
11. — — The duplex nature of the retina of nocturnal gecko as reflected in the electroretinogram. J. gen. Physiol. **44**, 1145—1160 (1961 b).
12. — and J. B. WALTHER: Photopic sensitivity mediated by visual purple. Experientia (Basel) **14**, 142 (1958 a).
13. — — Electroretinographic evaluation of the gecko's visibility function. XVth Intern. Congr. Zool., London (1958 b), Paper 40.
14. DOWLING, J. E., and G. WALD: Nutritional night blindness. Ann. N. Y. Acad. Sci. **74**, 256—265 (1958).
15. ELENIUS, V.: Recovery in the dark of the rabbit's electroretinogram. Acta physiol. scand. **44**, Suppl. 150 (1958).
16. — u. J. HECK: Vergleich zwischen der b-Wellen-Amplitude und dem Verlauf der Sehpurpurregeneration bei Achromaten und Gesunden. Ophthalmologica **136**, 145—150 (1958).
17. GAUPP, E.: Ecker's und Wiedersheim's Anatomie des Frosches III/2. Braunschweig 1904.
18. GRANIT, R., A. MUNSTERHJELM and M. ZEWI: The relation between concentration of visual purple and retinal sensitivity to light during dark adaptation. J. Physiol. (Lond.) **96**, 31—44 (1939).
19. HAGINS, W. A., and W. A. H. RUSHTON: The measurement of rhodopsin in the decerebrate albino rabbits. J. Physiol. (Lond.) **120**, 61 P (1953).
20. HECHT, S.: Photochemistry of visual purple I. The kinetics of the decomposition of visual purple by light. J. gen. Physiol. **3**, 1—13 (1921).
21. HIMSTEDT, F., u. W. A. NAGEL: Die Verteilung der Reizwerte für die Froschnetzhaut im Dispersionsspektrum des Gaslichtes, mittels der Aktionsströme untersucht. Ber. Naturf. Ges. Freiburg i. Br. **11**, 153—162 (1901).
22. HOLMGREN, F.: Über Sehpurpur und Retinaströme. Untersuch. Physiol. Inst. Heidelberg **2**, 81—88 (1882).
23. KOHLRAUSCH, A.: Tagessehen, Dämmerungssehen, Adaptation. Handb. norm. path. Physiol. XII/2. Berlin 1931.
24. KRAUSE, W.: Die Anatomie des Kaninchens. Leipzig 1884.
25. KÜHNE, W.: Unters. Physiol. Inst. Heidelberg 1877—1882.
26. KUFFLER, S.: Neurons in the retina: Organization, inhibition and excitation problems. Cold Spr. Harb. Symp. quant. Biol. **17**, 281—292 (1952).
27. LE GRAND, Y.: Light, colour and vision. New York 1957.
28. LEWIS, D. M.: Regeneration of rhodopsin in the albino rat. J. Physiol. (Lond.) **136**, 624—631 (1957).
29. MÜLLER, H. K.: Über den Einfluß verschieden langer Vorbelichtung auf die Dunkeladaptation und auf die Fehlergröße der Schwellenbestimmung während der Dunkelanpassung. Albrecht v. Graefes Arch. Ophthal. **125**, 624—642 (1930).
30. RIGGS, L. A.: Dark adaptation in the frog eye as determined by the electrical response of the retina. J. cell. comp. Physiol. **9**, 491—510 (1937).

31. Rushton, W. A. H.: The difference spectrum and the photosensitivity of rhodopsin in the living human eye. J. Physiol. (Lond.) 134, 11—29 (1956).
32. — Visual pigments in man and animals and their relation to seeing. Progr. Biophys. 9, 239—283 (1959).
33. — F. W. Campbell, W. A. Hagins and G. S. Brindley: The bleaching and regeneration of rhodopsin in the living eye of the albino rabbit and of man. Opt. Acta 1, 183—190 (1955).
34. Schouten, J. F., and L. S. Ornstein: Measurements of direct and indirect adaptation by means of a binocular method. J. Opt. Soc. Amer. 29, 168—182 (1939).
35. Schultze, M.: Zur Anatomie und Physiologie der Retina. Arch. mikrosk. Anat. 2, 175—286 (1866).
36. Segal, J.: Mechanismus des Farbensehens. Jena 1957.
37. Tansley, K.: Some observations on mammalian cone electroretinograms. Bibl. Ophthalm. 48, 7—14 (1957).
38. — The retina of two nocturnal geckos, Hemidactylus turcicus and Tarentola mauritanica. Pflügers Arch. ges. Physiol. 268, 213—220 (1959).
39. Wald, G.: Retinal chemistry and the physiology of vision. Nat. Physical Lab. Symposion on visual problems of Colour. Teddington 1957.
40. Walls, G. L.: The visual cells of the white rat. J. comp. Psychol. 18, 363—366 (1934).
41. Zewi, M.: On the regeneration of visual purple. Acta Soc. Sci. Fenn. N.S.B. 2, No. 4 (1939).

Diskussion s. S. 94.

Vergleichende Elektrophysiologie der Retina*

Von

H. Bornschein

Mit 1 Abbildung

Die in den letzten Jahren von zahlreichen Neurophysiologen unternommenen Versuche, mittels Mikroelektroden die komplexe elektrische Antwort der Retina zu analysieren und die strukturelle Zuordnung sowie die funktionelle Bedeutung der einzelnen Komponenten zu klären, haben vorläufig noch keine gesicherten Ergebnisse gebracht. Wenn es auch kaum einem Zweifel unterliegen dürfte, daß der in dieser Richtung eingeschlagene Weg der zweckmäßigste ist, so sollten dennoch die mitunter interessanten Aspekte nicht vernachlässigt werden, die sich auf den nicht direkt zum Ziele gerichteten Nebenwegen darbieten. Vergleichende Untersuchungen dürften zwar kaum eine Lösung der eingangs erwähnten Probleme bringen, sie liefern jedoch wichtige Details wie z. B. hinsichtlich der Gültigkeit tierexperimentell gewonnener Ergebnisse für die Humanphysiologie sowie hinsichtlich prinzipieller Fragen wie der Duplizitätslehre. Allerdings darf die Möglichkeit, Beziehungen zur Ökologie der betreffenden Tierart herzustellen, nicht zu einer teleologischen Betrachtungsweise führen, wie später am Beispiel der Eule gezeigt werden soll.

Die Frage, ob die bei den üblichen Laboratoriumstieren erhobenen Befunde auch für den Menschen Gültigkeit besitzen, ist insofern von einer gewissen Bedeutung, als bestimmte Probleme (direkter Vergleich mit empfindungsanalytischen Werten) nur beim Menschen untersucht werden können, während andererseits schädigende

---

* Aus dem Physiologischen Institut der Universität Wien, Österreich.

Einflüsse im allgemeinen auf den Tierversuch beschränkt bleiben müssen. Hinsichtlich der auch klinisch interessierenden Frage der Überlebens- und Wiederbelebungszeit der Netzhaut konnten in jüngster Zeit vergleichende Daten gewonnen werden, die vor allem das Elektroretinogramm betreffen. Bei menschlichen Augen, die trotz relativ geringen Funktionsausfalls wegen bösartiger Neubildungen enucleiert werden mußten, waren die positiven Komponenten des ERG 2 min nach der Enucleation komplett ausgelöscht, während die negative Komponente (a-Welle) mit einer Halbwertszeit von 3—5 min wesentlich langsamer abnahm (2). Die gemessenen Werte entsprachen dabei durchwegs dem in zahlreichen Versuchen beobachteten Verhalten der Katzenretina. Die Ausdehnung dieser Versuche zur Feststellung der Wiederbelebungszeit der menschlichen Retina hat bisher in 2 Fällen ergeben, daß nach kompletter Ischämie der Retina (vorübergehende intraoculare Drucksteigerung auf 200 mm Hg) von 20 bzw. 22 min Dauer eine vollständige Erholung der Sehfunktion eintritt. Das ERG war zwar schon 60 sec nach Freigabe der retinalen Zirkulation wieder nachweisbar, benötigte aber zu seiner Normalisierung mehrere Tage, während die am Tage nach dem Druckversuch kontrollierten subjektiven Funktionen völlig normale Werte ergaben. Die Befunde bestätigen nicht nur die von WEGNER (1928) angegebenen, überraschend hohen Wiederbelebungszeiten der menschlichen Retina (zwischen 22 und 45 min), sondern decken sich auch weitgehend mit den Ergebnissen der von POPP (1955) beim Kaninchen durchgeführten analogen Untersuchungen.

In diesem Zusammenhang ist ferner noch die Tatsache erwähnenswert, daß durch komplette retinale Druckischämie beim Menschen schon nach 6 sec jede echte visuelle Wahrnehmung blockiert wird; es folgt eine intensive entoptische Helligkeitsempfindung, die erst nach etwa 40—60 sec erlischt (21). Die Spontan- und Belichtungsaktivität des N. opticus der Katze erscheint schon wenige Sekunden nach Beginn einer kompletten retinalen Druckischämie reduziert, um innerhalb 60 sec völlig zu verschwinden (5).

Ein weiteres vergleichend untersuchtes Problem ist entwicklungsgeschichtlicher Natur. Bekanntlich ist das ERG des Menschen in den ersten Lebenstagen nur mit hohen Reizintensitäten auszulösen und benötigt zu seiner vollen Entwicklung nahezu das ganze erste Lebensjahr (26, 13). Bei verschiedenen bisher untersuchten Tierarten (Kaninchen, Hund, Katze) war das ERG erst zwischen 6. und 21. Lebenstag nachweisbar und erreichte nach 40—90 Tagen seine volle Größe (9, 16, 27, 15a). Im Gegensatz hierzu fand sich bei wenigen Stunden alten Meerschweinchen ein vollständig ausgebildetes ERG, das nur bei schwachen Reizintensitäten eine signifikant niedrigere Amplitude aufwies als das ERG der erwachsenen Tiere (7). Die hohe allgemeine Reife des neugeborenen Meerschweinchens spiegelt sich also auch im ERG wider, dessen photopische Komponenten im Zeitpunkt der Geburt voll entwickelt sind, während die skotopischen Komponenten noch einen gewissen Entwicklungsrückstand aufweisen.

Für vergleichende Untersuchungen in Hinblick auf das Duplizitätsprinzip erscheinen vor allem solche Tierarten geeignet, deren Aktivität in extremer Weise an bestimmte Beleuchtungsbedingungen gebunden ist und deren Netzhäute charakteristische Strukturunterschiede aufweisen. Es sei in dieser Hinsicht an die klassischen ERG-Untersuchungen von PIPER (1905, 1911), v. BRÜCKE und GARTEN (1907) sowie KOHLRAUSCH und BROSSA (1914) erinnert. In neuerer Zeit hat vor allem Dodt (1954) mit der Flimmerreiztechnik aufschlußreiche Ergebnisse erhalten. Er konnte zeigen, daß hohe Flimmerverschmelzungsfrequenzen stets mit Zapfen-, niedere dagegen meist mit Stäbchenaktivität in Beziehung stehen. Wird die ERG-Fusionsfrequenz als Funktion der Reizintensität aufgetragen, so ergibt sich bei gemischten Netzhäuten eine unstetige Kurve, die sich aus zwei durch einen Knick getrennten Abschnitten (skotopische bzw. photopische Funktion) zusammensetzt. In einer ergänzenden Studie konnte gezeigt werden, daß die reine Zapfennetzhaut des europäischen Ziesels *(Citellus citellus)* eine einfache Fusionskurve liefert, wobei die maximalen Fusionswerte mehr als 100/sec betragen (6). Das ERG des Ziesels weist auch sonst alle charakteristischen Merkmale auf, die eine reine Zapfennetzhaut erwarten läßt (*1, 3, 22*). Neben geringer Adaptation und hoher Intensitätsschwelle ist dabei vor allem die Tatsache hervorzuheben, daß sich die Beziehung zwischen Reizintensität und Gesamtamplitude des Einzel-ERG als eine stetige Kurve von auffallender Steilheit darstellt. Das hohe zeitliche Auflösungsvermögen der Zieselretina zeigte sich auch in Versuchen mit Doppelblitzen. Als Nebenbefund ergab sich dabei, daß der zeitliche Verlauf der photopischen Einzelantwort von der Reizintensität praktisch unabhängig ist.

Die bei einem extremen Tagtier (Ziesel) erhaltenen Ergebnisse legten es nahe, analoge Untersuchungen auch bei einem extremen Nachttier durchzuführen. Dabei ergaben sich bei der Sumpfohreule *(Asio flammeus)* Befunde, die zunächst überraschten (*7a*). Die Methodik war die gleiche wie bei den Untersuchungen von Zieseln und Meerschweinchen. Ferner wurde zu Vergleichszwecken die Taube (Tagvogel) mituntersucht, deren Flimmer-ERG übrigens bereits von Dodt und Wirth (1953) eingehend studiert worden ist. Das Einzelblitz-ERG der Eule zeigt eine wesentlich niedrigere Schwelle als das ERG der Taube, unterscheidet sich aber von letzterem praktisch nur durch einen langsameren Verlauf. Die Beziehung zwischen Reizintensität und Gesamtamplitude des Einzel-ERG ist bei beiden Tieren eine stetige Funktion, welche jedoch bei der Taube wesentlich steiler verläuft als bei der Eule. Die maximale Flimmerverschmelzungsfrequenz der Eule liegt mit 65—70/sec überraschend hoch, wenngleich sie die Werte der Taube (>100/sec) nicht errreicht. Die Fusionsfrequenzkurve als Funktion der Reizintensität zeigt bei der Eule einen angedeuteten Knick, der bei einer schwachen, für das Tauben-ERG unterschwelligen Reizintensität liegt. Ein weiterer Unterschied ergab sich bei Doppelblitzversuchen. Bei hohen Reizintensitäten erscheint die Anwort der Eulenretina auf den zweiten Reiz stark verkleinert, nicht aber die Anwort der Taubenretina. Aus den Ergebnissen war daher der Schluß zu ziehen, daß sich das ERG des Nachtvogels nur in bestimmten quantitativen Aspekten (Intensitätsschwelle, zeitlicher Verlauf), nicht aber in prinzipieller Weise vom ERG des Tagvogels unterscheidet. Es sei in diesem Zusammenhang darauf hingewiesen, daß die hochentwickelten Netzhäute der Vögel nach Kolmer (1936) eine wesentlich geringere Variation des Stäbchen/Zapfen-Verhältnisses zeigen als die Säugernetzhäute. Nach älteren histologischen Untersuchungen (s. b. Kolmer, 1936) enthält die Eulennetzhaut Zapfen in reichlicher Anzahl, ein Befund, der bei der untersuchten Sumpfohreule verifiziert werden konnte (*7a*). Ebenfalls älteren Datums sind übrigens zahlreiche verstreute Literaturangaben (s. b. Walls, 1942), wonach die Eulen im Gegensatz zu einer weitverbreiteten Meinung ein ausgezeichnetes Tagessehvermögen besitzen und die Tagessehschärfe eines Uhu jene des Menschen übertreffen soll.

Die Retina nächtlich lebender Reptilien *(Hemidactylus turcicus* und *Tarentola mauritanica)* weist nach den parallel durchgeführten elektrophysiologischen und histologischen Untersuchungen von DODT und WALTHER (1959) bzw. TANSLEY (1959) Besonderheiten auf, die eine eindeutige Klassifizierung einer photopischen bzw. skotopischen Funktion erschweren. Neben Merkmalen, die für ein hohes Auflösungsvermögen sprechen, findet sich eine auffallend hohe Lichtempfindlichkeit, für deren Erklärung eine große Sehpigmentdichte, vor allem aber der extraretinale Faktor einer besonderen Lichtstärke der Dioptrik in Betracht gezogen wurde. Von Interesse werden in diesem Zusammenhang vergleichende Untersuchungen bei verwandten tagaktiven Arten sein.

Extreme Nachtsäugetiere stellen die Fledermäuse dar, von denen eine spät fliegende Art, das Großmausohr *(Myotis myotis)*, orientierend untersucht wurde. Die Versuche, das ERG zu registrieren, schlugen zunächst bei einigen Tieren fehl, bis sich ergab, daß erst nach einer mindestens 3stündigen kompletten Dunkeladaptation eine langsame Antwort von niedriger Amplitude zu erzielen ist. Histologisch fand sich eine Stäbchenretina mit auffallend großer Konvergenz, wobei die innere Körnerschicht auf eine bloße Doppelreihe von Zellen reduziert erscheint und die Ganglienzellen äußerst spärlich sind. Bekanntlich orientieren sich diese rasch und sicher fliegenden Tiere nach dem Echolotprinzip, während das bei fehlender oder extrem schwacher Beleuchtung wertlose visuelle System keine zeitlich-räumliche Differenzierung erlaubt, aber offenbar noch eine allgemeine Unterscheidung von Hell und Dunkel ermöglicht. Die Retina der Fledermaus stellt mit der dürftigen Entwicklung ihrer neuralen Schichten einen Sonderfall dar, während bei der ebenfalls vom Stäbchensystem beherrschten Retina des Kaninchens innere und äußere Körnerschicht etwa gleiche Breite besitzen; die Retina des Ziesels ist nicht nur durch das völlige Fehlen von Stäbchen, sondern auch durch eine mächtige Ausbildung der neuralen Schichten gekennzeichnet, wobei die Zahl der nachgeschalteten Neurone jene der Receptoren übertrifft (Abb. 1). Das hohe Differenzierungsvermögen der Zieselretina findet nicht nur in der schon erwähnten hohen Flimmerverschmelzungsfrequenz ihren Ausdruck, sondern auch in ihrem Verhalten bei Änderung der Reizanstiegssteilheit. Systematische Untersuchungen über den Einfluß dieses Reizparameters auf das ERG wurden bisher nur beim Menschen durchgeführt. Dabei haben RONCHI und GRAZI (1956) sowie BORNSCHEIN und GUNKEL (1956) in unabhängigen Untersuchungen festgestellt, daß die Höhe des skotopischen on-Effekts durch die Verlängerung der Anstiegszeit eines Dauerreizes nicht beeinflußt wird, selbst wenn der Reizanstieg 230 bzw. 280 msec beansprucht. Die Antworten zeigen lediglich einen verlangsamten Verlauf, wobei die Gipfelzeit der b-Welle die Anstiegszeit stets übertrifft und mehr als 300 msec betragen kann. Während also das skotopische System des Menschen ein weitgehend integratives Verhalten aufweist, reagiert das rein photopische System der Zieselretina in stark abweichender Weise *(7b)*. Mit Verlängerung der Anstiegszeit von 7 auf 180 msec sinkt die Amplitude des positiven on-Effekts linear auf etwa die Hälfte ab. Die vom Reizbeginn gemessene Gipfelzeit zeigt bei Verlängerung der Reizanstiegszeit eine wesentlich geringere Verlängerung, so daß bei einer Anstiegszeit von mehr als

120 msec der Gipfel des on-Effekts bereits vor Ende des Reizanstiegs auftritt. Im reinen Zapfen-ERG des Ziesels entspricht daher die Höhe des on-Effekts dem Differentialquotienten des Reizanstiegs nach der Zeit. Analoge Untersuchungen über das Verhalten des beim Ziesel besonders stark ausgeprägten off-Effekts sind im Gange.

Wenn die vorliegende Übersicht nur das Wirbeltier-ERG betrifft und in erster Linie teilweise unveröffentlichte eigene Untersuchungen besprochen wurden, so

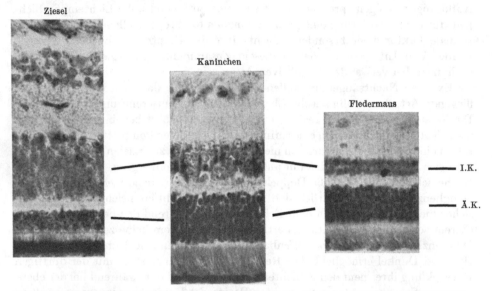

Abb. 1. Histologischer Aufbau der Netzhäute von Ziesel, Kaninchen und Fledermaus. Heidenhains Eisenhämato-xilin, gleiche Vergrößerung. *I. K.* Innere Körnerschicht. *Ä. K.* Äußere Körnerschicht

geschah dies lediglich mit Rücksicht auf die nur beschränkt zur Verfügung stehende Zeit. Es sollte das Thema einer vergleichenden Elektrophysiologie der Retina zur Diskussion gestellt und an Hand einiger Beispiele gezeigt werden, daß diese Arbeitsrichtung interessante Ergebnisse zu liefern vermag, wenn sie durch exakte histologische Untersuchungen gestützt und der Ökologie eine zwar nicht entscheidende, aber doch beratende Funktion zuerkannt wird.

Summary

Comparative electrophysiological studies on the retina are reported and their value in the treatment of a number of problems is stressed. Some recent investigations as well as unpublished work along these lines are reviewed. It concerns retinal survival and revival time, ontogenetic development of the mammalian retina and experiments on animals with highly specialized retinal organization (souslik, owl, bat).

Literatur

1. ARDEN, G. B., and K. TANSLEY: The spectral sensitivity of the pure-cone retina of the souslik (Citellus citellus). J. Physiol. (Lond.) **130**, 225—232 (1955).
2. BÖCK, J., H. BORNSCHEIN u. K. HOMMER: Die Überlebenszeit der a-Welle im Elektro-retinogramm des Menschen. Albrecht v. Graefes Arch. Ophthal. **161**, 6—15 (1959).

3. Bornschein, H.: Elektrophysiologischer Nachweis einer I-Retina bei einem Säuger (Citellus citellus L.). Naturwissenschaften 41, 435 (1954).
4. — and R. D. Gunkel: The effect of rate of rise of photic stimuli on the human electroretinogram. Amer. J. Ophthalm. 42/2, 239—243 (1956).
5. — Spontan- und Belichtungsaktivität in Einzelfasern des N. opticus der Katze. I. Der Einfluß kurzdauernder retinaler Ischämie. Z. Biol. 110, 210—222 (1958).
6. — u. Gy. Szegvari: Flimmerelektroretinographische Studie bei einem Säuger mit reiner Zapfennetzhaut (Citellus citellus L.). Z. Biol. 110, 285—290 (1958).
7. — Zur postnatalen Entwicklung der Netzhautfunktion. Vergleichende elektroretinographische Untersuchungen. Wien. klin. Wschr. 71, 956—958 (1959).
7a. — u. K. Tansley: Elektroretinogramm und Netzhautstruktur der Sumpfohreule (Asio flammeus). Experientia, in Druck.
7b. — Der Einfluß der Reizanstiegszeit auf die Belichtungsantwort der reinen Zapfennetzhaut. Pflügers Arch. ges. Physiol., in Druck.
8. Brücke, E. Th. v., u. S. Garten: Zur vergleichenden Physiologie der Netzhautströme. Pflügers Arch. ges. Physiol. 120, 290—348 (1907).
9. Demirchoglian, G. G., u. V. S. Mirzoian: Die Entwicklung der elektrischen Reaktion der Retina bei der Ontogenese (Russisch). Dokl. Akad. Nauk. SSSR. 90, 371—374 (1953).
10. Dodt, E., and A. Wirth: Differentiation between rods and cones by flicker electroretinography in pigeon and guinea pig. Acta physiol. scand. 30, 80—89 (1953).
11. — Ergebnisse der Flimmer-Elektroretinographie. Experientia (Basel) 10, 330 (1954).
12. — u. J. B. Walther: Über die spektrale Empfindlichkeit und die Schwelle von Gecko-Augen. Elektroretinographische Untersuchungen an Hemidactylus turcicus und Tarentola mauritanica. Pflügers Arch. ges. Physiol. 268, 204—212 (1959).
13. Heck, J., u. B. Zetterström: Analyse des photopischen Flimmerelektroretinogramms bei Neugeborenen. Ophthalmologica 135, 205—210 (1958).
14. Kohlrausch, A., u. A. Brossa: Die photoelektrische Reaktion der Tag- und Nachtvogelnetzhaut auf Licht verschiedener Wellenlänge. Arch. Anat. Physiol. 1914, 421—431.
15. Kolmer, W.: Die Netzhaut. In W. v. Möllendorf: Handbuch der mikroskopischen Anatomie des Menschen 3/2, 295—467 (1936).
15a. Noell, W. K.: Differentiation, metabolic organization, and viability of the visual cell. A.M.A. Arch. Ophthalm. 60, 702—731 (1958).
16. Parry, H. B., K. Tansley and L. C. Thomson: Electroretinogram during development of hereditary retinal degeneration in the dog. Brit. J. Ophthalm. 39, 349—352 (1955).
17. Piper, H.: Untersuchungen über das elektromotorische Verhalten der Netzhaut bei Warmblütern. Arch. Anat. Physiol. 1905 (Suppl.), 133—192.
18. — Über die Netzhautströme. Arch. Physiol. 1911, 85—132.
19. Popp, C.: Die Retinafunktion nach intraocularer Ischämie. Albrecht v. Graefes Arch. Ophthal. 156, 395—403 (1955).
20. Ronchi, L., and S. Grazi: The dependence of the human electroretinogram on the shape of the stimulus as a function of time. Opt. Acta 3, 188—195 (1956).
21. Schubert, G.: Ein entoptisches Hypoxie-Phänomen. Z. Biol. 110, 232—235 (1958).
22. Tansley, K.: Some observations on mammalian cone electroretinograms. Bibl. ophthal. (Basel) 48, 7—14 (1957).
23. — The retina of two nocturnal geckos Hemodactylus turcicus and Tarentola mauritanica. Pflügers Arch. ges. Physiol. 268, 213—220 (1959).
24. Walls, G. L.: The vertebrate eye and its adaptive radiation. Cranbrook Inst. of Science, Bloomfield Hills, Michigan 1942.
25. Wegner, W.: Die Funktion der menschlichen Netzhaut bei experimenteller Ischaemia retinae. Arch. Augenheilk. 98, 514—564 (1928).
26. Zetterström, B.: The clinical electroretinogram. IV. The electroretinogram in children during the first year of life. Acta ophthal. (Kbh.) 29, 295—304 (1951).
27. — The effect of light on the appearance and development of the electroretinogram in newborn kittens. Acta physiol. scand. 35, 272—279 (1956).

Diskussion s. S. 94.

Stoffwechsel und Funktion der isolierten Netzhaut*

Von

WERNER SICKEL

Mit 5 Abbildungen

Die Netzhaut erfaßt einen Bereich von Reizparametern, der von den für das Verständnis dieser biologischen *Funktion* herangezogenen Modellen nicht ohne weiteres verarbeitet werden kann. Tatsächlich schließen sich allerdings extreme Leistungen wie die Erfassung kleinster Leuchtdichten und schnelles zeitliches oder auch räumliches Auflösungsvermögen gegenseitig aus, und es bedarf, um diese Möglichkeiten auszuschöpfen, eines zeitfordernden Umstellungsprozesses, der Adaptation. Diese beinhaltet weiterhin neben einer spektralen Verschiebung (Purkinje-Effekt) eine Verlagerung des optimalen Intensitätsauflösungsvermögens in denjenigen Leuchtdichtebereich, auf den adaptiert worden ist, weshalb in einer Kritik zum Weber-Fechnerschen Gesetz die Adaptation von RANKE (*38*) als *Bereichseinstellung* im technischen Sinne beschrieben worden ist.

Bemerkenswerterweise sind die Adaptationsumstellungen dieser verschiedenartigen Sehleistungen offenbar immer in Gemeinschaft betroffen. Jedenfalls scheinen keine pathologischen Befunde vorzuliegen, die etwa den isolierten Ausfall des Purkinje-Effektes bei erwartungsgemäßem Gang der Schwellenwerte aufwiesen. Eine derartige Verkoppelung erhellt ebenfalls aus dem gleichsinnigen Einfluß des Adaptationszustandes, beispielsweise auf Flimmerverschmelzungsfrequenz und Sehschärfe. Aus einer großen Zahl von Publikationen mit der Fragestellung: photochemische und nervöse Faktoren des Adaptationsprozesses geht hervor, daß eine rein photochemische Beschreibung unzureichend ist, man vielmehr „eine Umstimmung der gesamten Netzhaut" (z. B. *20*) zu interpretieren hat.

Obwohl die *Stoffwechsel*sonderstellung der Netzhaut — höchste Umsatzgröße mit einem vermutlich auch unter physiologischen Bedingungen bemerkenswerten aeroben Glykolyseanteil (*48, 49*) — bekannt ist, sind die Angaben der Literatur über Zuordnung von Sauerstoffverbrauch, Säurebildung u. a. zu dem Adaptationszustand widersprüchlich (s. *37*).

Es hat dies offensichtlich methodische Gründe. Ein Teil der Befunde ist unter Bedingungen erhoben worden, die außerhalb des Funktionsbereiches der Netzhaut liegen (z. B. Indicatorzusätze zur pH-Bestimmung) und daher nicht notwendig die gewünschte Zuordnung erlauben. Bei anderen wieder ist damit zu rechnen, daß die geprüften Stoffe noch unter der Aufarbeitung nicht kontrollierbare Reaktionen (z. B. Gleichgewichtseinstellungen, Resynthesen) eingehen, wenn man nicht etwa durch Anwendung tiefer Temperaturen dem vorgenannten Einwand begegnen will. Schließlich sind indirekte Schlußfolgerungen aus Toleranzermittlungen und Einwirkungseffekten auf die im Verband befindliche Netzhaut mit einer gewissen Zurückhaltung zu werten, solange man nicht die am Ort ablaufenden Prozesse übersieht. Sauerstoffmangel wird an der Netzhaut beispielsweise erst nach Erschöpfung des Hämoglobin-Speichers (Dissoziationskurve) wirksam (*1; 27*); bei toxischer Sauerstoffwirkung konnte ebenfalls eine protektive Kreislaufwirkung wahrscheinlich gemacht werden (*2*), Azetaldehyd wirkt an der Netzhaut mehrfach stärker toxisch, wenn ihm der Transport auf dem Blutweg erspart bleibt (*19*), usw.

---

* Aus dem Physiologischen Institut der Universität Leipzig.

Eine Konfrontierung eines durch die adaptierende Lichtwirkung bestimmten Funktionszustandes mit der Stoffwechselsituation erfordert daher ein zwar funktionstüchtiges, jedoch Messungen des bzw. Eingriffen in den Stoffwechsel zugängliches Präparat, an dem sowohl bezüglich der Licht- als auch der Stoffwechselsituation unter steady state-Bedingungen gearbeitet werden kann: es empfiehlt sich das Präparat der umströmten Netzhaut (39; 27).

Als Funktionskriterium wird das von HOLMGREN 1865 als Modulation des Bestandsstromes beschriebene Elektroretinogramm vorgeschlagen. Bereits von KÜHNE und STEINER (23) ist festgestellt worden, daß es sich bei diesem mehrphasischen Kurvenverlauf nicht um wandernde Potentiale, sondern um ortsgebundene, in ihrer Intensität zeitlich sich ändernde Potentialbildungen handelt (s.a. 36), die offenbar die Resultante mehrerer einfacher Komponenten sind. Unter zahlreichen Differenzkonstruktionen hat sich die von GRANIT (16) vorgeschlagene bewährt, da die Komponenten im Experiment isoliert dargestellt werden konnten.

Der Einfluß der (Hell-) Adaptation kommt im Elektroretinogramm zum Ausdruck durch

1. schnelleren Ablauf der Prozesse,
2. Überwiegen der negativen Komponenten,
3. Akzentuierung der off-Antwort gegenüber der on-Reaktion.

Durch optische wie nichtoptische Beeinflußbarkeit (Lit. s. 33) erweist sich das Elektroretinogramm für das vorliegende Vorhaben besonders aufschlußreich und geeignet. Es ist jedoch festzustellen, daß es auch gegenwärtig beträchtliche Schwierigkeiten bietet, die mit Makroelektroden ableitbaren Belichtungspotentiale in die Kette des Sehprozesses einzuordnen. Ihrem zeitlichen Ablauf nach sind sie von den Erstuntersuchern (23) mit elektrischen Erscheinungen an Drüsen verglichen und als Sekretionsströme beschrieben worden. Sie mögen Beziehungen haben zu den langsamen corticalen Potentialschwankungen. Jedenfalls ist es bislang ebenso wenig wie dort für das Elektroretinogramm gelungen, die kausalen Beziehungen zu den mit Mikroelektroden aus verschiedenen Netzhautlagen ableitbaren Potentialschwankungen schlüssig aufzuzeigen.

Die verwendete Methodik erlaubt bei nur unwesentlicher Abwandlung die Registrierung von spike-Aktivität (Registrierbeispiel Abb. 1c) als Beleg dafür, daß auch die Ganglienzellen als vermutlich empfindlichstes Glied funktionstüchtig sind. Da aber die zu kombinierenden Analyse- und Einwirkungsverfahren sich auf das gesamte Präparat beziehen, vor allen Dingen aber der zu untersuchende Prozeß die Netzhaut als Ganzes betrifft, ist es sinnvoll, als Kriterium eine Summenantwort zu wählen.

Das Elektroretinogramm bietet weiterhin den Vorzug, daß es mit gleichem Informationswert vom gleichen Untersuchungsobjekt bei verschieden weit eingreifender Präparation erhoben werden kann. Schließlich läßt sich die Untersuchung auf isolierte Netzhäute beliebiger Species einschließlich der des Menschen (43) ausdehnen.

Methodik

Das Präparat: die umströmte Netzhaut. Die Untersuchungen wurden vornehmlich an Teilen isolierter Netzhäute von rana temp. und esc. durchgeführt.

Zur Sicherung gegen präparationsbedingte Artefakte wurden die mitgeteilten Befunde soweit angängig an weniger weit isolierten Präparaten überprüft. Über das Vorgehen bei der

ERG-Ableitung vom intakten Tier (*2*), von dem isolierten, an Luft (*1*) bzw. in Flüssigkeit (*42*) befindlichen Bulbus ist an anderem Ort berichtet worden. Der Feststellung der Verallgemeinerungsfähigkeit der in der Froschnetzhaut erzielten Resultate dienten Untersuchungen von Netzhäuten anderer Species, besonders Warmblütern. Die dabei angewandte Technik unterscheidet sich von der im folgenden mitgeteilten nur insoweit, als von den meist größeren Augen nach Eröffnung mit einem Trepan Fundusstücke in der für die vorhandene Anlage passenden Größe ausgestanzt wurden.

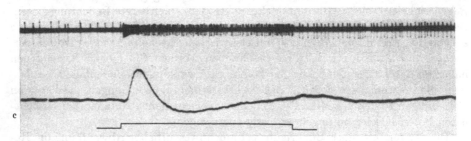

Die Versuchstiere wurden in der Regel 2 Std. dunkeladaptiert, um eine schonende Lösung des Pigmentepithels zu erzielen. Die weitere Präparation erfolgte im allgemeinen bei Rotlicht. Es ist dies nicht erforderlich, erspart jedoch im eigentlichen Versuch Zeit zur Erreichung stationärer Adaptationsverhältnisse. Nach Enukleation wurden die Bulbi unter Verzicht auf subtiles Vorgehen in einer Halterung von einer mit Federkraft geführten Rasierklinge äquatorial eröffnet. Dadurch werden mechanische Insulte weitgehend vermieden, vor allem aber durch Zeitersparnis die Entstehung eines wesentlichen Sauerstoff-Defizits bis zur Freilegung

Abb. 1 a—c. Plexiglas-Kammer für die umströmte Netzhaut. a Schema: Netzhaut — in der Mitte — gehaltert von Maschengewebe mit Zu- und Abfluß sowie Ableitelektroden; Lichteinfall von oben oder unten; b Ausführungsbeispiel mit Umschalthahn und Glaselektrode; c Registrierbeispiel: Simultanableitung mit Makro- (ERG) und Mikro-(Spike-Aktivität) Elektroden auf punktförmigen (0,3 mm) Lichtreiz (Marke 1 sec; 100 bzw. 30 μV)

der Netzhaut. Die Netzhaut wird der hinteren Bulbushälfte unter Flüssigkeit entnommen, wobei gegebenenfalls mit feinen Pinzetten an der lose anhaftenden Chorioidea manipuliert, und — zweckmäßig jedoch noch vor Eröffnung des Bulbus — der Opticusstumpf nach innen gedrängt werden kann. Anschließend wird die Netzhaut auf einen mit Perlon- (Strumpf-) Gewebe bespannten Plexiglasring von etwa 10 mm äußerem Durchmesser aufgenommen und (nötigenfalls in einer verdunkelten feuchten Kammer unter Luftzutritt aufbewahrt und praktisch beliebig später) in der vorbereiteten Elektrodenkammer in den Versuch genommen.

Die Kammer. Prinzip: Die Netzhaut befindet sich nahezu unbeschwert und im freien Stoffaustausch mit einem beiderseits strömenden Medium, lediglich gehaltert von zwei Maschengeweben, inmitten eines Kammerraumes in günstiger Position zu den beiden in geringem Abstand angeordneten Elektroden, einer Lichteinwirkung frei zugängig (Schema: Abb. 1a).

Abbildung 1b zeigt ein Ausführungsbeispiel: Der Kammerraum wird von zwei Plexiglasblöcken mit symmetrisch profilierten Ausarbeitungen gebildet, die nach dem Beschicken verschraubt werden. Sie enthalten die Ausführungen der bis auf ihren freien Querschnitt isolierten Silberableitelektroden, die in genormten Steckverbindungen endigen, sowie Zu- und Abfluß des kleinvolumigen Kammerraumes. In den Zufluß ist mit kurzem Totweg ein Umschalt-hahn eingearbeitet, der wahlweise eine von zwei Vorratslösungen durch den Kammerraum leitet und die andere im Bedarfsfall gleichzeitig durch Extraauslaß bis in den Hahn hinein aus-zutauschen gestattet. Im Ausfluß ist als Beispiel eines Meßwertgebers eine Glaselektrode ge-zeichnet.

Zur simultanen Messung des Sauerstoff-Verbrauches findet eine prinzipiell gleichartige Anordnung Verwendung, die jedoch zur Erreichung der Nachweisgrenze mehrere (2×8) in Serie liegende Netzhäute aufnimmt. Für Arbeiten bei beschränktem Flüssigkeitsvolumen kann die Bewegung des Mediums auch durch ein magnetisches Rührwerk unterhalten werden. Durch eine kleine Öffnung des Oberteiles oder durch Austausch des Ausflußteiles gegen einen Überlauf bei freier Zugänglichkeit des Präparates von oben können Mikroelektroden in verschiedene Lagen der Netzhaut eingeführt werden.

Ein Beispiel simultaner Registrierungen mit Makro- (ERG) und Mikro- (spike-Aktivität) Elektroden von der umströmten Netzhaut zeigt die Abb. 1 c.

Die Reizeinrichtung vereinigt zwei Strahlengänge (Reiz- und Dauerlicht) mit Farb- und Graufiltern sowie Photoverschlüssen. Definierte Lichtlücken konnten mit einem entsprechend umgebauten Compurverschluß geboten werden. Soweit nicht anders vermerkt, betrug die Reiz-dauer 1 sec, das Intervall zwischen zwei Reizen 3 min.

Die Verstärkung und Aufzeichnung der Elektroretinogramme erfolgte mit direktschreiben-dem Elektroencephalographen (System Schwarzer, München). Die RC-Verstärker (Zeitkon-stante 1,0 sec) bieten zwar keine absolut getreue Wiedergabe der Netzhautaktivität, liefern aber bei erstrebenswerter Nullpunktkonstanz hinsichtlich der im Elektroretinogramm ent-haltenen Frequenzen hinreichend Informationen und können bezüglich der auszuwertenden on- und off-Effekte als zweckmäßig angepaßt gelten. Ergänzende Untersuchungen zur Kontrolle der ERG-Konfiguration bei Gleichspannungsverstärkung wurden mit einer Tönnies-Apparatur (Freiburg/Br.) vorgenommen. Vornehmlich diente diese Anlage jedoch der Re-gistrierung von Mikroelektrodenableitungen mit 3 m KCl gefüllten Glascapillarelektroden.

Milieukontrolle. Als Standardlösung zur Umströmung der Netzhaut wurde eine modifi-zierte Tyrodelösung mit Phosphat als Puffersystem verwendet. Der p_H-Wert wurde im Bereich von 7,2—8,1 variiert. Äquilibrierung mit Gasgemischen auch unter Überdruck war möglich. Im allgemeinen wurde bei Zimmertemperatur gearbeitet. Ein Heizmantel in einer der Zuleitun-gen erlaubte, die zimmertemperierte oder vorgekühlte Lösung auf abweichende Temperaturen zu bringen. Kontrolle erfolgte durch Thermoelement im Ausfluß.

Sauerstoffverbrauchsmessungen wurden in der strömenden Flüssigkeit, d. h. bei stationä-rem Angebot mit der tropfenden Quecksilberelektrode vorgenommen. Ein Verfahren zur Messung der Säureproduktion durch fortlaufende Titration im Ausfluß befindet sich in Ent-wicklung.

Ergebnisse

1.

Für eine in ein flüssiges Medium verbrachte Netzhaut, deren Stoffaustausch nicht mehr auf flüchtige Substanzen beschränkt ist, gelten — wie allgemein bei derartigen Untersuchungen an überlebenden Präparaten — eine Reihe von Be-dingungen, deren Gegebenheit im vorliegenden Fall an Hand mehrerer Kriterien überprüft werden kann:

1. Optimale Potentialausbeute (z. B. Höhe der b-Wellen),
2. Konfiguration der Reizantworten (ERG-Formen, on/off-Relation),
3. Konstanz der Antworten über längere Zeit (steady-state).

In umfangreichen Voruntersuchungen wurden die Auswirkungen von Milieu-änderungen mit dem Ziel der Ermittlung von Standardbedingungen geprüft. Von den Ergebnissen sei auszugsweise mitgeteilt:

Isotonie. Hypotone Lösungen (90 mM NaCl) mindern den 2. Anteil des von SMIT (*45*) beschriebenen doppelten off-Effekts, werden aber im übrigen relativ gut toleriert. Hypertone Lösungen (150 mM NaCl) verringern die b-Welle und führen zu einem Anstieg des zweiten trägen off-Anteils.

Substrat und Sauerstoff-Versorgung. Unter den gewählten Bedingungen war eine Strömungsgeschwindigkeit von 2—3 ml/min erforderlich, die nicht durch Angebotserhöhung kompensiert werden konnte. Limitierend ist offensichtlich der CO_2-Abtransport (geringerer Strömungsbedarf bei geöffnetem Oberteil). Andererseits war dabei der O_2-Bedarf durch Zimmerluftsättigung gedeckt. Reiner O_2 wirkt bei geringer Glucosekonzentration bereits toxisch. Ein protektiver Glucoseeffekt macht nennenswerte endogene Energiequellen unwahrscheinlich. Andererseits führt osmotisch noch nicht wirksame Erhöhung der Glucosekonzentration zu Potentialminderung.

Spezifische Ionenwirkung. Kaliumüberschuß (20 mM KCl) führt zu stationärer Ausbildung der negativen Komponente (PIII), Kaliummangel (0,2 mM KCl) zu progressivem Potentialverlust. Negative Komponenten sind auch — nach Durchlaufen übernormaler, später träger Stadien — als Folge eines Calciummangels zu erhalten. Unter verringerter Calciumkonzentration (0,1 mM $CaCl_2$) ist ein Calcium-Magnesium-Antagonismus an der on/off-Relation zu erkennen.

Puffer. In ungepufferter Lösung sind von der umströmten Netzhaut anfangs Retinogramme zu erhalten, die den an Luft gewonnenen gleichen. Sie unterliegen aber einem rapiden Verfall. Dieser Zeitgang ist aufzuhalten durch Pufferzusatz (Carbonat, Borat, Phosphat). Es besteht ein spezieller Phosphatbedarf, besonders für Dunkeladaptation (10 mM/l). Über den p_H-Wert siehe unten.

Temperatur. Im allgemeinen brachte Temperaturerhöhung keinen nennenswerten stationären Potentialgewinn (in Abhängigkeit vom Adaptationszustand s. u.), auch nicht an den bisher untersuchten Warmblüternetzhäuten. Latente Noxen (Sauerstoffüberdruck; *41*) treten dann in Erscheinung in Form einer trägen off-Reaktion als Schädigungssymptom, besonders unter Rot-Reizen.

Spezielle Zusätze (Makromoleküle). An Warmblüternetzhäuten (Schwein, Mensch; nicht bei Meerschweinchen und Kaninchen) erwies sich zur Erzielung normal konfigurierter Elektroretinogramme ein Plasmazusatz als erforderlich. Dieser war auch noch nach mehrstündiger Versuchsdauer in proteinfreiem Medium (PIII-Formen) wirksam.

2.

Die on/off-Relation (Abb. 2).   a) Löst man unter konstanten Adaptations- und Milieubedingungen Elektroretinogramme durch Lichtreize von 1 sec Dauer und steigender Intensität aus (schematisch am oberen Bildrand), so steigt die b-Welle und erreicht schließlich einen konstanten Endwert. Der off-Effekt wächst zunächst ebenfalls, fällt jedoch bei höheren Reizintensitäten wieder ab. Die Sättigungscharakteristik der b-Welle zeigt im mittleren Bereich einen etwa linearen Anstieg bei logarithmischer Reizlichtsteigerung. Der insgesamt mit Änderung der b-Wellenhöhe beantwortete Reizlichtintensitätsbereich umfaßt jedoch nicht mehr als 2—3 log-Einheiten (s. *10*). Die Höhe des off-Maximums wächst bei steigender Reizlichtdauer. Der anschließende Abfall ist von HARTLINE (*18*) am Limulusauge beobachtet und als Hemmung beschrieben worden.

b) Erzeugt man den Potentialzuwachs nicht durch höhere Intensität, sondern durch längere Dauer des Lichtreizes, so erreicht die b-Welle noch unterhalb 1 sec ihren Endwert. Der off-Effekt steigt jetzt jedoch mit wachsendem zeitlichen Abstand vom on-Effekt weit über das eben gezeigte Maximum und strebt schließlich ebenfalls einem Endwert zu. (Zwischen der Erhebung der einzelnen Meßwerte wurde durch einen Testreiz die Konstanz des Adaptationszustandes überprüft und entsprechende Intervalle eingelegt. Konstante Adaptationsverhältnisse sind an der Konstanz der b-Wellenhöhe zu erkennen.)

c) Läßt man den off-Effekt nicht einer b-Welle folgen, sondern erzeugt ihn als erste Reizantwort, d. h. arbeitet man mit Lichtlücken, so strebt der off-Effekt

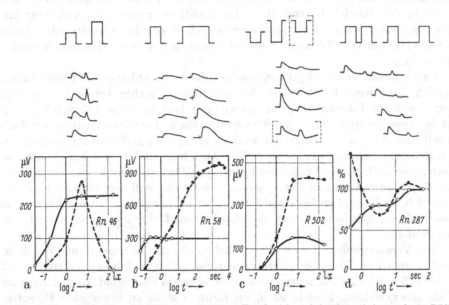

Ab. 2 a—d. Die on/off-Relation im ERG der umströmten Froschnetzhaut bei (schematisch am oberen Bild): a Lichtreizen steigender Intensität; b Lichtreizen wachsender Dauer; c Lichtlücken zunehmender Leuchtdichtedifferenz; d Doppelreizen wachsenden Intervalles (2. Antwort in Prozent der ersten). Mitte: Original-ERG; unten: Auswertung der b-(———) und d-(— — —) Wellenhöhen

ebenfalls einem Endwert zu. Die b-Welle durchläuft jetzt — nicht sehr ausgeprägt — einen Höchstwert. Deutlicher wird dieser Sachverhalt an den beiden unteren Original-Elektroretinogrammen: Läßt man bei der Lichtlücke nämlich eine gewisse Grundhelligkeit bestehen, so verringert sich erwartungsgemäß der off-Effekt. Aber die b-Welle, für die der Reiz ebenfalls kleiner geworden ist, ist unter diesen Bedingungen vergleichsweise höher.

d) Bei Doppelreizen wachsenden Intervalls fällt die zweite b-Welle zunächst kleiner aus und erreicht in dem gezeigten Zeitverlauf bei etwa 1 min-Abstand vom ersten Reiz den Ausgangswert. Der nach einer Sekunde auftretende off-Effekt ist jedoch größer als der vorausgegangene. Bei wachsendem Intervall fällt der off-Effekt zunächst in dem Maße wie die b-Welle ansteigt und durchläuft, bevor er nach 1 min ebenfalls den Ausgangswert erreicht, ein Minimum.

Diese Befunde lassen eine Funktionsbegrenzung bezüglich der Reizintensität erkennen, die für on- und off-Reaktion in gleicher Größenordnung liegt (a, c), d. h. das System arbeitet nach logarithmischer Transformation etwa linear. Oberhalb einer bestimmten Belastung (a, c, d) besteht ein reziprokes Verhalten von on und off als Ausdruck der Konkurrenz um die gleiche Energiequelle. Die zeitliche Summationsfähigkeit ist für die b-Welle bei etwa 1 sec erschöpft, die Lichtwirkung dauert jedoch an, wie aus dem off-Zuwachs bis über 15 min (b) zu ersehen ist.

3.

Als Ausdruck der Änderung des Funktionszustandes der Netzhaut tritt unter geänderten Adaptationsbedingungen eine Verschiebung der on/off-Relation ein (Abb. 3a). Mit zunehmender Grundhelligkeit werden die b-Wellenkurven nach rechts in den Bereich höherer Reizlichtintensitäten verschoben, und zwar annähernd parallel, wobei die Sättigungswerte auch absolut keine wesentlichen Änderungen erfahren. Die off-Maxima treten ebenfalls nach rechts und werden beträchtlich erhöht.

Es wird also der Punkt größter Steilheit der b-Wellenkurve sinngemäß in den Bereich der jeweils herrschenden Adaptationsleuchtdichte verschoben, so daß dort das beste Intensitätsauflösungsvermögen besteht. Eine prinzipiell gleichartige Verschiebung der Intensitätscharakteristik kann stationär unter festgehaltenem Adaptationslicht durch eine Änderung des p_H-Wertes der umströmenden Flüssigkeit erzeugt werden (Abb. 3b). Auch hier handelt es sich nicht um eine Empfindlichkeitsminderung bei geringerem p_H-Wert, die durch eine Verflachung der Kurve zum Ausdruck käme, wie es unter Sauerstoffmangel tatsächlich der Fall ist (s. a. *4*), sondern um einen Prozeß, der als kompetetiv zu bezeichnen und damit als am gleichen Ort wie die adaptierende Lichtwirkung angreifend ausgewiesen ist.

Die Veränderungen der off-Effekte liefern die zur Kennzeichnung der Reiz *und* Adaptations-Situation ausstehende Information und lassen erkennen, daß unter hellerer Grundbeleuchtung wie unter höherem Säuregrad die Netzhaut am Ende der gewählten 1 sec-Reize in verstärktem Maße zu neuerlicher Potentialbildung fähig ist und diese Fähigkeit erst bei entsprechend höherer Reizlichtbelastung erschöpft ist.

Die darin zum Ausdruck kommende schnellere Reaktionsweise der Hell-Netzhaut ist aber bereits im on-Effekt erkennbar (Abb. 3c, d): Bei doppeltlogarithmischer Auftragung der Dauer (Abszisse) und Intensität (Ordinate) des Lichtreizes verbindet die Gerade unter 45° diejenigen Wertepaare, die bei Gültigkeit des Reizmengengesetzes konstante Effekte — hier b-Wellenhöhen — zeitigen. Die Gültigkeit dieses Gesetzes, d. h. die Summationsfähigkeit ist jedoch nach langen Reizzeiten hin begrenzt, die Effektgröße wird schließlich unabhängig von der Zeit, d. h. die Kurve läuft abszissenparallel aus. Interpolation beider experimentell gut faßbarer gerader Kurvenstücke ergibt einen Zeitgrenzwert als Nutzzeit. Entsprechend dem Diagramm (c) ist für 10 lux Adaptationsleuchtdichte oberhalb 0,1 sec eine Intensitätsminderung nicht mehr durch längere Reizdauer kompensierbar, sehr wohl jedoch bei 0,4 lux. Eine entsprechende Verschiebung der Summationsgrenze nach längeren Zeiten ergibt sich bei konstanter Adaptationsleuchtdichte, wenn man den p_H-Wert der die Netzhaut umströmenden Lösung erhöht (*17*) (d).

Der längeren Nutzzeit der dunkel bzw. alkalisch gehaltenen Netzhaut entspricht andererseits der längere Zeitbedarf für eine folgende Reizantwort (s. Abb. 5a). Es sind damit oberer und unterer Zeitgrenzwert festgelegt, so daß die Ergebnisse den üblicherweise durch Ermittlung der Flimmerverschmelzungsfrequenz erhobenen Sachverhalt ausweisen.

Schließlich läßt sich zeigen (Abb. 3 e, f), daß auch eine Verschiebung der spektralen Reizwerte in gleicher Weise durch Licht- und p_H-Einflüsse hervorgerufen werden kann: In drei Versuchen (Dreieck, Viereck, Kreis) wurden zunächst von

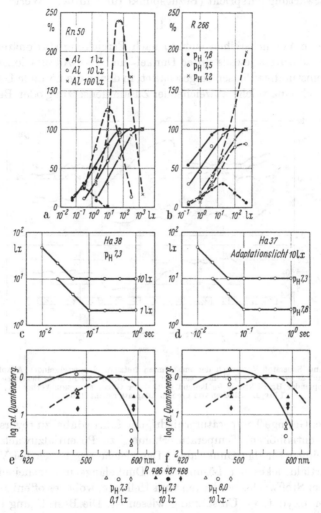

Abb. 3 a—f. Bereichsverschiebung der Intensitäts- (*a*, *b*), Zeit- (*c*, *d*) und Spektral- (*e*, *f*) Charakteristik des ERG der umströmten Froschnetzhaut; links (*a*, *c*, *e*): durch Adaptationslicht; rechts (*b*, *d*, *f*): durch p_H-Änderung des Mediums. Erläuterung siehe Text

blauen, grünen und roten Spektrallichtern die für gleiche b-Wellenhöhen erforderlichen Quantenbeträge unter dunklem Adaptationslicht und relativ saurem p_H-Wert bestimmt (offene Zeichen links). Danach wurde das Adaptationslicht erhöht und die so bewirkte spektrale Reizwertverschiebung ermittelt (gefüllte Zeichen links = rechts), die dann durch Erhöhung des p_H-Wertes wieder rückgängig gemacht wird (offene Zeichen rechts). Im linken Teil der Abbildung sind die durch Adaptationslicht, rechts die durch p_H-Änderung bewirkten Verschiebungen dargestellt. Die eingezeichneten Kurven stellen die spektrale Absorption von Sehpurpurlösungen (DARTNALL, ausgezogene Linie) sowie die phototopische Dominatorkurve (GRANIT, unterbrochene Linie) entsprechend einem Vorgehen von DONNER und RUSHTON (*11*) dar und zeigen, daß das Ausmaß der Verschiebung in beiden Fällen der Erwartung entspricht (Bezugspunkt für sämtliche Werte: 534 nm).

4.

In mehreren Versuchsreihen wurden nach Erreichung stationärer Antworten auf einen Standardreiz jeweils unter Dunkel- und Hell-Adaptationsbedingungen einhalb- bis einstündige Phasen eingeschaltet, in denen die normale Umströmungsflüssigkeit durch eine solche abweichender Zusammensetzung oder Beschaffenheit

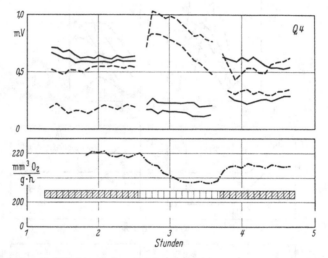

Abb. 4. ERG und Sauerstoff-Verbrauch der umströmten Netzhaut bei wechselnder Adaptation. Oben: *b*-(———) und *d*- (— — — — —) Wellenhöhen der 2. und 15. von 16 in Serie liegenden Retinae; unten: simultan mit tropfender Hg-Elektrode fortlaufend bestimmter Gesamtsauerstoff-Verbrauch; Reize: Lichtreize 1 lux, Lichtlücken von 1 sec im Adaptationslicht (100 lux)

ersetzt wurde. Geringe Temperaturerniedrigung führte dabei zu reversibler Minderung der Potentialhöhen, Temperaturerhöhung zu Potentialzuwachs, und zwar beides ausgiebiger für das Dunkelauge. Das gleiche ergab sich bei Variation des Sauerstoffpartialdruckes der Lösung. Das Dunkelauge unterscheidet sich somit auch in seinem Stoffwechselverhalten vom Hellauge, wobei es offenbar in höherem Maße auf den oxydativen Umsatz angewiesen ist. Die Bestätigung liefert das in Abb. 4 wiedergegebene Versuchsprotokoll: In der Mehrfachkammer wurden 16 in Serie liegende Netzhäute unter Dunkeladaptationsbedingungen durch Lichtreize von etwa 1 lux in 5 min-Abständen auf ihren Funktionszustand geprüft. Dargestellt sind zwei beliebige (vom Anfang und Ende der Reihe) herausgegriffene *b*- und *d*-Wellenverläufe sowie der im Ausfluß fortlaufend ermittelte Gesamtsauerstoffverbrauch. Eine Stunde nach Erreichen konstanter Werte (Einstellphase nicht gezeichnet) wurde ein Dauerlicht von etwa 100 lux geboten, das in 5 min-Abständen durch kurze Lichtlücken (1 sec) zur Erhebung der off- und on-Antworten unterbrochen wurde.

Es zeigte sich, daß in der Hellphase der Sauerstoffverbrauch abfällt, um in der anschließenden Dunkelphase wieder anzusteigen. Noch nicht abgeschlossene Versuche mit einem fortlaufenden Titrationsverfahren ergaben unter gleichen Bedingungen in der Hellphase eine erhöhte Bildung nicht flüchtiger Säuren.

Aufschluß über die Rolle der Glucose neben der des Sauerstoffs ergeben Untersuchungen der Restitutionskinetik, d. h. des zeitlichen Verlaufs der Wiederherstellung der Reizantwort mit Hilfe von Doppelreizen. Unter Hellbedingungen erreicht die Antwort (b-Welle) auf den zweiten Reiz in wenigen Sekunden fast die

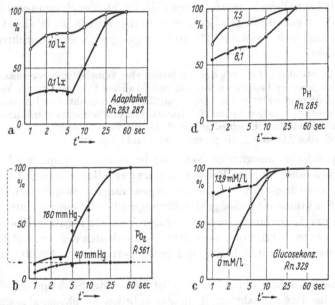

Abb. 5 a—d. Restitutionskinetik der b-Welle (Doppelreize: b-Wellenhöhe auf 2. Reiz als Prozent der ersten). a unter Hell- und Dunkeladaptation; b unter Dunkeladaptation bei verschiedener O₂-Versorgung; c unter Helladaptation mit und ohne Glucoseversorgung; d bei c.p. geändertem pH-Wert der Umströmungsflüssigkeit

volle Höhe der ersten (Abb. 5a). Unter Dunkeladaptation dagegen vergehen mehrere Sekunden, in denen die b-Welle auf einem niedrigeren Wert bleibt, um danach in deutlich abgesetztem Zeitverlauf dem Ausgangswert zuzustreben. Es sind demnach für die Beseitigung der Reiznachwirkungen zwei einander folgende, jedoch abgrenzbare Prozesse maßgebend, die für Dunkel- und Hellauge in verschiedenem Maße bedeutsam sind.

Aufschluß über den zweiten dieser Prozesse gibt der folgende Versuch (Abb. 5b). Nach Aufnahme einer Restitutionskinetik unter Dunkelbedingungen wird der Sauerstoffpartialdruck auf etwa 40 mm Hg erniedrigt und die Einstellung konstanter b-Wellenhöhen auf einem niedrigeren Niveau (Pfeil) abgewartet. Eine Wiederholung der Doppelreizserie zeigt, daß dieser Wert im schnellen Zeitverlauf erreicht wird. Unter Sauerstoffmangel fehlt demnach der zweite Anteil der Restitution. Wird andererseits (Abb. 5c) unter Helladaptation die Glucoseversorgung unterbrochen, so führt dies zum Absinken des ersten Teiles der Restitutionskurve.

Die beiden Anteile der Restitution zeigen also alternativ eine Glucose- (1. Teil) bzw. Sauerstoff- (2. Teil) Empfindlichkeit, und es kommt offenbar durch Veränderung des pH-Wertes (Abb. 5d) ebenso wie unter der adaptiven Lichtwirkung zu einer anteiligen Verschiebung des Einflusses beider Teilschritte.

Besprechung der Ergebnisse

Die Möglichkeit, Elektroretinogramme von der isolierten Netzhaut zu erhalten, ist seit den grundlegenden Arbeiten von Kühne und Steiner (1882) bekannt, ihr Stoffwechselverhalten durch das klassische Werk Otto Warburgs und seiner Schule. Eine Verbindung beider Methoden und Fragestellungen ist bisher nicht unternommen worden[1]. Die Möglichkeiten eines solchen Vorgehens liegen darin begründet, daß sämtliche Voraussetzungen, die für Stoffwechseluntersuchungen an Gewebsschnitten gelten (5), gegeben bzw. erfüllbar sind (z. B. intakte Oberfläche, Schichtdicke und weiter siehe S. 83) und ein geeignetes Funktionskriterium zur Verfügung steht.

Es weist eine spezifische Leistung eines einfachen aber kompletten Systems aus und ist bei verschieden weitgehender Isolation sowie von verschiedenen Species einschl. Mensch zu erhalten, d. h. es ist repräsentativ. Es liefert quantitative und qualitative Informationen über den Funktionszustand verzögerungsfrei, fortlaufend und mit beträchtlicher Empfindlichkeit[2], und ist schließlich in technisch befriedigender Weise auf dosierbare physiologische Reize artefaktfrei in gradueller Abstufung mit geringem Aufwand zu gewinnen.

Am Präparat der umströmten Netzhaut ist es unter adäquaten Milieubedingungen möglich, über Stunden Reizantworten zu erhalten, die nach Erscheinungsbild und funktionellem Verhalten den in situ gewonnenen entsprechen. Beeinträchtigung des Funktionszustandes geht mit progressivem Schwund und/oder einer Verformung der Elektroretinogramme (träger Verlauf; negative Phasen) einher, wobei Stadien extremer Adaptationszustände durchlaufen werden. Auf die Ähnlichkeit der Hellantwort mit Schädigungsformen hatte bereits Fröhlich (13) hingewiesen.

Nach biochemischen Befunden (26) ist das erste Schädigungszeichen eine Tangierung der Pasteurreaktion, d. h. des subtilen — phosphatgesteuerten — Abgleiches der beiden — glykolytischen und oxydativen — Teilschritte energieliefernder Reaktionen. Als eine Überforderung dieses Abgleiches ist der potentialmindernde Effekt eines Mißverhältnisses von Kohlenhydrat- bzw. Sauerstoffangebot zu betrachten, wobei die Grenzen geradezu austitriert werden können.

Warburg (1957) (49) weist neuerdings darauf hin, daß eine meßbare Glykolyse bei normalen Geweben grundsätzlich als Schädigung aufzufassen ist, da sie sich in Serum beseitigen — bei der Netzhaut zumindest zurückdrängen — läßt. Dem entspricht, daß zur Erzeugung normaler Elektroretinogramme bei Warmblüternetzhäuten im allgemeinen ein Plasmazusatz erforderlich ist[3].

Als ein System zur Aufrechterhaltung der „retinalen Homöostase" wird von Noell (34) und von Svaetichin (46) auf Grund elektronenmikroskopischer (47) sowie histochemischer (24; 29) Befunde das über die gesamte Netzhaut ausgedehnte und die nervösen Elemente lückenlos einhüllende System der Müllerschen Zellen angesprochen. Nach fermentativer Ausstattung sowie Glykogengehalt dürften ihm die hier herausgestellten Aufgaben zufallen.

---

[1] Über vergleichbares Vorgehen an anderen Organen: s. z. B. (25, 32).

[2] Beurteilt an der Reversibilität von O_2-Mangel-Einwirkung ist die Sauerstoff-Verbrauchsgröße weit widerstandsfähiger (8).

[3] Waterhouse u. Witter (50) wiesen im menschlichen Plasma einen die DNP-Entkopplung hemmenden Faktor nach; es erscheint aussichtsreich, einem wirksamen Prinzip mit der hier beschriebenen Methodik nachzugehen.

Die Existenz eines lichtgesteuerten retinalen Mechanismus zur Bereichseinstellung hinsichtlich Intensitäts-, Zeit- und spektraler Reizcharakteristik konnte aufgezeigt und dieser stofflich — durch p_H-Einstellung — nachgebildet werden. Die Wirksamkeit von Fluorid, Jodacetat und Dinitrophenol (40) sowie der aufgezeigte Bedarf an dem für Phosphorylierungsprozesse (12) wichtigen Kalium weisen auf die Beteiligung des Adenylsäuresystems und die zugehörigen Energiecyclen bei der Entstehung der Elektroretinogramme hin.

Tabelle 1

Stofflicher Prozeß (Embden-Meyerhof/Krebs-Cycl.)		*Elektrischer Effekt* (Elektroretinogramm)
Glykolyse (schnell verfügbar; 12) Endoxydation (ergiebig)	1. Teilschritt 2. Teilschritt	Glucose- empfindlicher Restitutions-Sauerstoff- prozeß (Abb. 5)
Pasteur-Effekt (30) ("O₂ hemmt Glykolyse") Crabtree-Effekt (6) (Glucose hemmt O₂-Verbrauch)	O₂- und Glucoseangebot	O₂-Mangel: b-Wellenhöhe korrel. zu O₂-Verbrauch (1) O₂-Überdr.: 2-phas. Potentialabf. (41) Glucose: protektiv b. O₂-Überdr. potentialmindernd bei geringem O₂-Druck
erhöhte Endoxydation (7) Schädigungsglykolyse (49)	Alkohol- bzw. Acetat-Einspeisg.; Entkoppelung (?) (durch Serum zu beheben)	b-Wellen (PII)-Steigerung ("Dunkelformen") (3; 19) b-Wellen-Minderg. PIII persistiert (43)
bes. unter O₂-Mangel (u. Dunkeladaptation!):	spreading depression (15)	on/off Verschiebg. nach off (b-Wellenminderung)
Massenwirkungs-Beziehung "Respiratorische Kontrolle" (28): Oxydation n. Maßgabe des anfallenden ADP begrenzter ADP-ATP-Pool K-Ionen halten [ATP] hoch Ca-Ionen (entspr. ADP): oxydationsfördernd (7) Mg-Ionen oxydationsmindernd (tightly coupled (7))	Reizwirksamkeit des Lichtes	log. Reizabhängigkt.; b-Steigerg. ≙ Latenzminderung Funktionsbegrenzung (Abb. 2): b-Wellengröße als Funktion der Reizgröße reziprokes on-off-Verhalten ("Erschöpfung") K-Wirkg: isol. PIII; off erst bei längerer Reizdauer Ca-freie Lösg.: b-Verlust, PIII Komp. Ca-Mg-Antagonismus
erhöhter O₂-Verbrauch (21) erhöhte Bildung nicht-flüchtiger Säuren (9; 22; 35) Koppelungsgrad (respiratory control rate) (Oxyd. m. ADP: Oxydat. ohne ADP)	Adaptationswirksamkeit des Lichtes Dunkeladaptation (Abb. 4) Hell-Adaptation	b-Wellen-Steigerg. (b. Latenzverlängerung) schnell-reagierend (Lit.: 33) "Bereichseinstellung" (Abb. 3)
loosely coupled (44): Oxydat. nicht mehr (ADP-bzw.) phosphat-limitiert vermindert. DNP-Effekt auf O₂-Verbrauch	p_H-Steigerung	entspr. Dunkeladapt. (39; Abb. 3) gleichsinnige p_H- u. Phosphat-Wirkung (40) geringere DNP-Wirkung bei Dunkeladapt. (40)

Da verschiedenartige Eingriffe in den Stoffwechsel und dieser selbst (O_2-Verbrauch) sich als adaptationsabhängig darstellen, ist eine auf dem Wege über pH-Verschiebungen a priori anzunehmende Verschiebung von Stoffwechselabläufen als Folge adaptiver Lichtwirkung als gegeben anzusehen.

Offenbar (Lit. s. *34*) spielt für die Netzhaut der Warburg-Horecker-Dickens-Pentose-Phosphat-Shunt keine wesentliche Rolle, wenngleich durch die Freisetzung beträchtlicher Energiebeträge bereits in den ersten Teilschritten sich dieser Abbauweg zur Interpretation der schnelleren Reaktionsweise wie auch der geringeren Jodacetat-Empfindlichkeit (*40*) der Hell-Netzhaut anbietet. Entsprechungen zwischen den Teilschritten des klassischen Embden-Meyerhof-Cyclus (Glykolyse) mit nachfolgendem oxydativen Endabbau und dem Verhalten des Elektroretinogramms sind in Tab. 1 zusammengestellt.

Unter Heranziehung von Befunden mit schnell auflösender Methodik (*7*) über „Antwort-Verhalten" des Stoffwechsels (O_2-Verbrauch) auf Zugabe geeigneter (Phosphat-Acceptor)-Substanzen (ADP) sind die Gegenüberstellungen über die beschriebenen homöostasierenden Phänomene (oberer Teil der Tab. 1[1]) hinaus versuchsweise fortgeführt worden. Es ergibt sich daraus (mittlerer Teil der Tab. 1) die Vorstellung, daß das einzelne ERG unmittelbarer Ausdruck energieliefernder Prozesse ist. Seine Konfigurationsänderung unter adaptiver Lichtwirkung (unterer Teil der Tab. 1) resultierte dann aus einer variablen Kopplung (*44*) der oxydativen Prozesse an vorausgehende energiezehrende (= ADP-bildende) Prozesse.

Als Quelle für die ableitbaren Potentialschwankungen — wie möglicherweise auch für vergleichbare bioelektrische Erscheinungen (*14*; *32*) — dürften daher elektrisch wirksame Teilschritte, etwa das Redoxverhalten beteiligter Kofermente, in Betracht kommen.

Summary

The technique of the perfused retina is described. It was used to study the relationship between electrophysiologically tested specific function and metabolic processes as simultaneously manifested in the measurable action upon the medium continuously passing the retina. The results report mainly the total response of the frog's retina but other species may be used, and microelectrode studies can be done with a similar experimental setting.

The results suggest that the electroretinogram represents the properties of a metabolic pool, fed by energy yielding processes and consumed by stimulation induced activity. The balance can be shown to be governed by phosphate controlled regulatory mechanisms combining need and supply. The change in the functional state of the retina caused by adaptation through light can be described as a zero level shift. This can be imitated by a shift in the pH-value of the surrounding medium as demonstrated for the intensity, time and spectral response patterns. The transition from one adaptation state to another involves a shift in metabolic pathways bringing into play fast and energy yielding reactions alternatively.

A tentative interpretation of the slow potentials is given by applying the analogy of biochemical findings of the respiratory control: the electrical response is assigned to the acceptor behavior and adaptational changes to a change in the control rate.

---

[1] Vgl. ergänzende Bemerkungen in Gruppendiskussion (S. 63).

Literatur

1. BAUEREISEN, E., H.-G. LIPPMANN, E. SCHUBERT u. W. SICKEL: Bioelektrische Aktivität und Sauerstoffverbrauch isolierter Potentialbildner bei Sauerstoffdrucken zwischen 0 und 10 atm. Pflügers Arch. ges. Physiol. **267**, 636 (1958).
2. BAUMANN, CH.: Sauerstoffüberdruck und b-Welle vom Elektroretinogramm des Froschauges in situ. Diss. Leipzig 1959.
3. BERNHARD, C. G., and C. R. SKOGLUND: Selective suppression with ethylalcohol of inhibition in the optic nerve and of the negative component PIII of the electroretinogram. Acta physiol. scand **2**, 10 (1941).
4. BORNSCHEIN, H.: Der Einfluß der Reizintensität auf die Überlebenszeit des skotopischen ERGs. Pflügers Arch. ges. Physiol. **270**, 184 (1959).
5. BURCK, H. C.: Tissue slices, incubation fluid, electrolyt content. In: Membran transport and metabolism. Symposion Prag 1960.
6. BURK, D.: A colloquial consideration of the Pasteur and Neo-Pasteur-effects. Cold Spr. Harb. Symp. quant. Biol. **7**, 420 (1939).
7. CHANCE, B.: Quantitative aspects of the control of oxygen utilization. CIBA Foundation Symp. on the Regulation of Cell Metabolism. S. 91. London: J. and A. Churchill, Ltd. 1959.
8. DETTMAR, P.: Der Sauerstoffverbrauch des isolierten Froschauges bei niedrigen Sauerstoffdrucken. Diss. Leipzig (1959).
9. DITTLER, R.: Die chemische Reaktion der isolierten Froschnetzhaut. Pflügers Arch. ges. Physiol. **120**, 44 (1907).
10. DODT, E.: dieses Symposion.
11. DONNER, K. O., and W. A. H. RUSHTON: An effect of a coloured adapting field on the spectral sensitivity of frog retinal elements. J. Physiol. (Lond.) **149**, 288 ff. (1959).
12. ELLIOT, K. A. C.: Brain tissue respiration and glycolysis. In: The biology of mental health and disease. New York: P. B. Hoeber 1950.
13. FRÖHLICH, F. W.: Beiträge zur allgemeinen Physiologie der Sinnesorgane. Z. Sinnesphysiol. **48**, 28 (1913).
14. GANGLOFF, H., D. PETTE and H. MONNIER: Action of pH, K and Na on the electrical activity of cortex, rhinencephalon and thalamus in the anesthetized rabbit. Acta physiol. pharmacol. nederl. **6**, 755 (1957).
15. GOURAS, P.: Spreading depression of activity in amphibion retina. Amer. J. Physiol. **195**, 28 (1958).
16. GRANIT, R.: The components of the retinal action potential in mammals and their relation to the discharge of the optic nerve. J. Physiol. (Lond.) **77**, 207 (1933).
17. HANITZSCH, R.: Die Summationsfähigkeit der isolierten Froschretina in Abhängigkeit von Adaptationszustand und Wasserstoffionenkonzentration. Diss. Leipzig (1960).
18. HARTLINE, H. K.: The response of single optic nerve fibers of the vertebrate to illumination. Amer. J. Physiol. **121**, 400 (1938).
19. HASCHKE, W., u. W. SICKEL: Das Elektroretinogramm der umspülten Froschretina unter Einwirkung von Methyl- und Aethyl-Alkohol sowie deren Oxydationsprodukten. 26. Tgg. dtsch. Physiol. Ges.; Pflügers Arch. ges. Physiol. **272**, 73 (1960).
20. HECK, J.: Der off-Effekt im menschlichen Elektroretinogramm. Acta physiol. scand. **40**, 113 (1957).
21. JONGBLOED, J., u. A. K. NOYONS: Sauerstoffverbrauch und Kohlendioxydproduktion der Froschnetzhaut bei Dunkelheit und bei Licht. Z. Biol. **97**, 399 (1936).
22. KOBAKOWA, J. M.: Änderung des Netzhaut-pH des Froschauges. Physiol. Z. UdSSR **32**, 385 (1946).
23. KÜHNE, W., u. J. STEINER: Über das elektromotorische Verhalten der Netzhaut. Unters. Physiol. Inst. Heidelberg **3**, 387 (1880); **4**, 64 (1881).
24. KUWABAVÁ, T., D. G. COGAN, S. FUTTERMANN and J. K. KINOSHITA: Dehydrogenases in the retina and Müller's fibres. J. Histochem. Cytochem. **7**, 67 (1959).
25. LARRABEE, M. G., and D. BRONK: Metabolic requirements of sympathetic neurons. Cold Spr. Harb. Symp. quant. Biol. **17**, 245 (1952).
26. LASER, H.: The metabolism of the retina. Nature (Lond.) **136**, 184 (1935).

27. LIPPMANN, H.-G., u.W. SICKEL: Die isolierte Retina als Präparat für objektiv sinnesphysiologische und stoffwechselanalytische Untersuchungen. 25. Tgg. d. dtsch. Physiol. Ges.; Pflügers Arch. ges. Physiol. **270**, 30 (1959).
28. LOOMIS zit. nach CHANCE, B.
29. LOWRY, O. H., N. R. ROBERTS and C. LEWIS: The quantitative histochemistry of the retina. J. biol. Chem. **220**, 879 (1958).
30. LYNEN, F.: Phosphatkreislauf und Pasteur-Effekt. 8. Koll. d. Ges. f. Physiol. Chem. in Mosbach (1957). Berlin-Göttingen-Heidelberg: Springer 1957.
31. MATSUMOTO, J., K. TSUKIYAMA, K. HIRAOKA and N. YOSHII: Redox-potential of the cerebral cortex and an interpretation of the electrocorticogram. Med. J. Osaka Univ. **6**, 867 (1956).
32. MCILWAIN, H.: Electrical influences and speed of chemical change in the brain. Physiol. Rev. **36**, 355 (1956).
33. MÜLLER-LIMMROTH, W.: Elektrophysiologie des Gesichtssinnes. Berlin-Göttingen-Heidelberg: Springer 1959.
34. NOELL, W. K.: The visual cell: electric and metabolic manifestations of its life processes. Amer. J. Ophthal. **48**, Part II, 347 (1959).
35. OGUCHI, T.: zit. nach MÜLLER-LIMMROTH. Acta Soc. Ophth. jap. **1937**, 2029.
36. PILZ, A., W. SICKEL u. R. BIRKE: Lokale Entstehung und Ausbreitung des Elektroretinogramms der isolierten Froschnetzhaut. Pflügers Arch. ges. Physiol. **265**, 550 (1958).
37. PIRIE, A., and A. v. HEYNINGEN: Biochemistry of the eye. Oxford: Blackwell 1957.
38. RANKE, O. F.: Die optische Simultanschwelle als Gegenbeweis gegen das Fechnersche Gesetz. Z. Biol. **105**, 224 (1952).
39. SICKEL, W.: Der Einfluß der Wasserstoffionenkonzentration auf das Elektroretinogramm des Frosches. 24. Tgg. d. dtsch. Physiol. Ges.; Pflügers Arch. ges. Physiol. **268**, 49 (1958).
40. — Über die on/off-Relation im Elektroretinogramm. 26. Tgg. d. dtsch. Physiol. Ges.; Pflügers Arch. ges. Physiol. **272**, 20 (1960).
41. — E. BAUEREISEN u. H.-G. LIPPMANN: Sauerstoff-Überdruck und b-Welle des Elektroretinogramms vom isolierten Froschauge. Pflügers Arch. ges. Physiol. **266**, 219 (1958).
42. — u. H.-G. LIPPMANN: Elektroretinogramm vom submersen Froschbulbus. Naturwissenschaften **45**, 67 (1958).
43. — — W. HASCHKE u. CH. BAUMANN: Elektrogramm der umströmten menschlichen Netzhaut. Ber. d. dtsch. Ophthalmolog. Ges. **63**, 316 (1960).
44. SLATER, E. C., and W. C. HÜLSMANN: Control of rate of intracellular respiration. CIBA Foundation Symp. on the Regulation of Cell Metabolism. S. 58. London: J. and A. Churchill, Ltd. 1959.
45. SMIT, J. A.: zit. nach GRANIT, R.: Sensory mechanisms of the retina. Oxford: Univ. Press 1947.
46. SVAETICHIN, G.: dieses Symposion.
47. VILLEGAS, G.: dieses Symposion.
48. WARBURG, O., E. NEGELEIN u. K. POSNER: Versuche an überlebendem Carcinomgewebe. Klin. Wschr. **3**, 1062 (1924).
49. — K. GAWEHN u. A. G. GEISSLER: Manometrie der Körperzellen unter physiologischen Bedingungen. Z. Naturforsch. **12b**, 115 (1957).
50. WATERHOUSE, CH., and R. F. WITTER: The inhibitory action of human plasma on dinitrophenol uncoupling of oxidative phosphorylation. Arch. Biochem. **85**, 1 (1959).

Diskussion zu DODT, BORNSCHEIN und SICKEL

Mit 1 Abbildung

E. BAUMGARDT: Den Ergebnissen von Herrn Dr. DODT und Herrn Dr. BORNSCHEIN entnimmt man, daß eine erhebliche Helladaptation ohne meßbare Verringerung der Konzentration der betreffenden Sehpigmente existieren kann, und zwar bei den verschiedenartigsten Organismen. Wenn lange Zeit hindurch (und heute noch aller Evidenz zum Trotz von G. WALD) der Adaptationszustand als rechnerisch von der Konzentration der Sehpigmente ableitbar betrachtet wurde, so existieren doch zahlreiche psychophysische Beobachtungen, die auf eine bedeutende nervöse Komponente hinweisen. Aus Messungen der Pigmentkonzentration in situ, sowie aus der Berechnung der Konzentrationsänderungen infolge Belichtung (die Zahl der Sehpurpurmoleküle pro Stäbchen ist bekannt, daher auch die obere Grenze der Konzentrationsverminderung pro Zeiteinheit der Belichtung errechenbar) ergibt sich, daß photochemische Adaptation z. B. beim Menschen erst bei mittleren photopischen Leuchtdichten meßbar wird — Größenordnung 1000 asb. So ergibt sich folgendes Bild des Adaptationsvorganges:

1. Adaptation durch Verkleinerung der Pupillenöffnung, beim Menschen zwischen 10^4 und 10^3 asb bereits meßbar.

2. Adaptation durch Verringerung des Durchmessers der funktionellen, quasi unabhängigen retinalen Einheit. Dieser Prozeß entspricht der lateral inhibition und wird beim Menschen bereits im skotopischen Bereich deutlich meßbar.

3. Adaptation durch Verringerung der Höchstdauer eines Reizes, welche eben noch seine Totalsummation zuläßt. Beim Menschen beträgt diese Konstante an der absoluten Schwelle 0,1 s, bei mäßiger Helladaptation nur 0,03 s.

4. Das Gesetz von BOUGUER-WEBER, welches die Konstanz von $\varDelta I/I$ ausdrückt, beginnt im mittleren photopischen Bereich gültig zu werden (für große Testflächen sogar schon nahe seinem Beginn). Dem entspricht eine schlechtere Ausnützung der Lichtquantenabsorptionen, welche im ERG und in der Impulsfrequenz zum Ausdruck kommt. Es sieht aus, als ob eine stetig wachsende Zahl von Absorptionen nötig sei, um denselben elektrischen Effekt zu erzielen, der an der Schwelle der Absorption von 2 Lichtquanten entspricht.

5. Photochemische Adaptation, die erst bei erheblichen Leuchtdichten einen wesentlichen Beitrag liefert.

W. SICKEL (zu DODT): Nach Verhaltensbefunden von BIRUKOW und eigenen Untersuchungen an der umströmten Retina tritt der Purkinje-Effekt beim Frosch im Bereich von 0,1—10 lx auf. Oberhalb ist die spektrale Empfindlichkeit stabil, jedoch wird die Intensitätscharakteristik auch weiterhin im Sinne einer Bereichsverschiebung (RANKE) verlagert.

(Zu BORNSCHEIN) Die Veränderungen des ERG bei Hemeralopie weisen auf das Bestehen einer Stoffwechselanomalie hin — beurteilt nach vergleichbaren ERG-Formänderungen der isolierten menschlichen Netzhaut bei inadäquaten Milieubedingungen.

W. BEST: Aus den Vorträgen von Herrn DODT und Herrn BORNSCHEIN haben wir gesehen, daß wir den Vorgang der Dunkeladaptation nicht allein mit der Zunahme der Sehpurpurkonzentration erklären können. Auch die räumliche Summation, deren Bedeutung zuerst von CRAIK und VERNON erkannt wurde, kann nicht der allein wesentliche Faktor bei der Zunahme der Lichtempfindlichkeit im Dunkeln sein. Der Gecko z. B. hat eine sehr gute Dunkelanpassungsfähigkeit, aber nur eine geringe räumliche Summationsfähigkeit. Ich glaube, daß neben den genannten Faktoren auch eine Adaptation der Ganglienzellen eine Rolle bei der Dunkeladaptation spielt.

M.MONJÉ: Meine Mitarbeiterin Fräulein TÖNJES hat den Zusammenhang zwischen der Intensität der Helladaptation und der Geschwindigkeit der anschließenden Dunkeladaptation geprüft und ist dabei zu Kurven gekommen, die mit denen von Herrn JESSEN völlig identisch sind. Auch wir fanden, daß die Anfangsschwellen nach intensiver Helladaptation höher lagen und steiler abfielen als nach schwächerer. Trägt man die Resultate in ein Koordinatensystem ein, in dem nicht nur die Ordinatenachse, sondern auch die Abszissenachse logarithmisch geteilt ist, so sieht man, daß sich die Werte nach stärkerer Vorbelichtung um 2 Gerade, die miteinander einen Winkel bilden (Kohlrauschscher Knick), scharen. Die 1. Gerade verschiebt sich bei weniger starker Vorbelichtung nach unten und steiler abfielen als nach schwächerer. Der Winkel zwischen beiden Geraden wird stumpfer, bis schließlich die 1. Gerade bei einer Vorbelichtung von etwa 100 Lux in die 2. Gerade übergeht. Das Zustandekommen der 1. Geraden wird ausführlich diskutiert. Die 2 Geraden streben einem gemeinsamen Punkt zu, der nach etwa 50 min erreicht werden müßte und unabhängig von der vorausgegangenen Helladaptation ist. Die Anpassung erfolgt demnach um so schneller, je intensiver die vorausgegangene Helladaptation ist.

E. DODT (zu BAUMGARDT): Vergleichen wir die Ergebnisse an der Ratte mit den von Herrn Dr. BAUMGARDT genannten Faktoren, so läßt sich eine Verminderung der Sehpurpurkonzentration erst für eine adaptive Beleuchtung errechnen, die etwa dem 10^4-fachen der absoluten

Schwelle entspricht. Für Lichtreize von 0,1 sec wäre dieses Intervall noch etwas größer, da die Reizschwelle für 40 msec im dunkeladaptierten Zustand etwa doppelt so groß ist wie für 100 msec. Die Konstanz von $\Delta I/I$ innerhalb eines weiten Bereichs adaptiver Beleuchtung gilt nur für elektrische Antworten bis etwa 150 μV, für größere Potentiale ist ein stetig zunehmendes ΔI notwendig, um den gleichen elektrischen Effekt zu erzielen. Da die Pupillenweite im vorliegenden Falle konstant war, dürfte die Erhöhung der Reizschwelle bis zum Eintreten photochemischer Adaptation Ausdruck *nervöser Faktoren*, möglicherweise der *lateral inhibition* sein.

(Zu Sickel) Prüft man beim Froschauge die Reizwerte für 462 und 605 mμ bei verschiedener adaptiver Beleuchtung, so entspricht der von Dr. Sickel für die Purkinje-Verschiebung genannte Bereich von 2 Dekaden etwa einem 80%igen Übergang der skotopischen zur photopischen Helligkeitsverteilung. Von einer konstanten Verteilung der Reizwerte farbiger Lichter kann jedoch weder unter- noch oberhalb dieses Beleuchtungsbereichs gesprochen werden. So weicht die relative spektrale Empfindlichkeit für langwellige Reize bereits bei Adaptation an ein Reizlicht vom 10fachen der absoluten Schwelle von der Dunkelempfindlichkeitskurve ab, und bei sehr hoher adaptiver Beleuchtung (10^6 mal Dunkelschwelle) entspricht die Empfindlichkeitskurve nicht dem photopischen Dominator, sondern dem Rotmodulator (Abb. 1).

(Zu Best) Bekanntlich besitzen die Ratten relativ wenige, die nächtlichen Geckos dagegen sehr zahlreiche Retinaganglienzellen. Für die absolute Schwelle ist dies offenbar ohne größere Bedeutung, im dunkeladaptierten Zustand ist die Reizschwelle für beide Tiere etwa die gleiche. Ganz anders während Dunkeladaptation: hier sieht man beim Gecko innerhalb weniger Minuten eine Senkung der Reizschwelle auf $^1/_{1000}$, während die Ratte bei gleicher retinaler Beleuchtung hierzu eine 20mal längere Zeit braucht. Es besteht kein Grund anzunehmen, daß dieses Verhalten auf einer unterschiedlichen photochemischen Adaptation beruht.

(Zu Monjé) Sinnesphysiologische Messungen des Adaptationsverlaufes sind echte Schwellenbestimmungen, meist für einen umschriebenen Netzhautbezirk. Elektroretinographische Messungen der Dunkeladaptation betreffen dagegen immer einen größeren Netzhautbezirk. In der Mehrzahl der bisherigen Untersuchungen wurde nicht die Schwellenenergie, sondern

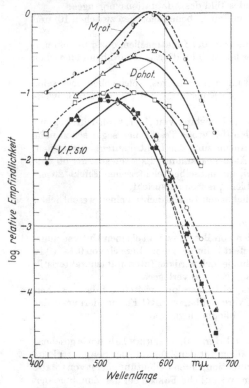

Abb. 1. Relative spektrale Augenempfindlichkeit des Frosches zwischen 418 und 673 mμ, erhalten durch Messung der für Einzelreiz-Elektroretinogramme konstanter Amplitude (20μV) notwendigen Energie, bezogen auf ein Spektrum gleicher Quantenzahlen. Erste Messung nach 12 Std. Dunkeladaptation (gefüllte Kreise), dann während stufenweise gesteigerter adaptiver Beleuchtung mit weißem (Xenon-) Licht: 0,84 Trolands = gefüllte Quadrate; 13 Trolands = gefüllte Dreiecke; 105 Trolands = offene Kreise; 840 Trolands = offene Quadrate; 6600 Trolands = offene Dreiecke; 52000 Trolands = halbgefüllte Kreise. Linien: V. P. 510 = Lythgoe's (1937) Sehpurpurabsorption, für λ_{max} 510 mμ umgezeichnet; $D_{phot.}$, M_{rot} = Granit's photopischer Dominator und Rotmodulator des Frosches. (Nach Dodt und Jessen, Vision Research 1961)

die Amplitude des Retinogramms bei konstanter Stärke des Testreizes registriert. Unter der Voraussetzung, daß die bei verschiedenem Adaptationszustand gemessenen Amplituden-Intensitätskurven der b-Welle einen parallelen Verlauf zeigen, lassen sich aus solchen Kurven bei geeigneter Stärke des Testreizes nachträglich die Veränderungen der Reizschwelle errechnen. Tatsächlich besteht z. B. bei Kaninchen und Ratten relativ gute Parallelität der bei verschiedenem Adaptationszustand erhaltenen Amplituden-Intensitätskurven der b-Welle bis zu einer bestimmten Potentialhöhe. Bei anderen Augen verlaufen die Amplituden-Intensitätskurven im photopischen Bereich (bis zum Knick der Dunkeladaptationskurve oder bei sehr hoher adaptiver Beleuchtung) etwas steiler als im skotopischen Bereich (nach dem Knick oder bei schwacher adaptiver Beleuchtung). Dies ist z. B. beim Eichhörnchen, Frosch und Gecko der Fall. Bei Mensch und Katze wird das Umgekehrte beobachtet; hier verläuft die Amplituden-Intensitätskurve im photopischen Bereich sehr viel flacher als im dunkeladaptierten Zustand, wodurch der Anfang der Dunkeladaptationskurve in eine fatale Abhängigkeit von der zur Schwellenbestimmung benutzten Potentialhöhe gerät. Ein Vergleich zwischen sinnes- bzw. verhaltensphysiologischen und elektroretinographischen Reizschwellenkurven bei verändertem Adaptationszustand ist daher bei einigen Netzhäuten, darunter leider auch beim Menschen, nur in begrenztem Umfange möglich.

H. Bornschein (zu Baumgardt und Best): Es ist zu hoffen, daß durch weitere vergleichende Untersuchungen von Netzhäuten mit extrem differenter Struktur Aufschlüsse über die verschiedenen Adaptationsmechanismen erhalten werden. Hinsichtlich der Frage, ob der Receptortyp oder die neurale Organisation den Ausschlag gibt, sagen die bisher erhaltenen Ergebnisse derartiger Untersuchungen insofern nichts aus, als beide Faktoren stets in bestimmter Weise verknüpft erschienen.

(Zu Sickel) Die erwähnten Formänderungen des ERG bestehen in einem Überwiegen der negativen Komponenten und konnten in Ischämieversuchen beim Menschen in einem Stadium bereits eingetretener Amaurose beobachtet werden. Das ebenfalls vorwiegend negative ERG bei bestimmten Hemeralopieformen ist durch einen selektiven Ausfall der skotopischen b-Welle charakterisiert, während die x-Welle ebenso erhalten ist wie das Tagessehvermögen. Soferne der Hemeralopie also eine Stoffwechselstörung zugrunde liegt, dürfte sie nur bestimmte retinale Prozesse skotopischer Natur betreffen.

Impulse Discharges from the Retinal Nerve and Optic Ganglion of the Squid[1,2]

By

E. F. MacNichol jr. and W. E. Love

With 4 Figures

The papers of Dr. Dodt and Dr. Bornschein amply demonstrate the value of the comparative approach to the study of retinal function. The availability of cone-type or rod-type retinas, which otherwise are essentially similar in their anatomical features, has permitted the differences in their responses to be attributed to differences in the receptors themselves. However, a direct study of receptor response would be more satisfactory if a suitable preparation could be found in which recordings could be made from single isolated receptor cells. Thus far no such vertebrate preparation has been found, and the search for an invertebrate preparation has been, till now, nearly as unsuccessful.

In those invertebrate species, such as the clam and earthworm, which have scattered single receptors, it is possible to locate the receptors easily only in fixed and stained material, so that it is difficult if not impossible to probe them with a

[1] From the Thomas C. Jenkins Laboratory of Biophysics, The Johns Hopkins University, Baltimore, Maryland, USA, and the Marine Biological Laboratory, Woods Hole, Massachusetts, USA.

[2] The research described in this paper was supported by National Science Foundation Grant No. G-7086 and by a grant (No. A 2528) from the National Institutes of Arthritic and Metabolic Diseases, U.S. Public Health Service.

microelectrode. In organisms such as insects, the receptors are so small and so closely packed that it is very difficult to record from single units.

For a time, it appeared that the horseshoe crab, Limulus, afforded a single receptor preparation. It is easy to record from the large nerve fibers coming from the ommatidia of the large coarsely faceted compound lateral eyes, and much work has been done with the preparation since HARTLINE's original experiments (1). Although it was at first thought that the fibers from which recordings were made were the axons of the receptor cells, it now appears that they are in fact axons of second order neurons. Furthermore mutual inhibitory interaction between ommatidia was demonstrated to occur (2). Thus the Limulus preparation is far from a simple one.

The molluscs offer some interesting possibilities. HARTLINE (3) has succeeded in recording from the optic nerve of the scallop, Pecten, which appears histologically to be composed of the axons of primary sense cells. He recorded an "on" discharge from the fibers coming from the proximal retinal layer and an "off" discharge from the axons of the cells of the distal retinal layer. However, the whole structure is small and the fibers are very short so that this eye does not appear to be suitable for extensive studies.

In the cephalopod molluscs such as Nautilus, Octopus and the squid the eyes are large, and some retinal nerve fibers are nearly a centimeter in length. Although some anatomical studies (4) have indicated that there are synapses between the sense cells and other cells which in turn give rise to the retinal nerve fibers, recent work with the light microscope (5) and especially with the electron microscope (6) indicates that the fibers of the retinal nerve are in fact the axons of the receptor cells.

Electroretinograms of the cephalopod molluscs have been studied for over 50 years, starting with the work of PIPER (7) and FRÖHLICH (8). Recently WAGNER and HAGINS (9) have demonstrated clearly that a large amplification of electric current takes place in these retinas. However no one has reported any impulse activity in the optic nerve although serious attempts have been made to determine whether or not it exists (10).

This leads to the interesting and attractive possibility that a large potential change, of which the E.R.G. is a sign, is generated in the receptor cells and conducted electrotonically by their axons in the retinal nerve. The currents flowing from the synaptic terminals of these axons would then excite the second order neurons in the optic ganglion either directly or by causing the release of a transmitter substance. Since the space constant in those invertebrate nerves that have been measured is in the range of 5 to 6 mm (11) and since approximately one tenth of the initial generator potential would appear at a distance of two space constants and one twentieth at a distance of three space constants there should be sufficient potential at the end of a short nerve fiber to fire the second order neuron. Thus it may not be necessary for a short axon to produce a propagated spike discharge in order to exert its influence on a second neuron or effector organ. Although this mode of operation is plausible it apparently has been demonstrated in only one instance. WATANABE and BULLOCK (12) were able to influence the firing rate in the posterior cells of the cardiac ganglion of the lobster by changing the internal polarization of the anterior cells even when the applied current was below threshold for firing the axons of these cells. As far as we are aware the electrotonic mode of conduction has not been demonstrated to be effective in any sensory neuron, although at one time it appeared to be demonstrable in the ocellar nerve of some insects (*13*). However, further investigation proved that under more nearly normal conditions propagated impulses arose in the fibers of this nerve (*14*). Thus the demonstration that a non-propagated response, rather than an all or northing spike, in the retinal nerve fibers of cephalopods causes a discharge in the neurons of the optic ganglion would be of great theoretical significance, not only in the physiology of vision, but also in that of the whole nervous system.

The negative results of experiments which sought to demonstrate an impulse discharge in the retinal nerve could indicate one of two possibilities: Either impulse conduction does not take place, or the experimental procedure destroyed normal function. (The animals were decapitated and the heads opened to expose the retinal nerve; or the eye was completely excised together with the retinal nerve and optic ganglion.) The experiments to be described were planned to distinguish between these two alternatives.

Experimental Design. It is well known that sharp, well insulated metal microelectrodes will record impulses both from nerve fibers and neuron somata. If a squid can be kept alive and in good condition although restrained it should be possible to insert microelectrodes into the optic ganglion and pick up from the ganglion cells discharges which are modified by stimulating the retina with light. Response of the ganglion cells to retinal illumination would indicate that the animal is in fact in sufficiently good condition for the visual system to be functional as far as the optic ganglion. Insertion of the microelectrode into the retinal nerve would then indicate the presence or absence of a spike discharge in the individual fibers.

Methods. The preparation was made as described in a preliminary report (*15*). Briefly: the animals were placed on their backs and their mantles wrapped in a sheet lead jacket. Two plastic tubes were inserted into the mantle on either side through the valve just behind the head. Seawater at about 17° C flowed through these tubes into the mantle and out through the syphon. Somewhat similar techniques have been used by other investigators to study the properties of the giant axon in vivo (*16*).

A squid in good condition would make normal breathing movements and eject water, and sometimes ink violently through the syphon when any part of the integument was stimulated sufficiently. Rapid synchronous changes in the melanophores over the whole body and motion of the tentacles also ensued. A marked pupilary reflex in response to light was also present. In short, the squid gave every indication of being "conscious". It was possible to keep animals in this condition for several hours and return them to the aquarium in an essentially undamaged state. Only animals in good condition would give the electrical responses to be described. Under suitable illumination the retinal nerve and optic ganglion could be seen through the transparent cartilaginous "skull" through which a strong, steeply tapered microelectrode could be inserted manually with negligible damage to the animal.

It was also possible to dissect away a portion of the skull, the muscle and other tissue overlying the back of the eye, retinal nerve, and ganglion to permit placing the electrode in the nerve, or ganglion under visual control. The records of Fig. 1 were taken under these latter conditions. When the top record was made the electrode was in contact with a bundle of fibers near their point of emergence from the back of the eyeball. At the start of the record there is a latent period of about 0.05 sec. after which there is a train of large amplitude oscillations (Fröhlich waves) which die out rapidly. The slow components of the electroretinogram are not recorded because a short time constant (0.001 sec.) was used in the amplifier circuit. Spike discharges of various amplitudes can easily be seen in the record. They presumably represent the non-synchronous discharges of a number of nerve fibers. Thus it appears that the retinal nerve fibers conduct impulses in a quite normal fashion. It is unlikely that the impulses originate elsewhere than in the retinal nerve since the overlying muscle was removed in this experiment; and slight motion of the electrode tip made a large difference in the amplitude of the spikes.

The second record was taken when the tip of the microelectrode was placed on the surface of the optic ganglion in a region where the nerve fibers entered it. As can be readily seen, both the Fröhlich waves and spike discharges were obtained.

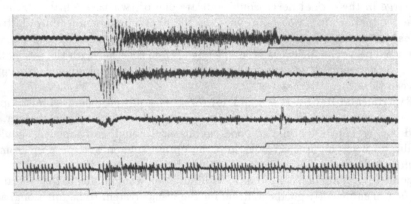

Fig. 1. Electrical activity of the retinal nerve and optic ganglion of the squid. A glass coated, platinized, platinum 30 percent iridium microelectrode was applied directly to the surgically exposed nerve and ganglion. (Top Trace) Electrode on nerve at point of emergence from retina; (2nd Trace) electrode on surface of ganglion; (3rd Trace) electrode penetrating ganglion; (Bottom Trace) electrode deep in ganglion. The bottom line in each trace shows the signal from a photoelectric cell used to monitor the stimulus; downward deflection indicates light on. Duration of stimulus 0.51 second; amplifier coupling time-constant, 0.001 second; amplitude of spikes in top record, approximatelly 500 μv

The third trace was taken with the electrode thrust part way into the ganglion. Here an "off" burst was found upon cessation of illumination. This was presumably due to some second or higher order neurons.

The bottom record was taken with the electrode thrust deeply into the ganglion. Here spontaneous activity was present although the response frequency was also affected by illumination. The spikes were of large amplitude, slow, and of opposite polarity to the nerve fiber discharges. They were presumably recorded from near the cell bodies of some higher order neurons. At this level tactile responses were also present and the activity was greatly increased when the animal struggled. It appears that much more than purely visual activity is present in the two optic ganglia, which form by far the largest part of the central nervous system of this animal.

It might be argued that the spikes recorded from the optic nerve fibers do not originate in them but are conducted electrotonically from the second order cells with which they synapse. Although no direct experiments were done to test this hypothesis there is some indirect evidence against it. In the first place the amplitude of the spikes that could be recorded from the optic nerve with a given electrode was independent of whether the electrode was at the eye end or the ganglion end of the nerve. In the second place the latency of the impulses was fairly short and nearly independent of intensity. Fig. 2 shows a series of records taken in order of decreasing intensity. Each lower record was taken at an intensity approximately a factor of 4 less than the one above it; the relative intensities between the first

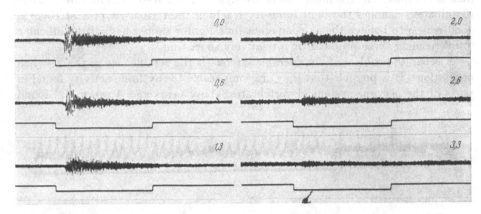

Fig. 2. Electrical response of the retinal nerve of the squid to flashes of variable intensity. Numbers indicate negative logarithm of light intensity; microelectrode inserted through skull. Other experimental conditions the same as for Fig. 1

and last record being about 2000 to 1. Yet impulses were produced even at the weakest intensity and the latency was little affected. The Fröhlich waves disappeared completely when the intensity of the stimulus was $1/_{16}$th of the maximum available and yet there was still a vigorous discharge of impulses. Apparently these waves are not necessary for the initiation of impulses, which are elicitable over a very wide range of stimulus intensities as in other eyes.

The discharge of impulses also shows considerable adaptation to light (which would be expected from work on other eyes), as is shown in Fig. 3. The preparation was dark adapted after which 0.55 sec. flashes were presented at 1.76 sec. intervals. The records show the responses to the first and to every 6th stimulus thereafter. As can readily be seen both the Fröhlich waves and the spike frequency adapt to light.

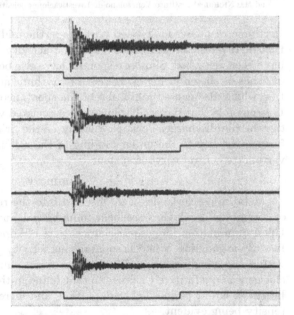

Fig. 3. Effect of light adaptation on the responses of the retinal nerve. Eye dark adapted before upper record was taken. Flashes 0.55 sec. in duration were repeated at 1.76 sec. intervals. Records show response to first and every succeeding 6th flash

Because of technical limitations, no quantitative experiments with the discharges from single units were attempted. Before this can be done it will be

necessary to immobilize the head of the animal sufficiently well to permit micro-
manipulation of the electrode to obtain and keep large discharges from an individual nerve fiber. The iris must also be paralyzed or removed since its closure upon
illumination changes the light intensity reaching the retina. At present there is
good reason to believe that a competent investigator should have little difficulty
in overcoming these problems in a relatively short time.

A separate problem of considerable interest is the significance of the Fröhlich
oscillations. It is possible that they are comparable to rhythmic activity found in
parts of the nervous system of vertebrates. Many years ago ADRIAN (17) found

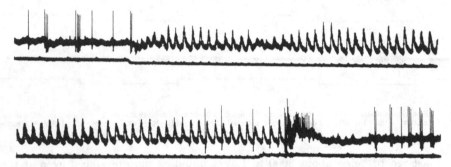

Fig. 4. Oscillatory potentials and impulse discharges recorded from a microelectrode inserted into the ganglion cell
layer of the isolated retina of a fish (Centropomis). Impulses from unit discharging spontaneously in dark and inhibited by illumination of retina; slow waves of undetermined origin present only during illumination. Downward
deflection of lower trace indicates illumination; time marks 0.1 sec. From unpublished experiments of SVAETICHIN
and MacNichol at Instituto Venezolano de Investigaciones Scientificas, Caracas, Venezuela, March 1959

rhythmic responses in isolated portions of the mid brain of the goldfish and since
then many other examples of rhythmic activity in the central nervous system
have been described. Similar responses have also been found in the isolated retinas
of fishes as shown in Fig. 4. Here slow rhythmic activity was caused by illumination which also caused inhibition of the spontaneous discharge of a ganglion cell.
It is possible that the oscillations were associated with the process causing inhibition of the discharge. Perhaps a study of the origin of the Fröhlich waves will
furnish the key to the understanding of the role played by slow rhythms in the
vertebrate central nervous system.

Summary

Metal microelectrodes were inserted into the retinal nerves and optic ganglia
of living squid which were held immobilized but otherwise in good condition.
Upon illumination impulse discharges were obtained from the nerve and the surface of the ganglion. Whereas spontaneous activity and "off" discharges were found
within the ganglion, no "off" responses were found in the nerve. The nerve discharge was qualitatively similar to that found in the optic nerves of other inverte-
brates; a latent period, light adaptation, and increase in frequency with light intensity being evident.

References

1. HARTLINE, H. K., H. G. WAGNER and E. F. MacNichol jr.: The peripheral origin of nervous activity in the visual system. Cold Spr. Harb. Symp. quant. Biol. 17, 125—141 (1952).
2. — — and F. RATLIFF: Inhibition in the eye of Limulus. J. gen. Physiol. 39, 651—673
(1956).

3. — The discharge of impulses in the optic nerve of Pecten in response to illumination of the eye. J. cell. comp. Physiol. 11, 465—478 (1938).

4. CHALAZONITIS, N., and A. ARVANATAKI: Réparation de quelques catalyzeurs respiratoires dans la retine de Sepia. Arch. Sci. physiol. 6, 163—191 (1952).

5. SNODGRASS, A.: Personal communication.

6. PALAY, S.: Personal communication.

7. PIPER, H.: Das elektromotorische Verhalten der Retina bei Eledone moschata. Arch. Anat. Physiol. (Leipzig) 453—474 (1904).

8. FRÖHLICH, F. W.: Beiträge zur allgemeinen Physiologie der Sinnesorgane. Z. Sinnesphysiol. 48, 28—165 (1913).

9. WAGNER, H. G., and W. A. HAGINS: The absolute magnitude of the membrane current in photoreceptors of the squid. Paper 02, Annual meeting of the Biophysical Society, Pittsburg, 1959.

10. HARTLINE, H. K., H. G. WAGNER and M. L. WOLBARSHT: Personal communications. Also experiments by one of us (E. F. M., jr., unpublished, 1949).

11. HODGKIN, A., and W. A. H. RUSHTON: The electrical constants of a crustacean nerve fibre. Proc. roy. Soc. 133 B, 445—479 (1946).

11a. — J. Physiol. (Lond.) 106, 305—318 (1947).

12. BULLOCK, T. H.: Neuron doctrine and electrophysiology. Science 129, 997—1002 (1959).

13. PARRY, D. A.: The function of the insect ocellus. J. exp. Biol. 24, 211—219 (1947).

14. HOYLE, G.: Functioning of the insect ocellar nerve. J. exp. Biol. 32, 397—407 (1955).

15. MacNICHOL, E. F., jr., and W. E. LOVE: Electrical responses of the retinal nerve and optic ganglion of the squid. Science 132, 737—738 (1960).

16a. LAPIQUE, L., et M. LAPIQUE: Chronaxie de l'innervation motrice du manteau chez le calmar. C. R. Soc. Biol. 102, 626—629 (1929).

16b. THIES, R. E.: Electrical recording in the living squid. Biol. Bull. 113, 333—334 (1957).

16c. HODGKIN, A.: Proc. roy. Soc. 148 B, 1 (1958).

16d. MOORE, J. W., and K. S. COLE: J. gen. Physiol. 43, 961 (1950).

17. ADRIAN, E. D.: The mechanism of nervous action. Chap. 5, pp. 78—94. Philadelphia: University of Pennsylvania Press 1932.

Discussion

H. BORNSCHEIN: Durch Lichtreize ausgelöste oscillatorische Potentiale können auch beim *Wirbeltier-ERG* beobachtet werden. Im menschlichen ERG sind sie der a- und b-Welle überlagert und zeigen eine Frequenz von etwa 120—140/sec.

R. JUNG: Da wir die Sehvorgänge bei niederen Tierformen in unserem Symposion nicht behandeln, bleibt MACNICHOLs Studie beim Squid, der durch seine Riesenfasern großes Ansehen in der allgemeinen Neurophysiologie hat, der einzige Beitrag von Nichtvertebraten. Obwohl die Frage der rhythmischen Potentiale von allgemeinem Interesse ist, müssen wir auf eine ausführliche Diskussion verzichten.

Wie Sie wissen, hat FRÖHLICH seinen Studien über Empfindungszeit und Nachbilder elektrophysiologische Ergebnisse am Cephalopodenauge zu Grunde gelegt und darauf eine Oscillationstheorie aufgebaut, mit der er seine Deutung von Erregungs- und Hemmungsvorgängen im visuellen System begründet. Da wir heute die Neuronentladungen im Auge und Hirn der Vertebraten besser kennen, wollen wir auch die subjektive Sinnesphysiologie FRÖHLICHs erst mit diesen Neuronenvorgängen diskutieren.

B. Geniculatum Laterale

Terminal Degeneration and Trans-Synaptic Atrophy in the Lateral Geniculate Body of the Monkey*

By

Paul Glees

With 6 Figures

The aim of this study was the re-investigation of the termination of optic fibres in the monkey (*10*), and our attention was directed more especially to the examination of three points. First, the possible somatotopic difference in the termination of crossed and uncrossed optic fibres, both in the laminated central portion of the lateral geniculate body, and in the coalescent peripheral portions; second, whether there is a difference in the synapses of optic fibres which end on large geniculate cells and those which end on small cells; and thirdly, what degree of trans-synaptic cell atrophy could be established when the optic nerve is cut.

Material. The material used for this investigation consisted of 18 macaque monkeys (11 Macaca mulatta and 7 Macaca nemestrina) and 5 baboons (Papio papio), but in the following account of the histological examination the species will not be specified, since there was no difference in the results.

For the purposes of our investigation the left eye was removed and the animals were killed between two and ninety-six days afterwards. They were then immediately perfused with formol-saline or formol-saline-acetic acid (*3, 4, 5*). This method is preferable to fixation by immersion for any material in which measurements are to be made, since it avoids the inevitable artificial variability in the size of cells for which immersion is responsible.

The material was then stained with the Marchi method or with the Glees or Nauta silver methods (*1*); we also used gallocyanine (*6*) to stain cells, and the Klüver method (*12*) to stain both cells and fibres.

Histology. Marchi sections cut in the plane of the optic tract show that the optic fibres enter the lateral geniculate body from the convexity of the layers, and that the fibres penetrate the more rostral layers to terminate in the caudal layers. This means that the interlaminar layers cannot be formed exclusively by optic fibres but must be mainly composed of the post-synaptic axones of geniculate neurones. Marchi sections also show that the large calibre fibres, whether crossed or uncrossed, can be traced to the layers containing large cells (layers 1 and 2). The Marchi degeneration which fills the layer affected by severance of the optic tract indicates that the optic fibres are myelinated right up to their terminal arborisation.

* From the University Laboratory of Physiology, Oxford, Great Britain. Present address: Institut für Histologie und experimentelle Neuroanatomie der Universität Göttingen, Germany.

Sections stained with the Nissl method show a distinct trans-synaptic atrophy after as little as four days (*10*, *13*). These changes are often called degenerative, but they are not due to any direct interference with the cell itself and are much more in the nature of functional atrophy; the cells are not fundamentally different from normal cells except that they are shrunken. The time course of this shrinkage has been investigated by MATTHEWS, COWAN and POWELL (*13*), who found that in the

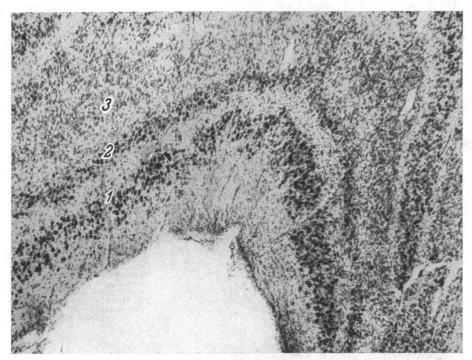

Fig. 1. Transverse section through the left lateral geniculate body of a Macaca nemestrina monkey 20 days after the left optic nerve had been cut. Ipsilateral layers 2 and 3 show distinct signs of transneuronal atrophy

first few months the cytoplasm shrinks proportionately more than the nucleus and nucleolus. They also observed that the atrophy appeared to begin earlier in those layers which receive crossed optic fibres: in these layers it could be seen at four days, whereas cells in the layers which receive uncrossed fibres did not reach this stage until the eighth day. There are several possible explanations of this — a) the difference in length and diameter between crossed and uncrossed fibres could determine the time course of the degeneration; b) the terminals of crossed and un-crossed fibres may be morphologically or chemically different; c) fibres from sources other than the retina may terminate in the uncrossed layers and therefore keep those geniculate cells activated to some extent and delay the atrophy. However, this difference in the time course of the atrophy cannot be regarded as fully estab-lished for unfortunately only two animals were used in this investigation, and there is also little doubt that many of the shrunken cells which appear in the pictures accompanying the report are the result of fixing the material by immersion and not necessarily solely a consequence of trans-neuronal atrophy (Fig. 1).

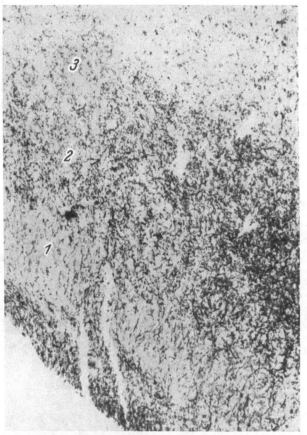

Fig. 2. Nauta section of right lateral geniculate body 20 days after cutting the left optic nerve. Heavy preterminal degeneration in layers 2 and 3. Compare with Fig. 3

Fig. 2

Fig. 3. Transverse section through lateral geniculate body. Marchi stain. Marchi degeneration is present over the whole of the lateral geniculate body after the contralateral optic nerve is cut but fine degeneration is more pronounced in layers 4 and 6. Note that degenerated optic nerve fibres penetrate all layers

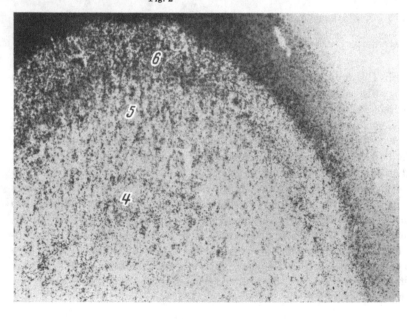

Fig. 3

Silver preparations. The two silver methods used stain different portions of a disintegrating nerve fibre, the Nauta method primarily the stem fibre and pre-terminals, the Glees method the preterminal and terminal fibres (2). They also show the degeneration at different periods of survival; EVANS and HAMLYN (7) found that the ter-minals of degenerated optic fibres in the tec-tum opticum of the chicken could be stained with the Glees technique at the seventh day, whereas the Nauta degeneration picture be-came fully established only after twenty-eight days, when the Glees degeneration products had practically disappeared (Fig. 2).

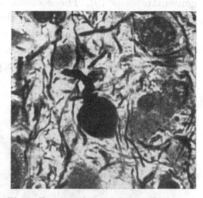

Fig. 4. Terminal degeneration in the lateral geniculate body 12 days after severance of the optic nerve. Note the large terminal swelling attached to a preterminal fibre

The material stained with the Nauta method had a survival time of either 7 days or 20 days, and the histological picture agrees with the remarks of EVANS and HAMLYN, for at 7 days only degeneration of the stem fibres can be seen, a picture similar to a Marchi stain at 12 days (Fig. 3). At 20 days the affected layers were filled with the debris of preterminal fibres, at which time no degenerated terminals could still be seen in a Glees preparation.

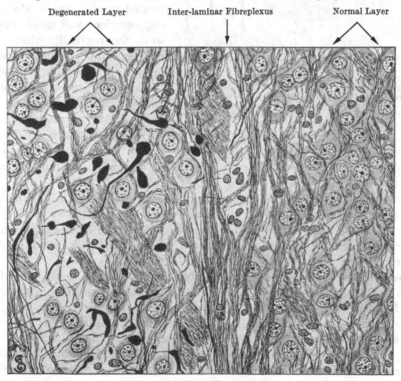

Degenerated Layer   Inter-laminar Fibreplexus   Normal Layer

Fig. 5. Terminal degeneration is sharply limited to layer 6 when the contralateral nerve is cut. The degenerating terminals in the left field are indicated by arrows. The normal layer 5 is to the right half of the figure, separated by an interlaminar plexus

The first sign of terminal changes can be seen in Glees sections after two or three days, when very small discs (0.5 μ in diameter) appear in contact with the geniculate cells (9). These continue to enlarge until on the 12th day they are 10—12 μ in diameter (Fig. 4, 5); they are then bulb-like structures, usually with a little tail attached to them which makes them resemble tadpoles, and it is reasonable to assume that they are degenerating synaptic rings. (2). The greatest amount of swelling however occurs at the point where the stem fibre branches off into a number of terminals, and in the later stages of degeneration there appears an oblong bulge at this point.

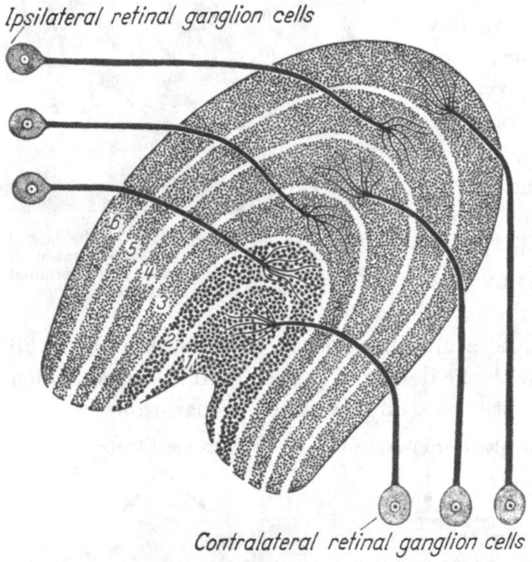

Fig. 6. Diagram of a transverse section through the right lateral geniculate body. The layers are numbered from ventral to dorsal. 1 and 2 are the large layers, 3, 4, 5, and 6 the small layers. Contralateral fibres project onto layers 1, 4, and 6 and ipsilateral fibres onto layers 2, 3, and 5 (based on experiments on terminal degeneration)

Comments

This investigation has again produced evidence that the contralateral and ipsilateral optic fibres terminate in different layers of the lateral geniculate body, for the degeneration when one optic nerve is cut is always confined to three of the six layers. Our previous work on this matter was limited to the earliest stages of degeneration, and there was always the possibility that overlapping fibres might degenerate more slowly, but at 14 days — the longest survival time for the Glees stained material in the present study — there was still no sign of any overlap of crossed and uncrossed fibre terminations, and it may be said with certainty that contralateral fibres end in layers 1, 4, and 6, and ipsilateral fibres in layers 2, 3, and 5 (see Fig. 6).

How far the lamination of the lateral geniculate body is vital to its functional organisation is however uncertain, for the study of degeneration has shown that the terminations of ipsilateral and contralateral fibres are also separate in the coalescent peripheral portions of the lateral geniculate body which are not laminated (14).

Nevertheless, there remains the question of the difference in the size of the cells in the several layers, layers 1 and 2 containing cells of considerably larger size than the other four layers. This argues some possible difference in function. It is likely that this difference lies in the projection of the cell rather than in the type of fibre which terminates on it. No evidence could be seen of any difference — in quality or quantity — of the synapses on large and on small cells. All terminals appeared to be in contact with the cell body and not with dendrites; this was the more obvious in the case of small cells whose dendrites are very short, but no synaptic degeneration could be seen on the much large dendrites of the cells in layers 1 and 2 either. Assuming that the conspicuous bulbous swellings are degenerative enlargements of synapses, it may be said that the number of terminals which synapse onto one cell is very small and possibly even only one terminal (Fig. 6).

Our examination of trans-synaptic cell atrophy was limited to a survival period of at most 96 days, at which time the atrophy was severe but there was no sign of an actual decrease in the number of cells. It would be interesting to establish at what stage and by what process a cell loss occurs: this is a question which awaits further investigation.

Acknowledgements

I would like to thank Miss F. Greene, Miss A. G. Smith and Mr. B. Sheppard for technical assistance. This investigation was supported in part by Grant No. 259 from the National Multiple Sclerosis Society.

Summary

1. Histological study of 23 monkeys following sectioning of one optic nerve with the silver methods of Glees and Nauta and maximal survival times for these methods show a distinctly separate termination of crossed and uncrossed fibres in the lateral geniculate body. This difference is not limited to the laminated portions of the lateral geniculate body but extends into the coalescent portions of this nucleus.

2. The mode of optic fibre termination is the same in large and small cell layers and there is no difference in crossed and uncrossed fibres.

3. The degree and time course of transneuronal atrophy can only be assessed accurately in perfused preparations.

4. All available evidence of terminal degeneration studies and transneuronal atrophy is against binocular fusion at the level of the geniculate body in the monkey.

References

1. Adey, W. R., A. F. Rudolph, I. F. Hine and N. J. Harritt: Glees staining of the monkey hypothalamus: a critical appraisal of normal and experimental material. J. Anat. (Lond.) 92, 219 (1958).
2. Bowsher, D., A. Brodal and F. Walberg: The relative values of the Marchi method and some silver impregnation techniques. Brain 83, 150 (1960).
3. Bywater, J. E. C., and P. Glees: The effect of the mode of fixation and the interval between death and fixation on monkeys' motoneurones. J. Physiol. (Lond.) 149, 3 P (1959).
4. — — Binuclear motoneurones in the monkey. Psychiatr. et Neurol. (Basel) 139, 285 (1960a).
5. — — Der Einfluß der Fixationsart und des Intervalles zwischen Tod und Fixation auf die Struktur der Motoneurone des Affen. Verh. Anat. Ges., Jena, 106/107, 194 (1960b).
6. Einarson L.: Notes on the morphology of the chromophil material of nerve cells and its relation to nuclear substances. Amer. J. Anat. 53, 141 (1933).
7. Evans D. H. L. and L. H. Hamlyn: A study of silver degeneration methods in the central nervous system. J. Anat. (Lond.) 90, 193 (1956).
8. Glees, P.: Die Endigungsweise der ipsilateralen und kontralateralen Sehfasern im Corpus geniculatum laterale des Affen. Verh. Anat. Ges., Jena, 55. Vers. p. 60 (1959).
9. — Analyse von Faktoren, welche die Darstellung der Terminaldegeneration beeinflussen, mit einem Hinweis auf die Pyramidenbahn. Verh. Anat. Ges., Jena, 56. Vers. 106/107, 187 (1960).
10. — and W. F. Le Gros Clark: The termination of optic fibres in the lateral geniculate body of the monkey. J. Anat. (Lond.) 75, 295 (1941).
11. — and W. J. H. Nauta: A critical review of studies on axonal and terminal degeneration. Mschr. Psychiat. Neurol. 129, 74 (1955).

12. Klüver, H., and E. Barrera: A method for the combined staining of cells and fibres in the nervous system. J. Neuropath. exp. Neurol. **12**, 400 (1953).
13. Matthews, M. R., W. M. Cowan and T. P. S. Powell: Transneuronal cell degeneration in the lateral geniculate nucleus of the Macaque monkey. J. Anat. (Lond.) **94**, 145 (1960).
14. Walls, G. L.: The lateral geniculate nucleus and visual histophysiology. Univ. Calif. Publ. Physiol. **9**, 1 (1953).

Discussion

R. L. de Valois: I would like to comment briefly on our physiological studies of the macaque lateral geniculate, the study of which was stimulated by conversations with Dr. Glees. With regard to the projection of the two eyes to the various LGN laminae, our physiological studies completely confirm that the contralateral projection is to the layers 1, 4, and 6, and the ipsilateral projection to layers 2, 3, and 5. Further we find no evidence for binocular interaction in the monkey lateral geniculate (although we do find it in the cat). Not only does every LGN cell fire only to one eye, but its response to this eye is also not modified by stimulation to the "wrong" eye. With regard to the question of interneurones in the monkey LGN we have on occasion recorded from two cells simultaneously which were mirror images in regard to their spectral response of each other. We have sometimes wondered if interneurones like Renshaw cells were involved here.

There has been a big problem on the optic tract lateral geniculate connections which has been made even worse by your recent experimental findings. That is the fact that you have optic tract fibres ending up on to 30 LGN cells and with each LGN cell receiving from only one fibre. This would imply that there must be 10—30 times as many LGN cells as optic nerve fibres. But many separate cell or fibre count studies have reported roughly the same number of optic nerve fibres or ganglion cells as LGN cells. Something is grossly wrong here.

P. Glees: I am glad to see that the histology of the monkey's geniculate is in agreement with the results of Dr. de Valois, namely that there is no binocular fusion. His paper raises the question of interneurones, although there is no direct evidence for such cells: All geniculate cells show rapid transneuronal atrophy and are in contract with degenerating optic boutons. I will, however, pay further attention to this problem. Concerning the number of geniculate cells in contract with one optic fibre I would like to refrain from any definite statement until I have collected more data. I am certain, however, that one optic fibre is in contact with more than one geniculate cell and probably more than 5 cells. The limited number of degenerating boutons suggests no overlap of neighbouring optic nerve fibres. I am as puzzled as Dr. de Valois about the numerical relationship and eventually I hope to have more definite information than I have at present.

Binocular Interaction in the Lateral Geniculate Body of the Cat*

By

Marianne Fillenz

With 4 Figures

The problem of the significance of the lateral geniculate body in the visual pathway has aroused considerable interest lately. From the evidence available so far it seems that this role is likely to be different in different animal species. In the cat there is evidence to suggest that the lateral geniculate body is an important integrative centre (*3, 4, 9, 14*).

I want to discuss only one of the transformations which occur in the lateral geniculate body of the cat: interaction of impulses coming from the two eyes.

* From the University Laboratory of Physiology, Oxford, Great Britain.

I shall first describe briefly the results of some electrophysiological experiments (carried out with Dr. ERULKAR and to be published in full elesewhere (9)) which initiated the neurohistological work to be described below.

Dr. ERULKAR and I recorded the activity of units in the lateral geniculate body. The cats were anaesthetised with Nembutal and dark adapted, the microelectrodes were metal filled glass pipettes with tip diameters between 2—10 μ and they were introduced under direct vision, since the overlying cortex had been removed by suction. The stimulus consisted of white flashes of light, delivered to the two eyes. We were careful to screen the two eyes from each other.

We isolated single units, most of which showed firing in darkness. We then stimulated each eye with light flashes. As the microelectrode passed down into the lateral geniculate body we found that the units were arranged in 3 zones, 2 zones containing units which responded to illumination of the contralateral eye, separated by a middle zone which responded to illumination of the ipsilateral eye. We isolated 66 units, each one of which we subjected to light stimulation of the two eyes. Only seven units could be activated from each eye separately: the rest responded only to either the ipsi- or the contralateral eye. In the seven units which responded to both eyes, the responses to the two eyes were different.

These seven units were such a small proportion of the total that it was difficult to see what their functional significance could be.

We then tried a different approach: after separate stimulation of the two eyes we tried various combinations of binocular stimulation. When we came to analyse the records we found that out of 19 units for which we went through this procedure, there were 13 units where illumination of only one eye produced a response but illumination of the other eye, even though by itself it produced no response, modified the response of the unit to illumination of the first eye. Figure 1 shows the responses of such a unit. Stimulation of the ipsilateral eye produced an "on" response, the latency of which is indicated by the solid black bars. The cross-hatched bars show the response latencies when the ipsilateral eye stimulation is closely followed by stimulation of the contralateral eye. In spite of the variation within each group there is no overlap between the groups. Figure 2 shows the responses of a unit which gave a series of brief bursts in response to contralateral eye stimulation. When a light was applied to the ipsilateral eye, all the bursts following this stimulus were delayed. This effect is the more marked the earlier the ipsilateral stimulus occurs.

Our findings fit in well with those of P. O. BISHOP and his co-workers using electrical stimulation of the optic nerves (3, 4). They also found that 10% of lateral geniculate neurones could be fired by separate stimulation of the two optic nerves, but that a much greater proportion are discharged by only one optic nerve, but are indirectly affected by stimulation of the other optic nerve.

The failure of GRÜSSER and SAUR (11) to find binocular interaction in the cat's lateral geniculate body may be due to the difference in their experimental conditions.

The anatomical evidence for binocular convergence at the level of the lateral geniculate body in the cat is still inconclusive. Earlier anatomical studies, using the Marchi stain for degenerating myelinated fibres (2) or a Nissl stain to show transneuronal degeneration (1, 7, 8, 15) described a trilaminar lateral geniculate body with complete segregation of fibres coming from the two eyes. These methods however cannot provide an answer to the problem of binocular overlap: the Marchi method does not stain the fine terminal ramifications, which are all unmyelinated, and in a nucleus where there is normally a wide range of cell size, transneuronal degeneration can only reveal gross overall changes.

In 1958 Hayhow (*12*) reinvestigated the problem of the distribution of optic nerve fibres in the cat's lateral geniculate body using the method of Nauta and Gygax which stains degenerating axons. His results indicated a much more complicated lamination in the cat's lateral geniculate body: besides the three classical layers A, A$_1$, and B, each receiving optic tract fibres from only one eye, he described two interlaminar layers, which in Nissl stained sections were found to contain large cells and which received the terminal ramifications of fibres coming from both eyes.

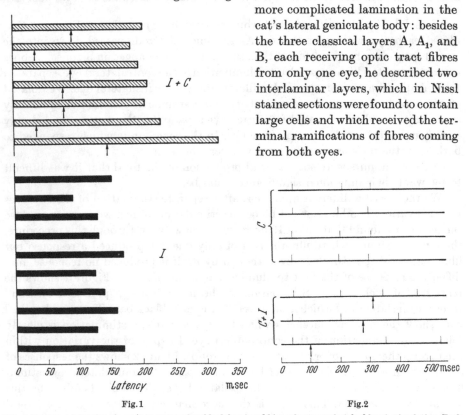

Fig.1   Fig.2

Fig. 1. Response latencies of a unit to monocular (black bars) and binocular (cross-hatched bars) stimulation. Each bar represents one response latency. *I* stimulation of ipsilateral eye alone. *I + C* ipsilateral eye stimulation followed by contralateral eye stimulation (at arrow)

Fig. 2. Multiple burst responses of a unit to monocular and binocular stimulation. Each vertical line represents one burst of impulses. *C* stimulation of contralateral eye alone. *C + I* stimulation of contralateral followed by ipsilateral eye stimulation (at arrow)

The disadvantage of the Nauta method is that it does not stain the fine preterminal fibres or the synaptic endfeet (*5*) and also that it selectively stains degenerating axons whose relation to normal structures can therefore not be seen on a single section. Hayhow (*13*) also used the Glees and Bielschowsky silver methods, but could get no clear cut results with them.

I have reinvestigated the problem of optic nerve fibre distribution in the lateral geniculate body using the Glees silver method on three types of animal: normal cats, cats surviving for 3—7 days after removal of one eye and cats surviving for 57—315 days after eye enucleation.

In a normal cat, stained with the Glees silver method, the lateral geniculate body in sagittal section shows three laminae, separated by two fibrous plexuses. Under the high power these two fibrous plexuses are seen to contain some large darkly staining cells and I shall refer to them as interlaminar A_1B and interlaminar A_1A layers. Under oil immersion, besides axons and fine preterminal fibres, numerous rings are seen in all layers (except layer B where they are very few in number) which are generally accepted as being synaptic endfeet (6).

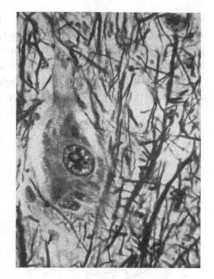

In cats surviving for 3—7 days after eye enucleation, the fibres and synaptic terminals of one optic nerve are seen in the process of degeneration (10). At 3 days degenerating synaptic terminals are very conspicuous. They are club shaped, black and have a stalk or tail (Fig. 3). Their distribution is much more easily visible in sagittal section, because in transverse sections of the lateral geniculate body many fibres are cut across. I shall therefore discuss only sagittal sections taken through the middle third of the lateral geniculate body, where the layers are most clearly visible. In such a sagittal section degenerated boutons are found in layers A and B on the contralateral side, layer A_1 on the ipsilateral side, and in interlaminar layers A_1B and A_1A on both the ipsi- and contralateral side. Occasional aberrant degenerated endings are sometimes seen in contralateral layers B and A_1 and ipsilateral layer A. The distribution of degenerated synaptic terminals is shown diagrammatically in Fig. 4.

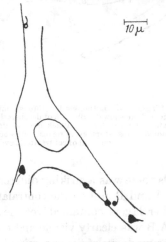

$10\,\mu$

This distribution is quite clear cut and visible under the high power without oil immersion, but only at 3 days. At 5 days most of the degenerated boutons have disappeared and it is the fibres now which are showing signs of degeneration (swelling curling). This appearance is not sufficiently striking and characteristic to enable one

Fig. 3. Large cell in interlaminar layer A_1A with a normal synaptic ring and a number of degenerating synaptic terminals. Two microphotographs at different focal depths. Glees silver impregnation at 3 days after contralateral eye enucleation

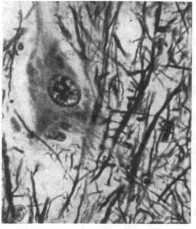

to map the distribution of degeneration. At 7 days the fibres are beginning to break up and there are numerous black bodies visible, but these again are of no use in mapping degeneration. This may account for Hayhow's results with the Glees silver stain, since most of his animals were killed between 5—7 days after eye enucleation.

The great advantage of the Glees silver method is that at 3 days the relation of the degenerating boutons to structures such as the A_1B and A_1A interlaminar layers can be clearly determined on a given slide. But unfortunately the problem of whether optic tract fibres from the two eyes converge on to the same lateral geniculate neurone can still not be answered: the presence of a degenerated bouton and a normal ring on the same cell is not at all uncommon (Fig. 3). But it is impossible to show that this normal ring belongs to an optic nerve fibre coming from the other eye.

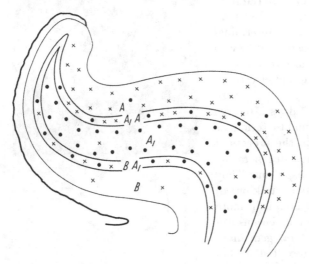

Fig. 4. Diagram of sagittal section through middle third of lateral geniculate body to show distribution of degenerating synaptic terminals 3 days after eye enucleation. Black dots = degenerating terminals after removal of ipsilateral eye. Crosses = degenerating terminals after removal of contralateral eye

In the animals surviving for 57—315 days after removal of one eye, one optic nerve and its terminations had completely degenerated and disappeared. In these animals there was a striking difference between the layers. On the ipsilateral side layers A and B and on the contralateral side layer A_1 were rich in fibres, whereas the other layers contained very few fine fibres. On both sides the interlaminar layer A_1B was clearly visible and contained a large number of fibres. It therefore must be made up of fibres coming from both eyes. With layer A_1A this was much more difficult to decide, since it is never so conspicuous (not even in a normal cat): it stood out fairly clearly on the ipsilateral side, i. e. when layer A was undegenerated; but it was difficult to see whether the fibre rich layer A_1 on the contralateral side did or did not include interlaminar layer A_1A. Evidence from other experiments indicates that layer A_1A also receives contributions from both optic nerves, but rather more from the contralateral than the ipsilateral optic nerve.

Examination under high power of the lateral geniculate bodies in cats surviving for long periods after eye enucleation revealed some interesting findings. The non-degenerated layers were rich in synaptic rings and the distribution and presence of rings sharply delimited the boundary between degenerated and undegenerated layers. A careful examination of the degenerated layers showed that these also contained synaptic rings, perfectly normal in appearance, but very much less numerous. They were however more numerous than the aberrant degenerating boutons found at 3 days after eye enucleation.

It seems likely, therefore, that these normal synaptic rings in degenerated layers belong to a fibre system other than the retino-geniculate system and the origin of these fibres is at present under investigation.

Finally, I would like to put forward the suggestion that the lateral geniculate body of the cat is one of the most complex: it is intermediate between the non-laminated lateral geniculate of animals such as the rabbit, rat and sheep which have lateral, non-overlapping visual fields, complete or almost complete decussation of the optic nerves and no binocular vision; and the laminated lateral geniculate of the monkeys, apes and man, who have frontal eye fields, almost complete overlap of visual fields and 50% decussation in the optic chiasma. These animals, judging from their synaptic organisation, have little or no interaction occurring at the geniculate level and the binocular fusion is taking place at the cortical level.

The cat, with 60% decussation in its optic chiasma, shows the beginnings of binocular interaction, some or all of which, together with other integrative mechanisms, is however still taking place at the geniculate level.

Summary

The use of the Glees silver method in both normal cats and in cats surviving for varying periods after eye enucleation, has shown the existence in sagittal section of two interlaminar layers, called respectively A_1B and A_1A, in addition to the classical layers A, A_1 and B. These interlaminar layers consist of a fibre plexus containing optic tract fibres derived from both eyes. In cats where the fibres from one eye are in the process of degeneration, the presence of degenerating synaptic terminals in both interlaminar layers of both sides, demonstrates that these interlaminar layers with their large cells, contain synaptic terminations from both eyes. The presence of degenerating and normal synaptic terminals on these large cells of the interlaminar layers is suggestive but insufficient evidence for binocular convergence on to a given neurone. Such convergence, however, is implied by the electrophysiological findings.

Acknowledgements

I wish to thank Dr. P. GLEES for making available the operated animals and Miss LINDA BEELEY for assistance with some of the histological work.

References

1. BARRIS, R. W.: Disposition of fibers of retinal origin in the lateral geniculate body. Course and termination of fibers of the optic system in the brain of the cat. Arch. Ophthal. (N. Y.) 14, 61—70 (1935).
2. — W. R. INGRAM and S. W. RANSON: Optic connections of the diencephalon and midbrain of the cat. J. comp. Neurol. 62, 117—153 (1935).
3. BISHOP, P. O.: Discussion in Mechanisms of Colour Discrimination. Ed. Y. Galifret. Oxford: Pergamon Press 1960.
4. — W. BURKE and R. DAVIS: Activation of single lateral geniculate cells by stimulation of either optic nerve. Science 130, 506—507 (1959).
5. BOWSHER, D., A. BRODAL and F. WALBERG: The relative values of the Marchi method and some silver impregnation techniques. Brain 83, 150—169 (1960).
6. BOYCOTT, B. B., E. G. GRAY and R. W. GUILLERY: A theory to account for the absence of boutons in silver preparations of the cerebral cortex, based on a study of axon terminals by light and electron microscopy. J. Physiol. (Lond.) 152, 3 P (1960).

7. Cohn, R.: Laminar electrical responses in lateral geniculate body of cat. J. Neurophysiol. 19, 317—324 (1956).
8. Cook, W. H., J. H. Walker and M. L. Barr: A cytological study of transneuronal atrophy in the cat and rabbit. J. comp. Neurol. 94, 267—292 (1951).
9. Erulkar, S. D., and Marianne Fillenz: Single-unit activity in the lateral geniculate body of the cat. J. Physiol. (Lond.) 154, 206—218 (1960).
10. Glees, P.: The termination of optic fibres in the lateral geniculate body of the cat. J. Anat. (Lond.) 75, 434—440 (1941).
11. Grüsser, O.-J., and G. Saur: Monoculare und binoculare Lichtreizung einzelner Neurone im Geniculatum laterale der Katze. Pflügers Arch. ges. Physiol. 271, 595—612 (1960).
12. Hayhow, W. R.: The cytoarchitecture of the lateral geniculate body in the cat in relation to the distribution of crossed and uncrossed optic fibres. J. comp. Neurol. 110, 1—63 (1958).
13. — Experimental degeneration of optic axons in the lateral geniculate body of the cat. Acta anat. 37, 281—298 (1959).
14. Hubel, D. H.: Single unit activity in lateral geniculate body and optic tract of unrestrained cats. J. Physiol. (Lond.) 150, 91—104 (1960).
15. Minkowski, M.: Über den Verlauf, die Endigung und die zentrale Repräsentation von gekreuzten und ungekreuzten Sehnervenfasern bei einigen Säugetieren und beim Menschen. Schweiz. Arch. Neurol. Psychiat. 6, 201—252 (1920).

Discussion

O.-J. Grüsser: Gemeinsam mit Saur[1] wurden 87 Neurone im Geniculatum laterale der Katze registriert und auf ihre Reaktion auf ipsi- und kontralaterale Lichtreize untersucht. Eine Selektion postsynaptischer Neuronentladungen wurden vorgenommen. Als Kriterium einer postsynaptischen Entladung wurde das Bestehen von zwei Komponenten des extracellulären positiven Potentials angesehen ($\alpha\beta$-spike). Durch hochfrequente elektrische Opticusreize läßt sich die α-Komponente von der β-Komponente trennen, da ihr kritisches Reizintervall kleiner ist[2].

Die Versuchsbedingungen für die binokularen Lichtreizversuche waren: Encephale-isolé-Präparation, Helladaptation, diffuse Ganzfeldbelichtungen, „weißes Licht" (0,01—650 Lux), Mikroelektroden unter 1 μ. Sämtliche Neurone reagierten nur *entweder* auf die Belichtung des ipsilateralen (31) *oder* des kontralateralen (53) Auges. 3 Neurone reagierten nicht. Bei synchroner binokularer Belichtung mit gleichen oder verschiedenen Beleuchtungsstärken zeigten nur 8 Neurone eine statistisch signifikante Verminderung der Entladungsfrequenz im Vergleich zur Belichtung des monokular aktivierenden Auges. Bei allen anderen Neuronen ergab sich keine Differenz im Vergleich zur monokularen Belichtung. Die kritische Flimmerfusionsfrequenz war ebenfalls nur monokular determiniert. Die Differenz zu den Resultaten von Frau Dr. Fillenz ist möglicherweise durch die verschiedenartigen Versuchsbedingungen erklärbar. Ihre größeren Mikroelektroden begünstigten vielleicht eine Selektion der relativ großen Nervenzellen zwischen den Hauptzellschichten des Geniculatums. Diese Zellen koordinieren möglicherweise binokulare Erregungen schon im Geniculatum laterale.

D. Hurvich-Jameson: In looking for binocular interactions, I wonder if Dr. Fillenz has tried adding a stimulus of lower intensity to the other eye to see if the first monocular response might show a greater reduction. In humans, stimulation of one or both eyes produce little, if any, difference in the brightness response when the two eyes are stimulated equally in the binocular situation. However, if one eye is stimulated with a relatively intense light and then a less intense stimulus is added in the other eye, we get the well-known Fechner Paradox: the binocular impression is of distinctly lower brightness than that of the first eye alone. Perhaps the use of different intensities in the two eyes of the cat might also give rise to more obvious evidence of binocular interaction than does the use of equal intensities in the two eyes.

---

[1] Grüsser, O.-J., u. G. Saur: Monoculare und binoculare Lichtreizung einzelner Neurone im Geniculatum laterale der Katze. Pflügers Arch. ges. Physiol. 271, 595—612 (1960).

[2] Grüsser-Cornehls, U., u. O.-J. Grüsser: Mikroelektrodenuntersuchungen am Geniculatum laterale der Katze: Nervenzell- und Axonentladungen nach elektrischer Opticusreizung. Pflügers Arch. ges. Physiol. 271, 50—63 (1960).

A. Arduini: It is proposed that the binocular interaction on the geniculate be tested with steady light on one eye and flash on the other.

L. M. Hurvich: Dr. Fillenz believes that the cat may represent a step on the way to binocular vision of the more advanced type possessed by primates and that binocular vision may occur at the lateral geniculate level in the cat. I am puzzled about an interaction which increases the contralateral latency. What functional significance do you think this has for the cat's vision ?

M. Fillenz: I agree with the possible reasons given by Dr. Grüsser for the difference in our results.

To Dr. and Mrs. Hurvich I would like to reply that the electrophysiological experiments on binocular interaction were limited by the visual stimulators at our disposal. All these experiments show is that there is a mechanism available for binocular interaction in the cat's lateral geniculate body. With diffuse illumination of the two eyes, the two stimuli being of equal and fairly high intensity, the interaction seemed to be mainly of an inhibitory kind; other stimulus situations may give very different types of interaction.

Influence of Visual Deafferentation and of Continuous Retinal Illumination on the Excitability of Geniculate Neurons[1,2]

By

A. Arduini

With 5 Figures

The experiments reported in this article have been performed in collaboration with Dr. Hirao[3] from 1957 to 1959 and with Dr. Goldstein[4] during the academic year 1959—1960. All these investigations were concerned with the striking changes in the excitability of the lateral geniculate body brought about by two seemingly opposite causes, retinal inactivation and continuous retinal illumination. The earlier results have already been published in Archives italiennes de Biologie (1, 2, 3) while the results obtained with Dr. Goldstein are still awaiting publication.

Our research was started following an observation made while investigating the effects of visual deafferentation (1) on the spontaneous EEG activity. It turned out that ischemic retinal inactivation had striking effects on the EEG even when it was performed during dark adaptation. The absence of sensory stimulation can neither be considered as a state of visual deafferentation nor as a state of quiescence of the retina, and actually it is well known (see 2) that a strong tonic activity is going on in the dark adapted retina (the "dark discharge"). Hence, it

[1] From the Istituto di Fisiologia della Università di Pisa, Italia.

[2] The researches reported in this article have been sponsored jointly by the Office of Scientific Research of the Air Research and Development Command, United States Air Force, through its European Office, under Contract No. AF 61(052)-107 and by the Rockefeller Foundation.

[3] Rockefeller Fellow. Department of Physiology, University of Gunma Medical School (Japan).

[4] Science Faculty Fellow of the National Science Foundation (U.S.A.) on leave of absence from the Electrical Engineering Department, Massachusetts Institute of Technology, Cambridge (Mass.).

was concluded that the abolition of the dark discharge was likely to be responsible for the EEG observations made by Claes in 1939 (7) and for our own findings.

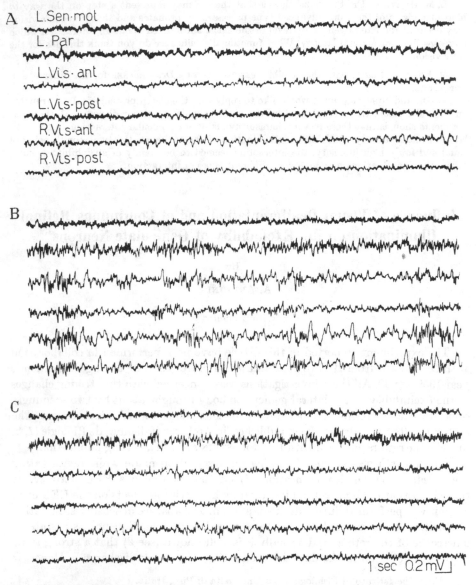

Fig. 1. Effects of visual deafferentation on the EEG of different cortical areas. Acute midpontine pretrigeminal cat. Cortical bipolar recording on ink-writing Electroencephalograph. A control record showing generalized activated patterns. B after 2 minutes of bilateral retinal anoxia (intraocular pressure 150 mm of Hg): trains of spindles are present in all leads, with the exception of those from the sensory-motor area. C immediately after the end of an ocular ischemia lasting 4 minutes. The sleep patterns have disappeared almost completely

The next problem was to investigate the central effect of the retinal dark discharge and, possibly, to understand its functional significance.

It will not be dealt in extent here with the consequences of interrupting the tonic flow of retinal impulses. The retinal ischemia which is known to abolish the impulse traffic in the optic nerve (5) is followed, in a few minutes, by EEG patterns of sleep (1) (Fig. 1).

That the sudden abolition of the tonic retinal outflow is followed by generalized EEG synchronization is not surprising, particularly in the pretrigeminal cat in which only the olfactory and the visual inputs are available. Much more surprising

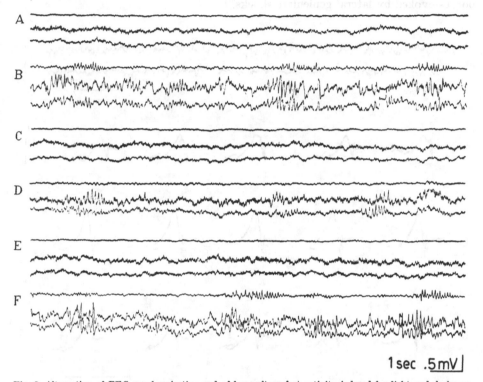

1 sec .5mV

Fig. 2. Alternation of EEG synchronization and of low voltage fast activity induced by light and darkness. C.R.O. recordings. A in darkness. B after 2 minutes of illumination with light at 90° angle. C after 5 minutes of darkness. D after 1 minute of illumination with light at 90° angle. E after 6 minutes of darkness. F after 2 minutes in light at 90° angle. In the order: L. frontal, L. visual, R. visual areas

is however that similar effects can be obtained during continuous retinal illumination (3) (Fig. 2).

The point we wish to stress is that both procedures, the subtraction of retinal activity as well as the continuous photic stimulation give rise to EEG patterns of sleep while, paradoxically, low voltage fast activity is present in the same animal during dark adaptation.

The striking similarity of the effects brought about by sustained light and by deafferentation was the base for the working hypothesis that continuous illumination of the retina might start a process leading to the suppression of the dark discharge, thus eliminating a major factor in the maintenance of low voltage fast activity, at least in a largely deafferented preparation as the pretrigeminal cat. It must be emphasized that the EEG synchronizing effects of continuous illumination may be obtained only with intensities and directions of light which reduce to a minimum the well known arousing effects of illumination. This point was already stressed upon in the original paper (3).

Another aspect of the problem raised by the presence of the dark activity of the retina, the one which will be dealt with extensively now, is represented by the influence that the dark activity exerts on the visual pathways. It was immediately apparent that our results had to be compared with those of CHANG, who in 1952 (6) demonstrated that steady illumination induces a potentiation of the cortical responses evoked by lateral geniculate shocks.

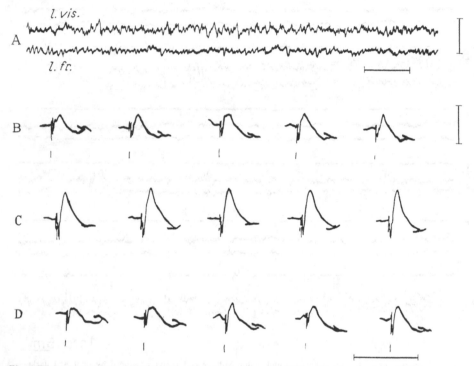

Fig. 3. Effect of steady retinal illumination of both eyes on the excitability of the visual system. A EEG activation patterns from visual and frontal areas. Cal. 300 μV, 1 sec. B responses from visual cortex to geniculate shocks (rectangular pulses, 1 msec, 5 V), in darkness. C same, during steady light. D back to darkness. Cal. B—D: 500 μV, 20 msec

The Chang effect can be reproduced in the midpontine pretrigeminal preparation (2), which we have utilized throughout our research (Fig. 3). The same phenomenon, that is the enhancement of the geniculo-cortical response, may be elicited not by light but also by reversible retinal inactivation performed in the dark adapted preparation (2) (Fig. 4).

Both light and deafferentation do not facilitate only the early part of the evoked response but they set up also an after discharge of slow, 4 to 6/sec waves, thereby modifying the cortical activity for a considerable time after the primary evoked response. We will be concerned, however, only with the earlier components of the response.

In conclusion, the suppression of the dark discharge by reversible retinal inactivation induces the same effects as the steady illumination also when we consider the cortical response to lateral geniculate shocks instead of the EEG waves. Thus the Chang effect might be attributed to decrease or complete blockade of the retinal discharge produced by continuous light impinging on the receptors. This however is purely a working hypothesis still awaiting crucial demonstration.

A problem now arises: which neural structures are played upon by the dark discharge? In view of the widespread synchronization of the EEG occurring during the retinal black-out one might be tempted to assume that the tonic retinal outflow exerts some kind of generalized energizing influence, not restricted to the visual pathways. This may be one aspect of the truth, although one must concede that the effects of visual deafferentation on the EEG are likely to appear more dramatic in the pretrigeminal cat, in which only two sensory inputs are available. However,

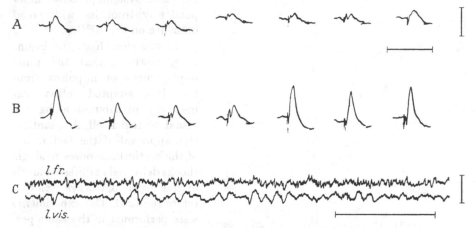

Fig. 4. Facilitation of evoked responses during retinal ischemia in the dark adapted animal. A responses of visual cortex to stimulation of lateral geniculate body (1 msec, 5 V) before retinal ischemia. B 4 minutes after the beginning of ischemia. Note enhancement with amplitude modulation of the evoked responses (Cal. A and B: 500 μV, 20 msec). C EEG records from frontal and visual areas during ischemia immediately preceding B. Note EEG synchronization in the visual cortex. Cal. 300 μV, 1 sec

the assumption that the retinal dark discharge influences, say, the ascending reticular system is not necessarily conflicting with the hypothesis of an influence on the specific functions of the visual system. A study of the cortical responses to geniculate shocks under the influence of either retinal deafferentation or continuous illumination is more likely to provide reliable evidence on this problem.

Either the continuous photic stimulation or the ischemic inactivation of one eye only are sufficient to bring about a potentiation of the geniculate responses on both visual areas (although unilateral visual deafferentation is not adequate to synchronize the EEG in the pretrigeminal cat). This is in line with the fact that the optic fibers in the cat are only partly crossing in the chiasma. On the other hand, however, a midline sagittal section of the chiasma, severing all crossed fibers, does not abolish the bilaterality of the effects obtained by operating on one eye at a time, although the potentiation thus obtained is far less conspicuous. The effect is particularly evident following unilateral increase of intraocular pressure, although pain is eliminated by the pretrigeminal section. The enhancement of the contralateral cortical response must be due to withdrawal of a tonic retinal influence, which is not exclusively mediated by the classical retino-geniculo-cortical paths.

Notwithstanding this fact, the potentiation remains localized to the visual areas. In a series of experiments (4) we have been unable to show a potentiation

of the response of auditory area I to medial geniculate shocks following bilateral
retinal black-out, although in these conditions EEG synchronization appears also
on the auditory cortex. We have been unable moreover to reproduce Chang's
results on the potentiation of the response of the auditory area to medial geniculate
stimulation during continuous retinal illumination, although our experiments were
performed not only in the midpontine cat but also in the intact animal under the
same kind of barbital anesthesia which was utilized by this author.

We should be inclined to conclude, therefore, that, at least in our experimental
conditions, the retinal dark discharge plays a major rôle within the boundaries of
the visual system, probably inde-
pendently from its widespread
influence on the EEG.

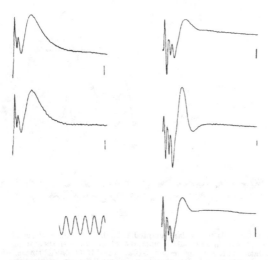

It was clear from the beginning, however, that the tonic
impingement of impulses from
the dark adapted retina was
unevenly distributed along the
visual system itself. A quantitative appraisal of the facilitation
of the cortical responses to single
shocks delivered at different levels
of the visual pathways was therefore required. The experiments
were performed in the same preparation. The main feature of
these experiments was the use of
the computer averaging technique
developed at the Massachusetts
Institute of Technology (see 8).
This method permits to work on
the average of a large number of
evoked responses. The results

Fig. 5. Different effects of visual deafferentation on the cortical
responses evoked from the stimulation of the anterior portion of
the lateral geniculate nucleus and of the optic tract. Averaged
responses from A.R.C. computer (8). Left column: responses to
stimulation of the anterior portion of the lateral geniculate
nucleus. From above: control, deafferentation. Right column:
responses to stimulation of the optic tract. From above: control,
deafferentation, recovery. Calibration: 50 μV, 200 cps

of this research have been published only in form of abstract (4), the analysis of
the data being still in progress. At this stage we can only state that when the stimulus is delivered to the optic tract the enhancement of the cortical responses, both
during continuous illumination and during retinal inactivation, concerns all the
components which have been described by previous authors, so that the voltages
of all positive spikes, as well as of the following negative wave, are increased,
although not uniformly (Fig. 5). Therefore, a first site of the facilitation is probably
represented by the geniculate neurons, without excluding a simultaneous effect on
the visual cortex. Further computer analysis of the data so gathered in a large
number of experiments will show how the potentiation is quantitatively distributed
among the different components of the response.

When the stimuli are delivered to the lateral geniculate the results indicate
that not all of the neurons are equally facilitated by the retinal illumination and
by visual deafferentation. On the base of routine histological controls of the
electrode position we have observed that only the cortical potentials evoked in

response to stimulation of the posterior three-fourth of the lateral geniculate body were increased, whereas the enhancement of the responses evoked from the anterior one-fourth of the nucleus was always much smaller. The interelectrode distance, more than one half of a millimeter, does not permit to discriminate easily between the different layers of the nucleus. On the other hand, the responses evoked by the stimulation of the optic tract, since it involved indiscriminately fibers to all parts of the nucleus, were consistently facilitated (Fig. 5).

The potentiation of the evoked cortical response produced by visual deafferentation or by continuous illumination must be in some way related with the physiology of vision rather than with unspecific effects of the retinal discharge. This statement is supported by at least three lines of experimental evidence: i) dissociation between EEG changes and effects on the evoked responses; ii) absence of any effect on the responses evoked in the auditory cortex by medial geniculate stimulation; iii) difference between anterior and posterior parts of the lateral geniculate body.

Since the only effect of intraocular compression in the dark adapted pretrigeminal cat can be the ischemic suppression of the retinal dark discharge one would be tempted to conclude that the excitability of the lateral geniculate neurons is in some way depressed by the tonic inflow of retinal impulses. Whether this depressing influence is an expression of true inhibition or is due to an occlusion phenomenon (a kind of "line busy" effect) must be left for further investigation. Work on this aspect of the problem is in progress.

Clearly, the functional significance of our findings is closely related with that of the retinal dark discharge, particularly if one concedes that continuous illumination acts by blocking this tonic activity of the retina. The problem is, however, too large to be dealt with in a few lines at the end of this report. Comments on the possible physiological rôle of the dark activity of the retina have been introduced in a previous paper (2) and discussed in connection with both the visual system (2) and the generalized EEG effects (3). Furthermore, experiments are still in progress and will form the object of further reports.

Summary

The suppression of the retinal dark discharge by reversible retinal inactivation is likely to be responsible for the EEG patterns of sleep in the midpontine pretrigeminal preparation. To the same mechanism is attributed the EEG synchronization obtained during continuous illumination of the retinae.

The suppression of the dark discharge induces the same effects as the steady illumination also when the cortical responses to lateral geniculate stimuli are considered instead of the EEG waves.

The potentiation of the evoked responses induced by retinal inactivation and by illumination, unlike the effects on the EEG activity, remains localized to the visual system.

It is concluded that the dark discharge exerts a constraining influence on the excitability of the geniculate neurones, although this influence is not evenly distributed within the geniculate nucleus.

References

1. ARDUINI, A., and T. HIRAO: On the mechanism of the EEG sleep patterns elicited by acute visual deafferentation. Arch. ital. Biol. **97**, 140—155 (1959).

2. —— Enhancement of evoked responses in the visual system during reversible retinal inactivation Arch. ital. Biol. **98**, 182—205 (1960).

3. —— EEG synchronization elicited by light. Arch. ital. Biol. **98**, 275—292 (1960).

4. — M.H.GOLDSTEIN: Localizzazione e meccanismo dell'effetto Chang. Boll.Soc.ital.Biol.sper. **36**, 1530—1532 (1960).

5. BORNSCHEIN, H.: Spontan- und Belichtungsaktivität in Einzelfasern des N. opticus der Katze. I. Der Einfluß kurzdauernder retinaler Ischämie. Z. Biol. **110**, 210—222 (1958).

6. CHANG, H. T.: Cortical response to stimulation of lateral geniculate body and the potentiation thereof by continuous illumination of the retina. J. Neurophysiol. **15**, 5—26 (1952).

7. CLAES, E.: Contribution à l'étude physiologique de la fonction visuelle. I. Analyse oscillographique de l'activité spontanée et sensorielle de l'aire visuelle corticale chez le chat non anesthésié. Arch. int. Physiol. **48**, 181—237 (1939).

8. Communications Biophysics Group of Research Laboratory of Electronics and William M. Siebert. *Processing neuroelectric data*. Cambridge, Massachussetts Institute of Technology, 1959.

Discussion

F. BREMER: One can say that this analysis of the Chang effect has led to an unexpected and almost baffling explanation of its mechanism. Yet ARDUINI's and HIRAO's conclusion that, in the experimental conditions they have chosen, the potentiation of the visual area response to a geniculate shock by retinal illumination is related to the suppression by light of the spontaneous activity of retinal neurons, the impulses of which exert a tonic inhibition on the thalamic and cortical visual structures, is corroborated by POSTERNAK, FLEMING and EVART's finding of the potentiation which results, for the response to an optic radiation stimulus, from the section of the optic nerves or destruction of the lateral geniculate bodies.

But one may ask — and ARDUINI and HIRAO have themselves considered this possibility — if in other experimental conditions, especially that of deep barbiturate narcosis where the existence of a spontaneous activity of retinal neurons is questionable, the potentiation of the response by light does not result, as in CHANG's original interpretation, from temporal and spatial summation of the conditioning retino-cortical impulses with the testing geniculo-cortical one. We have observed a clear Chang effect in deteriorated cerveau isolé preparations, where spontaneous cortical activity had completely disappeared. On the other hand, the light potentiating effect has shown, in our experiments, formal characteristics very similar to the reticular facilitation of the same visual area response, a facilitation which certainly is not the expression of a liberation phenomenon. Light, even dim one, potentiated the vestibular nystagmus of the pigeon (VAN EYCK, 1959) and also the response of the toad tectum, in recent experiment by CHANG and his associates (1959). Thus, in spite of my dislike for compromises, I am inclined to believe that the Chang effect may be an heterogenous phenomenon, having different possible mechanisms.

H. BORNSCHEIN: Die physiologische Natur der Spontanaktivität retinaler Neurone der Katze kann durch Mikroelektrodenableitung vom N. opticus (knapp vor dem Chiasma) bei intakter Retina gesichert werden. Temporäre retinale Ischämie durch vorübergehende intraoculäre Druckerhöhung auf 200 mm Hg bewirkt eine reversible Auslöschung dieser Aktivität.

A. ARDUINI: As Prof. BREMER has said, we also have considered the possibility of an active facilitation due to impulses elicited by retinal illumination. We can only say that in our experimental conditions the effects obtained with illumination are duplicated by retinal deafferentation. On the other hand the the striking effects obtained in our experiments by changing the direction of the light beam (as far as EEG synchronization is concerned) suggest that under continuous illumination there is an excitatory component counteracting and occasionally overwhelming the effects of the abolition of the dark discharge. If this assumption is true we might have an explanation of the presence of CHANG's effects under deep barbital anesthesia or in a deteriorated preparation, i. e. when the retinal dark discharge is likely to be absent.

I can only thank Dr. BORNSCHEIN for his statement confirming his previous results of the presence of a retinal dark discharge which is reversibly blocked by raising the intraocular pressure. We are also indebted to him for the technique of visual deafferentation.

Action of Afferent and Corticofugal Impulses on Single Elements of the Dorsal Lateral Geniculate Nucleus[1,2]

By

L. WIDÉN[3] and C. AJMONE MARSAN

With 3 Figures

During a study of the unit activity of the visual cortex our curiosity with regard to the problem of the existence of cortico-geniculate connections was aroused. Some of the old anatomists claim evidence for it, while others deny it, and the situation appears much the same among recent investigators: NAUTA and BUCHER (1954) found evidence for cortico-geniculate fibres in the albino rat and NAUTA (personal communication) has confirmed these findings also in the cat (more fibres, however, go to the ventral lateral geniculate nucleus than to the dorsal one), but KRUGER, using proton ray lesions of the visual cortex, has not been able to find such fibres (personal communication).

With strychnine neuronography, NIEMER and JIMENEZ-CASTELLANOS (1950) demonstrated a projection from area 17 (but not from perivisual association areas) to the dorsal lateral geniculate nucleus (LGD) in the cat, and JASPER et al. (1952) found that an after-discharge set up in area 17 in the monkey was conducted to a restricted part of the LGD.

Our series of experiments were performed in order to see whether we could find any evidence of corticofugal effects upon single elements of the LGD and, if so, to analyze the type of regulatory function exerted. By using very brief, single shocks for the cortical stimulation it should be possible to estimate accurately the latency of these effects, necessary prerequisites for differentiating orthodromic phenomena from antidromic.

Method. The experiments were performed on cats ("cerveau isolé" preparation), induced with pentothal, the anesthesia being discontinued as soon as the bilateral inter-collicular section had been completed. The cortex was stimulated with conventional silver ball electrodes. The afferent stimulation consisted of electric shocks to the optic tract in some experiments and in others photic stimulation with a Grass stroboscope. The unit activity of the LGD was re-corded with stereotaxically oriented electro-polished tungsten wires coated with a vinyl lac-quer, i. e. the type of microelectrode designed by HUBEL (1957). The microelectrode was in-troduced through the unopened arachnoid of the lateral portion of the middle suprasylvian

[1] From the Branch of Electroencephalography and Clinical Neurophysiology, National Institute of Neurological Diseases and Blindness, National Institutes of Health, Bethesda, Maryland, U.S.A.

[2] The results of the present investigation are presented in detail in the October issue of Exper. Neurol. 1960.

[3] Present address: Department of Clinical Neurophysiology, Serafimerlasarettet, Stock-holm, Sweden.

gyrus. The gross LGD response evoked by a shock to the optic tract has a very characteristic shape, the details of which have been analyzed in studies by, among others, G. H. and P. O. BISHOP and their groups. This response was used by us as a guide for localization of the nucleus.

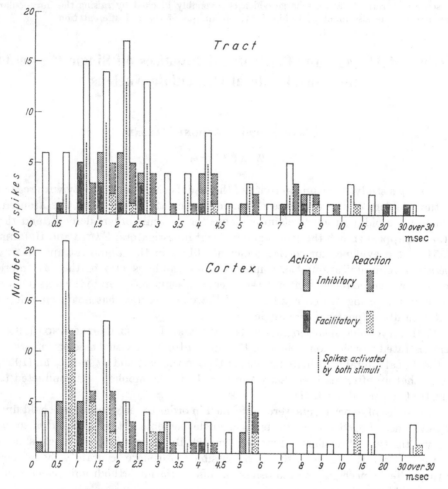

Fig. 1. Distribution of LGD spikes elicited by stimulation of the optic tract and of the cortex according to latency and a schematic display of their reciprocal effects. The height of the white columns represents the number of spikes in each group of latency value for the two types of stimulation (upper histogram: optic tract; lower histogram: cerebral cortex). The height of the dotted line in some of these columns indicates the number of spikes which could be activated by both stimuli (in such cases the latency values do not necessarily correspond and they refer to the main stimulation for which the spikes are plotted). The hatched and/or dotted column on the left of a white column indicates the number of spikes elicited by a tract stimulus (upper histogram) or a cortical stimulus (lower histogram) which, when employed as the conditioning stimulus, exerted an effect (inhibitory or facilitatory "action") on the test spike elicited by the other stimulus. Those on the right of the white column indicate the number of test spikes evoked by a tract stimulus (upper histogram) or a cortical stimulus (lower histogram) which were influenced (inhibitory or facilitatory "reaction") by the other conditioning stimulus. [This and the following illustrations are from LW and CAM, Exp. Neurol. (1960)]

Results. The activity of single units in the LGD of cat in response to photic or electrical stimulation has been described by, among others, TASAKI and collaborators (1954) and recently by HUBEL (1960). We shall therefore mention only a few points relevant to our problem. The unitary responses from the LGD to stimulation of the optic tract are presumably derived from three sources: a) fibres of the optic tract, b) cell bodies of the LGD (recording from dendrites with the type of microelectrode employed is unlikely) and c) axons of the optic radiation. Since with optic tract stimulation the conduction distance is only a few millimetres, the latency of the tract spikes should be very short.

As shown in the upper histogram of Fig. 1, only a small fraction of all the spikes elicited by tract stimuli (slightly over 5%) have a latency of less than 0.5 msec. Longer latencies would not be expected for presynaptic spikes, not even for those arising from the small fibres which, according to P. O. Bishop et al. (1953), have a mean conduction velocity of 18 metres per second. More than half of the number of spikes evoked by tract stimuli were found to have a latency of 0.5 to 3 msec. Monosynaptically transmitted spikes recorded from within the LGD or in its immediate vicinity could hardly have a longer latency than 1 to 1.5 msec. and therefore some of the spikes of this group are probably activated through disynaptic or polysynaptic pathways. The remaining later spikes (36) plotted in the same histogram are fairly evenly distributed in the various groups of latencies. The very long delays before activation of these units suggest rather complex neuronal pathways or, perhaps more likely, inhibitory effects.

LGD unit activity could also be elicited by single electrical pulses of a few tenths of a msec. applied to the cortical surface. The lower histogram of Fig. 1 shows the latency distribution of these spikes. Over half of them occurred with a latency of 2 msec. or less; some of these may very likely be antidromically activated. In an earlier work (1960) we found that impulses in geniculo-cortical fibres evoked by stimulation of the optic radiation close to the LGD and recorded with a microelectrode in the visual cortex or underlying white matter could in rare cases have latencies of 1.5 to 1.75 msec., but that the vast majority of such spikes occurred with less than 0.5 msec. latency. Thus, only exceptionally would antidromic spikes with latencies longer than 0.5 msec. be expected in the LGD with cortical stimulation. Consequently most of the spikes plotted with latencies longer than 0.5 msec. — and they are about 95% of all the spikes — should not be evoked by direct antidromic stimulation. We shall return to the problem of possible antidromic activation through recurrent collaterals in the discussion of the results.

In each experiment various regions within the visual cortex and surrounding areas were tested. The position of the two stimulating electrodes was mapped in all the experiments and it appears that: a) no significant corticofugal effects were elicited by stimulation of the area from which the maximum or best developed evoked responses were recorded and b) all the "active" points lay in a relatively restricted area between the middle and posterior gyrus lateralis and between the middle and posterior gyrus suprasylvius. This area covers about 7 to 8 mm^2; the posterior part of it is in the striate area 17, the anterior in a part of visual area II or area 21 according to the brain map of Gurewitsch and Chatschaturian (1928). Not all areas of the exposed cortex were tested and no systematic topographical study was attempted: it is therefore impossible to provide a more precise or detailed outline of this region or to state that this was the exclusive one from which corticofugal effects could be elicited.

Having repeatedly confirmed the possibility of activating LGD elements with cortical stimulation, the various interactions between corticofugal and corticopetal impulses at the LGD level were analyzed and are described in some detail in the following.

The most commonly observed effect of cortical stimulation upon unit discharges in the LGD evoked either by stimuli to the optic tract or photic stimuli was *inhibition*. In a of Fig. 2 a unit discharges repetitively in response to a flash of light which was placed at the very beginning of the sweep. When, in b, a cortical stimulus preceded the discharge, the interval being about 20 msec., the latter was completely abolished. In this case the unit would not be activated by the stimulus

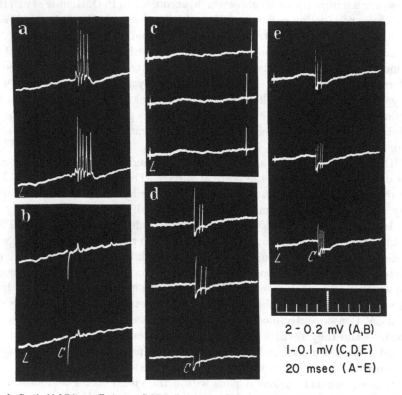

2 - 0.2 mV (A,B)
1 - 0.1 mV (C,D,E)
20 msec (A-E)

Fig. 2. a, b: Cortical inhibitory effects upon LGD spikes activated by photic stimulation. a. Two examples of photic stimulation (L) alone. b. Two examples of combined photic (L) and cortical (C) stimulation. Note inhibition of spikes. c—e: Photic facilitatory effects upon LGD spikes elicited by cortical stimulation. c. Three examples of photic stimulation (L) alone. d. Three examples of cortical stimulation (C) alone. e. The two stimuli are combined: the facilitatory effect exerted by the photic stimulus is manifested by a shortening of the latency, and higher tendency to repetitive firing, of the spike activated by cortical stimulation. — (Note that there is a reciprocal effect with abolition of the photically induced spike.) (In a and b the photic stimulus is synchronous with the beginning of the sweep, in c and e with the artefact.)

to the cortex. In the experiment illustrated in c through e, on the other hand, a unit was fired both by afferent (light) and corticofugal impulses. In c there is a late single discharge evoked by a flash of light, in d the response of the same unit to a shock to the cortex and in e the effect of a combination of the two stimuli: the response to light is blocked but the response to the cortical stimulation is facilitated in the sense that the latency is shorter and the tendency to repetitive firing somewhat greater.

Fig. 3, a through d, shows another example of corticofugal inhibitory influence on the afferent inflow. The spike-discharge evoked by a tract stimulus (a) is inhibited when preceded by a cortical stimulus (C) which did not trigger the unit (b).

However, the spike is not completely abolished; a small "prepotential", a graded response, was left: this is better shown in d with higher sweep speed and barely threshold stimulation.

In e through h of the same figure, from another experiment, a facilitatory corticofugal effect is instead demonstrated: a unit was activated by cortical (e) but not by a tract (g) stimulus. If the cortical stimulus was made subliminal (f) and then used as conditioning stimulus, it had a facilitatory effect and the unit responded to the test tract stimulus (h). This effect was still present with a shock interval of over 20 msec.

Whereas the corticofugal influences on the afferent impulses were most often inhibitory, the effect of the afferent inflow on the unit discharges evoked by cortical stimulation was slightly more often facilitatory. Otherwise, the behaviour was rather similar to that described in the preceding section with most of the effects taking place with subliminal (optic tract and/or photic) conditioning stimuli and within a wide range of interstimuli intervals.

The various results of reciprocal interactions between descending and ascending impulses at the LGD level are summarized in Fig. 1.

Comments. Before attempting any functional interpretation of our findings the

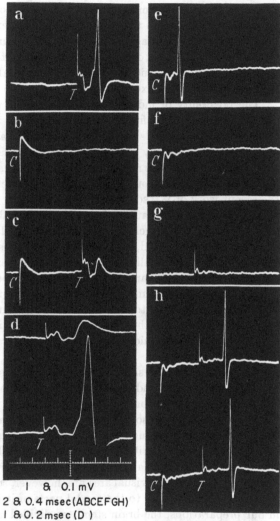

I & 0.1 mV
2 & 0.4 msec (ABCEFGH)
I & 0.2 msec (D)

Fig. 3. a—d: Cortical inhibitory effects upon LGD spike elicited by optic tract stimulation. Optic tract stimulation (T) alone in a (submaximal) and d (just liminal). Note presence of slow "prepotential" and different sweep speed in d. Cortical stimulation (C) alone in b: no visible response. Both stimuli are applied at about 9 msec. interval and an inhibitory effect is observed in c. e—h: Cortical facilitatory effects upon LGD spike elicited by optic tract stimulation. Cortical stimulation (C) is supraliminal in e and subliminal in f. Optic tract stimulus (T) is subliminal in g. A facilitatory action is observed in h (two examples) when the two stimuli are applied at about 7 msec. interval. Note that in this instance the same spike can be activated by the two stimuli (cf. e and h) though with different latency. These facilitatory effects were seen whether or not the conditioning stimulus produced a spike and could be observed with an inter-shock interval of more than 20 msec.

possibility of some of the corticofugal effects being the result of antidromic activation of optic radiation fibres or their recurrent collaterals should be discussed.

For reasons already mentioned, it is safe to conclude that only a negligible contingent of the corticofugal spikes with latencies longer than 0.5 msec., and they are about 95% of all the corticofugal spikes, could be antidromic. It should further be added that part of the cortical region from which centrifugal effects were elicited is an extra-striate area to which probably no direct geniculo-cortical fibres arrive. Still another argument against the effect being due to a direct antidromic activation is the fact that most of the effects upon afferent impulses could be demonstrated with cortical stimuli which were either subliminal for the unit tested or failed to activate it even when excessively strong.

The possibility of indirect antidromic effects through activation of recurrent collaterals cannot be definitely ruled out, but for the following reasons it appears unlikely that such effects should play any significant role: according to O'Leary's (1940) histological study of the LGD, the number of principal cells equipped with this type of collaterals is negligible and therefore cannot be of the same importance for the effects of antidromic stimulation as in the spinal cord. Finally, except for the recent work of Wilson (1959), no facilitatory action upon the motor neurons with antidromic stimulation of the recurrent collaterals has been described and as a rule the LGD principal cells, like the spinal cord motor neurons, would be expected to be inhibited, not facilitated, if exposed to this type of stimulation. Yet, about one fifth of all the tract spikes which exhibit a reaction are facilitated. It is true that Li (1958) and Phillips (1959) independently have described facilitatory phenomena in the motor cortex in response to stimulation of the pyramidal tract. They are inclined to interpret them as due to activity in recurrent collaterals of the Betz-cells but, as they themselves point out, it was not possible to exclude the possibility of orthodromic effects through collaterals leaving the pyramidal tract of the brain stem.

From what has been said, it seems justified to state that a considerable portion of our results actually indicates that the effects observed with cortical stimulation are the consequence of orthodromic stimulation.

The long latency of some of the corticofugal impulses might suggest that they have been relayed through multisynaptic pathways. Since a reticulo-geniculate pathway has been described, one may wonder whether some of the corticofugal effects are actually mediated through the brain stem reticular system. Projections to this system from the visual area are, however, scanty and, according to Brodal (1957), most of them go to the caudal parts of it in the pons and medulla. Since, in our preparations, the brain stem was divided at the mid-collicular level, practically only the thalamic and subthalamic parts of the reticular systems were left in functional connection with the cortex. According to Jasper, Ajmone Marsan and Stoll (1952) there are no projections from the primary visual area to the intralaminar and midline nuclei of the thalamus. Since the long-latency responses could be elicited also from the primary visual area, it seems less likely that the reticular system should be involved in their transmission. It would be possible, on the other hand, that some of the effects elicited by stimulation of the posterior suprasylvian region might be mediated through the cephalic portion of the reticular formation. However, we wish to point out that while most of the phenomena observed in the conditioning-test experiments could be demonstrated with relatively long interstimuli delays, the same were — as a rule — present also, if not more often, when the conditioning (cortical) shock preceded the test stimulus by only 2—3 msec. This observation makes very unlikely a cortico-reticular-geniculate pathway.

Our series of experiments provides some evidence for the existence of specific, probably extra-reticular, corticofugal mechanisms in the visual system in analogy to what has been suggested for other sensory systems. In the past few years a wealth of evidence has accumulated which emphasizes the role of the brain stem reticular formation not only in its ascending or motor descending influences but also in its control of sensory mechanisms. In fact, most of the described cortico-fugal (extramotor) systems have been interpreted as preferentially impinging upon the central core of the brain stem reticular formation and according to available data they would exert their influence at this level where most of the inter-actions with the incoming impulses from the different peripheral sources take place. Yet it is rather difficult to understand which, if any, functional role these cortico-reti-cular pathways might play in the mechanism of integration of the various percep-tual data. A structure such as the reticular formation where impulses from mul-tiple different sources converge and mutually occlude could hardly be selected as the site of perceptual integration. This concept was clearly expressed by BREMER (1955), who also concludes that one must look "in the neurophysiological study of the relations between cortex and specific thalamic nuclei" for the mechanism involved in perceptual integration. The present results might provide some ex-perimental evidence for this statement.

Summary

1. This study was undertaken to investigate whether any descending effects, other than antidromic, can be demonstrated in a sensory system. This was carried out by studying the effects of stimulation of higher levels (visual and para-visual cortex) upon lower sectors (unitary elements of the dorso-lateral geniculate nu-cleus — LGD) in the same sensory pathway.

2. "Corticofugal" effects on the LGD could easily be elicited by stimulation of a small area on either side of the borderline between area 17 and area 21, i.e. parts of visual areas I and II. No systematic study of other cortical areas was done.

3. The effects of cortical, optic tract and photic stimulation, singly and in various combinations, were analyzed.

4. With different combinations of shocks it was found that: a) A cortical con-ditioning stimulus may inhibit or facilitate a spike produced by an optic tract or photic test stimulus. Inhibitory effects generally predominate. b) An optic tract or photic conditioning stimulus may facilitate or inhibit LGD spikes elicited by a cortical test stimulus. In this situation facilitatory effects slightly predominate. c) Most of these interactions take place in the absence of any spike activation by the conditioning stimulus.

5. The nature of the corticofugal effects is discussed. The experimental evidence indicates that a large proportion of these effects is due to *ortho*dromic activation.

6. These findings provide some evidence for the existence of specific, probably extrareticular, corticofugal mechanisms in the visual system.

References

Bishop, P. O., D. Jeremy and J. W. Lance: The optic nerve. Properties of a central tract. J. Physiol. (Lond.) 121, 415—432 (1953).

Bremer, F.: Quelques aspects physiologiques du problème des relations réciproques de l'écorce cérébrale et des structures sous-corticales. Acta neurol. belg. 55, 947—965 (1955).

Brodal, A.: The reticular formation of the brain stem. Anatomical aspects and functional correlations. London: Oliver and Boyd, Ltd., 1957.

Gurewitsch, M., u. A. Chatschaturian: Zur Cytoarchitektonik der Großhirnrinde der Feliden. Z. Anat. Entwickl.-Gesch. 87, 100—138 (1928).

Hubel, D. H.: Tungsten microelectrode for recording from single units. Science 125, 549—550 (1957).

— Single unit activity in lateral geniculate body and optic tract of unrestrained cats. J. Physiol. (Lond.) 150, 91—104 (1960).

Jasper, H., C. Ajmone Marsan and J. Stoll: Corticofugal projections to the brain stem. Arch. Neurol. Psychiat. (Chicago) 67, 155—166 (1952).

Li, C.-L.: Activity of interneurons in the motor cortex, in The Reticular Formation of the Brain, edited by H. H. Jasper. Boston: Little, Brown and Company 1958.

Nauta, W. J. H., and V. M. Bucher: Efferent connections to the striate cortex in the albino rat. J. comp. Neurol. 100, 257—286 (1954).

Niemer, W. T., and J. Jimenez-Castellanos: Cortico-thalamic connections in cat as revealed by "physiological neuronography". J. comp. Neurol. 93, 101—123 (1950).

O'Leary, J. L.: A structural analysis of the lateral geniculate nucleus of the cat. J. comp. Neurol. 73, 405—430 (1940).

Phillips, C. G.: Actions of antidromic pyramidal volleys on single Betz cells in the cat. Quart. J. exp. Physiol. 44, 1—25 (1959).

Tasaki, I., E. H. Polley and F. Orrego: Action potentials from individual elements in cat geniculate and striate cortex. J. Neurophysiol. 17, 454—474 (1954).

Widén, L., and C. Ajmone Marsan: Unitary analysis of the response elicited in the visual cortex of cat. Arch. ital. Biol. 98, 248—274 (1960).

Wilson, V. J.: Recurrent facilitation of spinal reflexes. J. gen. Physiol. 42, 703—713 (1959).

Discussion

F. Bremer: I should like to mention, as an addition to the bibliographical information given by our colleague, that Desmedt and Mechelse work in our laboratory on the inhibition of the cat's cochlear nucleus and of auditory receptors by centrifugal, probably corticofugal fibers, represents clearly a case where the brainstem reticular formation is *not* the mediator of the inhibitory control.

R. Jung: Vielleicht gibt diese Erregungskonvergenz an Geniculatumzellen mit dem Nachweis rückläufiger cortico-fugaler Verbindungen und ihrer vorwiegend hemmenden Wirkung Hinweise auf die physiologische Funktion des Geniculatum und der 2. visuellen Area. Sonst haben weder neurophysiologische noch psychophysiologische Untersuchungen die Funktion des Geniculatumrelais zwischen Retina und Cortex klären können. Eine einfache Fortleitung unter Vermehrung der Neuronenzahl hat keinen rechten funktionellen Sinn und eine binokulare Koordination scheint nach Grüssers und Saurs Befunden zweifelhaft.

Wahrscheinlich sind Widéns cortico-fugale Impulse multisynaptische Verbindungen aus den peristriären Cortexfeldern und es handelt sich nicht um einfache doppeläufige Verbindungen zwischen Area 17 und Geniculatum, ähnlich den cortico-thalamischen Neuronenkreisen, wie sie Bishop und Hassler postuliert haben. Sonst müßten mehr cortico-fugale Ergebnisse nach Reizung des primären optischen Cortex zu erhalten sein. Ist neben dem 2. visuellen Gebiet und Area 21, von der die besten cortico-fugalen Ergebnisse erhalten wurden, auch Area 18 oder 19 beteiligt?

L. Widén: As Professor Bremer mentioned, the experiments of Desmedt and Mechelse which were published in 1957 certainly demonstrate the existence of extrareticular centrifugal inhibitory mechanisms.

In reply to Professor JUNG I would like to say that already the findings of both excitatory and inhibitory influences of afferent impulses on LGD cells would seem to indicate that this nucleus is not a simple relay station but an integrating centre. I agree that the demonstration of an input to the LGD also from cortical visual areas further emphasizes the role of this nucleus in the analysis and integration of visual perceptual data.

As I said, we have made no systematic study of the cortical areas from which centrifugal effects on the LGD can be elicited. We know that they can most easily be evoked by stimulation of a small area on either side of the borderline between areas 17 and 21, but also other cortical areas, e. g. areas 18 and 19, may very well be "active" in this respect even if in our preliminary trials we did not obtain any evidence for it.

Single Unit Activity in the Rabbit Lateral Geniculate Body during Experimental Epilepsy*

By

U. SÖDERBERG and G. B. ARDEN

With 3 Figures

Introduction

In many epileptic attacks the patients suffer from a variety of abnormal sensations or unconsciousness. Up to now, the attention seems to have been focused exclusively on those phenomena that precede or follow upon the generalized seizure, because they can tell about the localization of the lesion that has initiated the attack. Most of these events are probably of cortical origin. Since the well-known activation of epileptic processes with intermittent photic stimulation (11, 29, 34) also influences other cortical areas than the visual, the light-evoked responses must spread diffusely within the brain. That this is the case was shown by the extensive studies of HUNTER and INGVAR (23) who not only traced the "non-specific" visual responses in the brain stem and thalamus but also concluded that the visual cortex might control the conduction of the light-evoked responses in subcortical structures (24).

HERNÁNDEZ-PEÓN and co-workers (19—22) found that when gross electrodes are chronically implanted in the optic pathways of otherwise intact animals, the evoked potentials that can be recorded are modified if auditory and olfactory stimuli are presented together with the photic stimuli, and the response from, for example the lateral geniculate body, varies with the animal's state of attention. The underlying mechanisms have been further elucidated by ARDEN and SÖDERBERG (2, 3) who showed that the rabbit lateral geniculate body receives tonic influences from the reticular formation of the brain stem which thereby modulates the transfer of optic information.

SÖDERBERG (31) observed that animals treated with the convulsant agent bemegride were hypersensitive to particular stimuli of differing modalities. Some of them responded with high-voltage cortical evoked responses, irradiation and clonic jerks when subjected to flashes of light but did not react to auditory stimuli,

---

* From the Nobel Institute for Neurophysiology, Karolinska Institutet, Stockholm, Sweden.

whereas other animals were extremely sensitive to clicks and claps but showed no response to photic stimulation either behaviourly or as judged by the electroencephalogram (EEG). SÖDERBERG assumed that this effect of bemegride was caused by a selective action of the convulsant agent on different cortical areas. Today, it can be added that the bemegride might also have influenced those structures that are normally engaged in regulating the sensory input when the animal's attention is fixed in a particular direction. A similar situation might also exist in epilepsy, in particular in those cases when the seizure is maintained from or mediated by the "centrencephalic system" in the middle of the brain (27). Previously neither analysis nor description of events at the cellular level seems to have been attempted. With gross electrodes in the lateral geniculate body of barbiturate cats treated with Metrazol, HUNTER and INGVAR (23) found very small changes both of the shape and the amplitude of the light evoked responses. The present communication describes results obtained when recording from single cells of the rabbit lateral geniculate body with simultaneous EEG control under various states of wakefulness and during seizures. In one group of experiments on encéphale isolé rabbits, epileptic seizures developed "spontaneously" or after activation with flickering light or moderate hyperventilation. All these animals had cortical lesions caused by removal of part of the cortex by suction. For comparison, another group of rabbits were tested in which increasing doses of bemegride were administered until seizure activity developed in the the EEG.

Experimental technique

The method has been described in detail elsewhere (3). Three types of preparation were used: the classical encéphale and cerveau isolé of BREMER (8) and the midpontine cerveau isolé (5—7) in which the section is made just rostral to the entry of the trigeminal nerve leaving more of the rostral portion of the brain stem intact and in functional connection with the geniculate body and the cortex than is left in the classical preparation. Some of the animals were immobilized with Flaxedil. In some animals part of the cortex was removed by suction.

The eyelids were held open by stay sutures, and the pupil dilated. Local anaesthetics were used to block conduction of nociceptive impulses. In a few animals one eye was eviscerated. The activity in the remaining eye could be reversibly blocked by ischaemia that was caused by raising the intraocular pressure well above the arterial level.

The spike responses of single lateral geniculate cells were recorded with ordinary sodium chloride-filled glass micro-pipettes by filming a cathode-ray oscilloscope. The average firing rate was also recorded on paper in parallel with the electroencephalogram (EEG) by feeding the amplifier output onto a rate meter (EKCO), suitably biased to discriminate from baseline noise. The rate meter and EEG record fed into an Offner dynograph. The cathode ray record was used as a most necessary check of the rate meter discrimination, and enabled us to be sure that the same cell remained under the electrode during the period of observation.

The eyes were dark adapted. A flickering light could be focused into either of the eyes so that an area of approximately 15 degrees of visual angle was evenly illuminated. The light was obtained from a tungsten filament lamp, run at constant voltage. The maximum intensity of light was about 180,000 lux. Neutral filters were used to reduce the intensity.

Results

General properties of the rabbit lateral geniculate body. ARDEN and LIU (1) had observed that the average firing rate of the lateral geniculate cells in the encéphale isolé preparation is largely independent of the intensity of the light stimulus. This finding was further investigated by the present authors who found that the resting

activity was also maintained after removal of the optic tract input (3). Alterations in the state of arousal (as judged by the EEG), whether provoked or spontaneous, were paralleled by changes in the geniculate discharge rate, but even
when the EEG was fully "aroused", more stimulation (whistles or claps) altered
the geniculate discharge still further. This was true both in the presence and
absence of optic tract input. Light-evoked responses could often only be
distinguished from the resting discharge by their synchronization with the stimulus which was the closer the higher the light intensity. A rise of the average discharge rate, for example during an "arousal" reaction, could either lead to a more
regular response to light or to the appearance of "irrelevant" spikes in between the
evoked responses. The resting discharge of the geniculate body was very sensitive
to barbiturates and it also gradually disappeared when the preparation deteriorated.

Many spontaneously active geniculate cells in the *encéphale isolé* rabbit were,
as a rule, not greatly influenced by light and since it was difficult to find any active
cells a large proportion must have been silent. In the *cerveau isolé*, on the other hand,
almost all cells responded to light and the responses were regular and repro-
ducible, but in the dark or when the optic tract input was interrupted most cells
of this preparation were silent. The new modified *cerveau isolé* obtained by midpontine brain stem transsection was intermediate in its properties between the
classical *cerveau isolé* and *encéphale isolé* preparations. Electrical stimulation of the
rostral part of the reticular formation could still "arouse" the brain and influence
the geniculate firing. When the cortical "arousal" outlasted the period of stimulation there was also a similarly prolonged effect at the geniculate level.

Removal of the visual cortex bilaterally had only insignificant effects on the
geniculate activity. On the other hand, when a larger part of the cortex was removed, the correlation between cortical and geniculate activity was less obvious
and the EEG in the remaining cortex abnormal.

It is concluded from these results that the lateral geniculate body of the rabbit
receives an important "second input" from the brain stem reticular formation
which is responsible for most of the resting activity and for the changes in the
treatment of the impulses from the "primary input" of the optic tract. The
"second input" can cause both increased average discharge rate and improved
synchronization of the evoked spikes to the light stimuli in the single cell, i. e.
increase the information conducted in the optic messages. Similarly, if the discharge rate of the lateral geniculate cell decreases, one may speak of true inhibition
only if the resting rate and the evoked spikes are decreased in proportion. Decrease
in the second input may only lead to a reduced resting discharge, i. e. to fewer
"irrelevant" spikes in the evoked responses. This is the reverse of inhibition.
However, it was frequently seen that "arousal" caused true inhibition of single cells
in the lateral geniculate body. This does not necessarily mean that the over-all
efficiency of the nucleus is reduced but only that the cell recorded from was inhibited, for example as a consequence of the presence of a contrast mechanism.

Geniculate activity during periods of seizure caused by cortical lesions. In those
encéphale isolé rabbits in which part of the cortex was removed by suction seizure
activity was often observed in the EEG. A contributory cause was the flickering
light that was used routinely as a stimulus of the eye. In addition, respiratory

alkalosis could not always be avoided when the curarized animals were ventilated artificially without control of blood p_H. This explanation is strengthened by the recent finding by Jöbsis and Söderberg (unpublished) that cats subjected to moderate hyperventilation could show generalized convulsions if a small cortical lesion had been made.

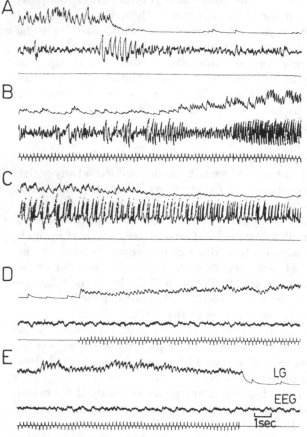

It was mentioned above that only a proportion of the lateral geniculate cells were active and could respond to light in the *encéphale isolé* rabbit. However, when seizure activity appeared in the EEG hardly any cells discharged either in the presence of absence of stimulation of the eye. Since we have only recorded the EEG from one channel at a time, it is difficult to give a precise correlation between the appearance of seizures and the inhibition of the cells of the lateral geniculate body. The most frequent finding was therefore a longlasting absence of geniculate activity during which the EEG showed fairly normal activity that was occasionally interrupted by episodes of "sharp waves", "spikes" or "spike and wave" patterns. These findings were obtained with an intact visual cortex as well as after its removal. When the seizure turned

Fig. 1. The relation of lateral geniculate activity to the EEG in periods of seizure activity (*A—C*) and after recovery from seizure (*D—E*). Each sample contains rate meter record of the firing of a single geniculate unit *(top)*, electrocorticogram of the contralateral striate cortex *(middle)*, and AC record of a photocell in the light beam *(bottom record)*. Downward deflection — light on. Upward — light off (horizontal straight line — no light). *A* shows the sudden beginning of the long-lasting inhibition of lateral geniculate activity simultaneously with the first appearance of sharp waves in the EEG. *B* and *C* illustrate the beginning and ending of a "grand mal" attack elicited by the flickering light. *D* and *E* show the normal pattern of geniculate activity about two hours after the seizures in *A—C*. The cell responds regularly to flickering light

into a "grand mal" attack the geniculate cells could again be brought into activity which was then correlated to the bursts of the EEG.

Since, in the presence of epileptic EEG activity, most records show a silent geniculate cell, it is difficult to find convincing illustrations. However, in Fig. 1 *A* from an experiment on an *encéphale isolé* rabbit in which the EEG was recorded from the visual cortex, we were lucky in recording what might be the very first sign of cortical epileptic discharges and the simultaneous beginning of a longlasting inhibition of the geniculate activity. From this moment we were unable for two hours to find any cells that responded normally to light. The EEG then recovered and the cells again behaved in a "normal" way as seen in records *D* and *E*. The animal also had a few "grand mal" attacks. One of those that started during a period when flickering light was presented to the right eye is reproduced in *B* and *C* which also shows the geniculate firing that is related in time to the "spikes" of the EEG. When the flickering light was turned off, before the beginning of *C*, the EEG discharges gradually decreased in amplitude and the geniculate cells ceased to fire. No real light response could be recorded from this cell, either during the period of "grand mal" when its firing was only related to the cortical activity, or afterwards when it was silent both in the dark and during flickering light stimulation.

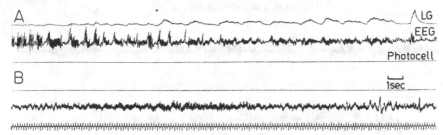

Fig. 2. Another type of seizure from the same rabbit as shown in Fig. 1. The cell is synchronized with the high-frequency bursts of the EEG but unresponsive to flickering light

Figure 2, from the same *encéphale isolé* rabbit as in Figure 1, also illustrated the relation between the geniculate discharge and the presence of an abnormal EEG pattern which, although quite different from the one of the previous Figure, is also characteristic of "grand mal" epilepsy (*15, 35*). Paroxysmal discharges in the EEG of "spikes" appearing at a rate of 24 per second in *A* are related to increased firing of the lateral geniculate unit. This geniculate cell was also unable to respond to light (*B*).

We have not seen any seizures in the *cerveau isolé* preparations. Since the operative technique was changed when we prepared the animals with high brain stem transsection, it is not possible to offer any explanation of the absence of seizures in these animals.

The effect of bemegride on lateral geniculate activity. Bemegride ("Megimide", 3-ethyl-3-methylglutarimide) was originally introduced as a barbiturate antagonist (*30*), but is was then found to resemble pentylenetetrazol ("Metrazol") yet with milder action and larger safety margin (*12—14, 28, 31*). Thus, in light anaesthesia a small dose of bemegride changes the pattern of EEG from "spindle bursts" to desynchronization but the amplitudes of the fast waves are usually higher than those of the true "arousal". In deep anaesthesia bemegride also increased the frequencies of the EEG to some extent but "arousal" cannot be obtained. There is good parallelism between the findings in the EEG and the behaviour of the animal.

In the lateral geniculate body (Figure 3) bemegride in moderate doses seems to excite the cells to increased discharge rates both in the dark and in the presence of light. In the case illustrated in the Figure, the dark rate had initially been reduced to zero with successive doses of Nembutal (altogether 120 mg) and the EEG had assumed a pattern of slow waves. The geniculate cell still responded to light, but with low firing rate (not reproduced in the Figure). Before *A* of Fig. 3, an intravenous injection of 10 mg bemegride had restored a pattern of "barbiturate spindles" in the EEG and a good response of the geniculate cell to illumination of the contralateral eye but there was no resting discharge in the dark. After further injection of 60 mg bemegride the resting activity in the geniculate cell also recovered and the light response was improved (*B*). The cell now also showed a faint response to illumination of the ipsilateral eye (not in the Figure). The firing could not be further increased by bemegride, and, in the EEG, additional injections were accompanied by "sharp waves" and "spikes". Strong noise, such as clapping, then

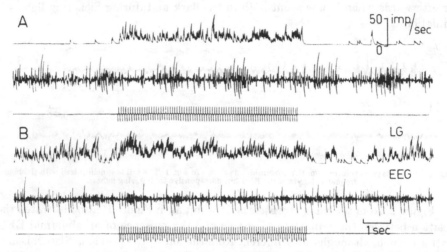

Fig. 3. *Encéphale isolé* rabbit anaesthetized with Nembutal until EEG showed slow wave activity and the geniculate cell responded with low firing rate to the flicker. Before *A* 10 mg bemegride had restored a pattern of "spindles" in the EEG and improved the geniculate response to light. A further injection of 60 mg bemegride before *B* gave further improvement of the light response and, in addition, evoked resting activity

induced high amplitude evoked responses but were without effect on the geniculate cell. In fact, there was no good temporal relation between the appearance of seizure potentials in the EEG and discharge in the lateral geniculate of the bemegride animals, in contrast to the finding obtained when seizures occurred "spontaneously" in the rabbits with critical lesions. In no instance, bemegride was found to inhibit lateral geniculate activity.

Comments

The finding of a "second input" to the lateral geniculate body from the brain stem which can modify the optic impulses before they reach cortical levels has already been discussed in detail elsewhere (*3*). In the present communication, the main results on which the conclusion was established have only been mentioned to provide a basis for the understanding of the seizure experiments.

In the two groups of animals with epileptic activity, the bemegride treated rabbits have as yet given surprisingly stereotyped results. The bemegride injections have only been followed by increased discharge rate in the geniculate body up to a maximum level which largely corresponds to the maximum rate obtained in unanaesthetized "aroused" animals. Both the resting discharge and light responses were influenced. Bemegride counteracted previously administered sodium pentobarbital. These results correlate well with some observations by Dr. CREUTZFELDT on the effect of bemegride on cortical neurones, described as a personal communication by SÖDERBERG (*31*), and there is also good agreement with the action of Metrazol on the light-evoked potentials of the lateral geniculate body (*23*). However, Metrazol administered in multiple small doses and photic stimulation of the Metrazol activated cortex have also been reported to cause cortical spreading depression in the rabbit (*32*).

The findings in the rabbits with "spontaneous" seizures seem to be more interesting although somewhat confusing, in particular when considering the anatomy of the visual pathways. The observation of strong inhibition of geniculate neurones throughout a period of seizure activity in the cortex indicates an inhibition mediated by the "second input". This is because the inhibition was largely the same, regardless of whether the visual cortex with any supposed cortico-geniculate pathways was removed or left intact, and this conclusion is also in full agreement with the finding that in animals with a normally functioning cortex the "second input" is capable of causing just the same sort of widespread geniculate inhibition. However, in "seizure rabbits" in which no spikes could be recorded from the lateral geniculate body, flickering light could still affect cortical activity even in the absence of the visual part of the cortex. According to the literature, it seems that when the striate area has been removed, the visual impulses are conducted to the brain stem over retino-collicular pathways (*4*). From the colliculus the impulses can then pass rostrally, for example in the tectothalamic tract that passes the nucleus centrum medianum (*9*).

Other pathways have also to be taken into account. Thus impulses conducted through the ventral portion of the lateral geniculate body can reach and influence the motor cortex even in animals in which the colliculi has been removed (*33*). Recently, BUSER et al. (*10*) have found that light-evoked responses can still be recorded from visual "association areas" in the cortex when the primary projection area has been removed. These "specific association responses" are relayed in the thalamus. INGVAR and HUNTER (*24*) also demonstrated visual responses in the thalamus of a decorticate cat in which the colliculi had been destroyed. Since in our experiments the lateral geniculate body was silent during the seizures, it does not seem likely that the impulses were relayed by geniculate cells. If they were, they must primarily have engaged small cells which we unintentionally might have failed to record from. There may also be other fibre systems to diencephalic structures which do not relay in the lateral geniculate body (*26*), and, in addition, in the rabbit the posterior accessory optic tract (*16, 17*) is large and its fibres are myelinated. This tract runs to a number of nuclei in the midbrain and subthalamus and has recently been studied with electrophysiological techniques (*18*).

INGVAR and HUNTER (*24*) when finding that the visual cortex could control the spread of light-evoked responses in the brain stem, suggested that the phylogenetically young geniculo-cortical system might, in general, control the visual functions of older parts of the brain, or in other terms, that the specific visual system is able to control the non-specific pathways. The present experiments and the work of HERNÁNDEZ-PEÓN et al. (*19—22*) and of ARDEN and SÖDERBERG (*3*) emphasize that the opposite is also true, i. e. non-specific events are of critical importance for the conduction of specific messages. However, it has to be remembered that in the rabbit those visual impulses that constitute part of the non-specific afferent inflow are not so important as the non-specific auditory and olfactory systems.

The nature of the inhibition of the lateral geniculate neurones in epilepsy has not yet been investigated. Since we have only recorded the EEG from one cortical area at a time, it has not been possible to examine whether or not there is a relation between the inhibition and the appearance of cortical spreading depression of LEAO (25). Very little is also known about the activity in subcortical structures when the cortical activity is depressed, but it seems possible that thalamic and geniculate inhibition might occur when epileptic activities or spreading depression can be recorded from the cortex (see 35).

Summary

The activity of single cells of the rabbit lateral geniculate body was studied and related to various states of wakefulness and to cortical seizures that developed "spontaneously", after activation with flickering light, moderate hyperventilation or after the administration of bemegride.

As has been analyzed in detail elsewhere, there is a remarkably good correlation between the average firing rate of the geniculate cells and the cortical activity as reflected in the electroencephalogram because of the presence of a "second input" to the lateral geniculate body from the brain stem.

The "second input" is also responsible for the presence of spontaneous resting activity in geniculate cells when the "primary input" from the eyes has been interrupted.

Bemegride increases the firing rate of geniculate cells both in the dark and when the retina is stimulated with flickering light. Bemegride counteracts the depressing effect of sodium pentobarbital. Even convulsive doses of bemegride have remarkably little influence on the lateral geniculate body. This is in agreement with previous findings with gross electrodes in Metrazol activated animals.

In "spontaneously" occurring epilepsy in encéphale isolé animals with acute cortical lesions, and after photic activation in these animals, there is a long-lasting marked inhibition of geniculate activity. This inhibition does not prevent flickering light from influencing cortical activity.

The findings are discussed in relation to previous investigations on the relation between specific and non-specific visual pathways.

The geniculate inhibition in a seizure may bear a relation to the reported loss in man of visual sensations which therefore need not necessarily be of cortical origin.

Note added during correction of proof: Since this paper was sent to the editor further support for the assumption that subcortical structures are influenced by cortical spreading depression has been presented by BUREŠ, BUREŠOVÁ and FIFKOVÁ in Arch. Ital. Biol. **99**, 23—32 (1961). Both increased and decreased rate of firing of bulbopontine reticular units could be observed as a consequence of cortical spreading depression. The reactions to homo- and contralateral spreading depression were similar.

Acknowledgement

The research reported in this document has been supported in part by the Office of Scientific Research of the *Air Research and Development Command, United States Air Force*, through its European Office under Contract AF 61(052)-119.

Dr. G. B. ARDEN held an Alexander Piggot Wernher Memorial Fellowship in Ophthalmology. His present adress is Institute of Ophthalmology, Judd Street, London W. C. 1, England.

References

1. ARDEN, G. B., and Y.-M. LIU: Some responses of the lateral geniculate body of the rabbit to flickering light stimuli. Acta physiol. scand. 48, 49—62 (1960).
2. — and U. SÖDERBERG: The relationship of lateral geniculate activity to the electrocorticogram in the presence or absence of the optic tract input. Experientia (Basel) 15, 163—164 (1959).
3. — — The transfer of optic information through the lateral geniculate body of the rabbit. In W. A. ROSENBLITH (Editor), Principles of sensory communication. Cambridge: Technology Press 1961.
4. BARRIS, R. W., W. R. INGRAM and S. W. RANSON: Optic connections of diencephalon and midbrain of cat. J. comp. Neurol. 62, 117—153 (1935).
5. BATINI, C., F. MAGNI, M. PALESTINI, G. F. ROSSI and A. ZANCHETTI: Neural mechanisms underlying the enduring EEG and behavioural activation in the midpontine pretrigeminal cat. Arch. ital. Biol. 97, 13—25 (1959).
6. — G. MORUZZI, M. PALESTINI, G. F. ROSSI and A. ZANCHETTI: Effects of completepontine transsections on the sleep-wakefulness rhythm: the midpontine pretrigeminal preparation. Arch. ital. Biol. 97, 1—12 (1959).
7. — M. PALESTINI, G. F. ROSSI and A. ZANCHETTI: EEG activation patterns in the midpontine pretrigeminal cat following sensory deafferentation. Arch. ital. Biol. 97, 26—32 (1959).
8. BREMER, F.: Cerveau "isolé" et physiologie du sommeil. C. R. Soc. Biol. (Paris) 118, 1235 to 1241 (1935).
9. BUCHER, V. M., and S. M. BÜRGI: Some observations on fiber connections of di- and mesencephalon in cat; fiber connections of tectum opticum. J. comp. Neurol. 93, 139—171 (1950).
10. BUSER, P., P. BORENSTEIN et J. BRUNER: Etude des systèmes associatifs visuels et auditifs chez le chat anesthésié au chloralose. Electroenceph. clin. Neurophysiol. 11, 305—324 (1959).
11. COBB, S.: Photic driving as a cause of clinical seizures in epileptic patients. Arch. Neurol. Psychiat. (Chicago) 58, 70—71 (1947).
12. COURJON, J., and H. BONNET: Comparative effects of Metrazol and Megimide in activation of epileptic patients. Electroenceph. clin. Neurophysiol. 8, 710 (1956).
13. DROSSOPOULO, G., H. GASTAUT, G. VERDEAUX, J. VERDEAUX and E. SCHULLER: Comparison of EEG "activation" by pentamethylenetetrazol (Metrazol) and Bemegride (Megimide). Electroenceph. clin. Neurophysiol. 8, 710—711 (1956).
14. FLODMARK, S., I. PETERSÉN and K. STENBERG: Activation with Megimide ($\beta\beta$-methylethyl-glutarimide) in electroencephalographic investigation of epileptic conditions. Electroenceph. clin. Neurophysiol. 9, 371—372 (1957).
15. GIBBS, F. A., and E. L. GIBBS: Atlas of electroencephalography. Cambridge: Addison-Wesley Press Inc. 1945.
16. GILLILAN, L. A.: The connections of the basal optic root (posterior accessory optic tract) and its nucleus in various mammals. J. comp. Neurol. 74, 367—408 (1941).
17. GUDDEN, B. VON: Über den Tractus peduncularis transversus. Arch. Psychiat. 11, 415—423 (1881).
18. HAMASAKI, D., and E. MARG: Electrophysiological study of the posterior accessory optic tract. Amer. J. Physiol. 199, 522—528 (1960).
19. HERNÁNDEZ-PEÓN, R.: In press in W. A. Rosenblith Editor: Principles of sensory communication. Cambridge: Technology Press 1961.
20. — C. GUZMAN-FLORES, M. ALCAREZ and A. FERNÁNDEZ-GUARDIOLA: Sensory transmission in visual pathway during "attention" in unanaesthetized cats. Acta neurol. lat.-amer. 3, 1—8 (1957).
21. — A. LAVIN, C. ALCOCER-CUARÓN and J. P. MARCELIN: Electrical activity of the olfactory bulb during wakefulness and sleep. Electroenceph. clin. Neurophysiol. 12, 41—58 (1960).

22. Hernámdez-Peón, R., H. Sherrer and M. Velasco: Central influences on afferent conduction in the somatic and visual pathway. Acta neurol. lat.-amer. **2**, 8—22 (1956).
23. Hunter, J., and D. H. Ingvar: Pathways mediating Metrazol induced irradiation of visual impulses. Electroenceph. clin. Neurophysiol. **7**, 39—60 (1955).
24. Ingvar, D. H., and J. Hunter: Influence of visual cortex on light impulses in the brain stem of the unanaesthetized cat. Acta physiol. scand. **33**, 194—218 (1955).
25. Leao, A. A. P.: Pial circulation and spreading depression of activity in the cerebral cortex. J. Neurophysiol. **7**, 391—396 (1944).
26. O'Leary, J.: Structural analysis of lateral geniculate nucleus of cat. J. comp. Neurol. **73**, 405—430 (1940).
27. Penfield, W., and H. H. Jasper: Epilepsy and the functional anatomy of the human brain. Boston: Little, Brown and Co. 1954.
28. Rodin, E. A., L. T. Rutledge and H. D. Calhoun: Megimide and Metrazol. Electroenceph. clin. Neurophysiol. **10**, 719—723 (1958).
29. Roger, H.: Thesis 1948. Quoted by Thiry, S.: Contribution à l'etude des effets de la stimulation lumineuse intermittante en électroencéphalographie. Mémoire pour le titre d'assistant étranger. Faculté de médecine de Paris, 1950.
30. Shulman, A., F. H. Shaw, N. M. Cass and H. M. Whyte: A new treatment of barbiturate intoxication. Brit. med. J. **1**, 1238—1244 (1955).
31. Söderberg, U.: Effect of Bemegride (Megimide) on cerebral blood flow and electrical activity of brain. Arch. Neurol. Psychiat. **79**, 239—249 (1958).
32. Van Harreveld, A., and J. S. Stamm: Cortical responses to Metrazol and sensory stimulation in the rabbit. Electroenceph. clin. Neurophysiol. **7**, 363—370 (1955).
33. Wall, P. D., A. G. Rémond and R. L. Dobson: Studies on the mechanism of the action of visual afferents on motor cortex excitability. Electroenceph. clin. Neurophysiol. **3**, 385—393 (1953).
34. Walter, W. G., V. J. Dovey and H. Shipton: Analysis of electrical response of human cortex to photic stimulation. Nature (Lond.) **158**, 540—541 (1946).
35. Winokur, G. L., S. A. Trufant, R. B. King and J. O'Leary: Thalamocortical activity during spreading depression. Electroenceph. clin. Neurophysiol. **2**, 79—90 (1950).

Discussion

R. Jung: Bei der Katze scheinen nach Baumgartners Untersuchungen mit Retina-Ischämie[1] die corticalen Neurone der Area 17 vorwiegend von der Pons aus aktiviert zu werden: cerveau-isolé-Katzen zeigen nach ischämischer Ausschaltung der spezifischen Opticusafferenz keine Spontanaktivität mehr, während sie bei encephale-isolé-Katzen erhalten ist. Beim encéphale-isolé können auch Schmerzimpulse über den Trigeminus bei Augendruck aktivierend wirken. Dies entspricht Söderbergs Untersuchungen am Kaninchen-Geniculatum, doch haben wir den Eindruck, daß bei der Katze die reticulären Afferenzen mehr zum Cortex laufen als zum Geniculatum.

A. Arduini: Two questions are raised:
1. Is the cerebellum intact? In this case in the pretrigeminal preparation impulses may bridge the gap through the cerebellum.
2. It is asked whether the intraocular pressure is made when the eye was dark or light adapted.

U. Grüsser-Cornehls: Die von Ihnen im Geniculatum des Kaninchens gefundenen nichtvisuellen Elemente stellen möglicherweise eine Eigentümlichkeit dieser Tierart dar, da sie im Geniculatum der Katze fehlen. In der visuellen Rinde des Kaninchens, die Kornmüller mit Hilfe von Makroableitungen abgegrenzt hat, konnten wir mit Mikroelektroden mehr als 50% nicht durch Lichtreize beeinflußbare Neurone registrieren. Man hat den Eindruck, daß diese sehr dicht mit visuellen Neuronen vermischt sind.

---

[1] Baumgartner, G., O. Creutzfeldt u. R. Jung: Microphysiology of cortical neurones in acute anoxia and in retinal ischemia. In J. S. Meyer and H. Gastaut: Cerebral anoxia and the electroencephalogram, pg. 5—34. Springfield: C. C. Thomas 1961.

U. Söderberg (zu Jung): Bei unseren Tieren waren die Schmerznerven der Augen entweder durchschnitten oder mit Lidocain („Xylocain") gelähmt. Die ischämische Ausschaltung der Opticusafferenz gab keine Veränderungen in Blutdruck, Pulsfrequenz oder im EEG. Beim Kaninchen wirken Schmerzimpulse am Geniculatum überwiegend inhibitorisch.

(To Arduini): The cerebellum was removed by suction in all the "pretrigeminal preparations". The brain stem transsection was then made through the posterior fossa which was closed afterwards with dental cement through which a thin rubber tubing was inserted as a drain. The rostral and caudal ends of the brain stem were separated by a thick piece of paper.

The answer of the second question is that all our rabbits were fairly well dark adapted.

(Zu Grüsser-Cornehls): Unsere „nicht-visuellen Elemente" sind von den Versuchsbedingungen abhängig, d. h. nach größerer Variation der Lichtreize ist die Zahl „nicht-visueller" Elemente kleiner, als wenn wir nur Flimmerlicht benutzen. Auch Reizstärke, Dunkeladaptation, Hirnstammdurchtrennung, Narkose usw. sind von großer Bedeutung.

C. Periphere und zentrale Grundlagen des Farbensehens

Opponent Chromatic Induction and Wavelength Discrimination[1,2]

By

LEO M. HURVICH and DOROTHEA HURVICH-JAMESON

With 5 Figures

One of the first concerns in any investigation of color vision, physiological, or behavioral, is whether or not the organism in question shows evidence of being able to respond differentially to different spectral wavelengths. The wavelength discrimination function for humans has been repeatedly investigated by psychophysical procedures (*13*), but little systematic evidence is available on the way this discriminatory capacity depends on the various parameters of stimulus conditions and physiological state.

This paper reports some experimental data showing the way in which wavelength discrimination varies with changes in chromatic adaptation and surround stimulation. Also, comparisons are presented between the experimental data and theoretically derived discrimination functions. The latter are based on the opponent-process theory of color vision and represent a continuation of our previous theoretical work (*6*), (*10*), (*11*).

To understand the way visual responses vary with varying pre-exposure and surround stimulation requires a consideration not only of the relatively simple adaptation processes but of induction processes and neural interactions as well. In our recent attempts to get at these mechanisms by analyzing the data of psychophysical experiments we have been measuring binocular — or more correctly — haploscopic color matching functions, for various adapting and surround stimuli. In such experiments, the surrounds of the test field (seen by the right eye) and the three-variable comparison field (seen by the left eye) are usually asymmetrical, that is, they are of different specified chromaticities (*8*). In determining color matches under such conditions it quickly becomes apparent that the observer's discriminative capacities change markedly with different surround chromaticities. For example, if with one surround the proportions of the three matching stimuli indicate that a clear-cut difference is perceived between, say, wavelengths 500 mμ

---

[1] From the Department of Psychology, New York University.

[2] The research project of which this study forms a part is being supported by grants G-4848 from the National Science Foundation and B-1721 from the National Institutes of Health.

and 510 mμ we find that merely by surrounding the same test stimuli with a field of different chromaticity, the new color equations indicate that 500 mμ and 510 mμ are now no longer differentiated by the observer. Clearly, the observer's discriminative capacities can be reduced by the presence of certain adapting and surround stimuli. This result reminds us, of course, of a large number of older papers by investigators like BURCH (3), ABNEY (1), and ALLEN (2), who were concerned with "selective fatigue" as a method for determining the "primary" sensations and regarded experimentally induced so-called "artificial color blindnesses" as analogues of congenital color disturbances.

If we examine the discrimination data in the enormous psychophysical literature on color vision, however, we find very little useful information on wavelength discrimination and chromatic adaptation and we know only two directly relevant studies.

LAURENS and HAMILTON did measure complete wavelength discrimination functions for different conditions of what they call "selective fatigue". In these experiments reported in 1923 (4), the discrimination measures were taken after periods of pre-exposure to chromatic stimuli. It was, incidentally, the normal, non-adapted data of LAURENS and HAMILTON that HECHT sought to fit with his quantitative theoretical color vision schema (5). Unfortunately, there is no indication in any of the LAURENS and HAMILTON work that stray light was controlled in their spectral apparatus. A more serious shortcoming is that the traditional "red", "green" and "blue" fatiguing lights they used were of different luminances. By using differently selective fatiguing lights at different luminances they confounded the effects of the wavelength and luminance variables. Regrettably, examples of similar confounding can still be found in the present-day literature on chromatic adaptation.

W. D. WRIGHT has also measured the effect of adaptation on the size of the discrimination step (16). Unfortunately, he did not record complete wavelength discrimination curves for a given state of adaptation. Instead, the discrimination step was measured at only three wavelengths 494 mμ, 530 mμ, and 580 mμ for three different adaptations: "white" (2800° K), a red, and a green. Although variations in intensity of adapting light were investigated, the intensity ranges were not comparable for the different adapting lights. The data are consequently insufficiently complete or systematic for our purposes. To interpret the discrimination changes he found WRIGHT merely restated his results in terms of deduced rates of change in three assumed sensations with respect to stimulus change for the different adaptations. Even at this qualitatively descriptive level, however, WRIGHT encounters a major theoretical difficulty. Adaptation to green produced an increase in the $\Delta \lambda$ for yellow (580 mμ) which was a positively increasing function of the adaptation brightness; with adaptation to red, on the other hand, there was (except for an initial increase) a progressive decrease in $\Delta \lambda$ for the same yellow test stimulus. In the traditional three color view which WRIGHT espouses, yellow discriminations should, of course, be affected similarly whether the adaptation is red or green.

We are currently obtaining some systematic information on wavelength discrimination in our own laboratory. Our purpose in measuring such functions is twofold: we want (I.) to supplement our haploscopic matching data for different

10

adapting-surround fields in order to facilitate their interpretation; we want (II.) to compare the discrimination functions obtained experimentally with the differently colored surrounds with theoretical functions predicted by the opponent-colors and opponent-induction hypotheses. In previous work we have made such comparisons for wavelength discrimination data measured at several different luminance levels in a dark surround (6).

Two Farrand prism monochromators placed at 90° to one another provide the spectral stimuli for the wavelength discrimination experiments. By means of appropriate prisms and lens system the observer sees a Maxwellian view of a bipartite field. The test and comparison areas making up the bipartite field are viewed monocularly and the total size (2°) is determined by an aperture stop in a non-selective diffuse reflector from whose surface the light of the adapting surround is reflected to the eye. The illuminated surround subtends about 35° in visual angle and its chromaticity is controlled by filtering a 2800° K, 6 volt microscope lamp that is suspended above the reflector surface.

After 10 minutes of preliminary dark adaptation to eliminate the effects of previous uncontrolled chromatic light exposure, the observer was given a three minute exposure to a given surround illumination. A series of threshold measures was then obtained throughout the spectrum. One such series was made in the short to long wavelength direction and a second series was taken in the opposite direction. In all instances, however, the threshold measure itself was obtained for comparison wavelengths longer than that of a given test stimulus. Initially, the experimenter presented the same wavelength in the test and comparison fields and, by adjusting the brightness of the comparison stimulus, the observer achieved a complete color match. The experimenter then introduced a considerable wavelength difference — the comparison field was changed to a longer wavelength — and the observer varied the comparison field luminance until brightness equality was reached. If the test and comparison fields were judged to be discriminable one from the other, the experimenter decreased the wavelength difference and the procedure was repeated until a non-discriminable comparison wavelength was reached. The wavelength difference was then increased again by small steps (the comparison luminance always adjusted to equality by the observer) until a color difference was again reported. At this point the wavelength difference between the comparison and test fields constitutes the just discriminable $\Delta \lambda$.

Experimental results for the one observer for whom we have so far obtained systematic data for a number of conditions are shown in Figure 1. The data are for two relatively desaturated surrounds, both at a fixed luminance of 10 mL, and for three different test luminances. The three levels of spectral test stimuli were 5 mL, 10 mL, and 20 mL, respectively, and discrimination measurements were taken at 20 mμ intervals. The data for the pale yellowish-red surround are designated in the figure by the number 30 (the Wratten filter designation); the data for the pale bluish-green surround are identified by the Wratten filter number 38A.

The changes that occur in the observer's discriminative capacity as the surround is changed from yellowish-red to bluish-green are marked; in the mid-spectrum the data for the bluish-green surround are on the whole lower than those for the yellowish-red surround, but in the long wave region the $\Delta \lambda$ tends to increase more rapidly than it does with the yellowish-red surround. Other systematic variations occur: for the blue-green surround the long wave minimum is higher than the short wave minimum at the lowest test luminance ($L_{0.5}$); with luminance increase there is a reversal and at the highest luminance (L_2) the short wave minimum is relatively higher than the long wave one. For the yellow-red adapted functions, on the other hand, the short and long wave minima tend to retain the same relative magnitudes at all luminances, but there is a progressive increase in sensitivity throughout the spectrum as the luminance increases. Furthermore, for the yellowish-red adapted functions there is a progressive shift of the mid-spectral maximum towards the longer wavelengths as luminance is increased. Finally, the difference between the discrimination functions for the two different adaptations are least at the highest test luminance. The latter result is consonant with the view that inductive effects produced in a test area by a surround of constant luminance are progressively less significant as the focal stimulation is increased in magnitude relative to that of the inducing stimulus (9) (12).

As we have shown in earlier papers (6), (7), by using the basic measures of the opponent-colors theory — the three functions expressing the relative distributions of whiteness, redness and greenness, and yellowness and blueness throughout the spectrum — we can derive percentage expressions for spectral hue and spectral saturation. Since wavelength discrimination depends on the rates of change in both hue and saturation throughout the spectrum, the percentage expressions for these two color attributes provide a basis for calculating the discrimination functions to be expected on the basis of theory. With changes in chromatic pre-exposure and surround, the spectral distributions of the three pairs of color responses are, of course, altered, and by postulating specific mechanisms of adaptation or opponent induction or both, quantitative predictions can also be made for the wavelength discrimination functions to be expected for specific experimental surround conditions. We have calculated such theoretical functions for the experiments of Figure 1, and compared them with the experimental functions for our one observer. With respect to the differences associated with the two surround chromaticities, the main features of the theoretical functions are essentially similar to those obtained experimentally. With the bluish-green surround, the $\Delta \lambda$ is predicted to be relatively small throughout the mid-spectral range but to increase rapidly at the longer wavelengths, whereas the $\Delta\lambda$ for the yellowish-red surround condition is predicted to be relatively large throughout the mid-spectral region, with better discrimination (smaller $\Delta \lambda$) at the long wavelengths. The predicted differences associated with change in test stimulus luminance are, however, of smaller magnitude than the differences measured experimentally.

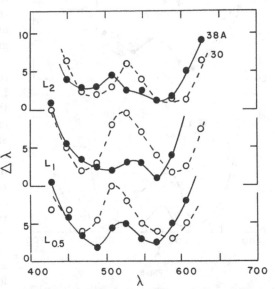

Fig. 1. Wavelength discrimination results for one observer for 2 pre-exposure/surround conditions. Open circles are experimental points for a yellowish-red (Wratten No. 30) surround and filled circles are experimental points for a bluish-green (Wratten No. 38A) surround. Surround luminance is 10 mL in all instances. (L_2), test:surround = 2:1; (L_1), test:surround = 1:1; and $(L_{0.5})$, test:surround = 0.5:1

Figures 2 and 3 show the experimental data obtained for more strongly saturated pre-exposure/surround stimuli. The yellowish-red surround (Wratten No. 29) and the green surround (Wratten No. 75) were of the same luminance (10 mL) as

10*

the previously described surround stimuli (Nos. 30 and 38A), and differed from them primarily in increased saturation. In each case two test luminances were used: one was $^1/_2$ the surround luminance of 10 mL and the other was twice this luminance. In Figures 2 and 3 the theoretically derived wavelength discrimination functions calculated for comparable conditions are shown in the lower half of the graph.

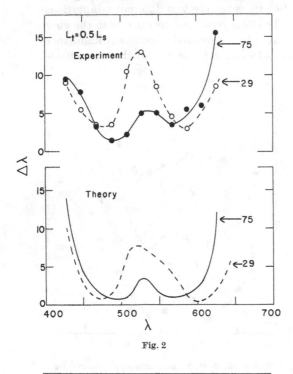

Fig. 2

In all instances, i. e., both for the relatively desaturated surrounds and for the more saturated ones, both the experimental data and theoretical functions point up an unexpected and paradoxical effect: without exception the observer is more sensitive in the longwave spectral region in the presence of a yellowish-red surround and more sensitive in the mid-spectral region in the presence of a green surround. (This generality depends, of course, on the spectral region examined. If we consider a test wavelength where the two discrimination functions intersect, then for this wavelength and luminance, both surrounds are equivalent in their effects.)

We consider this finding to be an especially significant one. The tendency is almost universal to argue that demonstrated deficiencies in discriminative capacity are due to an absence of specific receptor function or a decrease in specific receptor activity (*14*). In these terms, a decrease in long wave discriminative

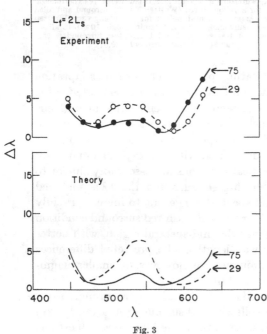

Fig. 3

Fig. 2. Wavelength discrimination for one observer for two relatively saturated pre-exposure/surround conditions at 10 mL luminance level are shown in the upper half of the graph and predicted functions based on the opponent colors theory are shown in the lower half of the graph. Open circles are experimental points for a yellowish-red (Wratten No. 29) surround and filled circles are experimental points for a green (Wratten No. 75) surround. Continuous and dashed lines in lower portion of graph are based on calculations for these surrounds and for a ratio of test : surround = 0.5:1

Fig. 3. Same as Figure 2. Ratio of test: surround luminance = 2:1

capacity, for example, would be taken to reflect a loss of red receptor activity. But our data show that with yellow-red adaptation, which presumably entails decreased yellow-red activity, discrimination among long wavelengths is not worse but rather better than for green adaptation. The same is true for mid-spectral discrimination: as we have already noted above, it is better with green adaptation than it is with yellow-red adaptation.

A brief outline of the procedures used in deriving theoretical predictions for the experimental data will at the same time show what lies at the root of this finding — one that is unexpected in terms of traditional theory.

The spectral distribution functions for the three paired responses of the opponent-colors theory that we have published in earlier papers (7) refer to a neutral condition of adaptation and a single level of stimulus luminance. As the stimulus luminance is increased or decreased, the magnitudes of the whiteness, redness or greenness, and yellowness or blueness responses at any given wavelength are altered relative to each other (this matter is discussed more fully in our second paper, see pp. 154), and the rates of change in hue and saturation throughout the spectrum are consequently modified. As discussed above, the least discriminable

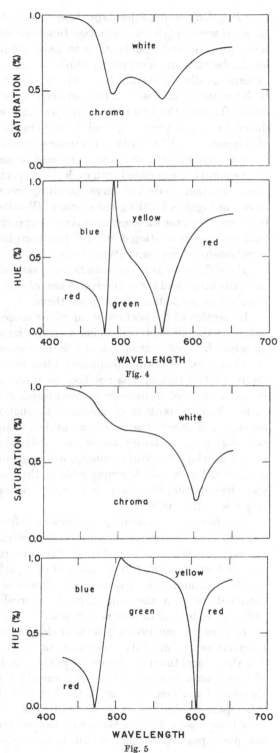

Fig. 4

Fig. 5

Fig. 4. Theoretical spectral hue and saturation coefficient curves calculated for a green surround (Wratten No. 75) and a spectral test luminance of $1/2$ the surround luminance

Fig. 5. Theoretical spectral hue and saturation coefficient curves calculated for a yellowish-red surround (Wratten No. 29) and a spectral test luminance of $1/2$ the surround luminance

wavelength difference depends on these rates of change, and consequently the precise forms of wavelength discrimination functions depend on the level of test stimulus luminance. In earlier publications we have compared theoretically predicted wavelength discrimination curves for different luminance levels with the data obtained experimentally by Weale (6), (15). In the present experiments we are varying both the test luminance and the chromaticity of the pre-exposure/surround stimulation. To take the latter effect into account, we assume that the excitation produced by, say, a green surround, induces in the focal test area a fixed magnitude of opponent "red" activity. This induced activity is assumed to be constant for a given surround stimulus, and is assumed to combine in additive fashion with the focal excitation associated with each given spectral test stimulus. The spectral hue and saturation coefficient curves resulting from such a theoretical treatment are shown in Figure 4 for the green surround (Wratten No. 75) and for the spectral test luminance of $1/_2$ the surround luminance. For comparison, Figure 5 shows the theoretical hue and saturation coefficient functions for the same test luminance but for a yellowish-red surround (Wratten No. 29).

The differences between both hue and saturation functions in the two instances are quite large, and these differences are, of course, reflected in the wavelength discrimination predictions based upon them.

Inspection of the coefficient functions makes it easy to see why poor discrimination in the mid-spectral region need not imply a deficiency of green response; likewise why poor discrimination in the long wave region need not imply a deficiency of red response. In our experiments, when the observer discrimates poorly in the green spectral region, it is not because there is a decrease in green activity but rather because of an increase in green response induced by the red surround, and with a high percentage of greenness throughout the mid-spectral wavelengths, the rate of change in hue from one wavelength to the next is relatively slow. A slow rate of change, the critical factor, may obviously occur when green activity is high as well as when it is low. Similarly, with a green surround inducing red excitation in the focal area, which simply adds to the focal red excitation aroused by long wave test stimuli, the observer becomes less capable of a differential wavelength response in this region.

One has to be extremely cautious therefore in concluding that an organism showing poor discrimination in a given spectral region is thereby demonstrating absence or decrease of a particular chromatic response, when poor discrimination may, in fact, be related to an excess of that particular response. The observer who fails to discriminate long wave stimuli from one another in the presence of a green surround may, at the same time, be marveling at the highly saturated deep yellowish-reds that he sees and reports.

In pursuing our investigations of the discrimination problem we plan both to extend the experimental measures and to explore the theoretical analysis more fully. The theoretical functions represent predictions for a group average, and we should, of course, have comparative data for more than a single observer. More basic to the theoretical analysis, however, is the fact that the predicted functions included in this report are derived on the basis of a simplified assumption that changes in induced response activities alone will account for the discrimination changes from one pre-exposure/surround condition to another. In these derivations we have ignored possible long term sensitivity reductions and photochemical light exposure effects. Such long term changes can be taken into account theoretically [as they have been in some of our earlier work (11)] by the application of the von Kries coefficient law, which assumes that, with adaptation, multiplicative sensitivity reductions occur in direct proportion to the excitation of a given system by the adapting stimulus. Changes of this latter sort may, of course, be involved in the current experiments together with the induced response changes. Other factors involved in the theoretical predictions that require further verification are: the assumed magnitude of the minimal difference in hue and saturation coefficients that determines the $\Delta \lambda$, and the assumed constancy of this value for the luminance range in question; the precise value of the induction factor (assumed to be 0.5 in the present study) which relates the magnitude of induced activity to the magnitude of the inducing (surround) activity; and, finally, the precise forms of the different response vs. intensity functions for the three paired response systems (assumed in the present study to be power functions differing one from the other by a 0.1 exponent difference). All of these specific assumptions required for quantitative prediction must be examined more closely and verified by further tests. Their specific validity or non-validity does not, of course, affect the opponent-colors model in its essential features as a useful and inclusive explanatory theory.

Summary

Experimental measures of wavelength discrimination were determined in a 2° foveal field with surrounds of four different chromaticities. The luminance level of the spectral test stimuli was also varied in three steps in different experiments.

The results show that wavelength discrimination is systematically dependent on both the hue and saturation of the pre-exposure and surround stimuli, and that it is further dependent on the test luminance for any given surround condition. With primarily red surrounds, discrimination is relatively poor in the mid-spectral region and relatively good in the long-wave spectral region, and the converse is true for primarily green surrounds. The differences are more marked for the more saturated surround stimuli, and for a given surround, they are more marked for the test luminance level that is lower than that of the surround. The particular discrimination changes that occur with particular surround colors are not consistent with the prevailing notion that poor discrimination in a given spectral region implies loss or reduction of a particular chromatic response activity.

Theoretical discrimination functions, based on the opponent-colors theory, are presented to show that the experimental results can be accounted for, to a first approximation, on the basis of opponent chromatic induction effects brought about by the presence of the chromatic surround activity in the visual field.

References

1. Abney, W. de W.: Researches in colour vision and the trichromatic theory. London: Longmans, Green & Co. 1913.
2. Allen, F.: Some phenomena of the persistance of vision. Phys. Rev. 28, 45—56 (1909).
3. Burch, G. J.: On artificial temporary colour-blindness with an examination of the colour sensations of 109 persons. Phil. Trans. B 191, 1—34 (1899).
4. Hamilton, W. F., and H. Laurens: The sensibility of the fatigued eye to differences in wave-length in relation to color blindness. Amer. J. Physiol. 65, 569—584 (1923).

5. Hecht, S.: Vision. II. The nature of the photoreceptor process. In C. Murchison (ed). Handbook of General Experimental Psychology, 704—828, Worcester, Mass.: Clark University Press 1934.
6. Hurvich, L. M., and D. Jameson: Some quantitative aspects of an opponent-colors theory. II. Brightness, saturation and hue in normal and dichromatic vision. J. opt. Soc. Amer. **45**, 602—616 (1955).
7. — — An opponent-process theory of color vision. Psychol. Rev. **64**, 384—404 (1957).
8. — — Further development of a quantified opponent-colours theory. In Visual Problems of Colour. II, 691—723. London: Her Majesty's Stationery Office, 1958.
9. — — Perceived color, induction effects, and opponent-response mechanisms. J. gen. Physiol. **43**, 63—80 (1960).
10. Jameson, D., and L. M. Hurvich: Some quantitative aspects of an opponent-colors theory. I. Chromatic responses and spectral saturation. J. opt. Soc. Amer. **45**, 546—552 (1955).
11. — — Some quantitative aspects of an opponent-colors theory. III. Changes in brightness, saturation and hue with chromatic adaptation. J. opt. Soc. Amer. **46**, 405—415 (1956).
12. — — Perceived color and its dependence on focal, surrounding, and preceding stimulus variables. J. opt. Soc. Amer. **49**, 890—898 (1959).
13. Judd, D. B.: Chromaticity sensibility to stimulus differences. J. opt. Soc. Amer. **22**, 72—108 (1932).
14. Miles, R. C.: Color vision in the squirrel monkey. J. comp. physiol. Psychol. **51**, 328—331 (1958)
15. Weale, R. A.: Hue discrimination in para-central parts of the human retina measured at different luminance levels. J. Physiol. (Lond.) **113**, 115—122 (1951).
16. Wright, W. D.: Researches on normal and defective colour vision. St. Louis: C. V. Mosby Company 1947.

Discussion see. pg. 161.

Opponent-Colors Theory and Physiological Mechanisms[1,2]

By

Dorothea Hurvich-Jameson and Leo M. Hurvich

With 5 Figures

Those who study the perceptual or psychophysical behavior of intact humans constantly raise questions about the implications of the psychophysical data for physiology, and, at this level, the answers to such questions are necessarily inferences, deductions, or hypotheses. For evidence that our inferences and hypotheses about underlying mechanisms are, at best, confirmable, or, at least, plausible, we look to the ever growing accumulation of information provided by the researches of physiologists and biochemists.

Our experience in the field of color vision has been that the wide variety of perceptual phenomena that have been investigated, both qualitatively and quantitatively, are most consistently encompassed within a theory of the visual mechanism that envisages three paired and opponent response systems underlying the three pairs of opponent phenomenal qualities: red-green, yellow-blue, and white-black (12). The most basic and necessary hypothesis of the opponent-colors

[1] From the Department of Psychology, New York University.
[2] The research project of which this study form a parts is being supported by grants G-4848 from the National Science Foundation and B-1721 from the National Institutes of Health.

theory is the postulated existence of two mutually opposed modes of response in the visual nervous tissue to correspond with the mutually exclusive perceptual responses to different kinds of light stimulation. For many years after HERING first proposed it (10), the opponent-process theory failed to receive serious attention in many quarters precisely because the physiological information then available provided no support for the fundamental assumption that a physiological response could occur in either of two mutually opposed modes. Stimulation was generally thought to produce activation in various degrees, or to leave the tissue in an inactive, quiescent state, and any other possibility seemed to many to be logically impossible, as well as experimentally unverified. In contrast to this earlier situation, however, we now know that the neural visual tissue may respond to light stimulation by either on- or off-discharge, by graded potential changes of either positive or negative polarity, by either excitatory or inhibitory events (2), (5), (6), (16), (21). The demonstrated existence of such opponent physiological processes thus fully justifies the basic postulate of the theory.

What of the assumption that such opponent activities differentiate the physiological responses associated with the paired color qualities, red-green, yellow-blue ? Positive evidence related to this assumption is only just beginning to accumulate, but during the past five to ten years we have learned that in certain preparations, electrophysiological measures of spectral response do show reversals when the spectral stimuli are varied from short to long wavelengths. Examples of relevance here are the reversal of polarity of slow potential response measures with change in stimulus wavelength for the mullet retina (18), the change from on-discharges to off-discharges in the ganglion cells of the goldfish (23), the comparable change from on- to off-discharges in some of the single cells of the monkey lateral geniculate (2), and the different on- and off-patterns recorded from the optic lobe of the pigeon (4).

Notwithstanding the rapid progress in this area in recent years, important and basic problems are still outstanding. We do not yet know in what structures the opponent responses originate or in what way they are generated by the receptor activities, nor do we know very much about the photochemistry of the retinal cones. Is the goldfish, whose retina shows evidence of a two-part color system, like a human dichromat in terms of visual discriminative capacities ? And what would behavioral indices of color discrimination show in the cases reported by SVAETICHIN of the three different species of fish which would be classified, in terms of the electrophysiological findings as monochromats, dichromats, and trichromats, respectively ? What perceptual significance should be attributed to the disproportionate increase with increase in intensity in long versus short-wave responses in the goldfish records if these responses are, indeed, not related respectively to scotopic and photopic receptor mechanisms ? (24).

A basic question still unanswered is the way in which the paired and opponent effects are specifically differentiated or coded to provide the necessary qualitative differentiation among the three paired color systems of the trichromatic individual. That some sort of tri-variate specificity must exist in the visual mechanism to account for the three-variable nature of human color experience seems self-evident. Whether this coding will ultimately be shown to be a matter of specific anatomical cells or cell layers (which seems to be the current bias among physiologists) or a subtler matter of biological process specificity (HERING's own original conjecture)

(*10*), is an important question, but not one that we can fruitfully pursue at this time. However, whatever the biological tag that codes red or green activity as different from yellow or blue activity, and this, in turn, from white or black activity, this biological differentation will probably involve, in addition to response differences in wavelength selectivity, other differences in physiological response characteristics in the three different systems. One such characteristic with which this paper is mainly concerned, is the function relating strength of physiological response to intensity of light stimulation.

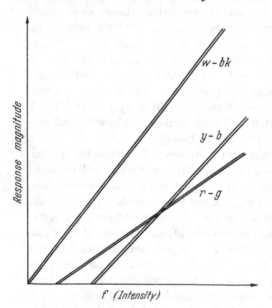

Figure 1 is an illustrative diagram in which the ordinate represents response, and the abscissa some unspecified function of stimulus intensity (*13*). The figure is intended to illustrate two differences in the characteristics of the three paired systems. One is a difference in threshold, with the achromatic system (w-bk) having the lowest threshold, the red-green system (r-g) the next, and the yellow-blue system (y-b) the highest threshold. Once the threshold has been reached, moreover, the rate of increase in response with increase in stimulus intensity is not the same for the three systems: it is most rapid for the achromatic system, somewhat slower for the yellow-blue system, and has a still lower slope for the red-green system.

Fig. 1. Schematic representation of the functional relations (unspecified) between the paired chromatic and achromatic response systems and stimulus magnitude

This illustrative diagram is consistent with the psychophysical data. The postulated threshold differences account for the so-called achromatic or photochromatic interval — the name given to the fact that the absolute light threshold, even in the fovea, is found at a lower intensity than the chromatic threshold at which spectral lights are first perceived as having hue (*1*). They are also consistent with the facts of so-called small-field dichromacy, a term which describes the condition of yellow-blue blindness found in normal color vision when very small stimulus areas of low intensity are observed (*3*), (*13*). The different slopes of the three functions are consistent with the change in saturation of spectral lights when luminance is varied at any given wavelength, and also with the changes in hue that occur with change in level of spectral light stimulation — the well-known Bezold-Brücke phenomenon. The different slopes are, furthermore, consistent with the changed forms of the spectral discrimination functions with changes in intensity under otherwise constant and standard conditions, that is, with the spectral hue and saturation discrimination data (*11*).

In a qualitative way, therefore, this illustrative picture is extremely useful in helping to account theoretically for some of the intensive phenomena of color perception. As soon as we wish to make the account quantitative, we must, of course, replace our very general f (Intensity) by explicit functional relations. What, specifically, are these functions ? Are they invariant, and if not, on what variables do they depend, and what is the nature of the dependence ? Remembering that the three functions will presumably be found to differ one from the other along the lines indicated above, let us examine more closely the achromatic response function — the one on which we should expect to find the most evidence, both from physiology and from psychophysical experiments.

Discussion of this relation usually starts with FECHNER, and his postulated logarithmic relation between psychological magnitude and physical stimulation, and FECHNER's relation would seem to find confirmation in terms of physiological response characteristics (5). Whether measurements are made of graded potentials or frequency of impulse discharge, the relation most usually found in electrophysiological studies tends to be described as one in which the electrical response index is logarithmically related to stimulus intensity. On the psychophysical side, scales of sensory magnitude which are synthesized by summing measured just-noticeable-differences along the intensity continuum are approximately logarithmic functions (22). The legitimacy of using this procedure for expressing sensory magnitude has been seriously questioned, however, and from as far back as FECHNER's own time, strong arguments have been brought forward to indicate that the proper psychophysical relation is a power function, rather than a logarithmic one (9). The case for the power function has most recently and forcibly been argued by STEVENS, who has marshalled an impressive amount of evidence from direct psychological scaling experiments in favor of this view (20). Our own inquiries of electrophysiologists on this matter have left us with the impression that it would be extremely difficult to determine from electrical indices whether the response vs. stimulus intensity function is more precisely approximated by a logarithmic or a power relation. A much reproduced graph of direct relevance to this problem is that originally presented by HARTLINE and GRAHAM in 1932 showing spike frequency vs. log intensity for the eye of the Limulus (7). This graph contains two curves, one which represents the frequency of the initial maximal discharge and which unquestionably shows a logarithmic dependence on stimulus intensity throughout most of the range. A second function represents the frequency of discharge in the same preparation and for the same stimuli, but measured 3.5 seconds after onset of illumination. This latter function is definitely not a simple logarithmic one, and our own test of the same data makes it clear that, in this case, the dependence of response frequency on stimulus intensity can be described quite well by a power relation with an exponent of 0.3, — the same exponent that STEVENS finds for brightness magnitude in the dark-adapted eye (20). If we wished to extrapolate from Limulus to human vision, we might venture the guess that whether the stimulus vs. response relation is logarithmic or a power function may depend on flash duration, but rather than forcing that parallel, let us look at some of the other parameters that might influence the psychophysical brightness-luminance relation.

Figure 2 shows some of our own brightness scaling data, obtained, not for the dark-adapted eye, but rather with a test stimulus in the presence of an illuminated surround. The data points are medians of brightness magnitude estimates made by a group of observers, and the figure shows log brightness as ordinate and log stimulus luminance as abscissa (14). The test stimulus is a narrow spectral band centered at 650 mμ seen within an illuminated surround of closely similar hue and saturation. The data plotted as open circles were obtained with a surround of low luminance, about 3 millilamberts, and the log-log relation is approximately linear. The results plotted as filled circles are numerical brightness estimates for the same series of test stimuli, but seen within a surround of higher luminance, i.e. about 30 millilamberts. The relative position of the two functions

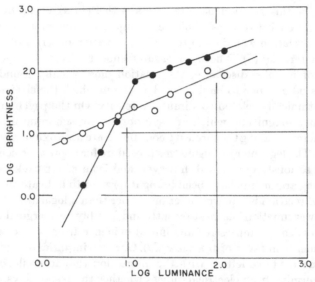

Fig. 2. Brightness scales. Test stimuli: 650 mμ. Open circles: surround luminance = 3 mL. Filled circles: surround luminance = 30 mL

with respect to the ordinate is arbitrarily determined. What we are interested in is the change in the form of the relation when the surround level is increased. The results for the higher surround luminance cannot be represented by a single linear function, and there is clearly a more rapid rate of change in apparent brightness for test stimuli at luminances lower than that of the surround, than for the test stimulus range above the surround level.

We have attempted to account theoretically for these changes on the basis of two assumed properties of the underlying physiological mechanism (14). First, we assume that the introduction of an increasingly bright surround may result in a general decrease in the sensitivity of the responding mechanism; and second, we assume that the excitation produced by the surround stimulus induces in the focal test area an opponent, response decrement, the magnitude of which is proportional to the magnitude of the surround activity. If sensitivity changes alone were operative, then the linear log-log relation obtained for the low surround level would remain unchanged except for a parallel displacement along the ordinate when the surround luminance is increased. On the other hand, if opponent interaction processes are operative, then the more intense surround will induce a larger decrement in the focal area brightness at all test intensities. Since this decrement will be constant for the constant surround, its quantitatively predicted effect on the brightness response function is to convert it to a curve which rises rapidly at the low levels of test luminance, and begins to approximate the slope of the original linear function at levels above that of the surround luminance (*14*). Only by taking opponent interaction into account can we explain the change in form of the psychophysical brightness response vs. intensity function with change in surround illumination.

The postulation of a physiological process of opponent interaction in the visual mechanism no longer need give any cause for concern. Not only is it necessary to account for the perceptual phenomena, but the numerous recent researches on various species showing evidence of such interacting excitatory and inhibitory effects resulting from spatially separate retinal stimulations provide a further basis for assuming such physiological opponent interaction processes for the human visual system. There are the receptive field studies by KUFFLER and his associates (*17*), the interaction effects in the Limulus eye reported by HARTLINE and his co-workers (*8*), and the demonstrations of physiological contrast in the optic tract and cortex of the cat by JUNG and his associates (*15*). For the scaling data that we have just been considering, moreover, the induced effects are fairly simple, and, to a first approximation, the measured psychophysical functions can be accounted for in terms of interactions as simple those described for two light stimuli interacting in the eye of Limulus (*19*).

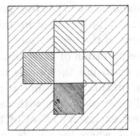

TEST STIMULUS PATTERN

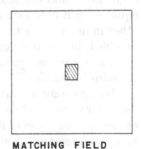

MATCHING FIELD

Fig. 3. Outline of stimulus test pattern and matching field. Striations of test pattern are used in the figure only to illustrate density differences of different individual areas

Psychophysical response vs. intensity functions are not always so simple as this, however, and it may be useful to examine the effects that occur when slightly more complex interactions are generated by a more varied stimulus array.

Figure 3 shows a stimulus pattern made up of equal areas of different density. In our experiments, this pattern was illuminated at each of three different levels through a range of 1.1 log units, and brightness matches were made to each of the square areas of the test pattern at each of the three levels of overall illumination. A successive matching procedure was used. The matching field is diagrammed in the lower right of the figure. It was a uniformly illuminated rectangle of continuously variable luminance, centered in a bright surround which was maintained at a constant luminance throughout the experiments.

Figure 4 shows the matching luminance data for each of the five square areas of the test pattern at the increasing levels of illumination. If there were a single relation of invariant form between brightness response and intensity of stimulation, that is, if the brightness of the given test area and the brightness of the matching field always depended on stimulus intensity in the same invariant manner, then each of the five matching luminance functions shown in Figure 4 would be represented by a straight line with 45° slope: the relation would be one of direct proportionality between test stimulus luminance and matching luminance. In contrast to this, the matching data actually measured for the lightest areas *1, 2* and *3* show only slight increases in matching luminance with increase in test luminance. For area *4*, the matching luminance is very nearly the same for all three test luminance levels: nearly perfect brightness constancy obtains for this part of the test configuration. Finally, for area *5* we have the paradoxical result that, as the illumination of the test pattern is *increased*, the luminance of the matching stimulus must be *decreased* in order to make it appear identical in brightness to this one area of the test pattern.

If our interpretation of these data is correct, then for area *5* the opponent induced effect, or to use the phrase more familiar to electrophysiologists, the inhibitory effect in this area, which is proportional to the excitatory magnitudes in the surrounding areas, grows with increase in luminance at a rate that is greater than the direct excitatory effect of the relatively weak focal stimulation in this area. For area *4*, where the results show approximate constancy, the focal excitatory effects and the induced inhibitory effects presumably increased by exactly equal magnitudes with increase in illumination and thus exactly cancelled each other in net visual effect. For the other three areas, induced effects are obviously involved, but their magnitudes relative to the magnitudes of the focal excitatory processes were not great enough completely to cancel the effects of increasing stimulus intensities.

An important question that arises at this point is what the matching luminance data of Figure 4 tell us about the actual perceived brightness of the test pattern at the various levels of illumination. It is safe to assume that when the matching luminance remains constant, the apparent brightness is also invariant, that when the matching luminance increases, so does the apparent brightness, and that when the matching luminance decreases, the perceived brightness must be decreasing. But to know what these changes amount to in units of perceived brightness instead of in units of stimulus luminance, additional information is required. We obtained this additional information by determining a direct brightness magnitude scale for the matching field itself, under the same conditions and for the same observers as in the matching experiments. The subjective brightness versus luminance function determined for this field shows a rapid rise throughout most of the luminance range and begins to be more gradual at the highest stimulus intensities at which the test luminance exceeds the surround luminance. The subjective brightness also approaches a limiting minimal value at the lowest stimulus intensities at which an appearance of maximal blackness is approximated. This is much the kind of function anticipated if opponent induction processes are operating, and when the intensity of the surround or inducing field is high relative to the range of test intensities (*14*).

We used these brightness scaling data for the matching field to convert the matching data shown in Figure 4 from units of matching luminance to units of perceived brightness, and the data converted in this manner are shown in Figure 5. Each one of the eight different functions shown in Figure 5 represents the psychophysical relation between stimulus intensity and visual brightness response. These eight different experimental functions hardly support the notion either of a single relation of the Fechnerian type, or a single power function with invariant exponent.

If we consider each of the three functions relating the five focal areas, then in each instance brightness increases with stimulus intensity, but neither the ordinate values nor the slopes remain invariant as the overall level of illumination is increased. Moreover, when we consider each individual area viewed at the different overall illumination levels, we find that visual brightness may even be inversely related to stimulus intensity.

It should be pointed out that, although the net effect of increasing the illumination may be algebraically not very different from zero for the pattern as a whole, this extra light is not at all wasted from a visual point of view. What does happen is that with increased illumination the difference in apparent brightness from the lightest area to the most dense one is appreciably increased: the relative luminance ratios are constant, but by putting more light on the scene we increase the apparent brightness contrast. Compare R_1 with R_3 in Figure 5. And wherever we find a situation of heightned visual contrast, whether of simple bright-dark, or

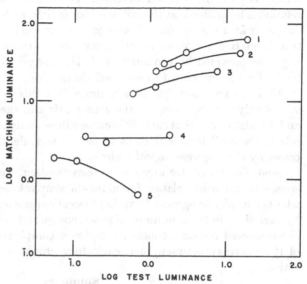

Fig. 4. Matching luminance data for each of 5 square areas of test pattern seen at increasing levels of illumination

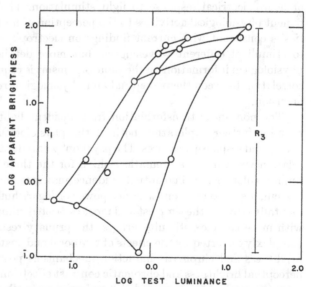

Fig. 5. Psychophysical relations between stimulus intensity and visual brightness response for complex stimulus array. Note variations in forms, slopes and signs of the 8 different functions

white-black relations, as here, or of comparable effects in perceived hue and saturation, we tend to look to physiological processes of opponent spatial and temporal induction as the most likely basis.

In conclusion, the evidence at hand suggests (a) that, for the simplest stimulating conditions, the relation between perceptual response magnitude and stimulus intensity is probably a power function. Whether the physiological correlate of this relation is logarithmic at the initial response time with a subsequent power relation emerging as a steady state is approached, or whether some other mechanism of transformation exists, we do not know, but we think the answer to this question might be provided by the analysis of electrophysiological response patterns over longer time intervals with continued stimulation.

b) The psychophysical data indicate that this intensity vs. response relation is probably not the same for the achromatic and the two paired color processes, and we might hope that such differences will be analyzed as carefully as wavelength selectivity itself in the attempt to isolate and identify chromatic response processes by electrophysiological techniques.

And, finally, (c) for any one response system, we should expect that the response vs. intensity relation found for the simplest conditions of light stimulation, whether in physiological or psychophysical experiments, will be radically altered by variations in the conditions of pre-exposure and surround stimulation, but that the measured response functions, however complex, will be analyzable in terms of the interplay between basic excitatory processes and opponent induced activities.

Summary

The essential hypotheses of an opponent-process theory of the visual mechanism are supported by electrophysiological evidence of the existence of opposite modes of neuro-electrical response to light stimulation. The postulated relation of opponent physiological activities to the perception of mutually exclusive color qualities is consistent with current findings on electrophysiological response reversals to stimuli of different wavelengths, but more detailed behavioral and electrophysiological information on the same organisms is required to establish the precise correlation between the perceptual and physiological responses with respect to color vision.

The non-linear transformation from incident light energy to visual response requires further exploration both of the physiological response indices and the perceptual response measures. The psychophysical data suggest that this non-linear relation will vary in systematic fashion for the three paired response systems of human color vision. Perceptual evidence indicates that, even for the achromatic system, a simple relation (whether power or logarithmic) will be measured experimentally only for the simplest and most restricted stimulating conditions, and that with more complex stimulus arrays, the primary response characteristics will be complexly distorted by the effects of temporal and spatial induction. The opponent brightness and chromatic induction mechanisms postulated to account for such perceptual brightness and chromatic contrast effects find a parallel in the inhibitory interaction phenomena recorded by physiologists. Because of these opponent inductions or inhibitory interactions, the relation of response magnitude to stimulus intensity is found in psychophysical experiments and predicted for electrophysiological experiments to be capable of assuming any of the following forms: an ascending function of stimulus intensity, a constant independent of stimulus intensity, or, finally, a descending function of stimulus intensity.

References

1. BOUMAN, M. A., and P. L. WALRAVEN: Some color experiments for red and green monochromatic lights. J. opt. Soc. Amer. **47**, 834—839 (1957).
2. DEVALOIS, R. L., C. J. SMITH, A. J. KAROLY and S. T. KITAI: Electrical responses of primate visual systems. I. Different layers of Macaque lateral geniculate nucleus. J. comp. physiol. Psychol. **51**, 662—668 (1958).
3. FARNSWORTH, D.: Tritanomalous vision as a threshold function. Farbe **4**, 185—197 (1955).
4. GALIFRET, Y. (Ed.): Mechanisms of Colour Discrimination. Pp. 116—117. New York: Pergamon Press 1960.
5. GRANIT, R.: Receptors and Sensory Perception. New Haven: Yale University Press 1955.
6. HARTLINE, H. K.: The neural mechanisms of vision. Harvey Lect. **37**, 39—68 (1941—42).
7. — and C. H. GRAHAM: Nerve impulses from single receptors in the eye. J. cell. comp. Physiol. **1**, 277—295 (1932).
8. — and F. RATLIFF: Inhibitory interaction of receptor units in the eye of Limulus. J. gen. Physiol. **40**, 357—376 (1957).
9. HERING, E.: Zur Lehre von der Beziehung zwischen Leib und Seele. I. Über FECHNER's psychophysisches Gesetz. S.-B. Akad. Wien, Math.-naturw. Kl. Abt. III. **72**, 310—348 (1876).
10. — Zur Lehre vom Lichtsinne. Wien: Carl Gerold's Sohn 1878.
11. HURVICH, L. M., and D. JAMESON: Some quantitative aspects of an opponent-colors theory. II. Brightness, saturation, and hue in normal and dichromatic vision. J. opt. Soc. Amer. **45**, 602—616 (1955).
12. — — An opponent-process theory of color vision. Psychol. Rev. **64**, 384—404 (1957).
13. — — Further development of a quantified opponent-colours theory. In Visual Problems of Colour. II, 691—723. London: Her Majesty's Stationery Office 1958.
14. JAMESON, D., and L. M. HURVICH: Perceived color and its dependence on focal, surrounding, and preceding stimulus variables. J. opt. Soc. Amer. **49**, 890—898 (1959).
15. JUNG, R.: Microphysiology of cortical neurons and its significance for psychophysiology. An. Fac. Med. Montevideo **44**, 323—332 (1959).
16. — u. G. BAUMGARTNER: Hemmungsmechanismen und bremsende Stabilisierung an einzelnen Neuronen des optischen Cortex. Pflügers Arch. ges. Physiol. **261**, 434—456 (1955).
17. KUFFLER, S. W.: Discharge patterns and functional organization of mammalian retina. J. Neurophysiol. **16**, 37—68 (1953).
18. MacNICHOL, E. F., jr., and G. SVAETICHIN: Electrical responses from the isolated retinas of fishes. Amer. J. Ophthal. **46**, 26—46 (1958).
19. RATLIFF, F., W. H. MILLER and H. K. HARTLINE: Neural interaction in the eye and the integration of receptor activity. Ann. N. Y. Acad. Sci. **74**, 210—222 (1958).
20. STEVENS, S. S., and E. H. GALANTER: Ratio scales and category scales for a dozen perceptual continua. J. exp. Psychol. **54**, 377—411 (1957).
21. SVAETICHIN, G.: Spectral response curves from single cones. Acta physiol. scand. **39**, Supp. 134, 17—47 (1956).
22. TROLAND, L. T.: The Principles of Psychophysiology. II. New York: Van Nostrand 1929.
23. WAGNER, H. G., E. F. MacNICHOL, jr., and M. L. WOLBARSHT: Opponent color responses in retinal ganglion cells. Science **131**, 1314 (1960).
24. — — — The response properties of single ganglion cells in the goldfish retina. J. gen. Physiol. **43**, (Suppl.) 45—62 (1960).

Discussion

W. JAEGER: Die sehr schönen und sorgfältigen Untersuchungen von Herrn und Frau HURVICH scheinen mir eine wichtige Bestätigung der Zonentheorie von VON KRIES zu sein. Obwohl die Kombination verschiedener Versuchsanordnungen die Ergebnisse schwer übersehbar macht, glaube ich, daß die Analyse jeden von uns überzeugt hat.

M. MONJÉ: Wir haben nach Anhaltspunkten für die Cluster-Hypothese von HARTRIDGE gesucht, indem wir die Empfindlichkeit der Fovea für verschiedene Reizfarben mit einer Reizmarke von 2,5 Bogenmin. Durchmesser an den verschiedenen Stellen der Fovea untersuchten. Dabei fanden wir, daß die Empfindlichkeit für die gleiche Reizfarbe an verschiedenen Stellen ungleich ist. An der gleichen Stelle ist die Empfindlichkeit unterschiedlich, wenn die Farbe verschieden ist. In der Umgebung des Fixierpunktes ist die Empfindlichkeit von dessen Farbe abhängig: Es dominiert stets die Empfindlichkeit der Farbe, die der Fixierpunkt hat. Dieser Befund scheint mir doch mehr für eine Theorie im Sinne von Helmholtz als von Hering zu sprechen.

U. Söderberg: I have two questions:

1. Can the different colour sensitivity of the peripheral visual field (used as large surround) distort the experimental results?

2. How far are eye movements distorting?

W. Sickel: Es wird auf die Kritik des Weber-Fechnerschen „Gesetzes" durch Ranke hingewiesen: Die von Fechner vorgenommene Integration ist für den Gesamt-Arbeitsbereich des Auges nicht zuverlässig, dieser wird vielmehr mit Hilfe der Adaptation (= Bereichsverschiebung) unter Wahrung des Intensitätsauflösungsvermögens umspannt. Für farbige Lichtreize zeigen die Intensitäts-Antwort-Kurven der b-Wellen an der umspülten Froschnetzhaut unterschiedliche Steilheit.

R. Jung: Frau Hurvich-Jamesons Ausführungen über die Grenzen logarithmischer und linearer Funktionsbeziehungen fand ich sehr einleuchtend. Sie sind auch durch neurophysiologische Befunde zu belegen. Zum Beispiel findet man die noch wenig beachtete "descending function" in der von mir und Baumgartner 1955 beschriebenen neuronalen Überlastungshemmung nach Flimmerreiz mit Lichtblitzen (bei steigender Flimmerfrequenz über 10/sec zunehmende Lichtmenge auf der Retina aber abnehmende Neuronentladung). Leider haben die Physiologen letztes Jahr bei Rosenbliths Symposion (on sensory communication) keine Verständigung mit Stevens erreicht, der an seiner linearen power function festhielt. Hurvichs psychophysische Ergebnisse bei verschiedenen Gegenfarbensystemen müssen auch von der Elektrophysiologie beachtet werden.

Die neuronale Grundlage simultaner und sukzessiver Kontrasphänomene haben wir zwar nur bei der Katze für Hell und Dunkel (Weiß und Schwarz) untersucht. Trotz unterschiedlicher psychophysischer Ergebnisse bei achromatischen und chromatischen Reizen sehe ich aber keine Schwierigkeit, ähnliche Neuronenkoordinationen auch für die Gegenfarben im Sinne Herings anzunehmen. Allerdings kennen wir ihren neuronalen Mechanismus bisher nur durch die Geniculatumuntersuchungen von De Valois bei Affen.

Neurophysiologisch sind alle Kontrastphänomene durch zwei antagonistische, sich reziprok hemmende und sukzessiv induzierende Neuronensysteme (für den Sukzessivkontrast) und außerdem durch laterale Hemmung synergistischer Neurone (für den Simultankontrast) befriedigend zu erklären. Baumgartner hat diese Mechanismen für den simultanen Hell-Dunkel-Kontrast experimentell sichergestellt.

L. M. Hurvich (to W. Jaeger): We wish to thank Dr. Jaeger for his appreciation of our work. Our formulation differs in one very important respect from v. Kries' zone theory. v. Kries postulated two zones in the visual system: a peripheral zone which was presumably a three-variable mechanism and a more central zone which was presumably a four-variable one. In this way v. Kries hoped to handle an ever increasing body of data resistant to explanation in simple Young-Helmholtzian terms. With the zone theory he sought to reconcile what he thought of as the Helmholtz three-color theory with the four-color concept that he attributed to Hering. We ourselves follow Hering more directly by assuming a three-variable mechanism at all levels. This is the reason that we have avoided v. Kries' term "four-color" theory, since the opponent-colors mechanism is assumed to be composed of three paired systems, namely, yellow-blue, red-green, and white-black. The fact that we, as well as any theorist (including Hering), assume that there are photochemical processes (Hering's „Empfangsstoffe") as well as neural processes (Hering's „Sehsubstanz") makes us all, of course, zone theorists but only in the sense that we have to conceive of photochemical absorption as different from neural processes.

To M. Monjé: Dr. Monjé cites experiments which demonstrate that for very small test stimuli, color sensitivity is not constant at different positions within the fovea. Moreover, sensitivity is greater for test spots that are the same color as the fixation point. The first point seems to me to further document the fact that the retina is not uniformly responsive throughout its extent, and that gradients of sensitivity exist, not only from fovea to parafovea to periphery, but also within each of these broadly delimited areas. The second point suggests that the stimuli used fell within the small limits of a retinal summation area. These results are important to have for understanding areal effects in vision, but I do not see that they argue for the validity of the Helmholtz theory. Small field studies do show, on the other hand, that a stimulus of any wavelength, if made sufficiently small at a moderate intensity is seen as either green or red in the fovea (small-field tritanopia); if made still smaller (or less intense) such spectral stimuli look white or achromatic. The paired loss of, first, blue and yellow, and second, red and green, is of course consistent with a theory of paired, opponent-color processes.

DOROTHEA HURVICH-JAMESON (to U. SÖDERBERG): 1. It is true that sensitivities vary in different parts of the retina but nevertheless homogeneous stimulus fields tend to be seen as uniform in appearance as if some sort of averaging process occurs. We would expect that surrounds of different sizes would yield different results both because of the sensitivity gradient and because of the effect of area *per se*. Thus we would consider surround size to be a relevant stimulus parameter. In the sense of "distorting" the results, however, this could occur only if we did not keep the surround image constant in comparisons of different surround chromaticities.

2. Eye movements certainly occurred in our experiments, and there is no question that different results are obtained when a "stopped-image" technique is used to compensate for involuntary eye movements and thus to keep the stimulus imaged on the same part of the retina. One of the major findings of the experiments utilizing stopped images is that there is a tendency for the test field to fade and eventually disappear. This artificial situation is more distorting with respect to normal vision than the one where involuntary eye movements do occur during fixation and where image clarity is maintained.

To W. SICKEL: We agree with Dr. SICKEL that the level of adaptation must be controlled in experiments that seek to determine the response vs. intensity relation whether the function is constructed from discrimination measures or measured directly. The relevance of adaptation level is seen in the work of CRAIK, MARSHALL and TALBOT, and HOPKINSON, among others. Our own subjective magnitude scales show the importance of adaptation level and surrounding stimulation for the form of the subjective brightness function.

The finding of different b-wave slopes for different stimulus wavelengths in the excised frog's eye provides an interesting lead, but to interpret the precise significance of this finding requires that we know more about the significance for vision of the various components of the ERG.

To R. JUNG: The finding of decreasing neural response with increase in stimulation in the flicker studies on cat is an excellent example that illustrates two of the main points that we have sought to make about the response versus intensity relation. It makes clear that in physiological studies as well as in psychophysical ones, experimental determinations of this function will show wide differences in form depending on the particular stimulating conditions used. Since this is so, it also illustrates why correlations between physiological and psychological measures should properly be restricted to the results of experiments in which the stimulating conditions are as closely similar as possible.

The Origin of "on" and "off" Responses of Retinal Ganglion Cells[1,2]

By

M. L. WOLBARSHT, H. G. WAGNER and E. F. MACNICHOL jr.

With 5 Figures

The complex train of neural events responsible for vision is initiated by the absorption of light in a photoreceptor cell, which in the vertebrate retina is but one

[1] From the Physiology Division, Naval Medical Research Institute, National Naval Medical Center, Bethesda, Maryland, and Thomas C. Jenkins Department of Biophysics, Johns Hopkins University, Baltimore, Maryland.

[2] The opinions or assertions contained herein are the private ones of the authors and are not to be construed as official or reflecting the views of the Navy Department or the naval service at large. The research was supported in part by National Science Foundation Grant G-7086.

unit of a highly organized structure containing many types of cells, nerve pathways and synaptic relationships. Very little is known regarding the role that each of the retinal structures plays in the transmission of information concerning the initial event of photoreception. We know that the various parameters such as intensity, hue, duration, shape, etc., must be encoded into the sequence of nerve impulses which leave the retina by way of the optic nerve. The ganglion cell is the final common pathway into the optic nerve through which the information regarding the stimulus must flow. In the complex pattern of the responses of this cell we can search for information on the controlling factors. Finding out the laws that govern the encoding of information by the retina is a basic step toward the understanding of the operation of the entire visual system.

It is well known from the work of HARTLINE (2), KUFFLER (4), GRANIT (1), and others that all vertebrate retinal ganglion cell response patterns may be fairly well fitted into three types according to whether evoked spike discharges occur during illumination ("on" type); or they appear following extinction of illumination ("off" responses); or at both times ("on-off" type). In addition to the "on" and "off" components of the response patterns, an inhibitory aspect can often be detected in the discharge patterns either as a suppression of any preexisting spontaneous activity, or as the abrupt termination of a prolonged "off" discharge by reillumination.

We consider that the response patterns and the presence of the three components can be explained on the basis of two independent processes acting on the ganglion cell. One is an excitatory influence tending to cause the ganglion cell to discharge spike potentials probably through a simple mechanism which depolarizes the cell membrane to the point of instability causing repetitive oscillations. The other process is an inhibitory influence which acts to prevent the ganglion cell from discharging spike potentials, perhaps by hyperpolarizing the cell membrane.

Since we assume that the membrane of the retinal ganglion cell is similar to those neural membranes whose electrochemical properties have been studied in detail, we would expect hyperpolarization of it by the inhibitory synapses to be followed by a post-inhibitory rebound or "off" discharge. This post-inhibitory rebound would be similar to the well known anodal break phenomenon and is consistent with the HODGKIN-HUXLEY model (3) of the nerve membrane. In this model, prolonged hyperpolarization decreases the potassium ion conductance and increases the rate of change of the sodium ion conductance when the membrane is subsequently depolarized. These changes in membrane conductance persist for some time after the hyperpolarizing current ends. Thus at the cessation of illumination when the hyperpolarizing influence is removed, the membrane potential of the ganglion cell falls toward the normal resting level. However, due to the decreased potassium ion conductance and the increased sodium ion conductance, the net ionic flux at the normal resting potential is inward. This results in still further depolarization of the membrane and the initiation of one or more impulses. Thus the inhibition and "off" components of the response are both the result of the same inhibitory process acting on the ganglion cell.

The evidence for the statement that the determinants of ganglion cell activity may largely if not exclusively depend upon the interaction of two simple opposed influences, one excitatory, the other inhibitory, is based on our studies on the isolated retina of the goldfish *Carassius auratus*. As will be shown, these results can be correlated with those obtained by others in different species and suggest strongly that the basic principles can be generalized to all vertebrate retinas.

The *experimental technique* used for the goldfish retina has been described in detail previously (*5, 6, 7*). The retinal ganglion cells have discharge patterns in re-sponse to illumination that de-monstrate the "on", the "off", and inhibitory components pre-viously mentioned. Figure 1, is a series of oscillographic represen-tations of the spike potential discharge patterns in response to illumination. This type of ganglion cell is of special interest since the response pattern underwent a change when the wavelength of the stimulus light was changed. "On" responses were excited by wavelengths from 400 mμ through 550 mμ but longer wavelengths (600 mμ through 700 mμ) gave pure "off" responses. The higher than usual spontaneous level of activity of this cell also demon-strates very clearly the inhibitory response during illumination. The two components, inhibition and the "off" discharge, are always found associated with each other.

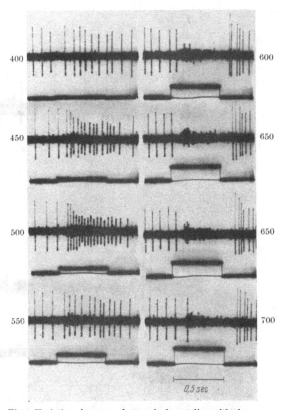

Fig. 1. Variation of response from a single ganglion with change of wavelength of a constant intensity stimulus (4 5 × 10⁻² μ watts/cm²). Wavelength of stimulus in mμ beside each record. The duration of the stimulus is indicated by the step in the signal tract at the base of each record. Impulses occurring before the onset of the stimulus are spontaneous in origin. Stimulation by wavelengths 400 mμ through 550 mμ causes increased activ-ity during illumination ("on" response) with a gradual return to the spontaneous level after illumination. The suppression of activity during illumination by the wavelengths 600 mμ to 700 mμ is attended by an increase in activity after illumination ("off" response)

Two classes of cells showing wavelength selectivity of their response patterns have been ob-served in the goldfish retina; those excited by short wavelength illumination and inhibited by long wavelengths, of which the cell in Figure 1 is an example; and a second class of cells which are excited by long wavelength light and inhibited by the shorter wavelengths.

The transition from excitation to inhibition as a function of wavelength is often quite abrupt. Figure 2 shows two records of the response patterns in a cell which made a complete shift from an "on" response to an "off" response with a change of only 10 mμ in wavelength of the stimulating light.

At certain wavelengths a change in intensity also will convert "on" responses into "off" responses. The top record in Figure 3 illustrates a pure "on" response. When the intensity was increased 15-fold, the response pattern as shown in the

middle record had both "on" and "off" components. A 50-fold increase in intensity
(lowest record) gave only an "off" response.

The sensitivity in different spectral regions for each of the components has been
plotted in Figure 4 for one of these ganglion cells. Each symbol represents the
threshold intensity necessary to evoke a constant response (usually one impulse)

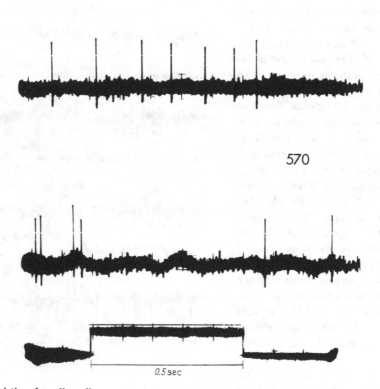

Fig. 2. Variation of ganglion cell response with a small change in wavelength. Wavelength of stimulus in mμ is in
upper right of each record. The duration of the stimulus is indicated by the step in the signal record at the base
of the series. Spikes occurring before the onset of the stimulus are "off" responses from preceding stimuli. Intensity
of stimulus 55 μ watts/cm²

for the "on" or the "off" component. For plotting the inhibitory component, the
criterion used was the intensity necessary to cause the complete suppression of all
activity during illumination.

These points have been joined with lines to establish spectral sensitivity functions for each component. The function for the inhibitory component closely follows that of the "off" response. The differences, particularly at the shorter wavelengths, are believed to represent interaction with the strong excitatory component
present. A more complete discussion of this point and the additional evidence for
considering the three components of the response as the result of just two processes: one excitatory, the other inhibitory are set forth in earlier papers (5, 6).

The two processes overlap from about 530 mμ to 610 mμ. In this region an
increase in intensity above that necessary to evoke the more sensitive process will,

in addition, evoke the opponent process also, and give rise to the "on-off" pattern. At still higher intensities the "on" response becomes less vigorous and above a critical level only an "off" discharge is seen.

The differential effect of light adaptation on the threshold sensitivities of the functions is perhaps the clearest indication that two processes, one excitatory, the

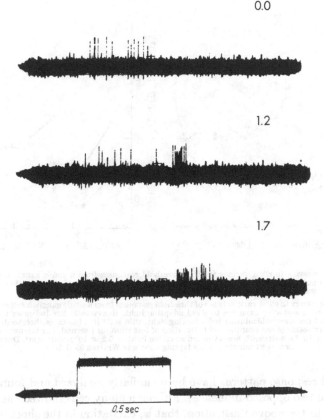

0.0

1.2

1.7

0.5 sec

Fig. 3. Variation of ganglion cell response with change in intensity of stimulus. Duration of stimulus is indicated by step in signal trace at base of the series. Log intensity of stimulus is in upper right of each record. 0.0 log units = 1.7 μ watts/cm^2

other inhibitory, arise from independent peripheral pathways or systems. Figure 5 shows the effect of selective chromatic light adaptation. A wavelength for the adapting light was chosen so that it would stimulate the inhibitory process strongly but the other process weakly or not at all. The heavy solid line defines the control thresholds of both components before adaptation. After several minutes of adaptation to red light, a new set of thresholds was obtained. The sensitivities of the two processes were different as indicated by the thin broken lines; the inhibitory process was only one-tenth as sensitive as before while the excitatory was actually more sensitive. It was possible to find thresholds for the excitatory process in all parts of the spectrum, including a region of the spectrum where no "on" thresholds were obtainable in the control situation. It was as if the excitatory process had been completely suppressed by the presence of the inhibitory process and that only when the latter was sufficiently weakened could the presence of excitation be demonstrated. Experiments on the same ganglion cell using blue light for adaptation showed that a similar decrease in the sensitivity occurred in the excitatory process while at the same time there was an increase in sensitivity of the inhibitory process. However, the effect was not nearly as marked as when red light was used.

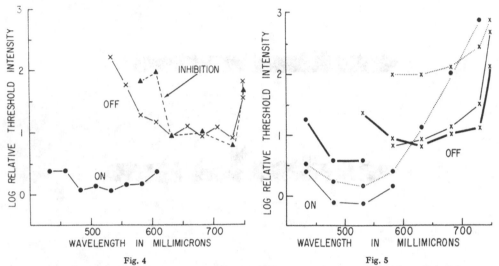

Fig. 4   Fig. 5

Fig. 4. Intensity necessary to elicit various types of threshold responses from a single ganglion cell at different wavelengths. Each point is an average of four determinations at one wavelength. The duration of the stimulus was 1.0 second; 0 log units = $5.5 \times 10^{-2}\,\mu$ watts/cm² for all wavelengths

Fig. 5. Intensity necessary to elicit various types of threshold responses from a single ganglion cell at different wavelengths before, during, and after exposure to a red adapting light. Heavy solid line indicates thresholds before adaptation, dotted lines, thresholds during red adapting light, thin solid line indicates thresholds approximately 10 minutes after extinction of the adapting light. Duration of test stimulus 1 second. For intensity of test stimulus 0 log units = $2.3 \times 10^{-2}\,\mu$ watts/cm². Energy of red adapting light = $5.2 \times 10^{3}\,\mu$ watts/cm². Duration of adaptation = 27 minutes. Red adapting light was Wratten 89 B filter

Other cell response patterns have been similarly analyzed and found to be the result of these two opposed influences. Although many cells showed the same basic pattern used in the above illustration, that is, excitation in the short wavelengths and inhibition in the long wavelengths; other cells showed just the opposite, that is, inhibition in the short wavelengths and excitation in the long wavelengths. Still other types were found to have no separation in the spectral sensitivities of the excitatory and inhibitory processes (5).

It now remains to be shown how these two influences can combine to produce the many response patterns observed. Conceptually, there must be at least two populations of photoreceptors differing in their spectral sensitivities: one with a maximum in the spectrum around 500 mμ, the second with a maximum around 650 mμ. The possible character of the photopigments within these systems has been dealt with in another paper (5). Each photoreceptor, when stimulated originates both an excitatory and an inhibitory influence. The actual site of origin of the dual influence cannot be located more specifically than somewhere in the conducting pathway between the ganglion cell and the photoreceptor. The influences after traveling separate neural pathways, and being subjected to dissimilar synaptic relationships with other retinal units will converge upon the same ganglion cell (as well as upon others). For the combinations of excitatory and inhibitory influences from red sensitive (R) and green sensitive (G) receptor cells, some fifteen possibilities exist as set forth in Table 1.

The preceding table does not reflect the possibilities of differences between the effectiveness of the excitation or inhibition on the ganglion cell which may well depend upon spatial, temporal, and other factors. All of these factors may be of considerable importance so the categorization in Table 1 should not be taken too literally.

The presence of excitation alone will produce a pure "on" response as in type V, VII and IX. Under certain conditions other types may be stimulated to give pure "on" responses. For example the wavelength of the stimulating light can be chosen to evoke an "on" response, and as will be shown later (8), the location of the stimulus on the retina will also have this effect. Pure "off" response patterns are similar in many respects to pure "on" responses. They represent either inhibition alone

Table 1

Type	Excitation	Inhibition
I*	R	G
II*	G	R
III*	R	R
IV	G	G
V	R	
VI*	—	R
VII*	G	—
VIII	—	G
IX	RG	—
X	—	RG
XI	R	RG
XII	G	RG
XIII	RG	R
XIV	RG	G
XV*	RG	RG

* Indicates that this type of response has actually been found in the goldfish retina.

as would occur in types VI, VIII and X, or where the excitatory process is suppressed due to weakness or delay in its arrival.

The "on-off" pattern is seen most commonly. Table 1 indicates that this variety in which both excitation and inhibition are present has the largest number of types. The "on-off" pattern implies that excitation is the first to arrive at the ganglion cell presumably because it has a more direct pathway. The ganglion cell gives a series of impulses which is terminated by the arrival of the inhibition with the result that there is only an "on" burst. The "on" burst may be short in duration, and of relatively high impulse frequency, if the time delay between the onset of the two processes is short and the stimulus is strong. The "off" burst is the result of post-inhibitory rebound when the inhibition is removed at the end of the illumination.

It will require considerably more experimental work before the above model could be said to be fully justified by the facts. In spite of the simplicity of the exciting influences, many functional varieties are possible. The significance of these patterns as related to the information coded in the optic nerve is not immediately apparent. Certain of the classes (I, II) appear to have an opponent color interpretation. It is probable that the effect of this opponent color antagonism may serve to sharpen the color differentiation mechanisms that are present.

Summary

The "on-off" response pattern of retinal ganglion cells can be analyzed into three components: "on", "off", and inhibition. The "on" component is generated by an excitatory influence, while an inhibitory process is responsible for both the inhibitory and "off" components. The "off" component is considered to be a post-inhibitory rebound phenomenon. The excitatory and inhibitory processes have their origin in at least two types of photoreceptors with differing spectral sensitivities. Each receptor type gives rise to both an excitatory and an inhibitory process. In the goldfish one of these photoreceptor types has its maximal sensitivity at about 650 mμ and another is most sensitive at about 500 mμ. Each can be light adapted inde- pendently of the other. Interaction at the ganglion cell level between the excitatory process from one receptor type and the inhibitory process from the other may have significance as an opponent color mechanism.

References

1. GRANIT, R.: Sensory mechanisms of the retina. London: Oxford University Press 1947.
2. HARTLINE, H. K.: The responses of single optic nerve fibers of the vertebrate eye to illumination of the retina. Amer. J. Physiol. 121, 400—415 (1938).
3. HODGKIN, A. L., and A. F. HUXLEY: A quantitative description of membrane current and its application to conduction and excitation in nerve. J. Physiol. (Lond.) 117, 500—544 (1952).
4. KUFFLER, S. W.: Discharge patterns and the functional organization of the mammalian retina. J. Neurophysiol. 16, 37—68 (1953).
5. MACNICHOL, E. F., jr., M. L. WOLBARSHT and H. G. WAGNER: Electrophysiological evidence for a mechanism of color vision in the goldfish. In W. D. MCELROY and H. B. GLASS: Light and Life. Baltimore: Johns Hopkins Press 1961.
6. WAGNER, H. G., E. F. MACNICHOL, jr., and M. L. WOLBARSHT: The response properties of single ganglion cells in the goldfish retina. J. gen. Physiol. 43 (6) suppl. 45—62(1960).
7. — — — Opponent color responses in retinal ganglion cells. Science 131, 1314 (1960).
8. WOLBARSHT, M. L., H. G. WAGNER and E. F. MACNICHOL, jr.: Receptive fields of retinal ganglion cells. This symposium.

Discussion see. pg. 175.

Receptive Fields of Retinal Ganglion Cells: Extent and Spectral Sensitivity[1,2]

By

M. L. WOLBARSHT, H. G. WAGNER and E. F. MACNICHOL jr.

With 3 Figures

In the preceding paper (9) the response patterns of certain retinal ganglion cells in the goldfish retina were shown to have several modalities; that is, under a given set of conditions the ganglion cell gave spike activity only during retinal illmunination (pure "on" response pattern), but if the conditions were slightly

[1] From the Physiology Division, Naval Medical Research Institute, National Naval Medical Center, Bethesda, Maryland, and Thomas C. Jenkins Department of Biophysics, Johns Hopkins University, Baltimore, Maryland.

[2] The opinions or assertions contained herein are the private ones of the authors and are not to be construed as official or reflecting the views of the Navy Department or the naval service at large. The research was supported in part by National Science Foundation Grant G-7086.

altered it responded only after extinction of the light (pure "off" response pattern), while intermediate circumstances would often evoke both ("on-off" response pattern). The conditions usually adequate to reveal these changes in behaviour were (a) a change in wavelength of the stimulating light, and (b) a change in intensity. One of the ways that the response patterns of these ganglion cells could be color coded was the following: when the wavelength of the stimulus was around 500 mμ there was a pure "on" response; a change to approximately 550 mμ gave an "on-off" response; and 600 mμ and longer wavelengths gave pure "off" responses. These same ganglion cells would also give a pure "on" response to low intensities of a stimulus of 550 mμ, and "on-off" response if the intensity was increased somewhat and a pure "off" response at still higher intensities. These patterns were explained on the basis that the response of the ganglion cell was being governed by two mutually antagonistic influences: one excitatory; the other inhibitory. Presumably these influences converge upon the ganglion cell through independent pathways which have their origin in separate receptor systems of different spectral sensitivities. The stimulus in all the above cases was diffuse illumination covering most of the retina. It is the purpose of this paper to discuss a third factor which also contributes to the bimodality of the response patterns. This factor is the spatial distribution of the stimulus. It will be shown that a systematic relationship exists, and that it must be considered among the determinants of the ganglion cell response pattern.

The ganglion cell of a vertebrate retina will respond only if illumination falls somewhere within a circumscribed area of the retina. HARTLINE (2), who first recognized the significance of this response area, termed it the receptive field of that ganglion cell. Later, KUFFLER (4) observed in the cat retina that the "on" and "off" components in the mixed response pattern could be separately evoked according to whether light fell in a central zone or in a peripheral zone. He termed these receptive fields either "on-center" or "off-center" fields according to which of the components was related to the central stimulation.

The goldfish retina also exhibits these phenomena. Figure 1 is a response pattern obtained from a single ganglion cell when a small sharply focused spot is used to stimulate each of a number of locations on the goldfish retina. The plot reveals a central area in which only "off" responses are evoked. This region is surrounded by an annular zone of mixed "on-off" responses and an outer ring of pure "on" responses. The symbols chosen in the figure do not reveal the quantitative vigor of the response patterns. Such a representation would have shown that the zone of mixed responses was a transitional one in which areas close to the center had strong "off" responses with weak "on" responses. Stimulation of more peripheral regions was accompanied by proportionately increased vigor of the "on" discharge and lessened "off" activity. The spatial representation in Figure 1 of the receptive field in its distinct separation into a central area and surround reflects the opposing influences on the ganglion cell. The presence of the transitional zone is of especial significance since it implies some interaction between the two influences.

The simplest explanation for the observed character of the "off-center" receptive field is that the central area consists of receptors which have an inhibitory influence on the ganglion cell and give "off" responses while the periphery contains receptors which excite "on" responses (4, 7). The transition zone would contain a mixture of both in varying degrees. However, as Kuffler (4) recognized and as we have confirmed, the character of the field can change markedly with dark or light adaptation. Receptors are fixed and cannot move laterally, and thus the explanation must be amended to show how receptors are functionally connected to the ganglion cells in one stage of adaptation but not in another.

The separation of the receptive field into "on" and "off" zones has an additional implication in the case of the type of ganglion cell shown in Figure 1. As has been mentioned above, the "on" and "off" responses of this type of ganglion cell are color coded; therefore the receptive field is also color coded. The separation of the "on" and "off" zones on the basis of chromatic selectivity has also been noticed by Motokawa et al. (6) in other fish, although no color separation of zones was found in the cat retina by Barlow et al. (1) who examined central and peripheral field relationships. The recent work of Hubel and Wiesel (3) indicates that color sensitive "on" and "off" ganglion cells are present, although rarely, in the spider monkey. It is probable that these will show the chromatic separation of the receptive field when examined.

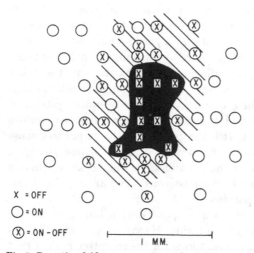

X = OFF

◯ = ON

Ⓧ = ON - OFF

I M.M.

Fig. 1. Receptive field response pattern of a color coded ganglion cell. Circular stimulus is of fixed intensity (18 μ watts/cm²), wavelength = 600 mμ, 153 μ in diameter, and 0.5 sec. duration. Each symbol represents a test location. The central area delineated in black gave only "off" responses. The outer zone gave only "on" responses. The hatched area represents a transitional zone of mixed responses in which the relative vigor of the separate components was proportional to the proximity to the respective "pure" response areas

However, the color sensitive ganglion cells offer a way to study the receptive fields of the "on" and the "off" processes, both independently, and with varying amounts of interaction; and thus to establish functional relationship between the receptive field and the ganglion cell. In Figure 1 the inhibitory process controlling the "off" response has its maximum spectral sensitivity at 650 mμ and the excitatory influence has its maximum sensitivity at 500 mμ. By using stimuli of these wavelengths the locations of the receptive field areas for each component can be plotted without interference with each other. Figure 2 shows this type of plot. The retinal fields eliciting "on" and "off" response patterns on the retina are enclosed by the two large circles which were drawn with the same reference to the position of the microelectrode and therefore may be considered to represent the same retinal areas. When the two circles are placed in register, it may be seen that the receptive areas for "on" and "off" responses are essentially identical. Each covers the entire area leaving no holes or gaps. The receptors controlling both the excitatory and inhibitory processes are present in all parts of the field.

Experiments such as this render untenable any premise that the receptive field is divided into three zones, two of which are exclusively responsible for the "on" or "off" components respectively, and a third which is a zone of the overlap. It becomes necessary to state that the receptive field is only relatively more likely to evoke an "off" (or "on") response in the center and an "on" (or "off") response in the periphery. This concept allows us to correlate this experiment with others which did not show the clear segregation of responses into "on" and "off" areas as seen in Figure 1. In these units, the entire field was often transitional. The relatively more "on" or more "off" areas included a few responses of the opposite type.

It is obvious that the excitatory and inhibitory processes causing the "on" and "off" response are activated unequally by stimulation of different parts of the retina. The most direct evaluation of their role is to measure their sensitivity.

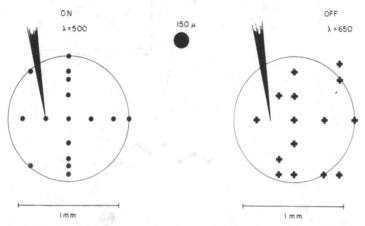

Fig. 2. Receptive field plots of the separate component responses of the same ganglion cell taken with stimuli of different wavelengths as indicated at upper right of each plot. The position of the microelectrode is symbolized in the upper left quadrant but should be interpreted as actually placed so that the axis is normal to the plane of the plot, intersecting with the tip in this illustration. Note that the tip is not located at the exact center of the response area. Stimulating spot was: 150 μ in diameter, with an intensity of 2.3 μ watts/cm² at 650 mμ and 1.5 μ watts/cm² at 500 mμ; and 0.5 sec. duration

Information concerning this has been obtained by determining the intensity necessary to produce a threshold response of each of the two types. The technique and criteria for these measurements were the same as used in earlier papers (7, 8).

Measurements were made at a number of retinal locations with the wavelength of the stimulus chosen to minimize interaction between the processes that give rise to the two kinds of response. From these measurements a profile of sensitivity for each of the two processes was constructed as a function of a single traverse through the center of the receptive field. Figure 3 is a plot taken from the data collected in this manner. In the upper right corner of this figure is a graph of the wavelength sensitivities of the "on" and "off" components to diffuse illumination. From these data 500 mμ and 650 mμ were chosen as the wavelengths to be used in testing the sensitivities of the separate processes. The ordinate value of the points in Figure 3 are the reciprocals of the log intensity for threshold responses. The abscissal values refer to the retinal distance measured from some arbitrary point (in this case, the approximate center of the receptive field). The plot represents the profiles of the sensitivities of the two processes.

One of the processes was very much more sensitive at the center but its sensitivity fell off very rapidly as the stimulus moved away from the center. The other component, although of lower sensitivity, seemed to be less affected by distance from the center. In the periphery it remained, as a consequence, more sensitive than the opponent process. All profiles of other units showing a clearly defined "on" or "off" center with a surrounding area giving a response of the opposite type were of this character.

The above data, together with what was previously know, are sufficient to offer a reasonable explanation for the color coded "off-center" type receptive field such as that represented in Figure 1 or its converse, the "on-center" field.

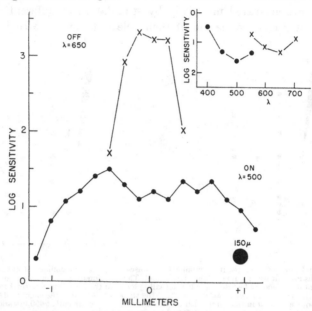

Fig. 3. Sensitivity profiles of the "on" and "off" component responses taken across the receptive fields of a color coded ganglion cell. Ordinate values are the reciprocal of the intensity necessary to evoke a threshold response. 0 log units = 12 μ watts/cm², diameter of stimulus spot = 150 μ, duration = 0.5 sec. Wavelength used for each response component indicated in the figure. Abscissal values = the displacements of the tested area from an arbitrary point near the center of the receptive field. The spectral sensitivity functions of the response components to diffuse retinal illumination are indicated in the upper right inset. For this plot 0 log units 0.2 μ watts/cm², stimulus duration = 0.5 sec

Whenever the stimulus contains spectral components which stimulate both processes, then the response observed will reflect the relative sensitivities and spatial contributions of the two processes at the point of stimulation. A stimulus of intermediate wavelength (around 550 mμ to 600 mμ) of supra-threshold intensity yields plots of the type shown in Figure 1. This stimulus, when restricted to the center of the field, will more effectively drive the inhibitory process than the excitatory one since the former is more sensitive. Therefore, no "on" response may be evoked because of the strong suppression present. In the peripheral locations an inverse situation is present. Here the excitatory process is most strongly driven. The "off" component never appears either because the inhibitory process is too insensitive or because it is suppressed by the process which causes the "on" discharge. At the intermediate distance the relative vigor of the two components would be determined by the relative strength of the two processes and their net interaction.

The response to diffuse illumination depends not only on the relative sensitivity of the two processes but also on the integrated contributions from receptors over the entire receptive field.

The above explanation for the organization of the receptive field has been based on the color coded type of ganglion cell. However, some ganglion cells in the gold-fish resemble those of the cat (4) in that there are "on-center" and "off-center" fields in which the inhibitory and excitatory processes have the same wavelength sensitivity. It is possible that these fields result from a convergence of inhibitory and excitatory influences on the ganglion cell from two groups of receptors of identical spectral sensitivity whose spatial organization is similar to those in the co-lor coded cells. Further study will no doubt suggest revisions of the theory.

Summary

The response pattern of the color coded ganglion cell of the goldfish is depen-dent upon the spatial location of the stimulus on the retina. The receptive areas for these ganglion cells show the separation of the components of the "on-off" pattern into three zones: a central area in which stimulation appears to evoke only one of the components, surrounded by a transitional area where a stimulus evokes both components, and a peripheral zone in which only the other component is evoked. There are "on-center" and "off-center" types. The inference that these zones represent the exclusive presence of one or the other component is shown to be wrong. When the processes that evoke the components are separately stimulated, the receptive field area for each component is essentially identical in size and lo-cation on the retina. Neither has any holes or unresponding areas. However, the sensitivity of the separate components is quite different. Sensitivity profiles for the separate components are plotted to show their relative relationship to each other. The excitatory and inhibitory processes are unequally activated at any point in the receptive field and the response pattern observed is the sum of the contribu-tions from each.

References

1. BARLOW, H. B., R. FITZHUGH and S. W. KUFFLER: Change of organization in the receptive fields of the cat's retina during dark adaptation. J. Physiol. 137, 338—354 (1957).
2. HARTLINE, H. K.: The response of single optic nerve fibers of the vertebrate eye to illumi-nation of the retina. Amer. J. Physiol. 121, 400—415 (1938).
3. HUBEL, D. H., and T. N. WIESEL: Unit responses in optic nerve of spider monkey. Physio-logist 3 (3), 83 (1960).
4. KUFFLER, S. W.: Neurons in the retina: organization, inhibition and excitation problems. Cold Spr. Harb. Symp. quant. Biol. 17, 281—292 (1952).
5. MACNICHOL, E. F., jr., M. L. WOLBARSHT and H. G. WAGNER: Electrophysiological evi-dence for a mechanism of color vision in the goldfish. In W. D. MCELROY and H. B. GLASS: Light and Life. Baltimore: Johns Hopkins Press 1961.
6. MOTOKAWA, K., E. YAMASHITA and T. OGAWA: The physiological basis of simultaneous contrast in the retina. This symposium.
7. WAGNER, H. G., E. F. MACNICHOL, jr., and M. L. WOLBARSHT: The response properties of single ganglion cells in the goldfish retina. J. gen. Physiol. 43 (6) Suppl., 45—62 (1960).
8. — and M. L. WOLBARSHT: Studies on the functional organization of the vertebrate retina. Amer. J. Ophthal. 46 (3) pt. 2, 46—55 (1958).
9. WOLBARSHT, M. L., H. G. WAGNER and E. F. MACNICHOL, jr.: The origin of "on" and "off" responses of retinal ganglion cells. This symposium.

Discussion

L. M. HURVICH (to the first paper): 1. In view of what we know of biological variability I am surprised that you would expect the transition wavelength from "on" to "off" responses to maintain a precisely fixed locus. On making psychophysical determinations of spectral

unique points, the pure blue, green or yellow in the spectrum, the wavelength locus is strongly
dependent on the immediate pre-exposure light even for short pre-exposure stimuli. The repetitive stimulation in your experiments will quite likely produce comparable displacements
and consequent variability.

2. To avoid confusion, Dr. Svaetichin should restrict the term "neutral point" to instances
of dichromatic color vision. For dichromats the transition point in the spectrum is indeed a
neutral, i.e. an achromatic one. For trichromatic systems however the transition point for one
system, say yellow-blue, is a point at which both the achromatic plus either red or green
systems are excited. Thus it is not a neutral point but a point at which a unique or pure hue is
seen. It might avoid confusion if we called these loci "transition points", or "equilibrium
points" rather than "neutral points", especially for electrical recordings on animals about
whose visual sensations we can, at the moment, say very little.

To the receptive field paper: 1. Some of the "on-off" responses that you record at a single
retinal level, i.e., ganglionic layer, you interpret as achromatic signals while others are taken
to represent color coding. For comparable polarity effects Svaetichin suggests two different
morphological loci, i.e., horizontal cells and Müller fibres. How is this specificity maintained
at the ganglionic level? What differentiates the achromatic "off" from the chromatic "off"
responses?

2. With respect to the question of the size of the receptive fields, it would be hard in
psychophysical experiments on humans to find any area stimulation of which would not be
shown to influence response to stimulation of any other area however widely separated the
two areas are.

H. Barlow: The finding that the goldfish has "on" and "off" receptive fields of different
sizes and different spectral sensitivities is extremely interesting, but I think one should not be
too hasty in concluding that the same arrangement will be found in frog or cat. With regard
to your suggestion that the cat's receptive fields may be colour coded, Kuffler, Fitzhugh,
and I had this idea in mind; obviously we cannot say that it never occurs, but we can say we
looked for it and did not find it. Instead we found that both central and peripheral zones of the
receptive field showed a Purkinje shift. We concluded that the duplex arrangement of the receptive field was not caused by the ganglion cell making different connections to rods and cones.
These experiments are reported in Journal of Physiology (1957) 137, pp. 327—337.

The arrangement of the receptive fields may differ in closely related species. I once repeated
some observations I had made on Rana Temporaria on Rana Esculenta. To my surprise I found
a difference; in Temporaria the "on" and "off" fields were of the same size, whereas in Esculenta they were frequently different — as in the goldfish. Where they are different you have
a Triplex, not a Duplex, arrangement of the receptive field, for outside the "on" and "off"
fields you have a zone of pure inhibition. Light falling in this region inhibits the "on" discharge
from light falling in the centre at "on", and inhibits the "off" discharge at "off", and it does
this at intensities such that, by itself, no discharge is evoked at "on" or "off". The same can
be shown in area/threshold curves, for with a large spot which includes this pure inhibitory
zone the threshold is higher, at both "on" and "off", than it is with a smaller spot[1]. I wonder
whether Wolbarsht and MacNichol have found this in goldfish?

R. Jung: Dr. Wolbarshts Ergebnisse sind ohne Schwierigkeit in die reziproke Struktur
der Rezeptormechanismen und Neuronenschaltungen einzuordnen, wenn man den Goldfisch
als Dichromaten auffaßt, der besser rot sieht.

W. Sickel: Aus Mikro-Ableitungen von der umströmten Froschnetzhaut ist ebenfalls die
Konvergenz mehrerer in verschiedenen Intensitätsbereichen wirksamer Generatoren an einer
Ganglienzelle zu erkennen. Es ist gleichzeitig zu entnehmen, daß bei hohen Spike-Folgen die
Amplitude der einzelnen Spike abnimmt und unter Helladaptation eine Stabilisierung eintritt.

A. Arduini: Is it possible to distinguish between central and peripheral fields on the
base of reciprocal influence? How large can be the diameter of the field of influence?

---

[1] See J. Physiol, 114, p. 80, fig. 8

G. BAUMGARTNER: Dr. WOLBARSHTs Darstellung der retinalen Ganglienzellaktivität als Folge excitatorischer und inhibitorischer Prozesse ist sicher richtig. Gegen seine Deutung der off-Aktivierung als einfaches rebound-Phänomen habe ich aber Bedenken. GERNANDT und GRANIT haben 1947 beschrieben, daß bei Gleichstrompolarisation des Auges durch Änderung der Durchströmungsrichtung die Lichtreaktionen der retinalen Ganglienzellen umgekehrt werden können. Unter dieser Voraussetzung könnte auch die verschiedene Richtung eines Generatorpotentials selektiv on- oder off-Reaktionen verursachen. Handelt es sich bei den R-C-Potentialen GRÜSSERs um Receptorpotentiale, so wäre durch sie, wie GRÜSSER annimmt, auch eine echte off-Aktivierung erklärbar, da das R-C-Potential nach Verdunklung einen von der Intensität abhängigen steilen Abfall, bei Belichtung einen nach Steilheit und Größe intensitätsabhängigen Anstieg zeigt. Ferner entstehen off-Aktivierungen auch nach ganz kurzen Lichtblitzen (< 1 msec), die wahrscheinlich zu keinen wesentlichen Elektrolytverschiebungen führen können, wie man dies bei längerer Hyperpolarisation eines off-Neurons durch eine Dauerlichtreizung diskutieren muß. Trotzdem halten auch diese Nacherregungen länger an, was für ein reines rebound-Phänomen ungewöhnlich wäre.

E. F. MacNICHOL (to L. M. HURVICH): It appears that color information is transmitted by specific ganglion cells which give "on" responses when stimulated by light in one of a pair of wavelength regions and "off" responses when stimulated by the other. In these cells white light is signalled by an "on-off" burst having an equal number of impulses in the "on" and "off" components. For unsaturated colors redness or greenness would perhaps be signalled by the *ratio of "on" to "off" impulses.* In addition some ganglion cells give on and off responses whose proportions do not vary with wavelength. These are presumably part of an achromatic or black-white system. Only these cells give the achromatic "off" responses to which Dr. HURVICH refers.

It is to be hoped that when more experimental data are available it will be possible to construct a mathematical model of the color and intensity coding system. This system would involve pairs of receptors having different wavelength sensitivities which would provide excitatory and inhibitory synaptic endings to a population of ganglion cells either directly or through a group of bipolar cells. Some cells would have mostly excitatory endings from a red or yellow sensitive system and inhibitory endings from a green or blue sensitive system, others would have the converse, and still others might have nearly equal numbers of excitatory and inhibitory endings from all the different kinds of receptors. More complete experimental data should permit assigning response functions to the receptors and to the synaptic system. Mutual interaction must also be provided for in any model.

M. L. WOLBARSHT (to L. M. HURVICH): The transition wavelength does not maintain a precisely fixed locus as it is the intersection of the sensitivity curves of the two processes. A shift of one curve relative to the other would move the transition wavelength.

To BARLOW: We have not seen any inhibitory surrounding of the receptive field similar to that described by BARLOW in which both "on" and "off" components of the response are inhibited. In a few of the experiments, we have examined the "on" and "off" processes separately and each appears to follow RICCO's law in the relation between area and intensity. A minimum value for the threshold intensity is reached as the area is increased. If the area is increased still further the threshold intensity remains constant. There is no rise in the intensity required such as BARLOW found in the frog with increased area.

To A. ARDUINI: We do not make a distinction between central and peripheral fields. Each process is maximally sensitive in the center of the field but the sensitivities of the two processes fall off at different rates as the periphery is approached. The diameter of the receptive fields may be as large as 2 millimeters.

To G. BAUMGARTNER: We can only speculate on the causes of retinal ganglion cell impulse activity until intracellular direct coupled recordings are obtained. However, in the goldfish retina, "off" responses are always connected with inhibition which suggests that "off" excitation is only a rebound phenomenon.

Single-Cell Analysis of the Organization of the Primate Color-Vision System*

By

R. L. DeValois and A. E. Jones

With 12 Figures

In order to determine the behavioral significance of various physiological responses to stimuli, it is obviously important to have a good idea of what sort of behavior the animal exhibits to these stimuli. Thus if one wants to determine if a particular type of ganglion cell response functions as part of the animal's color vision system one must first have some information about what sort of chromatic discrimination, if any, the animal is capable of making. Unfortunately, almost all of our evidence with regard to the psychophysics of color vision is from man, whereas most of our physiological evidence must inevitably be from other animals. One can minimize these difficulties by studying the physiology of color vision in an animal whose visual system is as similar as possible to man, or an animal on which there is considerable psychophysical data, or an animal from which it is fairly easy to obtain psychophysical evidence to correlate with the physiological findings. The macaque monkey actually satisfies all of these criteria: Its visual system anatomically, from the retina to the cortex, is essentially identical to that of man; it has been studied behaviorally a number of times and has been clearly shown to have a trichromatic color vision system which is in most regards the same as the human; and finally, it is comparatively easy to obtain psychophysical data from the monkey. For these reasons we have chosen to study the physiology of color vision in the macaque monkey.

Our recording site is the lateral geniculate nucleus (LGN) of the thalamus, the point at which the axons of the retinal ganglion cells synapse, and thus the 4th order neurons of the visual system. All indications are that responses to light recorded here are probably the same as would be recorded in retinal ganglion cells. Recording from the LGN we eliminate such problems as selective bias due to the varying size of ganglion cells, and possible disturbance of the retinal organization produced by stripping out the retina or inserting electrodes into the eye. However, our primary reason for choosing this recording site is the interesting lamination of the LGN which would indicate that there is a functional split of the visual system at this point.

Method

A small trephine hole is made in the skull above the LGN, with the monkey under barbiturate anesthesia. The 1—2 μ tip diameter, 3M KCl-filled micropipette is lowered under stereotaxic control through the intact brain to the LGN. The responses of single cells are fed through a conventional amplifying and audio-monitoring system and photographed with moving film from the face of a multiple-beam oscilloscope. At the termination of the experiment the brain is sectioned and the LGN layer from which a given cell response was recorded is determined from the electrode tracks.

---

* From Indiana University, Bloomington, Indiana, U.S.A.

The optical system consists of three beams from a single tungsten ribbon-filament light. The two primary beams, one for each eye, pass through a variable-duration shutter, are collimated to pass through interference and neutral density filters, and are then brought to a focus on the pupil so that the animal has a Maxwellian view of the light. The interference filters are adjusted with neutral density filters to equate them for physical energy. Movable aperatures or slides presenting patterns can also be introduced into these beams. The third beam can be combined with either or both of the primary beams just before the final lens and is used to present adaptation or bleaching lights. The animal is kept in a box which is light-tight except for the stimulating beams, and, except when otherwise indicated, the animal is in a dark-adapted state.

Results

The experiments to be reported here are an extension of those reported earlier (*1, 2, 3, 4*), which might be briefly summarized here.

The macaque LGN consists of six layers of cells in the caudal, foveally related portions of the nucleus. These layers are conventionally numbered 1 to 6 from ventral to dorsal. Anatomical studies, confirmed by our recordings, show that layers 1, 4, and 6 receive projections from the contralateral eye, and layers 2, 3, and 5 from the ipsilateral eye. This three-way split in the visual pathway at this level indicates a true functional division since each small part of the central retina projects to each of the three layers corresponding to that eye.

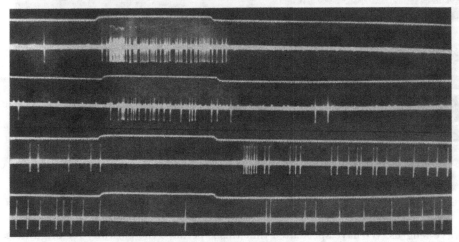

Fig. 1. Single cell records from cell in dorsal layer (top) and ventral layer (bottom) of LGN. Lower record in each pair is to lower intensity light flash. Top line on each of the four records is the signal marker with upward deflection indicating light on. Duration of flash: 500 msec

We have found that the different pairs of LGN laminae give different patterns of response to diffuse stimulation of the eye. Most (about 75%, from our single-cell recordings) of the dorsal layer (layers 6 and 5) cells give on-responses to light, with little or no inhibition to light of any wave-length (see Fig. 1 top pair of records). Most of the cells in layers 4 and 3, on the other hand, either increase or decrease their rate of firing when the eye is stimulated with light, depending on the wave-length (see Fig. 2). The large cells in the ventral layers 1 and 2 are inhibited by light of all wave-lengths and fire off-responses. (See Fig. 1, bottom pair of records.)

12*

The ventral layer inhibitory cells have been found to have broad spectral sensitivity curves, with peak sensitivity in the region of 510 mμ in the dark-adapted state. Some of these cells, when tested under conditions of light adaptation, have been found to show a Purkinje shift, with the peak sensitivity now at longer

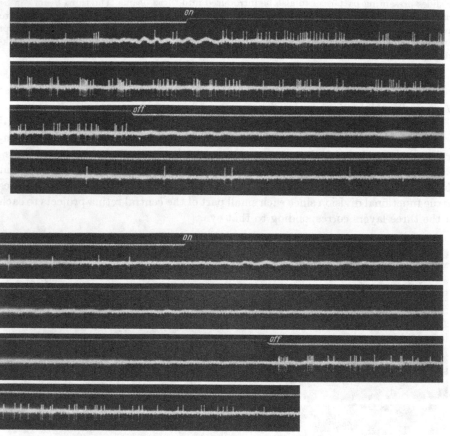

Fig. 2. Two records from a single intermediate layer LGN cell. Each record is to a single long light pulse and is cut into four parts. Top record: 650 mμ light. Bottom record: 500 mμ light

wave-lengths. We have speculated that this is perhaps the pathway for brightness information, separate from the pathways for color vision.

Almost all of the on-cells in the dorsal pair of layers, 6 and 5, on the other hand, have quite narrow spectral sensitivities; they respond to only a single narrow range of wave-lengths. We have reported that these color-selective on-cells fall into five spectral sensitivity categories, with the peak sensitivities of the various elements being found at about 440, 510, 550, 580, and 620 mμ.

The cells in the intermediate pair of LGN layers respond to various wave-lengths in an opponent manner, with excitation to one spectral region and inhibition to another spectral region being exhibited by a single cell. These cells were reported to be of two types: a red-on, green-off cell and a blue-on, yellow-off cell.

The presence of these two different varieties of cell responses, both of which seem to be related to color vision — the narrow-band on-cells of the dorsal layers, and the opponent on-or-off cells of the intermediate layers — suggest to us the possibility of two different color vision systems in the primate. It would appear that color-vision information is encoded in two different ways in the retinal nervous system, one in an essentially Helmholtzian manner, in the sense of independent paths for the various spectral regions, and the other in an essentially Hering-like manner with opponent relations between complementary spectral regions.

In the experiments to be reported here, we explore how these cells in the four most dorsal layers respond to various adaptation and contrast situations, and what their relation might be to receptor pigments.

Successive contrast situation. There are many after-effects of retinal stimulation, but perhaps the most prominent one is what is called the negative after-image. As far as the chromatic aspect alone is concerned, a flash of light of one color induces roughly the complementary color in the same area after the light has been turned out. Furthermore, this induced after-image will interact with lights presented to the retinal area during the period of the after-image just as in a color-mixing situation. Thus, for instance, if one observes a red light for a period of time and the light is then turned off, one will now see a green after-image. And if one looks from the red light not to a white surface but to a green spot, this spot will now appear more saturated, "greener", than if one did not have the preexposure to the red light. The green afterimage thus is summing with the response to the "green" spot to produce more of a chromatic effect than if the after-image had not been induced.

It is dangerous to jump to the quick conclusion that a physiological process is the mechanism for a given kind of psychophysical behavior on the basis merely of a rough sort of correspondence between the two. Such an identification must await more careful quantitative analysis, but a qualitative agreement is surely an important first step in understanding the situation.

If one looks at the after-effects of stimulation on these various elements, one immediately sees that the on-or-off cells give essentially the opposite type of behavior after a light has been turned off as they gave during the light (see Fig. 2). Thus an element that was excited by 620 mμ, is inhibited for a prolonged period of time at the termination of the light. And similarly, if it was inhibited by the light, it fires at the termination of the light. If one postulates, as we do, that each of these on-or-off units is carrying two sorts of information, inhibition signalling one color and excitation another, then this post-excitatory inhibition and post-inhibitory excitation could form the bases for negative afterimages.

In Fig. 3 can be seen the response of a red-on, green-off cell to successive stimulation by two roughly complementary lights (bottom record), as compared with the response to each alone (top records). As can be seen, there is a larger amount of excitation ("red") to the 650 mμ light when it had been preceeded by the 500 mμ light than when it had not. This is analogous to the larger perceptual effect a red light would have if it were preceeded by a green light than if it were not. What is happening, of course, is that the on-response to the 650 is summing with the off-response to 500. It is interesting to note, incidentally, that this addition of the two processes is roughly linear. We have shown that in the reverse sequence of presentation there is also summation of inhibition.

182   R. L. DeVALOIS and A. E. JONES:

The on-cells, on the other hand, exhibit little post-excitatory inhibition: the firing rate after the termination of the light does not differ very much from the spontaneous firing rate.

Simultaneous contrast. It is well known that if an achromatic area is surrounded by a chromatic area, the achromatic area is seen as colored, and of about the complementary color of the surround.

In a few preliminary experiments we have attempted to determine how various types of cells respond in such a contrast situation. The procedure is to explore the stimulus field with a small spot of light until the retinal area has been found which

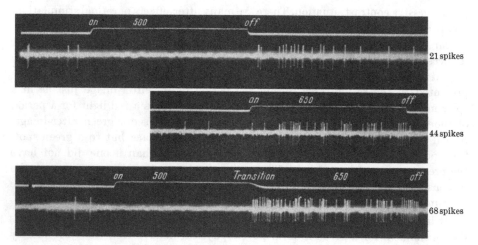

Fig. 3. Three records from a single on-or-off cell

best fires the cell. This area is then stimulated with a spot of white light with a chromatic surround and the resulting cell response compared to that produced by diffuse white and chromatic stimuli.

We have just begun these experiments and have nothing definitive to report as yet, but it is interesting to note that when these stimuli are presented to the eye while recording from on-or-off cells, we find behavior analogous to simultaneous contrast. For instance, a cell which fires on to "red" light and is inhibited by "green" and gives essentially no response to white light has been found to give an on-response to a spot of white light on a "green" surround. That is, it behaves here in the same manner as to stimulation with a "red" light. Such pronounced contrast effects have not been found with pure on-cells.

Spectral shifts with intensity. Describing the activity of color-selective cells by plotting spectral sensitivity curves — either size of response to an equal-energy spectrum, or intensity required for equal size response — is a common practice, and one that we have done ourselves. It is useful as a crude indication of the cell's behavior but the limitations of it should be understood. It is, of course, quite crucial to specify the adaptation conditions because quite different results can be obtained just as a function of achromatic, to say nothing of chromatic, adaptation. What we would like to point out here, however, is that the sort of curve one obtains is also a function of the intensitiy of the monochromatic stimuli used.

The spectral sensitivity curves shift as the intensity level changes so that equal response curves will vary as a function of the size of the response chosen as the criterion. This is true for both on and on-or-off cells, although the changes are more pronounced in the latter case. In Fig. 4 are two examples of these changes, one in the blue-on part of a blue-on, yellow-off cell, the other in a red-on cell. In each case the peak shifts away from the middle spectral range as the intensity is increased. These changes have been quite consistently found in cells of these types. In other cases the situation appears to be more complex and we would like to clarify the situation for ourselves before reporting about them.

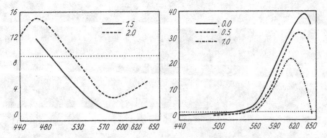

Fig. 4. Plots of the responses of two cells to different intensities and wavelengths of light. In each graph the dotted horizontal line is the spontaneous firing rate. The solid curve in each case is the highest intensity level.

We would do no more than suggest a possible relationship between these changes and the Bezold-Brücke-effect which relates hue changes to luminance. Above about 580 mμ one must increase the wave-length to maintain constant hue as luminance is increased. Correspondingly, we find in the red-on cells (or red-on phase of the red-on, green-off cells) that one must increase the wave-length to produce maximal response as the intensity level is increased. At the other end of the spectrum the changes, in the case both of the Bezold-Brücke-effect and our unit recordings, are toward the shorter wave-lengths.

Distinction between on and on-or-off cells. The above and our previously reported work would make it appear that the distinction between on-cells and on-or-off cells is a quite clear-cut one. Actually, even in the dark-adapted eye, this is not so. Some cells, in the dark-adapted state, are completely excitatory: that is, one can find no evidence of inhibition to any wave-length. Others have completely balanced inhibition and excitation to complementary spectral regions (and with no response to white light). But other cells lie in between these extremes, having large on-responses and yet some inhibition to light of certain wave-lengths. In other words, rather than two completely distinct categories, there is a continuous, but clearly bimodal, distribution.

Taking this into consideration, incidentally, we feel that the classification of the 550 on-cells should be changed. Having extended the spectral range of our stimuli, we have clearly found that these cells show strong inhibition to light from both of the ends of the spectrum. These cells, then, should probably be considered green-on, purple-off cells, particularly since these cells have turned out to be found predominantly in layers 3 and 4.

The basic similarity between these two types of cells is seen in the relationships among their peak spectral sensitivities. The peaks of the excitatory and inhibitory

184   R. L. DeVALOIS and A. E. JONES:

phases of the red-on, green-off cells correspond roughly to the 620 on and the
510 on-cells, being c. 630—650 and 500—530 mμ respectively. The crossover points,
i. e., the spectral point at which the transition occurs from excitation on one side

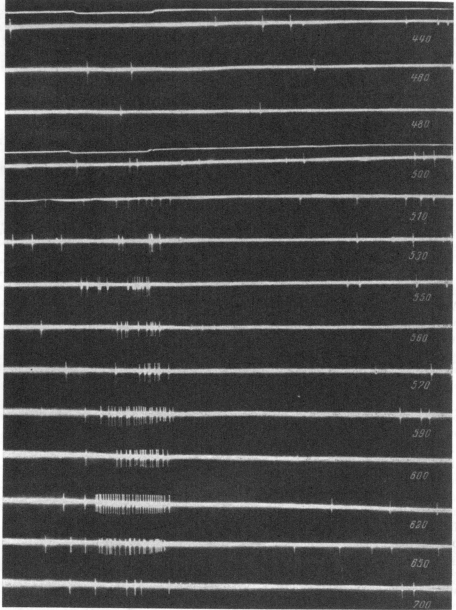

Fig. 5. Superimposed records of the responses of a single cell to different wavelengths of light, all equated for
physical energy. The signal marker can be seen on the top record

to inhibition on the other, vary from 560 to 600 mμ from cell to cell. In Fig. 5 and 6
can be seen two examples of these cells, one a red-on, the other a red-on, green-off cell.

The blue-on, yellow-off cells have their excitatory and inhibitory peak sensitivities at about 420 to 460 mμ and 560 to 600 mμ, corresponding roughly to the peak of the 440 and 580 on-cells. The crossover points in these cells are in the

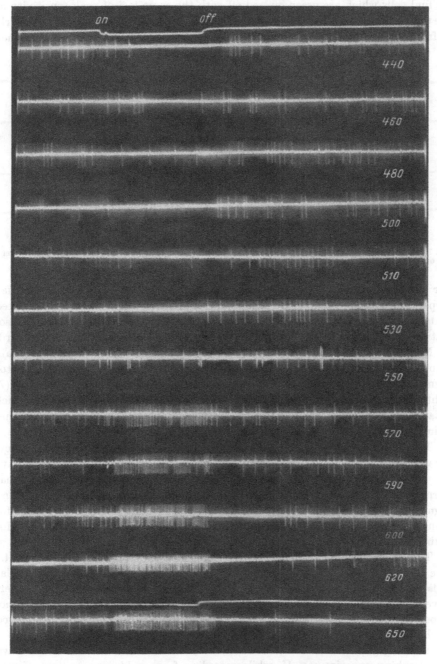

Fig. 6. Superimposed records of responses of a single cell to an equal energy spectrum

range of 490 to 520 mμ, varying from cell to cell. The green-on, purple-off cells have their peak excitation at c. 550 mμ, and crossovers at about 470 and 600 mμ.

On occasion we have found cells which are the mirror images of the afore-mentioned on-or-off cells, with inhibition and excitation reversed. For instance, we find cells which are green-on, red-off with the same loci of peak sensitivity as the red-on, green-off cells. These reversed cells, however, have not been found nearly as frequently as the others. An incidental finding is that on several occasions when

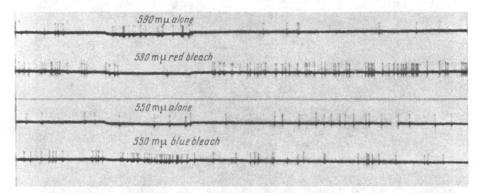

Fig. 7. Responses of a single LGN cell to conditions described in text (pg.187). In these records the signal marker is on the same channel as the recording and light on is indicated by the downward deflection of the baseline

our electrode picked up from two cells simultaneously, we have found that they respond in completely opposite fashion, one inhibiting when the other is excited and visa versa. We have at times wondered whether there is some sort of asso-ciation here similar to the Renshaw cells and motoneurons of the spinal cord.

Narrow or broad-band pigments. The spectral sensitivity curves which we obtain from LGN cells in the four dorsal-most layers are much narrower than any receptor pigments which have been extracted from eyes or measured with Rushtons (7) ophthalmalogical techniques. The same is true for the "modulators" which Granit (6) has found (or produced by selective adaptation) in a variety of other animals.

Two alternative hypotheses have been put forth to account for this discrepancy. Granit (6) has suggested that there may be narrow-band pigments which have not as yet been discovered. Donner (5), on the other hand, has argued that narrow-band modulators must be produced by neural interaction of broad-band pigments. The latter alternative would certainly be more attractive, both for being in better agreement with what is known about retinal pigments, and for fitting better the demands of psychophysical experiments on color-mixing.

The on-or-off cells are quite clearly related to two different retinal pigments. The receptors containing these different pigments must be connected to bipolar cells [if this is indeed the site of the slow potentials Svaetichin (8) and others have recorded] in such a way that one produces depolarization and the other hyperpolarization. The resulting excitation and inhibition is presumably relayed to the LGN.

That the pigments involved are broad rather than narrow band can be shown by bleaching experiments. If, while recording from a blue-on, yellow-off cell, we turn on an intense short wave-length bleaching light and then record the response to monochromatic lights across the spectrum, we find inhibition to all wave-lengths including those which previously produced excitation. With appropriate choices of wave-length and intensity of the bleaching light, the inhibition produced by longer wave-lengths of monochromatic lights is now also greater than in the dark-adapted state. The opposite result, that is, a great extension in the spectral range which will produce excitation, is produced by bleaching lights of long wave-length. It must therefore be that two broad band retinal pigments are involved here, each covering almost the whole spectrum. Producing opposite effects at some retinal site, they cause either excitation or inhibition or no response to any particular wave-length as a function of the algebraic summation of their effects.

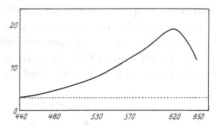

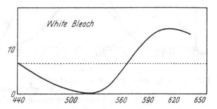

Fig. 8. Plot of the responses of a LGN cell when the eye is in the dark-adapted (top graph) and light adapted (bottom graph) state. Dotted horizontal line is the spontaneous activity level

Performing exactly the same bleaching experiments while recording from pure on-cells, we obtain the same results. When the responses to various spectral lights are recorded when the animal is dark-adapted, large on-responses are found to a certain spectral region and smaller or no responses elsewhere. No lights produce inhibition. But if a bleaching light of the wave-length to which the cell is most responsive is turned on and the experiment repeated, inhibition is now produced over most of the spectrum. Conversely, on-responses can be produced by wave-lengths which were previously ineffective if the eye is bleached with a light from the opposite end of the spectrum.

In Fig. 7 is seen an example of the results from such an experiment. These records are from a red-on cell which, as can be seen from top record of each pair, fired a sizable on-response to 590 mμ and gave little response to 550 mμ in the dark-adapted state. When a long wave-length bleach (bottom record, top pair) was turned on, however, 590 mμ now inhibited the cell, which also was inhibited now by shorter wave-lenths. If a short wave-length bleach was now used and the procedure repeated it was found that 550 mμ, which in the dark-adapted state produced no response, now produced a large on-response (bottom records, Fig. 7).

Occasionally it has been found that such shifts can be produced by achromatic as well as by chromatic adaptation. In Fig. 8 are the equal-energy curves for a red-on cell in the dark-adapted state (top curve) and in a light-adapted state (bottom curve).

Again the evidence quite clearly indicates that broad-band pigments are involved, and that even in the case of the pure on-cells there is an interaction between excitatory and inhibitory effects. It is this algebraic summation of opponent processes that results in the narrowness of the spectral response curves.

Relation to Rushton's pigments. With his ophthalmoscopic technique, Rushton (7) has found evidence for two broad-band cone pigments in the human eye. Although there may be some question about the results, particularly with regard to possible contamination with chromatic bi-products of bleaching, they are certainly the best evidence we have available on human cone pigments. In Fig. 9 are the absorption curves of these two pigments, plus a blue pigment which we have put in because Rushton's measurements did not extend to the lower wavelengths.

Let us assume that these three pigments are distributed among various cones, and that groups of cones synapse with a bipolar in such a way that, at a particular bipolar, the red cones produce depolarization and the green cones hyperpolarization. If we further assume that there are differences, among bipolars connected in this

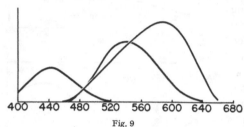

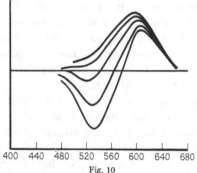

Fig. 9. Absorption curves of retinal pigments. Two long wavelength pigments are from Rushton's data; the short wavelength pigment is hypothetical

Fig. 10. Curves produced by subtracting Rushton's 540 pigment from the 590 pigment

fashion, in the proportion of red to green cones to which they are related, then we would find that the algebraic summation of the potentials would give curves similar to those in Fig. 10. In this figure the successive curves going from top to bottom have increasingly larger proportions of green acting in an inhibitory direction with respect to the red pigment feeding in its effect in an excitatory manner. The net result in the top case where there is relatively little green inhibitory connection is excitation or no response across the spectrum. On the other hand, in the bottom curve there is balanced inhibition and excitation to different spectral regions.

The qualitative similarities between the top and bottom curves and our red-on and red-on, green-off cells respectively are obvious. Worth noting is the shift in the red peak toward the longer wave-lengths in the balanced case as compared to the situation which is unbalanced in the excitatory direction. Our red-on, green-off cells correspondingly have their red excitatory peak sensitivities at longer wave-lengths than do the pure red-on cells.

The picture we now have of the organization of these two color vision systems is that of all of these cells being connected to receptors which interact at some retinal stage in an opponent manner. In some cases this interaction is such that there results balanced inhibition and excitation; in others the balance is shifted toward excitation. The former is the on-or-off system, the latter the on system.

In Fig. 11 and 12 are the averaged results of our on-or-off cells, and what would result from a particular interaction among Rushton's pigments. The gross qualitative agreement is clear. Attempting to go beyond this point without specific information on the cone pigments in macaques, as opposed to man, does not seem warranted.

Similar sorts of curves could be made for the on-cells. One problem that does arise here is how one could get a narrow band on-cell with a peak at 580 mμ,

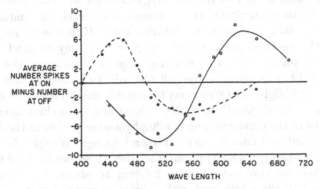

Fig. 11. Plot of the averaged results from our on-or-off cells

our yellow-on cells. A possibility that suggests itself, but which we have not as yet had an opportunity to explore, is that there could be a mixture of the red and green pigments in one class of receptors, which, after the log transformation, would be connected in the opposite direction in a bipolar with both red and green receptors. In other words, the resultant would be $\log (R + G) - \log R - \log G$.

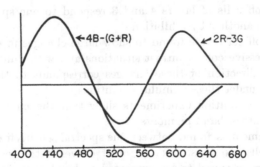

Fig. 12. Curves produced by subtracting the pigment curves in Fig. 9 from each other as indicated on the graph

Comments

Some people may perhaps be troubled with the idea we have been propounding of two separate (to an extent) color vision systems, two different ways in which the information from the color receptors is encoded, particularly since it appears that the on-or-off cells give a different sort of information than do the on-cells in color contrast situations, whether successive or simultaneous. It is, however, only a problem if it be thought that each single cell is carrying some absolute information about the chromaticity of the stimulus, without regard to what other cells are saying. This is absurd, and could not be true even if there were only one type of color vision system. Thus a red-on cell will give equal responses to the long wave-lengths or to white light if the relative intensities are appropriately adjusted. But these two stimuli will produce different responses in other cells, and the color seen will be a function of the type of activity going on in a number of different cells. The same is, of course, true for the on-or-off cells, any one of which will give the same response to a number of discriminably different wave-lengths.

Specifically with regard to the contrast situations we should remember that in the case of either simultaneous or successive contrast, the induced color is considerably less saturated than the inducing color. If, however, we observe the behavior of the on-or-off cells it would appear that they respond with almost equal responses under these two circumstances. For instance, the off-response to a "green" light, in a red-on, green-off cell, will be almost as large as the on-response to a "red" light, and vice versa for the inhibitory phases. In other words, they appear to "over-respond" to contrast situations, or to chromatic adaptation when compared to the corresponding psychophysical responses to these situations. On the other hand, the on-cells do not respond enough. We speculate, therefore, that the resulting percept is a compromise between these two kinds of information. In the simultaneous contrast situation referred to above, the on-or-off cell is signalling "red" to the white spot with a green surround, whereas the on-cells signal "white". What one actually sees in this situation is a very desaturated red.

Summary

1. Cells in the three pairs of lateral geniculate nucleus laminae give different patterns of response to light.

2. The on-cells of layers 6 and 5 respond to only one or another of four spectral regions in the dark-adapted state.

3. The on-or-off cells of layers 4 and 3 respond to one spectral region with excitation, and to another by inhibition.

4. The on-or-off cells were found to show large changes in response in simultaneous and successive color contrast situations and with different intensities of stimulation. The direction of these changes corresponds to the psychophysical changes observed under these stimulus conditions.

5. Chromatic adaptation experiments show that the modulator-like on-cells are connected to broad-band pigments.

6. Close agreement is found between the spectral sensitivities of these various types of LGN cells and RUSHTON's pigment curves if the receptors containing these pigments are assumed to be connected to bipolars in opposing excitatory and inhibitory fashion, and with variable proportions of excitation and inhibition in different cells.

References

1. DeVALOIS, R. L., C. J. SMITH, S. T. KITAI and A. J. KAROLY: Responses of single cells in different layers of the primate lateral geniculate nucleus to monochromatic light. Science 127, 238—239 (1958).
2. — — A. J. KAROLY and S. T. KITAI: Electrical responses of primate visual system. 1. Different layers of macaque lateral geniculate nucleus. J. comp. physiol. Psychol. 51, 662—668 (1958).
3. — — and S. T. KITAI: Electrical responses of primate visual system II. Recordings from single on-cells of macaque lateral geniculate nucleus. J. comp. physiol. Psychol. 52, 635 to 641 (1959).
4. — Color vision mechanisms in the monkey. J. gen. Physiol. 43, 115—128 (1960).

5. DONNER, K. O.: The spectral sensitivity of vertebrate retinal elements. In: Visual Problems of Colour. Nat. Phy. Lab. Sym. 8, 541—563 (1958).
6. GRANIT, R.: Receptors and Sensory Perception. New Haven: Yale Univ. Press 1955.
7. RUSHTON, W. A. H.: Kinetics of cone pigments measured objectively on the living human fovea. Ann. N. Y. Acad. Sci. 74, 291—304 (1958).
8. SVAETICHIN, G., and E. A. MACNICHOL: Retinal mechanisms for chromatic and achromatic vision. Ann. N. Y. Acad. Sci. 74, 385—404 (1958).

Discussion see pg 197

Some Findings on Central Nervous System Organization with Respect to Color[1,2]

By

MARGARET A. LENNOX-BUCHTHAL

With 5 Figures

Much is known about retinal mechanisms in color vision and about psycho-sensory phenomena. Less is known about how the retinal messages are trans-mitted to the brain — whether retinal mechanisms alone determine the psycho-sensory phenomena or whether and in what way the messages are altered in the nervous system. It has been established that there is ample anatomical basis for neuronal and receptor interaction in the retina (25) and that such interaction must account for the narrow spectral sensitivity curves of retinal ganglion cells (10, 13). Neuronal interaction in the retina must account, too, for the changes in off/on ratio with adapting lights of different colors (11) and for the differential on and off spectral sensitivity of single cells in goldfish retina according to whether the center or the periphery of the receptive field is stimulated (27).

The simplest question which can be asked is whether the spectral sensitivity of the gross response in visual centers corresponds to the spectral sensitivity of the retinal response. INGVAR (15) has studied this problem, defining the "spectral sensitivity of the cortical centers" as the reciprocal of intensity at equal amplitude. His illustrations show that the cortical spectral sensitivity curves differ sufficiently in degree (though there is a resemblance in kind) from the retinal spectral sensiti-vity that there is every reason to suspect that the signal is altered during trans-mission in the central nervous system. We, too, had found that the amplitude of the cortical response in cats did not mirror the amplitude of the retinal response to different colors (20), the discrepancy being greatest outside the primary visual receiving area (22). In fully dark adapted animals, however, the correspondence in primary optic cortex was very close (17).

LE GROS CLARK (6) made the stimulating proposal that color discrimination may be mediated by differences in the conduction velocity of the fibers subserving end organs of different spectral sensitivity. An additional postulate, that the

[1] From the Institute of Neurophysiology, University of Copenhagen.

[2] The research reported in this document has been sponsored by Air Force Research Division of the Air Research and Development Command, United States Air Force, through its European Office.

geniculate lamination is the anatomical mediator of this division, has been dis-proved (*5, 9*) as has the assignment of large fibers to blue sensitive units (*4, 20*).

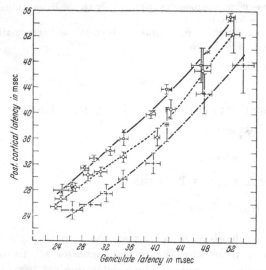

Fig. 1. Latency of responses to colored light flashes at posterior optic cortex (ordinate) and at lateral geniculate (abscissa). Mean of 21 experiments. Mean error is indicated by horizontal and vertical lines. Response latencies to: ● —— ●: blue flashes (445 mμ); × —— ×: green flashes (515 mμ); ○ —— ○: yellow flashes (578 mμ); + — · — · +: red flashes (over 600 mμ) (from *17*).

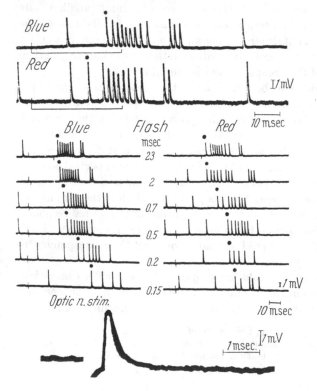

The primary postulate has, however, received support. In humans red is perceived sooner than blue of equal brightness (*24, 26*). The response evoked in the optic tectum of cat-fish consisted of an early and late component when the flash was red, of a component with an intermediate latency when the flash was blue or yellow (*3*). In cats Chang (*4*) found that the triple response to geniculate stimulation was enhanced by illumination of the eye, and that the first component was enhanced when the illumination was red, the third most when it was blue. We found in cats (*20*) that colored flashes equilibrated in intensity to evoke a retinal response of the same amplitude, evoked a cortical response of shortest latency for red. Furthermore, no adjustment of the intensity could be made such that the responses to the different colors were the same in amplitude and latency in

Fig. 2 (left). Example of on response of an on-off unit to blue and red flashes (above) and of change with decreasing flash duration (middle). Because of abundant spontaneous spikes, first spike of response as determined by its constancy with repeated flashes is marked with ●. Threshold of second burst is seen but that of initial discharge cannot be seen here as unit was still responding at shortest flash duration used; with constant flash duration and decreasing intensity, threshold intensity was 0.03 per cent for blue and 0.003 per cent for red flashes. Short latency response of same unit to optic nerve stimulation is shown at bottom. Positive is up. |⎴⎴⎴| and ⌐⎴⌐ indicate flash (from *18*).

contrast to the finding that the responses in *Limulus* (*12*) could be made identical to different colors by suitable adjustment of the intensity. Finally, comparing the response at geniculate and at cortex the same findings resulted: that the transmission time in the central nervous system was shortest in response to red flashes, intermediate to yellow and longest to blue and green (*17* and Fig. 1).

In an attempt to obtain additional proof that this difference in transmission time does indeed occur in the central nervous system and not in the retina, a single unit study was carried out recording from single optic tract fibers (*18*). In line with the evidence that cats have no (*14, 23*) or poor (*1*) color discrimination no units were found which responded only to red or to blue, the two equal-brightness colors used. The units did, however, differ in the intensity of the response to the two colors, and the briskness and latency of the response reflected the color sensitivity in those units whose threshold could be determined. Here again it turned out that the fibers with fast conduction velocity subserved red sensitive

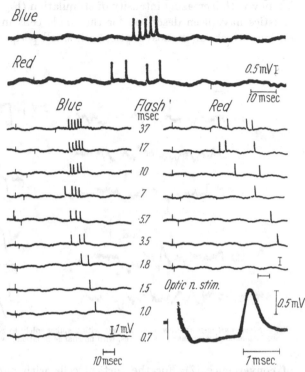

Fig. 3. Example of on response of a pure on unit to blue and red flashes (above) and of change with decreasing flash duration (below). Long latency response of same unit to optic nerve stimulation is shown at lower right. Positive is up. ⊥ indicates flash (from *18*)

composite segments in the retina (Fig. 2), whereas the slowly conducting fibers responded most actively when the flash was blue (Fig. 3).

In sum, it has been demonstrated in cat that the signal evolved in the retina undergoes transformation in the central nervous system and that the direction of the transformation in time depends on the color of the stimulating light. It has been argued that this fact, however interesting, has not been shown to have anything to do with color vision. The objection is justified for the experiments carried out on cats whose color vision is rudimentary at best (*1*). Findings in the same direction in cat-fish (*3*) are not subject to this objection.

This specific problem has not been answered in the monkey, which possesses full color vision, but there are two series of experiments in monkeys pertaining to central nervous organization with respect to color, one involving recordings from cortex (*19*) and the other from geniculate (*8, 9*).

More than half the single cortical cells responding to light did so with a restricted spectral responsiveness, responding to only one of the broad-pass filters with peak transmission at 450, 515, 587 and over 600 mμ (*19*, Fig. 4, 5). No unit was found which responded only to the filter with peak transmission at 560 mμ. The response of these units was with one or two spikes to a single flash at all intensities and after an interval which suggested that they were "on" responses. They responded in the same way to electrical stimuli delivered to the optic nerve and usually with no change in latency with increasing intensity of stimulation (Fig. 4, 5). These response charac- teristics have been described for the single cells in the cat's trigeminal sensory nucleus which are monosynaptic, with small peripheral fields and little evidence

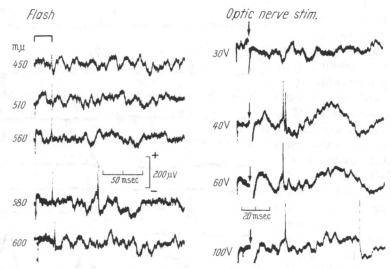

Fig. 4. *Single unit response from monkey cortex* with 2 spikes solely to *yellow* and of the same unit to *optic nerve stimulation* with one or two spikes, with no change in latency with increasing stimulus intensity

of convergence (*7*). For the cortical cells with narrow spectral responsiveness, then, there is evidence that the pathway between retina and cortex is one-to-one. The characteristic response to flash of single units in monkey geniculate (*8, 9*) [and in the cortex in cat (*16*)] consists of a burst whose number of component spikes and frequency of discharge depend on the intensity of the light. In some way, then, the response in cortex has been narrowed down, both in spike number and in spectral responsiveness, to a greater degree than in geniculate.

Such a "narrowing down" of spectral responsiveness, apparently due to neural interaction, has been demonstrated for single ganglion cells in the retina of frog (*10*) and cat (*13*) and such a narrowed responsiveness in the cortex by "partially shifted overlap" was postulated by LORENTE DE Nó (*21*) on the basis of anatomical and theoretical considerations to account for the fineness of visual acuity.

It is curious that on-off and off responses are so rarely seen at cortex as are responses to color pairs (*19*), the characteristic response of the cells of the middle geniculate layers (*8*). Off and on-off responses are seen, as are burst responses and responses to all colors, but not nearly as frequently as might be expected. One suspects that this information, too, has in some way been re-coded.

DE VALOIS and his collaborators (*8, 9* and see preceding article in this volume) have recorded from single cells in the geniculate and have demonstrated a very clear re-classification of information in that the cells in the dorsal layers responded to the onset of the flash and with rather narrow responsiveness, maximally to 450, 510, 550, 580 or 620; the responses in the middle layers were on-off to pairs of stimuli, that is on to blue and off to green-yellow or on to red and off to green;

in the ventral layers the responses were mainly off but the characteristics with respect to color are not reported.

Thus, in the geniculate there is already a classification of information received. All three types of information reach the same small area of cortex, for small cortical excisions cause small areas of atrophy including all six layers of the geniculate (25). Why then the single units in cortex have such different response characteristics and such different patterns of spectral responsiveness is not at all clear; — whether the information is "fed" on to the cortical cells in such a way that new patterns of response and new limits to spectral responsiveness appear, or whether the difference is due to different methods, though this seems rather unlikely. It seems likely that the information available to single cortical cells is in fact different from that sent out by the geniculate and that it is simpler. Such a recodification and simplification of the message can apparently be accomodated in a theory of human color vision (2).

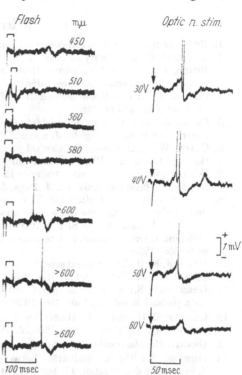

Fig. 5. *The response of a single unit in monkey cortex with one spike to three successive red flashes and the absence of a response to the other colors used.* The same unit responded similarly to stimulation of the optic nerve with constant latency with increasing intensity. It ceased to respond at a stimulus intensity about twice threshold

Summary

1. Evidence is reviewed that reorganization of visual messages with respect to color occurs in the central nervous system.

2. In man (24, 26), cat-fish (3) and cat (4, 17, 18, 20) blue and red stimuli of equal brightness appear to undergo temporal differentiation in that red stimuli are transmitted more rapidly than blue. This has not so far been confirmed for monkey.

3. In monkey cortex (the eye light adapted) more than half the single units responding to light did so with narrow spectral responsiveness. Different units responded to flashes through only one of four broad pass filters peaked at 450, 515, 587 or > 600 mμ. All single units with narrow spectral responsiveness to 560 mμ responded as well to one or two adjacent filters.

4. The response of the same cells to optic nerve stimulation suggested that they lay on a one to one pathway from optic nerve to cortex.

5. The different experimental conditions from those used in studies of monkey geniculate (8, 9) do not appear sufficient to explain the difference in results. It seems likely that the information available to single cortical cells is different from that at geniculate and that it is simpler.

References

1. BONAVENTURE, N.: Personal communication.
2. BOYNTON, R. M.: Theory of color vision. J. opt. Soc. Amer. 50, 929—944 (1960).
3. BUSER, P.: Analyse des réponses électrique du lobe optique à la stimulation de la voie visuelle chez quelques vertébrés inférieurs. pp. 162. Paris: Masson & Cie 1955.
4. CHANG, H. T.: Functional organization of central visual pathways. Ass. Res. nerv. Dis. Proc. 30, 430—453 (1952).
5. CHOW, K. L.: Failure to demonstrate changes in the visual system of monkeys kept in darkness or in colored lights. J. comp. Neurol. 102, 597—606 (1955).
6. CLARK, W. E. LE GROS.: Anatomical pattern as the essential basis of sensory discrimination. pp. 16. Oxford: Blackwell Scientific Publications 1947.
7. DARIAN-SMITH, I.: Neurone activity in the cat's trigeminal main sensory nucleus elicited by graded afferent stimulation. J. Physiol. 153, 52—73 (1960).
8. DE VALOIS, R. L., C. J. SMITH, S. T. KITAI and A. J. KAROLY: Response of single cells in monkey lateral geniculate nucleus to monochromatic light. Science 127, 238—39 (1958).
9. — — A. J. KAROLY and S. T. KITAI: Electrical responses of primate visual system: I. Different layers of macaque lateral geniculate nucleus. J. comp. physiol. Psychol. 51, 662—668 (1958).
10. DONNER, K. O.: The spectral sensitivity of vertebrate retinal elements. Visual problems of colour, II. 541—563. London: Her Majesty's Stationery Office 1958.
11. GERNANDT, B.: Selective adaption and the off/on-ratio of the retinal on/off-elements. Acta physiol. scand. 17, 150—160 (1949).
12. GRAHAM, C. H., and H. K. HARTLINE: The response of single visual sense cells to lights of different wave lengths. J. gen. Physiol. 18, 917—931 (1935).
13. GRANIT, R.: Mammalian colour modulators. J. Neurophysiol. 11, 253—259 (1948).
14. GUNTER, R.: The discrimination between lights of different wave lengths in the cat. J. comp. physiol. Psychol. 47, 169—172 (1954).
15. INGVAR, D. H.: Spectral sensitivity, as measured in cerebral visual centres. Acta physiol. scand. 46, suppl. 159, pp. 105 (1959).
16. JUNG, R., R. v. BAUMGARTEN u. G. BAUMGARTNER: Mikroableitungen von einzelnen Nervenzellen im optischen Cortex der Katze: Die lichtaktivierten B-Neurone. Arch. Psychiat. Nervenkr. 189, 521—539 (1952).
17. LENNOX, M. A.: Geniculate and cortical responses to colored light flash in cat. J. Neurophysiol. 19, 271—279 (1956).
18. — The on responses to colored flash in single optic tract fibers of cat: Correlation with conduction velocity. J. Neurophysiol. 21, 70—84 (1958).
19. LENNOX-BUCHTHAL, M. A.: Single units in monkey (Cercobus torgnatus atys) cortex with narrow spectral responsiveness. Vision Res., in press.
20. LENNOX, M. A., and A. MADSEN: Cortical and retinal responses to colored light flash in anesthetized cat. J. Neurophysiol. 18, 412—424 (1955).
21. LORENTE DE NÓ, R.: Studies on the structure of the cerebral cortex. II. Continuation of the study of the ammonic system. J. Psychol. Neurol. 46, 113—177 (1934).
22. MADSEN, A., and M. A. LENNOX: Response to colored light flash from different areas of optic cortex and from retina in anesthetized cat. J. Neurophysiol. 18, 574—582 (1955).
23. MEYER, D. R., R. C. MILES and P. RATOOSH: Absence of color vision in cat. J. Neurophysiol. 17, 289—294 (1954).
24. PIÉRON, H.: Les temps de réaction au chroma en excitation isolumineuse. C. R. Soc. Biol. (Paris) 111, 380—382 (1932).
25. POLYAK, S.: The vertebrate visual system. The University of Chicago Press 1957.

26. SCOTT, P., and K. G. WILLIAMS: The latency of visual perception in man to very brief coloured flashes of light. Vickers Group Research Establishment, Weybridge, Surrey, England: Report No. 50/1, 15, 1958.
27. WAGNER, H. G., E. F. MACNICHOL, jr., and M. L. WOLBARSHT: The response properties of single ganglion cells in the goldfish retina. J. gen. Physiol. 43, 45—62 (1960).

Discussion

K. O. DONNER: When the results of SVAETICHIN, WOLBARSHT and MACNICHOL and DE VALOIS are compared they agree in a general way, each of them showing some kind of antagonistic effects with different spectral sensitivities. Thus an interpretation in terms of an opponent-colour theory seems natural. There are, however, some points that makes one ask whether it is justified to make such a broad generalization:

1. In the experiments of DE VALOIS the antagonistic on-off-curves with impulse frequency plotted against wave-length for equal energy stimuli change shape as well as location of maxima under different states of adaptation. This does not seem to be the case in SVAETICHIN's experiments (C-response). If the potentials recorded by SVAETICHIN are somehow directly related to the generation of impulses, the impulse frequencies recorded would not be expected to follow the pattern observed by DE VALOIS.

2. In all these cases rod activity has not been well controlled, it is thus not clear whether some of the experiments refer to a rod-cone antagonism which may have nothing to do with colour vision.

3. In case of diffuse illumination of the whole receptive field in the cat's retina during dark-adaptation, impulse frequency for on and for off separately are related to intensity in a rather complicated and unpredictable way. In such a case the use of equal energy stimuli in different wave-lengths and plotting the impulse frequencies against wave-length, produces curves with different and rather variable maxima for on and off although the responses have been elicited only by rod activity.

G. BAUMGARTNER (zu R. L. DE VALOIS): Ich habe 3 Fragen:

1. Wie soll die Helligkeitsinformation durch ein lichtgehemmtes System übertragen werden? Wenn in den Schichten 1 und 2 vorwiegend off-responses vorkommen, würde nur Dunkel gemeldet.

2. Warum nehmen Sie an, daß durch Hemmung einer red-on-cell der Schichten 3 und 4 die Information „grün" übertragen wird? Haben Sie auch green-on-cells gefunden? Wenn sie existieren, ist in Analogie zu dem Hell-Dunkel-System der Katze folgende Funktionsdeutung möglich: Eine red-on-cell meldet immer rot, wenn sie aktiviert wird. Sie meldet nichts, wenn sie gehemmt wird. Gehemmt wird sie aber durch grün, welches eine green-on-cell aktiviert, die umgekehrt durch rot gehemmt wird.

3. Wenn on- und off-Zellen räumlich in verschiedenen Schichten getrennt sind, müßte eine gegenseitige Beeinflussung zwischen den Schichten für die reziproke Funktion des on- und off-Systems vorhanden sein. Sind hierfür physiologische oder histologische Grundlagen vorhanden?

P. GLEES (to R. L. DE VALOIS): Which results did Dr. DE VALOIS obtain from the large cell layers 1 and 2. Do they yield colour responses or brightness?

R. JUNG: DE VALOIS' opponent on- or off-responses einzelner Geniculatumneurone nach komplementärer Farbreizung sind die ersten objektiven Befunde über den sukzessiven und simultanen Farbkontrast im ZNS. BAUMGARTNERs on- und off-Umkehr der gleichen Neurone im simultanen Schwarz-weiß-Kontrast der wahrscheinlich farbblinden Katze ist wohl eine Parallele im Hell-Dunkelsystem.

Daß die Neurone in dorsalen Schichten mehr der Helmholtzschen und in intermediären Schichten der Heringschen Farbtheorie entsprechen, ist allerdings ein sehr überraschender Befund. Wenn die ventralen Schichten mit vorwiegenden off-Antworten ein Hell-Dunkelsystem darstellen, müßte man eine trinitarische Funktionstrennung der Schichten 1,2 gegenüber 3,4 und 5,6 annehmen?

Wenn eine Zellspezifität des Farbsystems mit kleineren Neuronen besteht, wie Svaeti-chin annimmt, dann müßten solche „Farbneurone" nur mit sehr dünnen Mikroelektroden re-gistrierbar sein. Fehlen farbspezifische Neurone in den großzelligen Geniculatumschichten 1 und 2 völlig und sind sie mit dickeren Elektroden über 1 μ seltener zu finden als Hell-Dunkel-neurone, die auf alle Spektralfarben antworten ?

M. A. Lennox-Buchthal: The fascinating study by Dr. de Valois correlating single unit finding in lateral geniculate with psycho-sensory data, is most stimulating. The results to date are solid and we look forward to what new experiments will yield.

There is still the disturbing discrepancy between findings at geniculate and at cortex. Psycho-sensory experiences are presumably determined at the cortical level. Why then can these findings not be confirmed when recording from cortical units ? Either the difference is an artefact due to differences in methods, or it is real, requiring re-evaluation of physiological and psycho-sensory correlations. There is probably no solution to this problem but the empirical one of experimentation.

R. L. de Valois (to K. O. Donner): 1. I find it hard to believe that a change in shape would not be produced by bleaching in any opponent-system. Clearly, if the two pigment curves did not completely overlap, the part of the composite curve produced by the non-overlapping portion would not be affected by bleaching the other pigment, whereas the overlap portion would be changed. Therefore a change in shape would result. Perhaps sufficiently quantitative data have not been presented to show these changes clearly.

2. The possible contribution of rod function to our results from the dorsal-layer cells is troublesome and we must investigate it further. But I should point out that we do not find the sensitivity differences among the various components which one might expect if some were being produced by rods and the others by cones. Furthermore, both the narrow-band on-cells, and the spectrally opponent on- or off-cells are found primarily in the foveally-related portions of the LGN.

One might also ask whether we understand enough about the make-up of the visual system to accept uncritically the traditional idea that rods have nothing to do with color vision.

3. We are well aware that plotting equal-response curves is better than studying the size of response to equal-energy stimuli. We have recorded equal-response curves from all of these different types of cells and have confirmed our results under those conditions. Variability of re-sponse, which you report finding in your experiments, cannot, I believe, account for our results. We find quite consistent curves from any given cell if adaptation conditions are maintained unchanged. All of the results we have presented have been from cells which we held long enough to replicate the curves. Furthermore, since we present our spectral stimuli in a random rather than spectral order, variability would lead to chaotic results from a given spectral sensitivity determination. This does not occur.

To G. Baumgartner: Your first two questions pertain to the problem of the significance of inhibition. I see no reason why information cannot be carried in the CNS through a decrease in rate of responding from the spontaneous level as well as by an increase in rate.

The only strong argument I can think of which would raise doubt about inhibition carrying information is that this would strongly limit the amount of information a cell can carry (a cell could increase its response from, say, 20 to 500/sec, but decrease it only from 20 to 0). Counter to this, I would make two points: (a) that one does not see these extremely rapid firing rates in response to flashes of light of an intensity corresponding to normal visual conditions. These are obtained only by blindingly bright lights or electrical stimulation. The system is thus not so asymmetrical as it would seem; (b) the extremely fine brightness or color discrimination of which a person is capable (implying many response steps) is based on an integration across hundreds of fibers and over long periods of time. Brightness discrimination becomes very poor with small fields and tachistoscopic flashes.

In favor of the notion that information is being carried by the inhibitory as well as the excitatory phase are the following: 1. economy. Everyone who records from single cells finds as much or more inhibition as excitation. It seems unlikely that all of this inhibitory in-formation is being discarded. 2. We find that the amount of decrease of firing is very systema-tically related to the stimulus parameters, whereas the off-response often is not. For instance we often find that the amount of inhibition during the light gives us a nice smooth sensitivity curve, whereas the succeeding excitation does not. 3. In many cells, the inhibitory phase is much more sensitive than the excitatory. One can often record quite clear inhibition during the light at one or more log units of intensity below the first discernable off-response at the termination of the light (see bottom record in Fig. 1, pg. 179). This last argument in particular appears to us to be quite convincing.

With regard to your third question, I would say that the interactions among the various systems occur in the retina (and presumably later in the cortex), but not at the LGN level.

To P. GLEES: The broad spectral sensitivity curves we record from layer 1 and 2 cells lead us to believe that these are brightness rather than color cells.

To R. JUNG: 1. The existence of three different systems, such as Prof. JUNG describes, would appear to be supported both by the anatomical and by our physiological evidence.

2. The idea that color information is carried by small cells, and brightness by large cells is, of course, supported by our results. The ventral layer (layers 1 and 2) cells are considerably larger than the dorsal layer (layers 3, 4, 5, and 6) cells, and our results point to the former as being concerned with brightness and the latter with color. But *within* any one layer, contrary to the situation in the retina and the cortex, there is only a small variation in cell size. Thus one does not have the problem of possible selective bias, with the electrode only isolating certain cells. The size of electrode needed to isolate single cell responses is a function not only of cell size, but of the distance between cells. Although by contrast to other thalamic nuclei the lateral geniculate cells are tightly packed, they are not nearly so close together as in the bipolar layer (or parts of the ganglion cell layer) of the retina. Thus it is quite possible to isolate the smallest cells with a 1μ electrode.

To M. A. LENNOX-BUCHTHAL: I don't think that it is possible, because of differences in technique, to tell whether her results and ours are discrepant or not. It is hard for me to understand how one can reliably differentiate on, on-off, and off-responses when only very brief flashes of light are presented, flashes which for the most part terminate well before any response is recorded. In the few experiments C. J. SMITH and I[1] ran on the monkey cortex using long light flashes, we on occasion recorded from cells which responded identically to our LGN cell types.

On the other hand, one would not, of course, expect all cortical cells to respond in the same manner as LGN or retinal cells. The information coming to the cortex obviously must be modified, analysed, changed in various ways rather than merely being relayed from cell to cell through the brain. So one should not be surprised at finding other cells which respond differently.

Subjektive und objektive spektrale Helligkeitsverteilung bei angeborenen und erworbenen Farbensinnstörungen*

Von

WOLFGANG JAEGER, PETER LUX, PETER GRÜTZNER und KARL-HEINZ JESSEN

Mit 4 Abbildungen

Einleitung

Bekanntlich gelingt es nur einem total Farbenblinden, durch direkten Vergleich zwei verschiedene Farben auf gleiche Helligkeit zu bringen. Der Farbentüchtige wird durch den Farbeindruck bei der Bestimmung des Helligkeitswertes zu sehr gestört. Höchstens in kleinsten Stufen bei jeweils sehr nahe beieinanderliegenden Farben ist für den Trichromaten und Dichromaten eine Bestimmung der

---

[1] SMITH, C. J., R. L. DEVALOIS and S. T. KITAI: Amer. Psychol. **13**, 387 (1958) and unpublished data.

* Aus der Universitätsaugenklinik Heidelberg.

Helligkeitsverteilung über das Spektrum möglich, der sogenannte Kleinstufenvergleich — eine sehr mühsame, zeitraubende und nur beim Geübten durchführbare Untersuchung.

Aus diesem Grunde hat die Physiologie schon lange nach Methoden gesucht,
auf psychophysischem und objektivem Wege die spektrale Helligkeitsverteilung,
die sogenannte Sensitivitätskurve, zu bestimmen.

Ein Teil dieser Methoden wurde hier in Freiburg entwickelt, weshalb die
Behandlung dieses Themas gerade hier an diesem Orte sich anbietet.

Methodik

a) Zunächst zu den subjektiven Methoden.

1. J. von Kries hat 1897 in Freiburg die Methode der *Peripheriewertbestimmung* angegeben. Die Farbe wird in der Peripherie der Netzhaut gezeigt, in einem Bezirk, in dem die
Netzhaut für die verwendete Flächengröße schon farbenblind ist. Der Farbreiz kann dann mit
einem farblosen Umfeld auf seine Helligkeit verglichen werden. Die ursprüngliche von Kriessche Methode arbeitet mit Spektralfarben. Sie kann aber auch auf Pigmentfarben übertragen
werden und ist dann die einfachste Methode der Bestimmung spektraler Helligkeitsverteilung
überhaupt (Demonstration).

Die Farbpunkte (jeweils Rot, Orange, Gelb, Grün und Blau) sind auf den Tafeln einer genormten Graureihe aufgeklebt. Man zeigt diese Tafeln in der Peripherie des Gesichtsfeldes,
wobei der Prüfling nur feststellen kann, ob der Punkt heller oder dunkler als das Umfeld ist. Die
Graustufe, auf der kein Punkt erkannt wird, gibt den Helligkeitswert der jeweiligen Farbe an
(Engelking).

2. Am Freiburger Physiologischen Institut hat 1907 Siebeck die *Minimalfeldhelligkeiten*
untersucht und als weitere subjektive Methode zur Bestimmung der spektralen Helligkeitsverteilung empfohlen. Die Verkleinerung des Farbobjektes wirkt auch im Gesichtsfeldzentrum
farbauslöschend. Es bleibt dann nur der Helligkeitswert, der mit dem eines farblosen Umfeldes
verglichen werden kann. Auch diese Methode ist ursprünglich für spektrale Farben ausgearbeitet worden, eignet sich aber auch für Pigmentfarben. Unsere genannten Grautäfelchen müssen
nur aus der nötigen Beobachtungsdistanz gezeigt werden: Die Farbe des Punktes ist dann nicht
mehr erkennbar, wohl aber ein Helligkeitsunterschied zum Umfeld. Die Graustufe, auf der
kein Helligkeitsunterschied angegeben wird, gibt den Helligkeitswert dieser Farben an.

Die Ergebnisse lassen sich kurvenmäßig darstellen. Die Graustufe, bei der Helligkeitsgleichheit angegeben wurde, wird gegen die Farbe aufgetragen.

Diese beiden Methoden sind zwar einfach, aber natürlich nicht sehr genau. Sie eignen sich
zur ersten Orientierung und in den Fällen, in denen keine andere Möglichkeit zur Bestimmung
der Sensitivitätskurven besteht.

3. Die psychophysischen Sensitivitätskurven, über die wir hier berichten wollen, sind mit
dem Flimmerphotometer nach Bechstein bestimmt. Die *Flimmerphotometrie* ist vom physiologischen und lichttechnischen Standpunkt die zuverlässigste Form der Bestimmung spektraler
Helligkeitsverteilung überhaupt. Wir haben uns dazu von Schmidt und Haensch ein etwas
modifiziertes Flimmerphotometer bauen lassen. Das Spektrum wird mit 32 Doppellinienfiltern durchlaufen, von denen etwa 25 in der Routineuntersuchung regelmäßig verwendet
wurden. Filter von Schott und Gen. Jedes Doppellinienfilter hat eine Halbwertsbreite von
etwa 9 mμ. Eine 500 Watt-Lampe mit der Optik eines Projektionsapparates bietet genügend
Intensität, um über das ganze Spektrum im photopischen Bereich untersuchen zu können.
Die relative spektrale Energieverteilung kann mit Hilfe eines geeichten Multipliers gemessen
und überprüft werden.

Die auf diese Weise erzielten Sensitivitätskurven entsprechen in etwa den IBK-Kurven
und den Kurven anderer Untersucher.

Soweit es sich um total Farbenblinde und annähernd total Farbenblinde handelte, war der
Direktvergleich für den Patienten einfacher als die Einstellung des Flimmerwertes. Der Direktvergleich wurde am gleichen Apparat mit den gleichen Filtern ausgeführt, lediglich das Prisma
im Photometerkopf befand sich in Ruhe und das Gesichtsfeld wurde von 2° auf 7° 42' vergrößert.
Mit dieser Methode wurden die Sensitivitätskurven der Achromatopsien ermittelt.

b) Nun zu den **objektiven Methoden** der Bestimmung der spektralen Hellig-keitsverteilung.

1. Die älteste objektive Untersuchung ist die *pupillomotorische Prüfung* nach C. von Hess. Sie hat seinerzeit ein weites Feld der vergleichenden Sinnesphysiologie eröffnet. Auch auf den Menschen ist sie angewendet worden. An der Freiburger Augenklinik hat Engelking vor 40 Jahren solche pupillomotorischen Sensitivitätskurven für Achromatopsien aufgenommen. Aber die Untersuchung ist noch mit erheblichen Ungenauigkeiten belastet. Namentlich läßt sie sich für den photopischen Bereich schlecht verwenden, weil der zugehörige Adaptations-zustand an sich schon eine enge Pupille mit sich bringt.

2. Aus diesem Grunde bedeutet es einen entscheidenden Fortschritt, daß mit Hilfe der *ERG* eine solche objektive Sensitivitätskurve aufgenommen werden kann. Namentlich auf dem Gebiet der Sinnesphysiologie der Tiere hat die ERG, soviel ich sehe, die Pupillometrie ganz abgelöst.

Für das dunkeladaptierte menschliche Auge sind die Sensitivitätskurven aus dem ERG schon lange bekannt (Piper 1910). Für das helladaptierte menschliche Auge kann man aber erst seit der Einführung des *Flimmer-ERG* nach Dodt brauchbare Sensitivitätskurven erhalten, die mit den psychophysischen vergleichbar sind. Erst seit der Entwicklung des Flimmer-ERG kann man sagen, daß subjektive und objektive Sensitivitätsbestimmungen gleichwertige, sich ergänzende Methoden sind.

Die Methode des Flimmer-ERG ist bekannt und braucht nicht genauer beschrieben zu werden. Auch unsere Apparatur ist in Anlehnung an die von Dodt gebaut worden.

Zur Herstellung der monochromatischen Lichter verwendeten wir 29 Doppelbandinter-ferenzfilter, von denen 14 in der Routineuntersuchung ständig angewendet wurden. Die Va-riation der Lichtintensität erfolgte durch Neutralfilter, deren optische Dichte für die jeweils benutzte Wellenlänge spektrophotometrisch bestimmt worden war. Die relative spektrale Energieverteilung wurde mit Vakuumthermoelement geeicht und laufend überprüft. Das Flimmerlicht ist konstant auf 31 Reize/sec mit Hilfe einer Sektorenscheibe eingestellt. Die Untersuchung erfolgt bei Adaptation auf 23 Lux.

Die Belichtungspotentiale wurden in der üblichen Weise mit Karpeelektrode abgeleitet, mit Differentialvorverstärker mit einer Zeitkonstante von knapp einer Sekunde verstärkt und photographisch mit Doppelkathodenstrahloszillograph registriert.

Die Auswertung erfolgte ebenfalls in der von Dodt angegebenen Weise: Die Höhe des Flimmerpotentials wird gegen die Lichtintensität aufgetragen und dadurch die für eine kon-stante Antwort notwendige Energie festgestellt. Nach den Angaben von Dodt bestimmten wir die Reizschwellen für 25 und 50 μV Potentialhöhe für die verschiedenen Wellenlängen. Die Sensitivitätskurven, die man erhält, sind sicher frei von skotopischen Einflüssen. Sie können mit den psychophysischen Kurven am Flimmerphotometer verglichen werden.

Bei den Achromatopsien läßt sich bekanntlich ein Flimmer-ERG nicht aufnehmen, weil sie keine photopischen Reizantworten geben. Es muß mit Einzelreizen bei Dunkeladaptation unter-sucht werden. An Stelle des Flimmerpotentials wird die Höhe der b-Welle gegen die Licht-intensität aufgetragen und daraus die Sensitivitätskurve berechnet.

Ergebnisse

a) Angeborene Störungen des Farbensinnes. Die Ergebnisse an den *angeborenen Störungen* des Farbensinnes (Proto- und Deuterostörungen) bringen über das, was Dodt, Copenhaver und Gunkel schon veröffentlicht haben, nichts Neues. Der Wert unserer Ergebnisse ist darin zu sehen, daß es wirklich *dieselben* Versuchs-personen sind, die mit fast den gleichen Spektralfiltern, am gleichen Ort, zu an-nähernd der gleichen Zeit mit subjektiven und objektiven Methoden auf ihre spektrale Helligkeitsverteilung untersucht wurden.

1. Blauüberhang. Die schon von Dodt, Copenhaver und Gunkel diskutierte Blaudiskrepanz oder, wie man es auch nennen könnte, der „Blauüberhang", kann auch in unseren Befunden eindrucksvoll gezeigt werden (Abb. 1).

Hier ein Beispiel der Deuterostörung (2 Deuteranomale und 2 Deuteranope) mit subjektiver und objektiver Sensitivitätskurve, wobei sich der bekannte Überhang der objektiven über die subjektive Kurve im Blau deutlich zeigen läßt. Auch wir sind der Meinung, daß der wichtigste Grund für diesen Überhang die Sensitivitätszunahme der „Blaureceptoren" in der Netzhautperipherie ist, denn die subjektive Sensitivitätskurve ist mit einer Reizfläche von 2°, die objektive Sensitivitätskurve dagegen mit einer Reizfläche von 40° ermittelt.

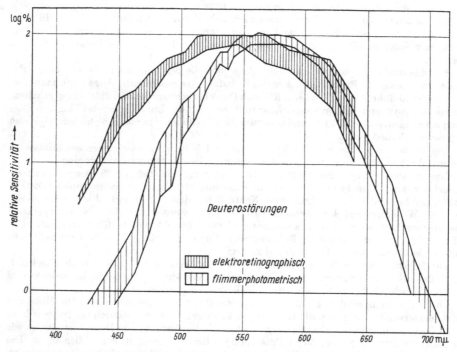

Abb. 1. Subjektive und objektive Sensitivitätskurven von Deuteranomalien und Deuteranopien. Subjektive Sensitivität gemessen mit Flimmerphotometer, objektive Sensitivität gemessen mit Flimmer-ERG

Diese Diskrepanz im Blau ist an sich schon lange bekannt als Differenz von Minimalfeldhelligkeiten und Peripheriewerten. Sie wurde nur früher nicht besonders betont, weil man der Heringschen Schule keine Nahrung zur Polemik geben wollte. Die Maculapigmentierung allein reicht zur Erklärung dieses Phänomens wahrscheinlich nicht aus, denn die Diskrepanz findet sich auch, wenn die Minimalfeldhelligkeiten knapp paramacular untersucht werden, also schon außerhalb des Maculapigments liegen. Weale hat dieses Phänomen untersucht und eine kontinuierliche Zunahme der Blausensitivität mit zunehmender peripherer Darbietung feststellen können.

2. Achromatopsie. Die Sensitivitätskurven der Achromatopsien waren überhaupt der Ausgangspunkt unserer Bemühungen. Man hat manchmal Zweifel an der Zuverlässigkeit der subjektiven Angaben der Achromaten, namentlich, wenn der Visus stark herabgesetzt ist. Wer viele dieser Achromatopsien untersucht hat, weiß, daß gelegentlich Patienten mit atypischer Helligkeitsverteilung darunter sind.

Namentlich die inkompletten Typen geben bei der psychophysischen Prüfung manchmal doppelgipflige Kurven oder Ausbuchtungen ihrer Kurven an. Es schien uns deshalb wünschenswert, diese Befunde objektivieren zu können. Über die *inkompletten* und *atypischen* Achromatopsien können wir heute allerdings noch nicht berichten. Die Zahl unserer Untersuchungen ist noch zu klein.

Zunächst sollen nur *Befunde an typischen Achromatopsien* gezeigt werden:

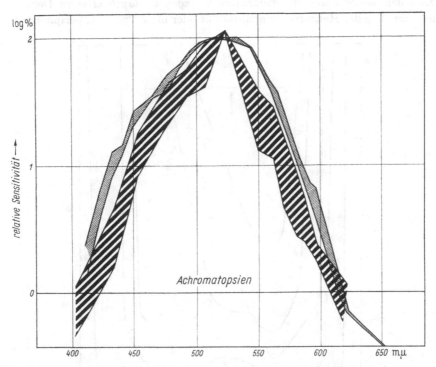

Abb. 2. Subjektive und objektive Sensitivitätskurve von Achromatopsien. Subjektive Sensitivität gemessen im Direktvergleich. Objektive Sensitivität gemessen mit ERG mit Einzelreizen

Hier objektive Sensitivitätskurven von 2 Achromatopsien (Abb. 2). Die ERG-Kurve ist etwas schlanker als die subjektive, zeigt also *nicht* die Diskrepanz, die wir bei den photopischen Kurven sahen. Vielleicht kann man das als Hinweis darauf nehmen, daß der Blauüberhang bei der photopischen Kurve wohl kaum von einer peripheren Stäbchenaktivität herrühren kann.

b) Erworbene Farbensinnstörungen. Wenden wir uns nun den erworbenen Farbensinnstörungen zu, also Farbenfehlsichtigkeiten, die durch eine Erkrankung der Netzhaut oder des Sehnerven hervorgerufen werden. Die reine Filterwirkung durch Gelbfärbung der Linse oder sonstige Medientrübungen können wir übergehen, weil sie über die Tatsache der Filterwirkung hinaus nichts Interessantes bietet.

Die erworbenen Farbensinnstörungen sind ein etwas vernachlässigtes For-schungsgebiet. W. D. WRIGHT sagt darüber in seinem Buch Researches on Normal and Defective Colour-Vision: "There is a big field here calling for more detailed investigation. Little published data is available on the luminosity curve, the colour mixture curves or the hue- discrimination curve in cases of acquired colour-blindness and measurements on these functions are likely to be rewarded with discoveries of both clinical and theoretical importance."

Das Problem der spektralen Helligkeitsverteilung bei erworbenen Farbensinn-störungen ist nicht immer der subjektiven *und* objektiven Untersuchung zugäng-lich (Lux).

Es fallen nämlich weg die *Farbensinnstörungen bei tapetoretinalen* Degenera-tionen vom Typ der Retinitis pigmentosa mit oder ohne Pigment, peripherer oder

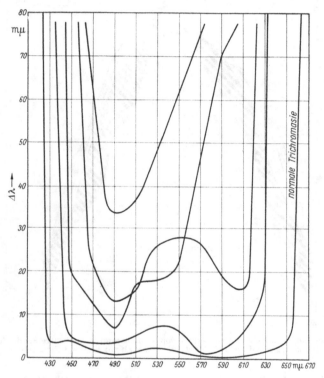

Abb. 3. Spektrale Unterschiedsempfindlichkeit bei Maculaleiden. $\Delta \lambda$ gemessen am Farbenmischapparat

macularer Lokalisation. Die objektive Methode versagt deshalb, weil das ERG bei diesen Patienten entweder ausgelöscht oder für diesen Zweck nicht meßbar ist.

Oft bestehen erstaunliche Diskrepanzen in der Schwere der verschiedenen Befunde: So z.B. bei einer 20jährigen Patientin mit tapetoretinaler Degeneration vom inversen Pigmentosa-Typ. Nur geringe Fundusveränderungen, Sehschärfe noch 5/7,5 jds., eben subnormale und verzögerte Dunkeladaptation. Blausinn-störung im Sinne einer herabgesetzten Unterschiedsempfindlichkeit für Farben-unterschiede in Grün und Blaugrün. Dagegen aufgehobenes ERG. Es handelt sich um eine gleichförmige Störung, die vier Geschwister der gleichen Familie betraf. Nur bei einem jüngeren Bruder war ein eben noch registrierbares Flimmer-ERG vorhanden, das aber auch für die Zwecke der Sensitivitätsbestimmung nicht mehr verwendbar war. Hier war es also nicht möglich, eine objektive Sensi-tivitätskurve aufzunehmen, um sie mit der subjektiv ermittelten zu vergleichen.

Dagegen können wir über eine Gruppe von erworbenen Farbensinnstörungen berichten, von denen wir zunächst eigentlich gar nicht erwartet haben, daß die elektroretinographische Untersuchung so ergiebig wäre: die *heredodegenerativen Macularleiden*. In gewisser Weise stellen sie das Gegenstück zur Pigmentdegeneration dar: Die Dunkeladaptation, also das skotopische System, ist praktisch nicht gestört. Der Prozeß betrifft in erster Linie das photopische System und damit auch den Farbensinn. Die *Art der Farbensinnstörung* wird wohl am besten durch die Kurve der Unterschiedsempfindlichkeit für Farbunterschiede charakterisiert

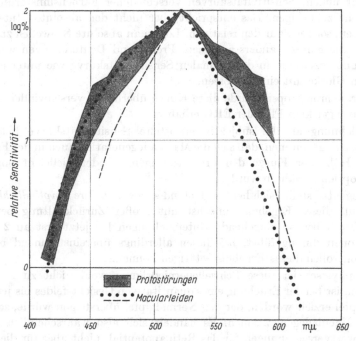

Abb. 4. Sensitivitätskurven von Protostörungen und Macularleiden gemessen mit dem Flimmer-ERG

(Abb. 3). In stark ausgeprägten Fällen wird ein Zustand erreicht, der dem einer Dichromasie entspricht, mit Verlust des Maximums in Gelb. Das äußert sich am Anomaloskop so, daß beide Grenzgleichungen anerkannt werden, und zwar mit einer Helligkeitsverteilung, die teils der Protostörung, teils sogar der angeborenen totalen Farbenblindheit entspricht (GRÜTZNER).

Dementsprechend ergibt die *Sensitivitätskurve am Flimmerphotometer* eine Verschiebung in Richtung zu dem kurzwelligen Ende des Spektrums. Die Kurven der Maculadegenerationen liegen — ähnlich wie die Protostörungen — zwischen dem Normalband und der Helligkeitsverteilung der Achromatopsie.

Eine *Sensitivitätskurve am Flimmer-ERG* ließ sich an unseren Fällen von Maculadegeneration ohne Schwierigkeit bestimmen (Abb. 4). In Übereinstimmung mit dem oben Gesagten und den subjektiven Ergebnissen fallen auch am ERG die Sensitivitätskurven der Maculadegenerationen mit denen der Protostörungen annähernd zusammen. Ohne ERG wäre man vielleicht geneigt anzunehmen, daß bei zunehmender Degeneration der Zapfen die Stäbchen auch unter Beleuchtungsbedingungen des Tagessehens die Sensitivitätskurve beeinflussen, wie sie das ja tatsächlich bei der Achromatopsie tun.

Das Flimmer-ERG beweist uns aber, daß es sich bei der Sensitivitätskurve der Maculadegenerationen um eine rein photopische Kurve handelt.

Auch ein anderer Befund macht es höchst unwahrscheinlich, daß das skotopische System an dieser Verschiebung der Sensitivitätskurve beteiligt ist. Man kann nämlich mit Hilfe des ERG eine *absolute Schwellenbestimmung* vornehmen. Es ist zwar üblich, Sensitivitätskurven verschiedener Farbensinnstörungen auf gleiche Höhe zu bringen. Das entspricht aber nicht den absoluten Intensitätsverhältnissen, sondern nur den relativen. Legt man absolute Schwellen zugrunde, so müßten die Kurven anders aussehen. Proto- und Deuterokurven wären viel niedriger und sozusagen in der normalen Sensitivitätskurve wie unter einer gemeinsamen Glocke mit eingeschlossen.

Bei der Achromatopsie würde diese Kurve überhaupt verschwinden, denn es läßt sich hier gar kein Flimmer-ERG erhalten.

In Anlehnung an die subjektiv ermittelte Sensitivitätskurve hatten wir ursprünglich angenommen, daß sich die Maculadegeneration auch in der Frage der absoluten Höhe der Kurve den Protostörungen — oder vielleicht sogar den Achromatopsien — nähern würde.

Das Gegenteil stellte sich heraus: Es fand sich eine *höhere Empfindlichkeit.* Natürlich muß dieses Ergebnis zunächst mit großer Zurückhaltung betrachtet werden. Wir haben so eingehende Untersuchungen bis jetzt erst an 2 Maculadegenerationen durchgeführt, bei diesen allerdings übereinstimmend bei zahlreichen Kontrollen dieses Ergebnis betätigen können.

Psychophysisch ist diese Schwellenerniedrigung wohl nicht zu realisieren. Bekanntlich ist bei der Erhebung eines quantitativen Gesichtsfeldes bis jetzt noch nie ein Gipfel erzielt worden, der den Normalgipfel übersteigen würde, schon gar nicht bei Maculadegenerationen. Es handelt sich also wahrscheinlich nur um Schwellenwertverschiebungen für das Retinapotential, nicht aber für die Sinnesempfindung.

Überraschend war das Ergebnis der Elektroretinographie bei Maculadegenerationen auch noch in anderer Hinsicht. Es zeigt nämlich, daß offensichtlich ein sehr großer Bezirk der Netzhaut verändert ist. Die beschriebenen Verschiebungen in den elektroretinographischen Sensitivitätskurven sind nämlich nur zu erwarten, wenn sich die degenerative Erkrankung auf mehr als nur die isolierte Macula bezieht. Tatsächlich zeigt eine genaue Untersuchung der Fundusperipherie auch hier gewisse Veränderungen in der Netzhaut, die kürzlich Mylius beschrieben hat. Demnach wäre der Name Maculadegeneration nicht ganz richtig, selbst wenn nur in der Macula selbst Pigmentverschiebungen zu finden sind. Man müßte wohl eher von einer Systemerkrankung der gesamten Netzhaut sprechen.

Zum Schluß seien als zusammenfassendes Ergebnis noch einige allgemeine Gesichtspunkte herausgestellt. Wenn man von reinen Filterwirkungen der brechenden Medien absieht, so läßt sich aus objektiven und subjektiven Bestimmungsmethoden bei angeborenen und erworbenen Farbensinnstörungen folgendes entnehmen:

Eine Farbensinnstörung, die mit einer Veränderung der Sensitivitätskurve einhergeht, scheint nur durch retinale Prozesse möglich zu sein.

Das gilt einmal für die *angeborenen Störungen.* Die Arbeiten von DODT, COPENHAVER und GUNKEL haben nachgewiesen, daß Proto- und Deuterostörungen sicher in der Netzhaut zu lokalisieren sind. Von der angeborenen totalen Farbenblindheit wußte man das schon lange.

Sehr wahrscheinlich gilt das Gesetz, wonach Veränderungen der Sensitivitätskurve nur durch retinale Prozesse möglich sind, auch für *erworbene* Farbensinnstörungen. Ob eine Opticusatrophie wirklich keine Veränderung der Sensitivitätskurve bewirken kann, wissen wir allerdings bis jetzt noch nicht genau genug. Wir wissen aber aus unseren Untersuchungen, daß degenerative Erkrankungen der Netzhaut Veränderungen der Sensitivitätskurve machen, und zwar subjektiv und objektiv.

Summary

In cases of congenital and acquired colour-defects psychophysical sensitivity curves and objective sensitivity curves were compared with each other. Measurements for psychophysical sensitivity curves were carried out with the Bechstein-Flicker-Photometer. The objective sensitivity curves were determined by Electroretinography (ERG): a) for the photopic vision using flicker-ERG (DODT), b) for the scotopic vision using single flashes.

In the different experiments the stimulus area of ERG was bigger than the stimulus area of Flicker-Photometer (ERG = 40°, Flicker-Photometer = 2°). Objective sensitivity curves of *Protanopia, Protanomaly, Deuteranopia and Deuteranomaly* showed an increase in short wave sensitivity compared with the psychophysical sensitivity measures of the same observers. We account for this discrepancy between psychophysical sensitivity measures and ERG-responses in terms of the different areas. The discrepancy seems to be caused by the increase of blue-sensitivity in the periphery of the retina (WEALE). Therefore in cases of congenital total colourblindness (Achromatopsia) no "blue-discrepancy" was found.

Further investigations were carried out with colour-defects, caused by acquired eye-diseases, especially with cases of *macular degeneration.* The maximum of sensitivity curves (the psycho-physical as well as the objective ones) is shifted in direction to short wave end of the spectrum. Sensitivity curves of macular degenerations in this way become similar to those of Protanopia and Protanomaly, sometimes even to those of Achromatopsia. In conclusion of these experiments not only the macular district, but also a bigger surrounding field must be involved.

Besides filtering effects of the ocular media — diseases of the retina alone seem to be able to elicit such shifting of sensitivity curves. It did not happen in experiments with diseases of the optic nerve or of the visual pathways.

Literatur

COPENHAVER, R. M., and R. D. GUNKEL: The spectral sensitivity of color-defective subjects determined by electroretinography. A. M. A. Arch. Ophthal. 62, 55—68 (1959).

DODT, E.: Cone electroretinography by flicker. Nature (Lond.) 168, 738 (1951).

— R. M. COPENHAVER u. R. D. GUNKEL: Photopischer Dominator und Farbkomponenten im menschlichen Elektroretinogramm. Pflügers Arch. ges. Physiol. 267, 497—507 (1958).

Engelking, E.: Über die Pupillenreaktion bei angeborener totaler Farbenblindheit. Ein Beitrag zum Problem der pupillomotorischen Aufnahmeorgane. Klin. Mbl. Augenheilk. **66**, 707 (1921).
— Farbtafeln zur klinischen Prüfung der Helligkeitsverteilung bei Farbenblinden. Ber. Dtsch. Ophthalm. Ges. Heidelberg 1951, 319.
Fincham, E. F.: Defects of the color-sense mechanism as indicated by the accommodation reflex. J. Physiol. (Lond). **121**, 570—580 (1953).
Grützner, P.: Typische erworbene Farbensinnstörungen bei heredodegenerativen Macula-leiden. v. Graefes Arch. Ophthal. **163**, 99 (1961).
Kries, J. v.: Abhandlungen zur Physiologie der Gesichtsempfindungen. Leipzig: J. Ambrosius Barth 1902.
Lux, P.: Elektroretinographische Befunde bei einer Familie mit Retinopathia pigmentosa centralis (sog. inverser Typ). Ber. Dtsch. Ophthalm. Ges. Heidelberg 1960, 322—326.
Mylius, K.: Über Fundusveränderungen außerhalb des Foveagebietes bei der Heredo-degeneration der „Macula". Klin. Mbl. Augenheilk. **126**, 539—546 (1955).
Piper, H.: Über die Netzhautströme. Arch. Anat. Physiol. **1911**, 85.
Weale, R. A.: Spectral sensitivity and wave-length discrimination of the peripheral retina. J. Physiol. (Lond.) **119**, 170—190 (1953).

Diskussion

M. Monjé: Nach unseren Untersuchungen ist die Absolutempfindlichkeit durch Farben-untüchtigkeit nicht gestört; eine Ausnahme bilden die Protostörungen, bei denen die Emp-findlichkeit im langwelligen Anteil des Spektrums herabgesetzt ist. Vielleicht liegt der Unter-schied zwischen den Proto- und Deuterostörungen darin, daß bei ersteren die Weißsubstanz verändert ist.

L. M. Hurvich: 1. The wave-length discrimination curve of one of your subjects looks like that of a tritanope. It reminds me of Fischer ten Doesschate and Bouman's case. Is this a case of acquired tritanopia?
2. Your case labelled "macular degeneration" shows a decrease in sensitivity. Since the filtering pigment is gone, ought we not to expect an increase rather than a decrease in sensi-tivity?
3. Your flicker-photometer spectral sensitivity functions for deuteranopes shows a slight increase in long wave sensitivity. Heath's experiments give evidence of much greater relative increases. I wonder what the difference can be attributed to? Of course, the flicker data in neither instance agree with the Graham and Hsia threshold data. What about this latter discrepancy?

D. Hurvich-Jameson: You have referred to the discrepancy between psychophysical sensitivity measures and electroretinogram responses in the short-wave end of the spectrum. You account for this discrepancy in terms of the different stimulus areas ordinarily used in the different experiments. There is, however, an observation reported by Armington and Biers-dorf in the Journal of the Optical Society of America (1956) which makes it clear that the dis-crepancy between perceptual and electrical responses in the human remains when there is no difference in stimulation. They obtained subjective reports of the appearance of the flash while measuring the electroretinogram, and learned that in the short-wave region of the spectrum, flashes that were not visible or just perceptible to the subject evoked electrical responses of large amplitude, whereas long-wave flashes that appeared very bright to the subject evoked elektrical responses of relatively small amplitude.

W. Jaeger (zu M. Monjé): Die „Absolutempfindlichkeit" bei Farbensinnstörungen ist sehr schwer zu messen. Unsere üblichen Schwellenwertbestimmungen (wie Gesichtsfeld, Be-stimmung der Schwellendistanz usw.) sind sicher dafür zu grob. Wenn man wirklich die abso-luten Schwellen messen will, so muß man sich, wie Hecht und Hsia das durchgeführt haben, in das Gebiet der Trefferstatistik im schwellennahen Bereich begeben. Bei diesen Untersuchun-gen von Hecht und Hsia ließen sich Unterschiede der Absolutempfindlichkeit finden: Der nor-male Farbensinn hat die höchste Empfindlichkeit, etwas niedriger liegen die Deuterostörungen und wesentlich niedriger die Protostörungen.

Zu L. M. HURVICH: Ad 1. Der gezeigte Fall ist tatsächlich eine erworbene Tritanopie. Bei Netzhauterkrankungen ist das gar nicht so selten, wie man bisher angenommen hat. Daß solche erworbene Tritostörungen so selten diagnostiziert werden, liegt daran, daß dazu ein spektraler Farbenmischapparat notwendig ist.

Ad 2. Bei der Maculadegeneration geht nicht nur das filternde Maculapigment zugrunde. Auch die in der Macula liegenden Photoreceptoren werden geschädigt. Deshalb ist es nur verständlich, daß eine geringere Empfindlichkeit besteht. Es entspricht dies auch dem langsamen Verfall der übrigen optischen Funktionen (Sehschärfe und zentrales Gesichtsfeld).

Ad 3. Die Unterschiede in der spektralen Helligkeitsverteilung zwischen normaler Trichromasie und Deuterostörungen können nicht sehr groß sein. Sie sind früher überhaupt nicht für signifikant gehalten worden. So wird z. B. in TRENDELENBURGs „Gesichtssinn" noch gelehrt, daß normale Trichromasie und Deuterostörungen dieselbe Sensitivitätskurve hätten. Unterschiedliche Ergebnisse sind zum Teil auch auf Unterschiede in der Größe der Reizfläche zurückzuführen. Eine Veröffentlichung meines Mitarbeiters GRÜTZNER wird darüber berichten.

Zu D. HURVICH-JAMESON: In unseren Experimenten hatten wir aus technischen Gründen keine Möglichkeit, gleichgroße Reizflächen für subjektive und objektive Prüfung zu verwenden. Ich kann deshalb zu den mir bekannten Ergebnissen von ARMINGTON und BIERSDORF aus eigener Erfahrung nichts sagen. Sie scheinen mir jedoch in Widerspruch zu stehen mit den Ergebnissen von DODT, COPENHAVER und GUNKEL sowie von COPENHAVER und GUNKEL. Könnte der Unterschied nicht damit erklärt werden, daß tatsächlich nur für das Flimmer-Elektroretinogramm mit der von DODT angegebenen Apparatur und Berechnungsmethode einen Rückschluß auf die photopische Sensitivitätskurve gestattet? Mit Einzelreizen erhält man die skotopische Komponente und damit natürlich verglichen mit dem subjektiven Helligkeitseindruck stets eine höhere Empfindlichkeit im kurzwelligen Bereich und eine niedrigere Empfindlichkeit im langwelligen Bereich.

D. Tectum Opticum

Gruppendiskussion

Introduction

By

D. WHITTERIDGE*

It is possible, but difficult, to obtain multiple responses from the superior colliculus in the monkey in response to a flash of light. In the Clarke Horsley plane the surface of the colliculus is so nearly vertical that the chances of hitting the superficial layers are much improved by bending the head at least 30° forward. P. M. DANIEL and I have recorded from the colliculus responses within 15−20° of the visual axis, checked in some experiments by simultaneous records from the posterolateral cortical surface on which the macular area is represented. It seems that the peripheral field has a very restricted representation. BROUWER and ZEEMAN (1926) failed to find signs of degeneration after macular lesions in the monkey, and the erroneous conclusion has been drawn that the macula is not represented on the colliculus (DUKE ELDER, 1931).

The superior colliculus of the cat has been elegantly mapped by APTER (1945). From her diagrams it is clear that the area centralis is represented at the anterior border, and that each degree has a larger representation anteriorly than posteriorly.

HAMDI and I obtained evidence of point to point representation on the colliculus in both goats and rabbits, but we did not obtain enough responses in any one experiment to begin quantitative mapping. The orientation of the visual field on the colliculus is approximately constant in all mammals with points anteriorly, i. e. in the long axis of the head represented anteriorly or anterolaterally, with the horizontal meridian running posteriorly across the middle of the colliculus, and with upper field represented near the midline, and lower field laterally.

In the submammalian vertebrates the arrangement of layers is quite different, the optic fibres reach the tectum in two bundles, medial and lateral, and spread over the surface as the stratum opticum. They turn down and end in layers 2−7 according to CAJAL (1952). A point to point representation of the retina in the pigeon was first described by HAMDI and WHITTERIDGE (1954), who pointed out that as the tectum enlarges in birds it rotates outwards through 90°, so that the horizontal meridian which crosses the greatest convexity in frogs and mammals lies horizontally on the tectum in birds. Recent work (unpublished) has shown that the fovea is represented on the lateral surface of the tectum and that its

---

* From the Department of Physiology, University of Edinburgh.

magnification factor is about 0,25 mm/°, whereas that of most of the peripheral field more than 30° out is only .04 mm/°. To this the anterior field just above the horizontal seems to be an exception, as here one obtains magnification factors of 0.8 up to 60° out. It seems that this may be a rudimentary special area in the pigeon, analogous to the second fovea which is found in a corresponding position in the retina in hawks and kingfishers.

The tectum has been used for the study of the lateral spread of potentials by CRAGG and HAMLYN (1953) and by ARMINGTON and CRAMPTON (1958) for the study of spectral sensitivity. The cells of layer 6 near to the terminations of the afferent fibres are only 6 μ in diameter and form a single layer packed as tightly as possible (CAJAL, 1952). The chances of leading from individual cells of this layer are at present slight.

Finally I should like to mention recent work on the frog's optic tectum. You are familiar with the work of LETTVIN et al. (1959) describing a point to point representation of the retina on the optic tectum, with perhaps four different afferent systems accurately in register. Recently JACOBSON (1960) has shown that there is an area of increased tectal representation in the midline above the mouth and probably corresponding with the target area of the tongue. He has drawn attention to the older descriptions of an area centralis in the frog's retina. A very interesting development from the technique of mapping the retina is the investigation by GAZE (1958) of the efficiency of restoration of tectal mapping which occurs during regeneration of a cut optic nerve. A good functional recovery as tested by optokinetic stimulation may be consistent with normal as well as anomalous areas of representation. This method now enables one to study the early stages and something of the mechanisms of retinal representation.

References

APTER, J.: Projection of the retina on superior colliculus of cats. J. Neurophysiol. 8, 123 (1945).

ARMINGTON, J. C., and G. H. CRAMPTON: Comparison of the spectral sensitivity at the eye and the optic tectum of the chicken. Amer. J. Ophthal. 46, 72 (1958).

BROUWER, B., and W. P. C. ZEEMAN: The projection of the retina in the primary optic neuron in monkeys. Brain 49, 1 (1926).

CAJAL, S. R.: Histologie du système nerveux. Madrid: Consejo Superior de Investigaciones Cientificas (1952).

CRAGG, B. G., and L. H. HAMLYN: Chicken's optic tectum: electrical responses. J. Physiol. (Lond.) 120, 52P. (1953).

DUKE ELDER, W. S.: Textbook of Ophthalmology, Vol. 1. London: Henry Kimpton 1931.

GAZE, R. M.: The representation of the retina on the optic lobe of the frog. Quart. J. exp. Physiol. 43, 209 (1958).

HAMDI, F. A., and D. WHITTERIDGE: The representation of the retina on the optic lobe of the pigeon and the superior colliculus of the rabbit and goat. J. Physiol. (Lond.) 121, 44P. (1953).

— The representation of the retina on the optic tectum of the pigeon. Quart. J. exp. Physiol. 39, 111 (1954).

JACOBSON, M.: The representation of the visual field on the optic tectum of the frog: evidence for the presence of an area centralis retinae. J. Physiol. (Lond.) 154, 31—32 (1960).

LETTVIN, J. Y., H. R. MATURANA, W. S. MCCULLOCH and W. H. PITTS: What the frog's eye tells the frog's brain. Proc. IRE. 47, 1940 (1959).

Rétinotopie au niveau tectal et réponses spectrales diencéphaliques chez le Pigeon*

Par

Y. GALIFRET

Avec 3 Figures

1. Rétinotopie tectale et stimulations colorées

La rétinotopie, étudiée en détail par le Professeur WHITTERIDGE, se traduit également dans les réponses de surface du tectum du Pigeon (le télencéphale ayant été enlevé par succion), par une variation en fonction de la longueur d'onde de la stimulation visuelle. En utilisant une stimulation rétinienne étendue, soit rouge, soit bleue, on peut mettre en évidence la projection fovéale au milieu du bord externe du lobe optique et la différencier de la projection périphérique sur le reste du lobe. La fig. 1 donne les tracés obtenus avec deux macroélectrodes (petites boules d'argent de 0,5 mm de diamètre) situées, l'une vers le milieu du bord externe du lobe (tracé inférieur de chaque cliché, électrode I sur le schéma), l'autre vers l'arrière de la convexité supérieure du lobe (tracé supérieur de chaque cliché, électrode S sur le schéma).

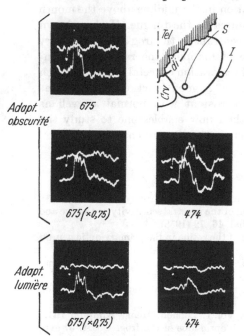

Adapt. obscurité — 675
675(×0,75) — 474
Adapt. lumière
675(×0,75) — 474

Fig. 1. En haut, à droite, schéma de la préparation vue de dessus avec le cervelet, le diencéphale, le télencéphale, partiellement enlevé et la convexité supérieure du lobe optique. Les chiffres indiquent a longueur d'onde stimulatrice. Le tracé supérieur correspond à l'électrode S et le tracé inférieur à l'électrode I. La stimulation est indiquée par un artefact sur le tracé supérieur. Durée totale du balayage: 180 ms

L'oeil étant adapté à l'obscurité, si l'on ajuste une stimulation bleue (filtre interférentiel, 474 mμ) et une stimulation rouge [filtre interférentiel, 675 mμ + filtre neutre de densité 0,4 : 675 ($\times$ 0,75)] pour obtenir sous l'électrode I des potentiels évoqués d'amplitude à peu près équivalente, on constate que, sous l'électrode S, seule la stimulation bleue provoque un potentiel évoqué, en retard (10 ms) sur le potentiel de I, mais de décours assez semblable, alors que la stimulation rouge ne provoque qu'un ressaut de la ligne de base à peine visible. Si l'on augmente l'intensité de la stimulation rouge en supprimant le filtre neutre, on obtient une notable augmentation du potentiel évoqué en I, sans pour autant provoquer de modification plus apparente en S (cliché supérieur). Si l'on passe en adaptation à la lumière (niveau de luminance du même ordre que celui de la stimulation bleue)

* Laboratoire de Neurophysiologie Générale, Collège de France, Paris.

on observe une diminution d'amplitude des réponses en I, plus marquée pour le bleu que pour le rouge et surtout un effondrement complet de la réponse au bleu en S.

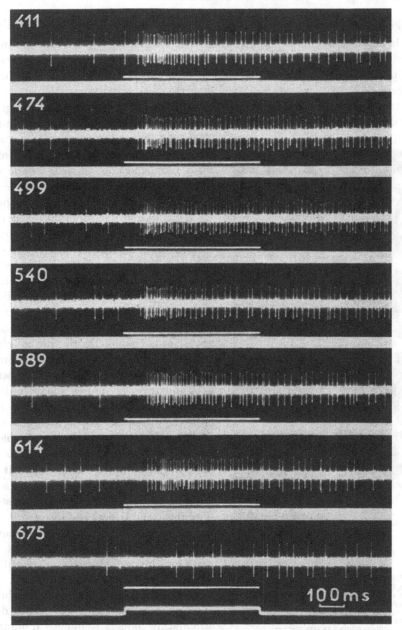

Fig. 2. Réponses d'une unité à diverses radiations spectrales. La longueur d'onde est marquée en mμ sur chaque tracé. En bas, réponse de la photocellule à la stimulation, répétée sur chaque tracé

Ainsi, il est possible, à la surface du tectum, de différencier la projection fovéale de la projection périphérique par le fait que la première répond à une stimulation

rouge extrême au contraire de la seconde et par le fait que le passage de l'adaptation
à l'obscurité à l'adaptation à la lumière affecte plus l'amplitude de la réponse
périphérique au bleu que celle de la réponse fovéale.

2. Réponses unitaires diencéphaliques à des stimulations monochromatiques

Si la majorité des fibres optiques aboutit au lobe optique, un certain contingent
se rend, cependant, aux formations diencéphaliques qui marquent la limite entre
diencéphale et mésencéphale le *nucleus geniculatus lateralis* et le *nucleus superficialis
synencephali*.

Cette constatation des anatomistes est confirmée par la possibilité d'enregistrement de réponses visuelles, au niveau de ces deux noyaux. Avec des microélectrodes de tungstène, nous avons recu-
eilli les réponses unitaires à des stimulations rétiniennes de longueur d'onde variable et d'énergie quantique égale. La
fig. 2 donne un exemple de telles réponses.

L'évaluation de l'efficience relative de
chaque radiation stimulatrice pouvait
être faite sur la base de la fréquence des
influx de la réponse. Il est apparu cependant que, dans le cas de la stimulation
rétinienne étendue (33°) que nous utilisons,
ce critère de la fréquence pouvait n'être
pas fidèle ainsi que le montre la fig. 3. On
voit dans la colonne de gauche, les réponses lentes sur lesquelles se superposent les
spikes, les chiffres indiquant la niveau de
la stimulation en unités logarithmiques.
Alors que l'amplitude de la réponse lente
croît régulièrement de − 3 à 0, le nombre
de spikes devient plus petit. Dans la colonne
de droite, l'activité du même élément a
été enregistrée après filtrage, on voit que
la fréquence des spikes croît de − 4 à − 2,
puis décroît ensuite jusqu'à 0. L'existence
d'inhibitions latérales, s'exerçant sur
la cellule étudiée, peut expliquer le
phénomène observé. Ces inhibitions sont
d'autant plus probables que nous utilisons
une stimulation rétinienne étendue.

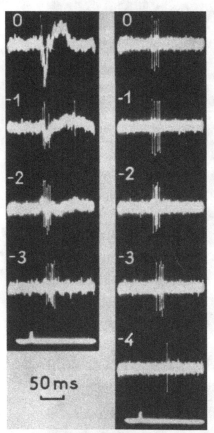

Fig. 3. Réponses unitaires à une stimulation achro-
matique d'intensité croissante. Les chiffres indiquent la valeur relative en unités logarithmiques,
0 correspondant à la stimulation maximale. A
droite, enregistrements faits avec filtre passe-haut,
éliminant la réponse lente. En bas, la réponse de la
photocellule à la stimulation

Cette constatation nous a conduit à
choisir comme indice de l'efficience d'une
stimulation, non la fréquence d'influx de
la réponse, mais *l'inverse de la latence*.
La latence, en effet, n'apparaît pas perturbée par les inhibitions latérales comme la
fréquence, et elle est plus facile à mesurer. En outre, si l'on compare l'évolution
en fonction du logarithme de la stimulation, d'une part de la fréquence des influx,

d'autre part de la rapidité de réponse (inverse de la latence), on constate que la seconde continue de croître quand la première a déjà atteint son palier. Nous avons vérifié ce fait sur nos résultats mais aussi sur ceux de nombreux auteurs et, en particulier, de HARTLINE (1), KUFFLER (2) et KENNEDY (3). La rapidité de réponse est donc également un indice plus sensible de l'efficience d'une stimulation.

En utilisant cet indice dans le cas de nos tracés nous obtenons un groupement des courbes de réponses, en fonction de la longueur d'onde, en trois familles admettant pour maxima respectivement 499, 540 et 589 mμ. S'agit-il là de la mise en évidence d'un mécanisme de discrimination chromatique, fondé sur le trichromatisme ? On pourrait le penser. Ce mécanisme n'est pas exclusif cependant d'un mécanisme à couples opposés, ayant comme support anatomique un autre noyau ou, dans les noyaux que nous avons étudiés, des cellules trop petites pour que leur activité soit enregistrée avec des microélectrodes de tungstène.

Bibliographie

1. HARTLINE, H. K.: The response of single optic nerve fibres of the vertebrate eye to illumination of the retina. Amer. J. Physiol. 121, 400—415 (1938).
2. KUFFLER, S. W.: Discharge patterns and the functional organization of the mammalian retina. J. Neurophysiol. 16, 37—68 (1953).
3. KENNEDY, D.: Responses from the crayfish caudal photoreceptor. Amer. J. Ophthal. 46, 19—26 (1958).

Remarks on the Optic Tectum*

By

R. W. DOTY

I am afraid Dr. KORNHUBER has asked me to say something about the tectum not because I know anything about it, but simply because I should. The implication, of course, is that the tectum may be playing a role in the visual pattern discrimination possessed by my kittens after neonatal removal of area striata. This possibility cannot be denied, but the tectum alone does not seem to be enough to sustain pattern vision in such cases. Thus animals with neonatal extirpations that include the middle and posterior ectosylvian gyri in addition to the marginal, splenial, postlateral and posterior suprasylvian are capable only of brightness discrimination.

The suspicion is prevalent that brightness discrimination in the absence of "visual" cortex is mediated by centers in the superior colliculus, but this has never been proven. Such discrimination proceeds in the absence of the superior colliculi if the area striata remains (e.g. 2).

An interesting possibility is raised by BLAKE (2) that the superior colliculus is somehow concerned in the discrimination of patterns. Her findings are puzzling since SPERRY, MINER and MYERS (7) obtained rather good pattern vision after lesions which destroyed the superior colliculi. In two of BLAKE's animals, however,

---

* From the Physiology Department, The University of Michigan, Ann Arbor.

with area striata intact, form discrimination and object recognition were apparently absent after destruction of the superior colliculi. Brightness discrimination and avoidance of obstacles showed that visual impulses were effective in some portion of the central visual system.

The latter fact is an important consideration in such experiments since removal of the colliculi destroys primary optic fibers and can lead to degeneration of retinal ganglion cells. GUDDEN (6) showed this clearly in operations on newborn kittens, and indeed was the first to show a "point to point" type of retino-collicular projection. Local lesions of the superior colliculus produced localized degeneration in the retina. Since great numbers of the fibers to the lateral geniculate body of the cat are collaterals of those passing to the tectum (1, 5), fiber degeneration following tectal lesions could seriously involve the lateral geniculate system.

Dr. INA SAMUELS, JOHN HOWELL, SARAH SOUTHWICK and I have begun an electrophysiological analysis of the superior colliculus of the cat, mostly with nembutal anesthesia, and can make some preliminary statements regarding it. We have consistently found that photically evoked potentials begin about 12 msec. later in the colliculus than in marginal gyrus. When secondary responses (4) are being recorded from the cortex, none appear in the colliculus; but a properly phased electrical pulse to the colliculus (or, for that matter, most any place in tectum and tegmentum) can greatly augment the secondary response. The "off" response of the colliculus is distinctly different from that at the cortex. It may not develop its full amplitude (equal to the "on", about 250 μV with bipolar electrodes in favorable locations) until the flash duration reaches 400 msec.

With electrical stimulation of the optic tract a small spike is seen in the colliculus a few tenths of a millisecond later than the first small spike (3) recorded from marginal gyrus. The conduction velocity of these faster fibers to the colliculus is of the order of 40 m/sec. A second much smaller spike following the first (total latency 0.9 msec.) indicates another group with a conduction velocity roughly half this. The next and major response of the colliculus does not develop until 3.5 msec after the optic tract stimulus, about 0.5 msec after the peak of cortical "spike" 4 (3) to the same stimulus. Stimulation from the same collicular electrodes evoked a single large monophasic spike in the optic tract. The cortical response in this case was the same as that seen to stimulation of the optic tract except that it began with "spike 2" (3) 1.1 msec after collicular stimulation and was of smaller amplitude. This appears to confirm the anatomical findings (1, 5) mentioned above and to show that antidromic central stimulation of a collateral branch can activate far-distant branches of the same fiber. Such antidromic activation of optic tract fibers has not been found in most regions of the colliculus and we are as yet unable to specify the exact region from which it is best obtained. Other potentials are evoked in many cortical areas by collicular stimulation, but the situation here is too complex for us to make any useful statements at this time.

References

1. BARRIS, R. W., W. R. INGRAM and S. W. RANSON: Optic connections of the diencephalon and midbrain of the cat. J. comp. Neurol. **62**, 117—153 (1935).
2. BLAKE, L.: The effect of lesions of the superior colliculus on brightness and pattern discrimination in the cat. J. comp. physiol. Psychol. **52**, 272—278 (1959).

3. CHANG, H.-T., and B. KAADA: An analysis of primary response of visual cortex to optic nerve stimulation of cats. J. Neurophysiol. 13, 305—318 (1950).
4. DOTY, R. W.: Potentials evoked in cat cerebral cortex by diffuse and by punctiform photic stimuli. J. Neurophysiol. 21, 437—464 (1958).
5. GLEES, P.: The termination of optic fibers in the lateral geniculate body of the cat. J. Anat. (Lond.) 75, 434—440 (1941).
6. GUDDEN, v. B.: Gesammelte und hinterlassene Abhandlungen. Wiesbaden: J. F. Bergmann 1889.
7. SPERRY, R. W., N. MINER and R. E. MYERS: Visual pattern perception following subpial slicing and tantalum wire implantations in the visual cortex. J. comp. physiol. Psychol. 48, 50—58 (1955).

Some Observations on the Superior Colliculi of the Cat by J. ALTMAN[1]

Communicated by

H.-L. TEUBER

With 3 Figures

The observations I should like to communicate to you in this discussion on the optic tectum were made by Dr. JOSEPH ALTMAN in the course of his work for a doctoral dissertation[2]. Dr. JOSEPH ALTMAN undertook these studies for three reasons:

1. Just as Professor DOTY, he believes that the optic tectum may play a greater role in the visually-guided behavior of carnivores and primates than has usually been assumed. His electrophysiological and subsequent anatomical studies were preliminary to behavioral experiments which are now in progress; his current work is concerned with changes in visual performance after removal of the superior colliculi and adjacent structures.

2. The superior colliculi raise a particular problem for correlating structure and function, because of their lamination. As WALLS (2) has pointed out, such lamination is found in neuroretina, superior colliculi, lateral geniculates and cortex; eventually, we should be able to account for the "purpose" of these laminar arrangements.

3. Lastly, there is the recurrent problem of the interaction which one assumes exists between superior colliculus and visual cortex. In his somewhat preliminary electrophysiological studies (in deeply barbiturized animals), Dr. ALTMAN found no direct signs of such interaction, but subsequent investigation of anatomical connections, by means of the Nauta stain, revealed a definite corticifugal pathway (ALTMAN and CARPENTER, in preparation). However, these recent studies with the Nauta stain did not disclose any corticipetal fibers from the cat's superior colliculus to its visual cortex.

---

[1] From the Department of Psychiatry and Neurology, New York University College of Medicine.

[2] This dissertation was cosponsored by Dr. LEONARD I. MALIS, Mount Sinai Hospital, New York City.

Now to the electrophysiological observations: They were all made on barbiturized cats with macroelectrodes, as well as tungsten microelectrodes prepared
according to HUBEL's method (tip diameter: 0.5 to 2 μ). I shall briefly describe
four of Dr. ALTMAN's findings, viz.: 1)
latency differences between superior colliculi and visual cortex; 2) differences in the
shape of evoked potentials in superior colliculus and visual cortex, respectively; 3)
evidence for some definite ipsilateral representation in the superior colliculus in addition to the well known contralateral projections; and 4) changes in the nature of
collicular responses when recorded from
progressively deeper lamina of this structure.

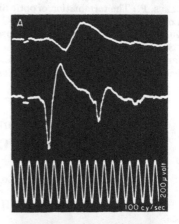

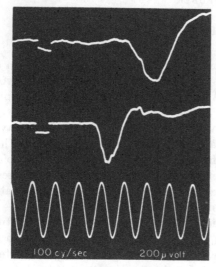

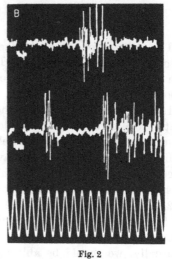

Fig. 1   Fig. 2

Fig. 1. Simultaneous recording of evoked response to a 5 msec. flash (as shown by stimulus artifact) to the cat's
eye. Upper trace: macroelectrode recording from superior colliculus; lower trace: corresponding recording from
lateral gyrus.

Fig. 2. Cortical and collicular response to light (5 msec. flash). A Simultaneous recording with macroelectrode
in both structures: upper tracing, collicular response, lower tracing, cortical responses (lateral gyrus). B Microelectrode recordings: upper tracing, collicular responses, lower tracing, cortical responses (lateral gyrus). Calibration
in B: 200 cy/sec.

1. Latency of collicular and cortical evoked potentials. In deeply barbiturized
cats, the mean onset latency of evoked potentials to light was 36.5 msec in the
superior colliculus and 27.0 msec in the cortex (see Fig. 1). The average difference
in latency (9.5 msec), between simultaneously recorded collicular and cortical
responses, was a constant which seemed independent of the absolute latencies of
the two kinds of response. When photic stimulation of the retina was replaced by
direct electric stimulation of the optic nerve, the results were essentially the same:
although absolute latencies were correspondingly decreased, the latency difference

between collicular and first cortical response remained around 7 msec. Apparently, the difference in latencies reflects a *slower conduction rate in retino-collicular fiber systems as compared with that in the retino-geniculo-cortical path.* This difference in conduction velocity must be considerable since the retino-geniculo-cortical pathway is much longer than the retino-collicular path, and interrupted by a synapse. A maximal conduction rate of 5 m/sec was calculated for the retino-collicular fibers. This conduction velocity is actually markedly lower than the

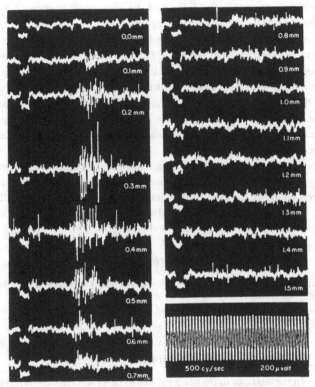

Fig. 3. Microelectrode recordings from increasing depths of superior colliculus. For details, see text.

lowest conduction velocity recorded by MARGARET LENNOX (*1*) in the optic tract after optic nerve stimulation.

2. Shapes of collicular and cortical evoked potentials. As fig. 2 shows, stimulation of the cat's eye by a single flash evoked a single potential in the colliculus, in contrast to the well known sequence of waves in the visual cortex. The average duration of the single wave in the colliculus was considerably longer (24 msec) than the duration of the initial cortical wave (10.8 msec).

3. Ipsilateral and contralateral representation in the superior colliculi. Macro- as well as microelectrode recordings revealed definite evidence for ipsilateral representation in the cat's superior colliculus. Evoked responses to stimulation of the contralateral eye were always larger in amplitude when recorded with macroelectrodes, indicative of the greater number of crossed representations.

However, there were evoked responses (recorded with macroelectrodes) as well as unit responses (obtained with microelectrodes) indicative of a sparse pathway from retina to ipsilateral colliculus.

4. **Changes in unit responses on penetration of superior colliculus.** As a micro-electrode traverses the colliculus from upper into lower lamina as shown in Fig. 3, one observes marked changes in the unit responses that can be obtained at the different depths indicated. Briefly, the most superficial electrode placements record the majority of unit responses that are modifiable by light presented to the eyes or by electric stimulation delivered to the optic nerve. These electrode placements seem to coincide with the stratum griseum superficiale. As is evident from Fig. 3, such responses are no longer found at greater depth, i. e., more than approximately one millimeter beneath the surface of the superior colliculus. Below this one encounters evoked potentials, but no individual units which could be driven by photic or optic nerve stimuli. This region may be identical with the stratum opticum. Still farther down one enters a region in which evoked potentials are shallow; at this depth one observes units that fire spontaneously, but there are no units whose activity could be modified by stimulating the eye or optic nerve.

In additional experiments, a tentative classification of collicular units has been established by Dr. Altman. In essence, he found five types of collicular cells that could be driven by light, namely units firing with short latency; units firing with long latency; units firing to light on only; units firing to light on and light off; and units inhibited by photic or optic nerve stimulation.

References

1. Lennox, M.: Single fiber response to electrical stimulation in cat's optic tract. J. Neuro-physiol. **21**, 62—69 (1958).
2. Walls, G. L.: The lateral geniculate nucleus and visual histophysiology. Univ. Calif. Publ. Physiol. **9**, 1—100 (1953).

Discussion

A. Arduini: In the relations to the observations of Doty that in cats deprived of the visual and of the association cortices the visual discrimination is destroyed, is reported a series of experiments performed in 1946—1947 by Arduini, Moruzzi and Zanchetti. Pigeons were tested for "fear reactions" to a menacing hand and it was observed that the fear reaction disappears after decerebration. However after a dilute strychnine solution was applied on one optic lobe the fear reaction reappeared when the menacing hand was presented to the eye contralateral to the optic lobe strychinized. It was concluded therefore, that the hemispheres in the pigeons had only a tonic energising influence. It is suggested that some similar mechanism might be present in mammals. This could explain the presence of visual discrimination in cats in which only the visual areas were destroyed in the immediate post-natal period.

W. Jaeger: Nimmt man heute nach den klinischen Erfahrungen noch an, daß das Tectum die vertikale Blickbewegung reguliert und Tectumläsionen eine Blicklähmung beim Menschen verursachen?

H. Kornhuber (zu Jaeger): Die physiologische Bedeutung des Tectum nimmt mit zunehmender Cerebralisation ab. Ob und welche Störungen beim Menschen durch Tectum-läsionen hervorgerufen werden, ist noch unbekannt. Falls er nach reinen Tectumläsionen überhaupt Störungen zeigt, sind diese wahrscheinlich gering. Der Lichtreflex der Pupille ist vom Tectum unabhängig (6). Auch die vertikale Blicklähmung, die man lange auf Tectumläsionen bezogen hat, ist ein Symptom der Mittelhirnhaube und Prätektalregion (1, 3, 5, 7). Wegen der Faserverbindungen des Tectum vom Occipitalhirn und zur Reticularis wären Störungen der optisch gesteuerten Blickbewegung oder der Fixation denkbar. Bei Affen fand sich aber nach bilateralen Tectumläsionen nur eine vorübergehende Verminderung des optokinetischen Nystagmus (2), und beim Menschen würde diese Störung vermutlich noch geringer sein. Dagegen zeigen Meerschweinchen nach einseitiger Tectumdestruktion einen Ausfall des optokinetischen Nystagmus zur Gegenseite (9). Die Untersuchungen von BLAKE an Katzen (4), die erhebliche Störungen des visuell kontrollierten Verhaltens nach Tectumläsionen ergaben, sind allerdings nur bedingt verwertbar, weil die operierten Tiere vertikale Blickparesen hatten, die Läsionen also offenbar — ähnlich wie in früheren Experimenten von anderen (8) — nicht allein das Tectum zerstört hatten.

References

1. ANGELERGUES, R., J. DE AJURIAGUERRA et H. HÉCAEN: Paralysie de la verticalité du regard d'origne vasculaire. Rev. neurol. **96**, 301 (1957).
2. BENDER, M. B., T. PASIK and P. PASIK: Effect of collicular lesions upon certain ocular functions in monkeys. Trans. Amer. neurol. Ass. **1957**, 19.
3. BENDER, M. B.: Pathways mediating vertical eye movements. Trans. Amer. neurol. Ass. **1959**, 159.
4. BLAKE, L.: The effect of lesions of the superior colliculus on brightness and pattern discriminations in the cat. J. comp. physiol. Psychol. **52**, 272 (1959).
5. JUNG, R., and R. HASSLER: The extrapyramidal motor system. In: Handbook of Physiology, Sect. Neurophysiology, Vol. 2. Washington, D. C., American Physiological Society, 1960.
6. MAGOUN, H. W.: Maintenance of the light reflex after destruction of the superior colliculus in the cat. Amer. J. Physiol. **111**, 91 (1935).
7. MUSKENS, L. J. J.: Das supra-vestibuläre System. Amsterdam, N. V. Noordhollandsche Uitgeversmaatschappij, 1934.
8. SCALA, N. P., and E. A. SPIEGEL: Subcortical (passive) optokinetic nystagmus in lesions of the midbrain and of the vestibular nuclei. Conf. neurol. (Basel) **3**, 53 (1941).
9. SMITH, K. U., and M. BRIDGEMAN: The neuronal mechanisms of the movement vision and optic nystagmus. J. exp. Psychol. **33**, 165·(1943).

E. Visueller Cortex

I. Retinale Projektion, binoculare Koordination und Spontanaktivität der Area 17

The Representation of the Visual Field on the Calcarine Cortex*

By

D. WHITTERIDGE and P. M. DANIEL

With 4 Figures

Since the work of HENSCHEN (1923), extended during the 1914−1918 War by HOLMES and LISTER (1916) and by PIERRE MARIE and CHATELIN (1914−1915), it has been generally accepted that localised wounds of the occipital cortex produce good evidence of point to point projection of the visual field on the occipital cortex. This has been strongly supported by the anatomical work of LE GROS CLARK and PENMAN (1934) and of POLYAK (1957), but there is not yet agreement even on the exact projection of the macular area on the cerebral cortex. The best physiological work which has been done is that by TALBOT and MARSHALL (1941), who have mapped the exposed postero-lateral surface of the occipital lobe in the monkey. In the present work we have used an essentially similar technique, but by introducing long steel needles we have mapped most of the cortex of the calcarine fissures and can give a quantitative account of the nature of the calcarine visual projection.

We have deliberately used large steel needles with points of about 10 μ, so that we have obtained responses due to a large number of cortical units. We have picked up a few single cortical units and these have confirmed conclusions drawn from multi-unit responses. To map the visual field on to the cortex it is essential to make as large a number of observations as possible on the same animal, and this also necessitated recording multiple responses rather than delaying to pick up single units. We have used spots of light down to 10′ diameter illuminated by 0.3−3 millilamberts and have concentrated our attention on the earliest cortical responses. These appear 30−50 msec after a flash and can be sharply localised. There are often a number of later responses to a flash after 70 m/sec and upwards. These show much less localisation and may even appear after flashes in the ipsilateral field [cf. DOTY (1958) on the cat]. We have synchronised the time base with the "on" or the "off" of longer lasting illumination, but have not found any difference in the optimal point giving "on" from that giving "off" effects.

---

* From the Department of Physiology, University of Edinburgh.

After our successful experiments in 1952, we had a number of failures almost certainly due to poor experimental conditions and especially to systolic blood pressures around 70–80 mm Hg. The last seven experiments on five baboons, a cynomolgus and a vervet monkey have all been successful. We have used penta-barbitone, hexabarbitone and chloralose successfully, but prefer chloralose which permits of a high blood pressure and gives excellent local conditions in the cortex. We have found no systematic difference in the localisation of responses under different anaesthetics in the monkey.

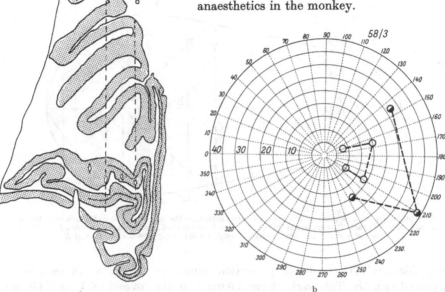

Fig. 1 a and b. *a* Parasagittal section of baboon's brain. Cortex identifiable as area 17 is marked by a black line. In the stem of the 'mushroom' there are four needle tracks made by needles slightly oblique to the plane of the section. Two of the tracks 3 and 6 of the series have been shewn as though projected on to the plane of the section. *b* The responses in the visual field from track 3 and track 6 (in *a*). Owing to the *S* bend of the 'stem' of calcarine cortex, track 3 gives responses from three points. Track 6 which crosses the head of the 'mushroom' gives responses from four points. (From GARLAND Lectures on Neurology Edinburgh: E. & S. Livingstone.)

Fixation of the eye always presents difficulty as there is much tonic activity in the extraocular muscles. We have used a ring sewn to the limbus, tubocurarine with artificial respiration and, in the later experiments, a fixed electrode on the cortical area of representation of the fovea, connected to a second amplifier. As long as responses are obtained from this electrode from a light at the centre of the perimeter, one can make observations with some certainty that the eye has not moved.

An electrode on the postero-lateral surface of the cortex will respond to a spot 10′ in diameter any where in a circle about 5°–6° diameter. Responses from points 20°–30° out may be obtainable from a circle about 10° in diameter. In one experiment in which a few single units were seen, consistent responses were obtained from a circle 5° in diameter, but in all cases the point giving the largest early responses could be determined to within about 1°.

A characteristic pattern of response has been the "reversal" – changing from a receptive area in the lower field to one in the upper field over 200–300 μ at a depth found later to correspond to the calcarine fissure. When the needle tracks passed more posteriorly across the folds which give a "mushroom-like" appearance with a head and a stem, more complex patterns appeared (Fig. 1a). At the end of the experiment the monkey was killed with nembutal and the brain perfused with 10% formol saline. After hardening, the brain was cut serially at 100 μ and the needle tracks identified.

By measuring angular distance along meridians in the visual field and distance between needle tracks in brain sections, it has been possible to determine cortical

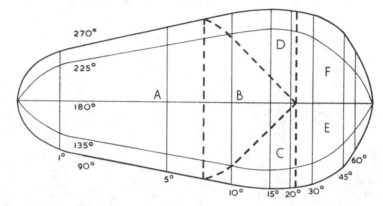

Fig. 2. A projection on to a plane of the reconstructed surface for the left hemisphere. Figures refer to the conventional perimeter chart. This surface is folded along the heavy dotted lines so that F touches E, that D and C touch B, and A folds round so that it touches and overlaps the deep surface of B

"magnification" M, the linear projection in mm on the cortex of each degree measured radially. This varies from 5.6 mm/° at the fovea to 0.1 mm/° 60° out. The magnification factor is also measured along arcs and is found to be equal to the local magnification factor measured on short distances along radii. Further, the magnification factor at all points on the same semicircle of latitude is the same. This simple state of affairs may be uncommon. It is not true of the representation of the visual field on the tectum of the frog (JACOBSON, 1960) nor the tectum of the pigeon (WHITTERIDGE, unpublished results). It does mean that calculation of the shape of the visual cortex in the monkey is comparatively simple. It was pointed out to us by Mr. DAVID KENDALL of Magdalen College, Oxford, that to arrive at the shape of the visual cortex we had only to calculate the lengths of the semicircles of latitude $- \pi$ r $\sin \theta -$ and to multiply each by the appropriate value of M and to set them further apart by distance between them $- (\theta_1 - \theta_2)$r where θ is measured in radians, and multiplied by the mean value of M. Such a process is most easily done by making wire semicircles of the appropriate length and spacing them apart on any meridian $-$ preferably along the horizontal meridian. Such a framework can be covered with papier maché and later casts made from it.

The calculated surface is 1320 sq mm, whereas LE GROS CLARK (1941) has measured area 17 in the monkey as 1450 sq mm. CHOW, BLUM and BLUM (1950) give a figure of 645 sq mm without allowance for shrinkage $-$ which is usually about 30% linearly. It is noteworthy that half the surface area is made up by the first 9°, and that the area for the peripheral field beyond 60° is very small.

It has been found by trial and error that if this surface is folded twice, once horizontally from 25° to 90°, and once vertically along the semicircle of latitude at 8° − 9°, the resulting surface (Fig. 2) closely resembles area 17 in the rhesus monkey and baboon (Fig. 1a). Parasagittal sections of the model and of the monkey's brain give similar patterns (Fig. 3a, b). The correspondence is so close that there is little doubt that the calcarine cortex in the monkey has been folded in development along horizontal and vertical lines in this way.

The monkey's visual acuity has been measured by GRETHER (1941) as 0.7′. This must mean that in the foveal area the minimal angle of resolution is projected on to 65 μ. This corresponds to about 6 cells in the densest part of layer III. We do not know the distribution of dendrites for the fibres of the visual radiation in the monkey, but in the cat these extend up to 500 μ (SHOLL, 1956). The corresponding figure for the projection of the minimal angle of resolution for the cortical representation of the cat's area centralis is 160 μ. The peripheral visual acuity of the monkey is not known and will be difficult to measure, but the curves for relative peripheral acuity in man and magnification factor in the monkey seem to fall off in a closely similar way (Fig. 4). If in fact peripheral acuity in the monkey falls off parallel to the magnification factor, it follows

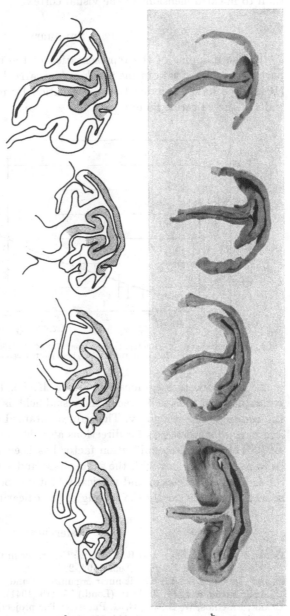

a   b

Fig. 3 a and b. *a* Parasagittal sections 2 mm apart of the baboon's brain. *b*. Parasagittal sections of a plasticine model made and folded as in Fig. 2. (From GARLAND Lectures on Neurology. Edinburgh: E. & S. Livingstone.)

that the minimal angle of resolution is always represented by 65 μ or thereabouts on the cortex for all parts of the visual field. In man the total area of visual cortex is about twice that of the monkey, but the cell density is about half. No doubt magnification factors should be related to cell density rather than to linear dimensions of the visual cortex.

Summary

1. The mapping of the representation of the macular field on the superficial part of the area striata in the monkey was carried out by TALBOT and MARSHALL (1941). We have extended their observation by mapping also the cortex of the walls of the calcarine fissure.

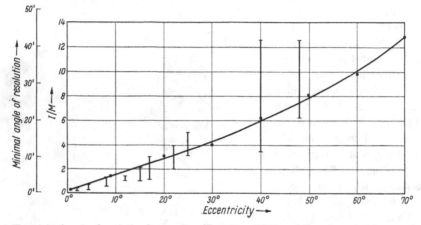

Fig. 4. The minimal angle of resolution for man from WEYMOUTH (1958), and the reciprocal of the magnification factor for the monkey, both plotted against eccentricity

2. The cortical magnification factor M, i.e. the distance in mm along the cortex devoted to each degree of the visual field, is found to fall off smoothly from the centre to the periphery. The values obtained are the same for all meridians and over short distances for directions at right angles to each other.

3. The cortical magnification factor has been used to distort the visual field so as to give a surface with the same shape and area as calcarine cortex.

4. With a horizontal and vertical fold it has been possible to fold this surface so as to resemble closely the folding of the calcarine cortex.

References

CHOW, K.-L., J. S. BLUM and R. A. BLUM: Cell ratios in the thalamocortical visual system of Macaca mulatta. J. comp. Neurol. **92**, 227 (1950).

CLARK, LE GROS, W. E.: The laminar organization and cell content of the lateral geniculate body in the monkey. J. Anat. (Lond.) **75**, 419 (1941).

CLARK, LE GROS, W. E., and G. G. PENMAN: The projection of the retina in the lateral geniculate body. Proc. roy. Soc. **B. 114**, 291 (1934).

DOTY, R. W.: Potentials evoked in cat cerebral cortex by diffuse and by punctiform photic stimuli. J. Neurophysiol. **21**, 437 (1958).

GRETHER, W. F.: A comparison of visual acuity in the rhesus monkey and man. J. comp. physiol. Psychol. **31**, 23 (1941).

HENSCHEN, S. E.: 40jähriger Kampf um das Sehzentrum und seine Bedeutung für die Hirnforschung. Z. ges. Neurol. Psychiat. **87**, 505 (1923).

HOLMES, G., and W. T. LISTER: Disturbances of vision from cerebral lesions, with specific reference to the cortical representation of the macula. Brain **39**, 34 (1916).

JACOBSON, M.: J. Physiol. (Lond.) (In Press).

MARIE, P., and C. CHATELIN: Les troubles visuels due aux lésions des voies optiques intracérébrales et de la sphère visuelle corticale. Rev. Neurol. **28**, 882 (1914—15).

POLYAK, S.: The vertebrate visual system. University of Chicago Press 1957.

SHOLL, D. A.: The organization of the cerebral cortex. London: Methuen & Co. Ltd. 1956.

TALBOT, S. A., and W. H. MARSHALL: Physiologic studies on neural mechanisms of visual localisation and discrimination. Amer. J. Ophthal. **24**, 1255 (1941).

WEYMOUTH, F. W.: Visual sensory units and the minimal angle of resolution. Amer. J. Ophthal. **46**, 102 (1958).

Discussion

L. M. HURVICH: In seeking to correlate the data of visual acuity with the topographical picture you have presented a set of visual acuity data taken presumably at a single level of intensity. Since visual acuity is known to vary with the intensity parameter one would have to be certain that the visual acuity-intensity function exhibits the same form at different retinal positions before accepting the correlation as generally valid. Should the acuity-intensity relationship vary differently at different field positions the correlation you present might be seriously affected.

R. W. DOTY: Dr. WHITTERIDGE has obviously made a superlative analysis of this difficult problem. Since his method circumvents certain of the objections that can be made to the anatomical analysis, I think his evidence is probably the most convincing yet offered for the discreteness and orderliness of the retino-cortical projection in primates, and it would not be profitable to dispute this basic scheme. However, perhaps because I am compulsively suspicious of simplicity in the CNS, I can't help wondering whether this precise arrangement is important in neural function, and asking what steps lie beyond this orderly projection. Dr. WHITTERIDGE's method of keeping a second electrode stationary on the cortical surface seems to answer any question about irradiation of the excitation to other retino-cortical sectors; although a final conclusion here will require the familiar microelectrode analyses in unanesthetized animals. Yet was there perhaps anything in the latencies, wave-forms, multiple and "off" responses which might indicate spatial elaboration of the evoked activity?

H.-L. TEUBER: I have several questions for Professor WHITTERIDGE: Does he consider his results compatible with the view that there is neither divergence nor convergence in the central visual pathway beyond the retina? I.e., does the primary visual projection system (the retinocalcarine system) at all levels (optic nerve, lateral geniculate, cortex) maintain a greater proportion of fibers in its central core, and a lesser proportion in the peripheral sectors? Furthermore, are his results, based on evoked potential maps, compatible with the cell counts now available[1]? Finally, does Professor WHITTERIDGE have recordings from the optic radiation? I am asking this because I believe that POLYAK's views on the optic radiation need considerable revision.

P. GLEES: Could we assume that there is a constant area of representation for each retinal ganglion cell in the visual cortex and that the macular region, having more ganglion cells, has greater magnification at cortical level for this reason.

If this were so, would it be permissible to compare the macula with a fine grain plate, allowing for enlarging and the periphery with a coarse grain photographic plate.

D. WHITTERIDGE (to L. M. HURVICH): The only figures for peripheral acuity at different light intensities which I have been able to find are those of MANDELBAUM and SLOAN (1947)[2]. At scotopic light intensities the curves show a peak at 4° out and are otherwise nearly flat, but the two photopic curves they give are of very similar shape. I do not think greater intensities would make much difference to the shape of the curve.

---

[1] CHOW, K. L., J. BLUM (SEMMES) and R. A. BLUM: Cell ratios in the thalamo-cortical visual system of Macaca mulatta. J. comp. Neurol. **92**, 227—240 (1950).

[2] MANDELBAUM, J., and LOUISE L. SLOAN: Peripheral visual acuity. Amer. J. Ophthal. **30**, 581—588 (1947).

To R. W. DOTY: Yes, the late responses can be obtained from a wider area of visual field and even from the uncrossed field on occasion. The sharply localised responses are the earliest responses. We have never found a different topographical localisation for the "off" responses in the monkey.

To Dr. H.-L. TEUBER: I have no systematic information on the optic radiation. I have no doubt that the whole primary visual projection system does maintain a greater proportion of fibres in its central core as opposed to the peripheral sectors. I have recalculated the figures of CHOW, BLUM and BLUM (1950) for the number of visual acuity units, measured as the solid angles corresponding to minimal angles of resolution, in the macular region, i.e. 0—5°, and the remainder of the peripheral field. On my figures the macular region has about 25% of the acuity units. This agrees very well with the figures they take from TALBOT and MARSHALL, which give the macular area as about 25% of the total surface of area 17.

To P. GLEES: I would agree entirely with Dr. GLEES, adding that the "grain" of the receptor surface at the cortex seems to be uniform all over, or nearly so. This also agrees with the cell counts of CHOW, BLUM and BLUM (1950).

Functional Significance of the Topographical Aspects of the Retino-Cortical Projection[1,2]

By

ROBERT W. DOTY

With 5 Figures

The existence of a spatial orderliness in the projection of sensory surfaces upon the cerebral cortex is well-established, and has offered a seemingly firm foundation for a wide variety of theories relating behavioral and perceptual phenomena to neural processes. The idea of spatial organization, with physical contiguity of the cortical neural components of the sensory systems, is equally prominent in Pavlovian physiology (35) and the Gestalt psychology of KÖHLER (see 22 for ref.), is utilized in an excellent theory of sensory acuity by MARSHALL and TALBOT (27), and to some degree in the theory of pattern discrimination proposed by PITTS and McCULLOCH (36); to cite but a few examples. Many questions remain, however, concerning the precision of the sensory projections to the cortex and, particularly, whether this topographical arrangement can be assigned any functional significance beyond that required for basic, inherited reflex patterns. It is, of course, exceedingly difficult to analyze the aspect of spatial arrangement as distinct from other aspects of cortical organization relating to cortical function. Nevertheless, the evidence reviewed below clearly suggests that topographical organization per se is of minor or no importance in the visual analysis of geometric patterns.

[1] From the Department of Physiology, University of Michigan, Ann Arbor, Michigan, U.S.A.

[2] New research reported here was begun in 1950 as a USPHS Postdoctoral Research Fellow in the laboratories of WARREN S. McCULLOCH. It was subsequently supported by United Cerebral Palsy Association, Inc. and by Research Grants B-938 and B-1068 from the National Institute of Neurological Diseases and Blindness of the National Institutes of Health, Public Health Service.

Anatomical and clinical evidence

The difficulty of even the "straightforward" anatomical problem is indicated by the fact that it took three generations of diligent effort to reveal the relation of the striate cortex to the lateral geniculate nucleus and visual processes. GUDDEN (*16*) greatly perfected neuroanatomical techniques, correlating behavioral and cellular changes subsequent to extirpation of neural tissue. He believed the "highest" visual center was the superior colliculus. His pupil, MONAKOW, in 1881, discovered the phenomenon of retrograde degeneration in the thalamus consequent to cortical destruction (see *33*), and could thereby trace out many cortico-thalamic relationships. He believed that the retina was rather diffusely represented in the cortex. In turn, his pupil, MINKOWSKI (*29*) in 1911 demonstrated in dogs a clear topographical relation of the lateral geniculate nucleus and striate cortex correlated with behavioral tests of visual defects. In subsequent years MINKOWSKI carefully elaborated these anatomical studies (*30, 31, 32*). A series of over 40 cats with various extirpations of striate cortex in our laboratories fully confirms Minkowski's anatomical findings and adds but a detail or two to his scheme of geniculo-cortical relations. POLYAK (*38*) has found the degeneration in the primate lateral geniculate nucleus to be extremely localized following small lesions of striate cortex. Thus this chapter seems closed.

Its meaning, however, is not entirely clear. No one can say specifically why some but not other types of neurons degenerate when their extensions are cut. It is thus premature to assume that the disappearance of a lateral geniculate cell following section of an unknown number of its collaterals signifies that it sent collaterals only to the restricted locus of injury. The cell might well send collaterals into widely separated cortical areas, and readily survive their separate loss; but degenerate upon removal of a more compacted group of branches. Such arrangement of branching would still leave a topographical projection, but would certainly alter its significance. Neurons do exist with widely divergent collaterals. The SCHEIBELS (personal communication) have observed neurons sending one branch subcortically and the other through the corpus callosum. The "sustaining projection" phenomen observed by ROSE and WOOLSEY (*43*) for the auditory system, wherein thalamic cells survive unless very extensive cortical ablations are made, also indicates a very wide, possibly diffuse projection zone for each cell. It thus seems unwise to infer solely on the basis of evidence obtained from studies of retrograde degeneration that the geniculo-striate system is exclusively a point to point projection, though this feature is undeniably present to some degree.

The studies of the central termination of optic tract fibers do not decide the issue. A topography of retinal quadrants ending within the lateral geniculate nucleus is demonstrable (*5, .39*), as is the separate ending there of the fibers from each eye (*32*, see *3* for review). POLYAK made exquisitely delicate, localized lesions in the retinae of monkeys, and interpreted his anatomical findings to indicate an extremely precise and orderly termination of retinal fibers within the lateral geniculate nucleus. His fine drawings of these experiments, do not, however, convince one of this fact, and indeed his Figure 203 (page 340, *39*) of MARCHI preparations following a 0.25 mm diameter lesion of the fovea would permit one to conclude this foveal area terminated throughout almost one-third of the lateral geniculate nucleus. The studies of GLEES (13) and of GLEES and CLARK (14) show the restricted termination of individual fibers required of a topographical arrangement, but of course, tell nothing of topography per se. For the monkey it appeared that each lateral geniculate cell received a bouton from only one optic tract fiber and each fiber innervated about five lateral geniculate cells (14). Yet something is distinctly wrong with this picture since no count of the numbers of optic tract fibers and lateral geniculate cells in monkey or man gives a ratio less than about 1:1 (7, 48).

One of the most interesting and surprisingly neglected findings of both GLEES (13) and of BARRIS, INGRAM and RANSON (2) is that the lateral geniculate nucleus of the cat is in large measure innervated by collaterals of fibers passing to the tectum. According to the electrophysiological experiments of APTER (1) the retinal representation in the colliculus is a topographical one. One might thus deduce that the topographical projection at cortex and colliculus represents the same neural system and function!

The clinical evidence on functional localization is almost as confusing as it is voluminous. Thirty-seven years ago HENSCHEN (17), in a vituperative, self-eulogizing essay on what he called the "40-year battle" over visual centers, reviewed evidence which would incontrovertibly prove the existence in man of an extremely precise point to point functional relation of the retina to the cortex. Yet HENSCHEN (18) could also believe "degenerated" cells survived in the visual system of people lacking eyes for 38 years, and use this to deny that fibers from the two eyes end in alternate layers of the lateral geniculate nucleus; publishing as he did so the histology, sent him by MINKOWSKI, which clearly showed this alternation. POLYAK's case of Dr. MALLORY (l.c. pages 735—747 in ref. 39) seems among the best to show that a small, lifelong scotoma arises consequent to a highly restricted lesion of area striata. Yet even POLYAK omits completely from consideration the possible relevance of the fact that Mallory in addition to the striate lesion had extensive loss of tissue involving the entire lingual gyrus. This gyrus presumably was mere peristriate cortex and of no concern in the etiology of the scotoma. Aside from this tendency to ignore all but the area striata in accounting for field defects, those favoring the point to point functioning of the visual system have also relied almost exclusively upon simple perimetry as their test for vision. POPPELREUTER (40) stressed the inadequacy of such a limited definition of visual function, and with more thorough and complex tests revealed many features of the visual deficit following occipital lobe injury which could not be explained on the basis of a point to point functioning. BENDER, TEUBER, BATTERSBY and their colleagues (e.g. 37 and TEUBER in this volume) have demonstrated that global diminution of certain visual functions generally accompanies visual deficits which appear highly localized upon simple perimetric examination. On the other hand, neither POPPELREUTER nor BENDER and his group supply adequate anatomical data to assure us that the more complex or global losses are not attributable to diffuse or widespread damage within the occipital area.

Electrophysiological evidence

Flashes of light which subtend most of the visual field evoke a remarkable series of oscillations in the optic tract of the cat and monkey. The oscillations range in frequency from 50 to 150/sec, varying in amplitude and frequency at various times throughout a flash of 500 msec duration. The entire complex series is exactly reproduced with each flash. These oscillating potentials can be seen in Fig. 1, but are much more prominent during the first hour or so after placing the electrode in the tract. It seems likely that these oscillations represent the continuing, synchronized discharge of retinal ganglion cells throughout the period of the flash. If this is so, then there must be some intraretinal mechanism capable of synchronizing cell discharges over widely separated regions of the retina.

Potentials can be evoked by flashes of light in regions of the cerebral cortex of the cat far beyond those included in the neuroanatomical definition of the cortical visual system (6, 11, 20, 28). The significance of these potentials for visual function is problematical. They can, for instance, be evoked in frontal cortex (20) or in anterior suprasylvian gyrus (11) following cortical extirpations which render the animal capable of making discriminations only of light intensity. Perhaps the potentials should suggest that these cortical regions participate in such intensity discriminations, but the question has never been examined. The potentials observed in the middle and posterior suprasylvian gyri themselves indicate little but, as is discussed below, are usually found in animals capable of visual pattern discrimination in the near or total absence of the geniculo-striate system.

The potentials evoked in cats by flashes or electrical stimulation of the optic nerve are much higher in amplitude in cortex adjacent to area striata than they are in it (11). It is probable that most of the studies of the electrophysiology of the cortical visual area of the cat have utilized this area on the central and lateral portions of the marginal gyrus giving the most impressive potentials to optic stimuli. The extirpation of this "high amplitude" region does not produce degeneration in the lateral geniculate nucleus (11). Continuing studies indicate no additional degeneration occurs when it is extirpated together with adjacent area striata. Probably no additional lateral geniculate cells survive when this "high amplitude" region remains and the striate area is removed, but this needs further study. Photically elicited activity appears to propagate into this region in the absence of direct connections with the lateral geniculate nucleus. In one cat following extirpation of all area striata save a strip of ventral splenial gyrus and perhaps a tag of marginal gyrus at the HORSLEY-CLARKE plane A-2, and with only a few scattered cells surviving in the anterior third of the lateral geniculate nucleus, 200 μV potentials of normal appearance were recorded as far as A-10 with a progressive delay suggesting a conduction velocity of 1 m/sec anteriorly from the A-2 focus.

Two other cats have been observed in which all connections to the marginal gyrus were severed save at the anterior or the postero-ventral ends. The background activity of the semi-isolated gyrus was low and abnormal. In one of these animals (DEH-104) a few cells in the anterior third of the lateral geniculate nucleus survived. From its anterior marginal gyrus photically elicited potentials propag at ed posteriorly for over 10 mm with an apparent velocity of 2 m/sec. The potentials of this chronically undercut cortex were highly abnormal but the amplitude difference between the middle portion of the gyrus and the medial border (area striata) was still maintained, as was a surprisingly normal cyto-

architecture even in the total absence of white matter. In the other animal
(DEH-103) the lateral geniculate nucleus was "totally" degenerated (*pars dorsalis*,
of course) and the only connections to marginal gyrus came through posterior
limbic cortex. Light flashes elicited a small surface negative potential with a
35 msec latency which about 30% of the time was followed in another 45 msec by
a 200 μV spike.

Thus, such little evidence as there is suggests: 1. that this "high amplitude"
region is inherently organized in such a way that it produces prominent potentials,
and 2. that this region can be extensively activated by intracortical conduction.
However, neither this nor the degeneration studies rule out the possibility that
it is normally also activated by collaterals from lateral geniculate neurons;
indeed, the lack of a latency difference in activation of this cortex and area
striata upon optic nerve stimulation strongly suggests that it is normally activated
by collaterals. Electrophysiologically it also shows a degree of topographical
relation with the retina (*11, 50*). It is almost impossible to gauge the origin and
extent of collaterals anatomically since the possibility always exists that the
branching occurs deep within the white matter. OCHS (*34*) has developed an in-
genious method of testing for the presence of such collaterals by direct stimulation
of the cortex at two points and observing at a third cortical locus the interaction
of these cortically elicited potentials and those elicited by optic nerve stimuli.
In the rabbit, where conditions are most favourable for this type of experiment,
OCHS's results indicate branching does occur in such a manner that the visual
afferents extend up to 10 mm in various directions over the visual cortex.

The decisive electrophysiological experiments on the question of topographical
relations should involve localized stimulation of the retina and the elicitation
of a localized response at the cortex. Unfortunately much of this is difficult to
achieve for purely technical reasons and the results are subject to various interpretations. The retinal area stimulated and the cortical region from which the
response is recorded each contributes uniquely to the characteristics of the
potentials observed, and the earliest response at a given cortical location may
also not be the largest. These factors make it difficult to decide on the basis of
amplitude and latency which cortical point is most closely related to which retinal
one. Nonetheless, certain retinal regions definitely activate certain cortical regions
better than others. TALBOT and MARSHALL (*51*) for the cat, and THOMPSON,
WOOLSEY and TALBOT (*52*) for the rabbit have emphasized this aspect. The retino-
cortical relations established electrophysiologically for the rabbit are in near
total disagreement with those established anatomically (*42*). The anatomy may
be indecisive in this case because of the MARCHI technique used by BROUWER
(see *5*) for retino-cortical relations and because of the irregular nature of the
cortical lesions used for retrograde degeneration studies; yet the electrophysiology
also appears to require an interpretative factor and is presented only as a "map"
of the cortex (*52*).

The data for the cat (*51*) agree with what is known of the anatomy (save for
the inclusion of extra-striatal areas as noted above), and the general features
of the electrophysiological results were readily confirmed (*11*). The fine detail
of point to point projection, however, should receive further study. The location
of a light flash within a few degrees affects the potential evoked from a selected

cortical point; but it similarly affects potentials over many millimeters of cortex. In arriving at their more specific delineations TALBOT and MARSHALL (51) and THOMPSON, WOOLSEY and TALBOT (52) have apparently discounted this diffuseness of the cortical response as being largely attributable to retinal excitation by light diffusion within the optic media. Such physical diffusion undoubtedly occurs, yet intraretinal and intracortical irradiation of the physiological response is also a possibility which should not be ignored.

My own experiments (11) are obviously deficient in this matter of light-scattering since they were done in the partially dark-adapted eye, and the cat, of course, has an extraordinarily sensitive eye with a highly reflective tapetum. Still, the light intensity employed was very near the limits of usability, just barely capable of eliciting a cortical response even when directed at the most favorable retinal locus, and did not show this presumed scatter effect in certain orientations (e.g. Fig. 11 in 11). The latency and amplitude of the "off" response were often reciprocal to those for the "on" response at cortex for various locations of retinal stimulation. This in itself makes the concept of point to point projection incongruous since the same criteria that establish the relations for the "on" system then yield antipodal locations for the "off" system. Nonetheless, in retrospect, it would have been desirable to have tried to balance out the possible effect of light-scattering by a background illumination. SUZUKI, TAIRA and MOTOKAWA (49) have just shown that the receptive fields of most geniculate and optic tract units in the cat become much smaller when a background illumination is used. However even under their conditions of highest background illumination it appears that a 40° field is common, although HUBEL and WIESEL (19) report fields at the cortical level which range only from 4° to 10° under other conditions. Again it is not certain how much of these differences in field size should be attributed to physical effects and how much to neurophysiological interactions.

To circumvent this problem of light-scattering Dr. FRANCES GRIMM and I (12) have utilized local electrical stimulation of the retina to evoke cortical responses This procedure has obvious difficulties of its own. The electrodes will excite fibers passing beneath them so that the cortical response observed represents a sector rather than a "point" of the retina. Stimulation through the sclera requires very high currents, so the cornea, lens and most of the vitreous humor were removed and the electrodes placed directly on the retina. For several hours potentials elicited at cortex by photic stimuli after opening the eye remained reasonably similar to those obtained with the intact eye. They were monitored throughout the experiment.

The electrical stimulation elicits two types of cortical response, both of which are depressed by antecedent flash stimuli. The "early" response is similar to that elicited by stimulation of the optic nerve save that it has a longer latency (3 to 5 msec), and is recorded from limited regions of cortex. By shifting the retinal electrodes progressively closer to the optic disc an intraretinal conduction velocity of about 5 m/sec can be estimated for this system, agreeing fairly well with the figures for the faster intraretinal fibers obtained by DODT (9) with a more accurate method. Figure 1 shows this early response appears farther anteriorly and medially on the cortex for stimulation of the more dorsal retina and is more posterior when the retinal stimulation comes closer to the horizontal meridian. There are thus

elements of a topographical organization for this early response and it was sometimes dramatically punctate in its cortical localization. Note, however, that in
Fig. 1 there is extensive overlap in the cortex activated from the "retinal sectors"
A and B. The response from both sectors is also most prominent in the "high
amplitude" strip of marginal gyrus, as can be seen by comparing the responses
to electrical and photic stimuli. For the entire dorsal retina this is invariably the
case. The only early responses detected on the exposed dorsal cortex to stimulation
of the ventral retina were found on the anterior-ventral edge of the postlateral
gyrus with electrodes in contralateral nasal retina 3 mm below the tapetum and
about 5 mm from the disc. It is our impression that the ventral retina is considerably less excitable than the dorsal.

The "late" response appears 20 to 100 msec after stimulation. Typically it is
similar in latency and form to responses elicited by photic stimuli, but there are
many variations and complexities (e.g. Fig. 1). It has a lower threshold than the
early response, but increasing stimulus intensity that develops an early response
at a particular cortical locus, causes the late response to diminish at that point.
The early and late responses thus tend to be mutually exclusive. A moderate
stimulus intensity evokes an early response in a restricted cortical area which is
surrounded by a large expanse of cortex in which the later responses appear. The
late responses are frequently found in both hemispheres. Evidence of a progressively delayed appearance of the late response at areas increasingly removed from
the cortical region of the early response (as between A-5 and A-1 for A in Fig. 1)
suggest a propagating phenomenon. This is not always true, however, and it is
uncertain, whether the propagation should be referred to retina or cortex or both.
A major portion of the late response originates in the retina since it is seen in the
optic nerve (Fig. 1). These results are obviously obtained under highly abnormal
conditions, but they are concordant with the experiments using punctiform
photic stimuli suggesting that an initially localized excitation spreads to occupy
major portions of the visual cortex.

The responses in area striata to a flash of light in acute experiments on unanesthetized monkeys are so complex and variable that analysis will be an extremely formidable task. Where surface-positive responses predominate in the cat, the
photic responses from monkey cortex are surface-negative or written on a slow,
surface-negative baseline shift. Irregular oscillations at a frequency of about 50/sec.
persist in the unanesthetized cortex throughout a flash of several hundred milliseconds and endure some 80 msec after nigrescence until interrupted by the
"off" spike. TALBOT and MARSHALL (51) found a topographical arrangement of
high precision for the monkey, but gave no details on the potentials observed.
From the anatomy one might expect a great elaboration of the cortical potential.
POLYAK (39) states: "... each particular point of the striate cortex is interconnected
both ways with a fairly large segment of cortex. According to a rough estimate,
the functional units of this kind may amount to at least one-sixth of the entire
striate area covering the external face of the occipital lobe of a monkey's brain."

Preliminary experiments with localized electrical stimulation of the peripheral retina in the monkey show several components traversing the optic nerve
for up to 30 msec after a 1- msec pulse and a response of about 35 msec latency
throughout much of one occipital lobe. Since no early response was found at the

cortex to correspond to the large early spike in the optic tract, it is conceivable that, as in the cat, this component may be highly localized and in inaccessible cortex in experiments to date.

JASPER, RICCI and DOANE (21) have shown flash stimuli affect unit activity in apparently all cortical regions in the monkey during behaviorally significant

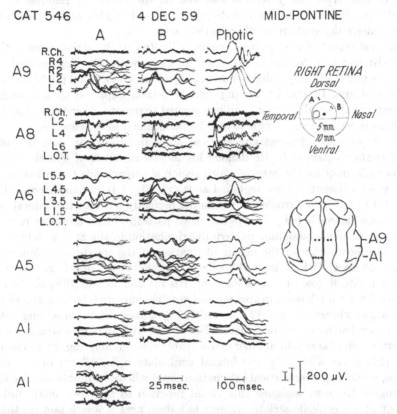

Fig. 1. Distribution of early and late responses at cortex to localized electrical stimulation of the retina and corresponding activity in optic tract. Right side of optic chiasm, R. Ch.; left optic tract, L.O.T.; cortex, R 4, L 2, etc signifying millimeters lateral to midline in Horseley-Clark planes A-1 to A-9, as shown on brain chart. Stimulation of exposed right retina with 1-msec 6-volt electrical pulses through electrodes at A (left column) B (middle column) or 160 msec light flashes (right column). Animal unanesthetized 11 hours after electrolytic transection of brain stem at mid-pontine level. Highest gain used for optic tract and chiasm, intermediate for cortex at A-9, lowest for other cortical records. Slower sweep speed for A-8 and lower A-1 record. See text. (R. W. DOTY and F. GRIMM, to be published.)

situations, but these findings are hard to relate to vision per se. In acute experiments potentials have so far not been found in cortex outside area striata even though temporal and frontal areas known to be associated with visual functions and eye movements are explored (11).

Evidence from behavior following cortical extirpations

The early efforts to identify the cortical visual area were very confused, and to some degree merited the scorn HENSCHEN (17) cast upon them. They had violated GUDDEN's dictum: „Zuerst Anatomie und dann Physiologie; wenn aber

zuerst Physiologie, dann nicht ohne Anatomie" (16). It was not until after MIN-
KOWSKI with behavioral and anatomical techniques had identified the cortical
visual system with the area striata that meaningful experimentation was possible.
LASHLEY brought this approach to fruition with precise measurement of both
behavior and anatomy, setting the methodological pattern for all future experiments of this type. Many reports followed on the effects of removal of "area
striata"; yet in no instance was extirpation limited to this region but included
very extensive destruction of other cortical areas.

The first report of extirpations precisely limited to the striate area is that of
DENNY-BROWN and CHAMBERS (8). Their monkeys with fully degenerated lateral
geniculate nuclei still responded to moving objects and had visual placing reactions.
Removal of area 18 and 19, leaving area 17 intact, impaired spatial judgment.
Thus important visual functions can be assigned to regions other than area striata,
and these functions can to some degree be maintained in its absence.

The importance of nonstriate cortical areas in vision can also be deduced
from LASHLEY's data (23). He defined his lesions in terms of FORTUYN's cyto-
architectonic map for the rat, on which region w corresponds to area striata and
region p an adjacent, lateral region. LASHLEY's Fig. 7 (23), summarizing lesions
which did not disturb pattern vision, almost perfectly outlines this lateral area p,
i.e. lesions which included p always disturbed pattern vision. LASHLEY recognized
this as a difficulty in assigning pattern discrimination to the area striata, but felt
it was the localization of the center of fixation in the striate area immediately
adjacent to area p which gave this effect. Yet the visual deficit is not entirely
correlated with degree of striate damage. His rat No. 39 had 72% of the striate
area intact yet with damage in area p could not discriminate triangles, and similarly
with No. 23; whereas rat No. 43 with only 37% of area striata remaining but with
area p intact had no visual disturbance. Rat No. 30 with all of area striata removed,
but with much of area p intact had considerable vision remaining. So too in a later
paper (24) a rat with only 700 lateral geniculate cells, 1/50th of the normal
number, remaining after cortical extirpation could still discriminate the orientation
of triangles. LASHLEY assigned this visual function to the very small unilateral
remnant of the geniculo-striate system; but since area p was intact on this side
the function might even more convincingly be assigned to it.

A laterally located cortical system which contributes to visual pattern discrimination after damage to area striata is certainly indicated in the cat (10).
In these experiments the animals were first trained to distinguish triangles from
circles of equal area. Three sizes were used, with areas of 3640, 910 and 400 mm^2.
These equal-area figures are hereafter designated problem A, B and C respectively.
The figures were transparencies mounted on plastic doors which the animal
pushed open to secure its freedom and a bite of food for a correct choice, or a
slight foot-shock for an error. Two errors or less in 20 daily trials was the criterion
for moving on to a more difficult problem. In the final tests the animal was
required to distinguish a triangle from squares, circles, and "diamonds" randomly
interchanged regardless of size. Adults were trained prior to surgery. Cortex was
removed by suction using full aseptic precautions. Extirpations were also performed
on more than 200 kittens within two days of birth. Most of these died of common
cat diseases in the laboratory after one to three months. Twenty-four that sur-

vived long enough for adequate testing were reared at home. Ordinarily the animals were kept together in a large pen that they might have opportunities for visuo-motor performance. Photographs, wax models and histological analyses were made of all brains, and in most the cortex was explored for photically evoked potentials at time of sacrifice. The following cases of over 80 in this series are representative of the results obtained.

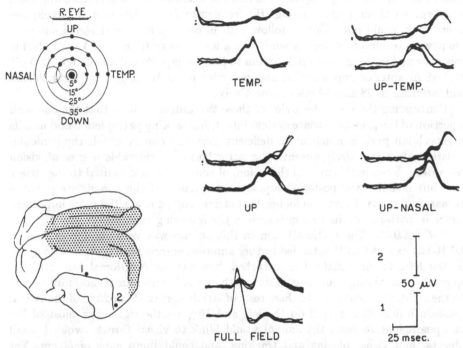

Fig. 2. Cortical responses of cat DEH-100 to simultaneous flashing of three 1° lamps from the four positions indicated in the visual field. Nembutal anesthesia. Upper trace, cortical point 2; lower trace point 1. Note variations in wave-form, amplitude and latency, and independence of these factors. The pattern seen at point 2 to full-field stimulation was also found in several other animals in this area. See text.

Cat DEH-127. Cortex overlying the tentorium, and the marginal, splenial and postlateral gyri were completely removed along with most of the posterior suprasylvian gyri. The lateral geniculate nucleus was fully degenerated. The large cells of the posterior nucleus were intact as were those, described by MINKOWSKI *(30)*, strewn in the tract and radiation. During eight postoperative months the animal was able to meet criterion on problem A with a total of 76 errors in 360 trials and consistently performed above chance levels on problem B with 580 errors in 2058 trials, without, however, attaining the criterion. Visual placing was poor, but present. The animal could jump a gap of 45 cm across and 20 cm up. She readily avoided a 3 cm. stick thrust suddenly athwart her path. Movement was quickly detected visually. Potentials evoked by full-field flashes were nearly identical to those shown in Fig. 2.

Cat DEH-134. Cortex was removed as in Cat DEH-127 plus the parasplenial and middle suprasylvian gyri. A small portion of cortex on the left tentorial aspect remained, however, and on this side about seven percent of the lateral geniculate nucleus survived. It was entirely degenerated on the other side. There was considerable degeneration in the pulvinar and most of the large cells of the posterior nucleus were missing. In six months of postoperative training this cat on two occasions made only three errors in twenty trials on problem A, but never reached the criterion. In 1460 trials on this problem he made 536 errors. Tests for visuomotor responses seemed to reveal a 20—30° island of central vision. He could detect movement of large objects such as a hand, blinked to their sudden approach and avoided them when running. He frequently failed, however, to avoid the 3 -cm stick, could not visually follow a 5-cm object and would strike out with his paw to reach a food dish when it was a meter away from him. Visual placing was poor and nothing would induce him to jump a gap. Potentials of 100—200 μV evoked in anterior suprasylvian and posterior ectosylvian gyri by light flashes had latencies of 38 and 50 msec respectively.

Contrasting the visual behavior of these two animals shows that the one with a portion of the geniculo-striate system intact, but lacking parasplenial and middle suprasylvian gyri, is much more deficient than the one in which the geniculo-striate system is entirely absent. The latter had a considerable degree of vision remaining. Even in this animal the lesion, of course, was not limited to the striate area but included the posterior suprasylvian gyrus and the non-striate portions of marginal gyrus. Further evidence that striate cortex is not the most important factor in pattern discrimination is seen in the following examples.

Cat DEH-25. The cortical lesion in this animal was very similar to that in DEH-127 except that it extended farther anterior, entering the postcruciate gyrus on the left. Tissue remained undisturbed, however, on the dorsal aspect of the splenial sulcus throughout most of its length on the left and for several millimeters on the right. Corresponding to these rests of striate cortex about 23% of the lateral geniculate nucleus survived on the left and 16% on the right. For most of her two postoperative years the animal would blink to visual threat, avoided small objects, had visual placing and tracking, and could jump gaps of 50 cm. Yet in 4000 trials on problem A she made 1834 errors, so that most of her performance was at the chance level and she never reached criterion. If the figures differed slightly in size she was readily able to differentiate them, and preoperatively had been an exceptionally clever animal on these visual problems. Flashes evoked 150 μV potentials around the posterior suprasylvian sulcus with a latency of 45 msec.

Cat EH-108. The entire lateral geniculate, pulvinar and adjacent nuclei plus a major portion of the internal capsule on the left were destroyed by electrolysis. The lesion on the right produced similar, but less extensive destruction and the posterior two-thirds of the lateral geniculate nucleus survived. Weil stains indicate the optic tracts were essentially intact. The striate cortex appears to be normal bilaterally. Throughout four months of survival this animal seemed totally blind, so no attempt was made to train it, as it was believed most of the optic tract had been destroyed. It "felt" its way along slowly, bumping objects in its path and never responded to moving objects. The pupils remained widely dilated, though they constricted and the eyes closed to light after a few minutes dark adaptation. The consensual pupillary reaction was equivocal. Photic stimulation of the left eye evoked potentials of normal latency and amplitude over the right postlateral and posterior suprasylvian gyri but responses to ipsilateral stimulation were restricted to the most ventral postlateral and posterior suprasylvian area.

Cat DEH-100. Cortical extirpation was restricted to marginal, splenial, post-lateral and lingual gyri. Some tissue deep in the most posterior part of the splenial sulcus escaped and about 12% of the lateral geniculate nucleus survived. During most of the postoperative period of 17 months, visual behavior was almost within normal limits. There was difficulty only in obtaining criterion performance on problem C, though performance was far above chance: 398 errors in 1810 trials. Subsequently however, this animal readily made criterion performances on figures of "random" size and discriminated a triangle of only 3.5 mm² from a square of the same area. The animal could track and catch small objects, had perfect visual placing, and jumped up and across gaps often and accurately. Potentials evoked by light flashes were found along both sides of the suprasylvian sulcus (e.g. Fig. 2). Photic responses were not evoked in posterior suprasylvian gyrus medial to a line extending the suprasylvian sulcus, probably because this cortex had been under-cut. Flashes subtending 1° and of about 1 millilambert intensity elicited potentials in the suprasylvian regions which varied greatly depending upon location of the stimulus. Technical difficulties with intensity control on the instrument used at that time prevented precise definition of the most favorable stimulus location for the two points shown in Fig. 2 (which yielded the highest amplitude potentials to full-field stimulation). Both points, however, appeared to be activated well from extensive areas of the retina. As in Fig. 2, flashes of single lamps also gave complex patterns in which the earliest response was not that of the highest amplitude and the effects tended to vary *pari passu* at the two widely separated cortical points. Thus the spatial location of the stimulus was definitely registered in the amplitude, latency and wave-form of the cortical response, but was dependent upon cortical as well as retinal location and not necessarily in a topographical manner.

Cat NDEH-59. The cortex overlying the tentorium, the marginal, splenial, postlateral and posterior suprasylvian gyri, as can be seen in Fig. 3 and 4, were removed within a few hours after the animal was born. Cortex corresponding to the lateral aspect of the marginal gyrus, normally within the depths of the lateral sulcus, was preserved on the left (Figs. 3 and 4). The histological patterns of the thalamus are particularly difficult to interpret in animals undergoing neonatal cortical excision. However, with 18 such brains now avaiable for comparison it is possible to state unequivocally that the many large cells (about 30 microns in diameter) seen in Fig. 5 scattered in the area normally occupied by the lateral geniculate nucleus do not indicate survival of any striate cortex. These cells were found in varying numbers bilaterally throughout the entire extent of the "nucleus" in this animal and there is no possibility of a corresponding survival of striate area. When tags of area striata were missed in such neonatal extirpations, the cells surviving in the lateral geniculate nucleus were readily recognizable as intact islands of cells similar to adult cases. These scattered cells (Fig. 5) have no definite relation to vision since they were present in neonatally operated animals with more extensive extirpation that had the full picture of "cortical blindness", and were absent in one animal (NDH-62) which had vision almost as perfect as this cat NDEH-59. These cells may possibly represent an expansion of the posterior nucleus or even lateral geniculate cells that have survived because of collateral connections, but do not seem to be the "scattered ganglion cells" or "Markganglien-zellen" of MINKOWSKI (30).

This animal thus had no geniculo-striate system; yet its visual abilities were indistinguishable from those of its normal litter mates. He tracked moving objects

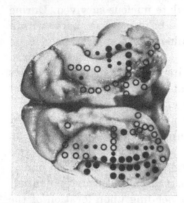

visually with high accuracy and jumped expertly with careful estimation of distance. He required only 243 trials to reach criterion on problem A; generalized immediately to problem B making only 18 errors in 120 trials and similarly with problem C, 52 errors in 329 trials to criterion; and with random interchanging of various sized figures made only 14 errors in 140 trials. His only apparent sign of cortical damage was an incessant hyperactivity. The photically elicited potentials (Fig. 3) were of normal latency and form, but were more widely distributed than is usual in the intact cat.

Fig. 3. NDEH-59. Distribution of electrical responses on brain of animal that had no geniculostriate system following cortical extirpation at birth. Visual behavior was essentially normal. Flashes were 160 msec, 0.3/sec. Flash to right eye: ● > 100 μV, ● < 100 μV, ○ no response.

GUDDEN (16) obtained similar results with neonatal operations on rabbits. His Tafel XXXVI (16) shows the brain of a rabbit which at the very most had only a periphe-

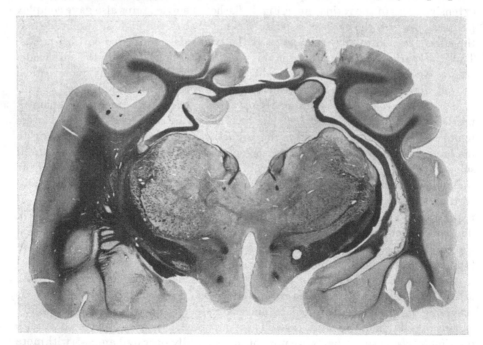

Fig. 4. Weil-stained section through brain of cat NDEH-59. Only the parasplenial gyrus remains medially on the right; a lateral edge of the marginal gyrus survives on the left.

ral tag of visual cortex as defined by THOMPSON, WOOLSEY and TALBOT (52), and on page 205 (16) describes the behavior of such animals: „Sie sahen, hörten, fühlten und bewegten sich anscheinend wie normale Kaninchen. . . . sie ohne alle und jede Spur von Sehsphäre sahen und ihr Sehen psychisch verwerteten."

It is not known what systems are responsible for pattern vision following extensive damage of the geniculo-striate system or in its absence. A cortical system seems to be required since pattern vision is lost with neonatal lesions which include parasplenial, posterior ectosylvian and middle suprasylvian gyri in addition to

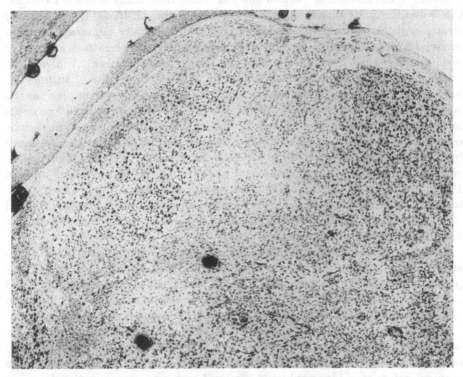

Fig. 5. Cat NDEH-59. Nissl-stained section through region which would normally contain the left lateral geniculate body. Scattered, large cells as shown were found bilaterally throughout the lateral geniculate area in this animal, but not in one other (NDH-62) which had comparably excellent pattern vision.

the tissue missing in NDEH-59. This, and the presence of photically elicited potentials, suggests the lateral areas may have particular significance for pattern discrimination. Yet in the presence of a nearly intact geniculo-striate system they do not appear to be essential since removal of middle and posterior suprasylvian gyri had no effect on visual performance (Cat DEH-87), nor did electrolytic destruction of about 90% of the pulvinar (Cat DH-90).

TALBOT (50) has reported that the visual system in the lateral part of the marginal gyrus and in the medial portion of the posterior suprasylvian gyrus is topographically organized, but he found no such organization for visual area III (52) which apparently corresponds to that along the suprasylvian sulcus. The anatomical pathway for visual impulses to the latter area, especially in the absence of the geniculo-striate system, is unknown. From its physiological characteristics such as variable location, highly differing wave-forms in different parts of the system (Fig. 2) and the discontinuous nature of loci yielding potentials in these lateral regions it seems unlikely that there can be a precise topographical retinal projection to this area. It is probable then that the cortical systems necessary for pattern discrimination in such cats as DEH-127, DEH-100 and NDEH-59 perform this function in the absence of any spatial mapping of the retinal stimuli on the cortical surface.

Additional support for the concept that the topographical arrangement is not germane to the function of pattern analysis comes from many sources. LASHLEY, CHOW and SEMMES (25) and SPERRY and his coworkers (45, 46, 47) have presented strong evidence and cogent arguments against tangentially organized function in visual cortex. The interdigitation of sensory modalities in somatosensory cortex and their columnar organization (41) does not suggest a tangential integration in that system. The comparable organization of visual "modalities" such as the various color functions, brightness functions, rod versus cone systems, etc., at the cortex has not been worked out, but it must be that "contour analysis" proceeds in and among these systems, seemingly without interaction. It must further be compounded with the presence of very extensive vestibular influences, as shown by the GRÜSSERS (15), and with the effects of the "nonspecific" systems as discussed in this volume by BREMER and by CREUTZFELDT. From the recent work of HUBEL and WIESEL (19) and of LETTVIN et al. (26) it appears that much of the topographical information has already been analyzed by retinal systems and is fed into higher centers as an abstract from which it would be pointless to reconstitute the original topographical relations.

Presence of the topographically organized visual cortex may in itself be insufficient for pattern discrimination, as shown above. BLAKE's report (4) that pattern vision is lost after excision of the superior colliculus even though the visual cortex is intact presents an even more striking example, though confirmation and extension of her experiments seems desirable. RIESEN and BAXTER (personal communication and 2a) also found with electrophysiological analysis in visually deprived cats that the cortical visual system is seemingly intact while the animal is incapable of pattern vision. A maturational or learning factor thus seems to be required before even topographically arranged cortex becomes functional.

The foregoing data and arguments are obviously stronger for the cat than for the primate. The monkey visual system is indeed so different from that of the cat that different principles of operation may be expected in it. Not knowing, however, what they may be, it seems prudent to abide by the evidence reviewed here and build theories of pattern discrimination upon statistical, "random net" principles, as begun by SHOLL and UTTLEY (44), rather than upon processes requiring spatial contiguity of the participating neurons.

Summary

It is argued that the topographical arrangement of the retino-cortical projection is in itself of minor or no importance in the visual analysis of geometric patterns.

1. The anatomical data, despite emphasis on point to point projection, are compatible with a system of extensive overlap and divergence. The clinical data appear indecisive.

2. Cortical responses to photic stimuli and to electrical stimulation of the retina in the cat suggest both a topographically organized process and a slower, more diffuse process, partly intraretinal, which activates major portions of the visual cortex following localized excitation.

3. Cortex other than area striata is necessary for visual pattern discrimination in cats after extensive damage to the geniculo-striate system. LASHLEY's data (*23, 24*) suggest a similar situation for the rat.

4. Normal visual abilities, including discrimination of shape, develop in the complete absence of the geniculo-striate system in cats from which area striata is removed at birth. Cortex in the suprasylvian and ectosylvian areas appears to be necessary in such cases and potentials can be evoked in these regions by photic stimuli. Evidence is scant, but the optic input to these regions is not likely to be organized in the topographic manner found for area striata.

References

1. APTER, J. T.: Projection of the retina on superior colliculus of cats. J. Neurophysiol. 8, 123—134 (1945).
2. BARRIS, R. W., W. R. INGRAM and S. W. RANSON: Optic connections of the diencephalon and midbrain of the cat. J. comp. Neurol. 62, 117—153 (1935).
2a. BAXTER, B. L.: An electrophysiological study of the effects of sensory deprivation. PhD. dissertation, Univerity of Chicago, 1959.
3. BISHOP, P. O., W. BURKE, R. DAVIS and W. R. HAYHOW: Binocular interaction in the lateral geniculate nucleus — a general review. Trans. ophthal. Soc. Aust. 18, 15—35 (1958).
4. BLAKE, L.: The effect of lesions of the superior colliculus on brightness and pattern discrimination in the cat. J. comp. physiol. Psychol. 52, 272—278 (1959).
5. BROUWER, B., and W. P. C. ZEEMAN: Experimental anatomical investigations concerning the projection of the retina on the primary optic centers in apes. J. Neurol. Psychopath. 6, 1—10 (1925).
6. BUSER, P., and P. BORENSTEIN: Observations sur les réponses corticales visuelles recueillies dans le cortex associatif suprasylvien chez le chat sous chloralose. J. Physiol. (Paris) 48, 422—424 (1956).
7. CHOW, K. L., J. S. BLUM and R. A. BLUM: Cell ratios in the thalamo-cortical visual system of macaca mulatta. J. comp. Neurol. 92, 227—239 (1950).
8. DENNY-BROWN, D., and R. W. CHAMBERS: Visuo-motor function in the cerebral cortex. J. nerv. ment. Dis. 121, 288—289 (1955).
9. DODT, E.: Geschwindigkeit der Nervenleitung innerhalb der Netzhaut. Experientia(Basel) 12, 34 (1956).
10. DOTY, R. W.: Effects of ablations of visual cortex in neonatal and adult cats. Abstracts Comm. XIX. Int. Physiol. Congr. 1953, p. 316.
11. — Potentials evoked in cat cerebral cortex by diffuse and by punctiform photic stimuli. J. Neurophysiol. 21, 437—464 (1958).
12. — and F. R. GRIMM: Cortical responses to local electrical stimulation of retina in the cat. (To be published.)
13. GLEES, P.: The termination of optic fibers in the lateral geniculate body of the cat. J. Anat. (Lond.) 75, 434—440 (1941).
14. — and W. E. LE GROS CLARK: The termination of optic fibers in the lateral geniculate body of the monkey. J. Anat. (Lond.) 295—308 (1941).
15. GRÜSSER, O. J., and U. GRÜSSER-CORNEHLS: Mikroelektrodenuntersuchungen zur Konvergenz vestibulärer und retinaler Afferenzen an einzelnen Neuronen des optischen Cortex der Katze. Pflügers Arch. ges. Physiol. 270, 227—238 (1960).
16. GUDDEN, B. VON: Gesammelte und hinterlassene Abhandlungen. 227 pp. Wiesbaden: J. F. Bergmann 1889.
17. HENSCHEN, S. E.: 40jähriger Kampf um das Sehzentrum und seine Bedeutung für die Hirnforschung. Z. ges. Neurol. Psychiat. 87, 505—535 (1923).

18. — Die Vertretung der beiden Augen in der Sehbahn und in der Sehrinde. Albrecht v. Graefes Arch. Ophthal. 117, 419—459 (1926).

19. HUBEL, D. H., and T. N. WIESEL: Receptive fields of single neurones in the cat's striate cortex. J. Physiol. (Lond.) 148, 574—591 (1959).

20. HUNTER, J., and D. H. INGVAR: Pathways mediating Metrazol induced irradiation of visual impulses. EEG clin. Neurophysiol. 7, 39—60 (1955).

21. JASPER, H., G. RICCI and B. DOANE: Microelectrode analysis of cortical cell discharge during avoidance conditioning in the monkey. The Moscow Colloquium on Electroencephalography of Higher Nervous Activity. Suppl. No. 13 to EEG clin. Neurophysiol. ed. H. H. Jasper and G. D. Smirnov, Montreal, 137—155 (1960).

22. KÖHLER, W., and D. W. O'CONNELL: Currents of the visual cortex in the cat. J. cell comp. Physiol. 49, suppl. 2, 1—43 (1957).

23. LASHLEY, K. S.: The mechanism of vision IV. The cerebral areas necessary for pattern vision in the rat. J. comp. Neurol. 53, 419—478 (1931).

24. — The mechanism of vision: XVI. The functioning of small remnants of the visual cortex. J. comp. Neurol. 70, 45—67 (1939).

25. — K. L. CHOW and J. SEMMES: An examination of the electrical field theory of cerebral integration. Psychol. Rev. 58, 123—136 (1951).

26. LETTVIN, J. Y., H. R. MATURANA, W. S. McCULLOCH and W. H. PITTS: What the frog's eye tells the frog's brain. Proc. IRE. 47, 1940—1951 (1959).

27. MARSHALL, W. H., and S. A. TALBOT: Recent evidence for neural mechanisms in vision leading to a general theory of sensory acuity. Biological Symposia VII Visual Mechanisms. ed. H. Klüver. 117—164. Lancaster, Penn.: Jaques Cattell 1942.

28. — — and H. W. ADES: Cortical response of the anesthetized cat to gross photic and electrical afferent stimulation. J. Neurophysiol. 6, 1—15 (1943).

29. MINKOWSKI, M.: Zur Physiologie der Sehsphäre. Pflügers Archiv. ges. Physiol. 141, 171—327 (1911).

30. — Experimentelle Untersuchungen über die Beziehungen der Großhirnrinde und der Netzhaut zu den primären optischen Zentren, besonders zum corpus geniculatum externum. Arbeit. Hirnanatom. Institut Zürich. 7, 259—362 (1913).

31. — Über die Sehrinde (Area striata) und ihre Beziehungen zu den primären optischen Zentren. Mschr. Psychiat. Neurol. 35, 420—439 (1914).

32. — Über den Verlauf, die Endigung und die Zentrale Repräsentation von gekreuzten und ungekreuzten Sehnervenfasern bei einigen Säugetieren und beim Menschen. Schweiz. Arch. Neurol. Psychiat. 6, 201—252, 7, 268—303 (1920).

33. MONAKOW, C. VON: Experimentelle und pathologisch-anatomische Untersuchungen über die optischen Zentren und Bahnen. Archiv Psychiat. 20, 714—787 (1889).

34. OCHS, S.: Organization of visual afferents shown by spike components of cortical response. J. Neurophysiol. 22, 2—15 (1959).

35. PAVLOV, I. P.: Conditioned reflexes. An investigation of the physiological activity of the cerebral cortex. 430 pp. Trans. by G. V. Anrep. London: Oxford Univ. Press 1927.

36. PITTS, W., and W. S. McCULLOCH: How we know universals: the perception of auditory and visual forms. Bull. Math. Biophys. 9, 127—147 (1947).

37. POLLACK, M., W. S. BATTERSBY and M. B. BENDER: Tachistoscopic identification of contour in patients with brain damage. J. comp. Physiol. Psychol. 50, 220—227 (1957).

38. POLYAK, S.: The main afferent fiber systems of the cerebral cortex in primates. Univ. of Calif. Publ. in Anatomy. 2, Berkeley: Univer. of Calif. Press 1932.

39. — The vertebrate visual system. Ed. H. Klüver. Chicago: Univ. of Chicago Press 1957.

40. POPPELREUTER, W.: Die psychischen Schädigungen durch Kopfschuß im Kriege 1914/16. Vol. I. Die Störungen der niederen und höheren Sehleistungen durch Verletzungen des Occipitalhirns. Leipzig: Voss 1917.

41. POWELL, T. P. S., and V. B. MOUNTCASTLE: Some aspects of the functional organization of the cortex of the postcentral gyrus of the monkey: a correlation of findings obtained in a single unit analysis with cytoarchitecture. Bull. Johns Hopk. Hosp. 105, 133—162 (1959).

42. PUTNAM, T. J., and I. K. PUTNAM: Studies on the central visual system I. The anatomic projection of the retinal quadrants on the striate cortex of the rabbit. Arch. Neurol. Psychiat. (Chicago) 16, 1—20 (1926).

43. ROSE, J. E., and C. N. WOOLSEY: Cortical connections and functional organization of the thalamic auditory system of the cat. Biological and Biochemical Bases of Behavior. 127—150. Ed. H. F. Harlow and C. N. Woolsey, Madison: Univ. of Wisconsin Press 1958.
44. SHOLL, D. A., and A. M. UTTLEY: Pattern discrimination and the visual cortex. Nature (Lond.) 171, 387 (1953).
45. SPERRY, R. W.: Neurology and the mind-brain problem. Amer. Scientist 40, 291—312 (1952).
46. — and N. MINER: Pattern perception following insertion of mica plates into visual cortex. J. comp. physiol. Psychol. 48, 463—469 (1955).
47. — — and R. E. MYERS: Visual pattern perception following subpial slicing and tantalum wire implantations in the visual cortex. J. comp. physiol. Psychol. 48, 50—58 (1955).
48. SULLIVAN, P. R., K. KUTEN, M. S. ATKINSON, J. B. ANGEVINE and P. YAKOVLEV: I. Cell count in the lateral geniculate nucleus of man. Neurology 8, 566—567 (1958).
49. SUZUKI, H., N. TAIRA and K. MOTOKAWA: Spectral response curves and receptive fields of pre and postgeniculate fibers of the cat. Tôhoku J. exp. Med. 71, 401—415 (1960).
50. TALBOT, S. A.: A lateral localization in the cat's visual cortex. Fed. Proc. I, 84 (1942).
51. — and W. H. MARSHALL: Physiological studies on neural mechanisms of visual localization and discrimination. Amer. J. Ophthal. 24, 1255—1264 (1941).
52. THOMPSON, J. M., C. N. WOOLSEY and S. A. TALBOT: Visual areas I and II of cerebral cortex of rabbit. J. Neurophysiol. 13, 277—288 (1950).

Discussion

L. M. HURVICH: Historically the Gestalt-movement in psychology was in essence a revolt against the analytical and atomistic approach which the Gestalters saw in the traditional content psychology of WUNDT and TITCHENER, for example. KÖHLER's now classic Gestalt-Psychology volume is, from one end to the other, an attack on atomistic point-for-point connectionistic psychology and physiology. The so-called "machine views" of traditional associationistic psychologists whether "mentalistic" or,, behavioristic" are contrasted throughout with the "dynamic" field theories favored by the Gestalters. I am therefore surprised to find that in your introductory remarks KÖHLER's isomorphic views and latter day experiments seem to you to typifiy the point-for-point topographical viewpoint.

F. BREMER: The potentials of long latency which are recorded outside the visual area of the unanesthetized (encéphale isolé) cat in response to an optic nerve or geniculate stimulus are regularly, and often strikingly, increased in reticular and sensory arousal. In agreement with BUSER and BORENSTEIN who studied them in the chloralosed cat, we found that they are not the expression of a cortico-cortical irradiation from the area striata response, although they may be influenced by such irradiation. Their spatial distribution corresponded rather well in our experiments with the cortical distribution of the potentials evoked by the stimulation of the lateralis-pulvinar complex. Recent observations by ALBE-FESSARD and ROUGEUL (1960) indicate that impulses issued from the n. centro-medianus may also be contributory to their evocation. The functional significance of these responses shares the obscurity of most electro-physiological data which concerns the neo-cortical associative areas.

A. ARDUINI: What is the functional state of the surviving cells in the lateral geniculate body after destruction of striate cortex ? It is suggested that the visual discrimination after decortication in the early days of life is performed through tectal mechanisms.

R. W. DOTY: To my knowledge no one has ever examined the degenerated lateral geniculate nucleus with silver stains to see what happens to the optic tract terminations after degeneration following cortical extirpation, or what type of connections are possessed by the cells which survive. Neither, I believe, has anyone looked carefully at the electrophysiology in such cases. There might be some surprises for us here.

The tectum certainly requires further analysis in relation to these experiments, although it alone is unable to support visual form discrimination.

M. Verzeano: Can you tell us what the latencies were in the area striata as compared with those outside area striata ? Would you think that longer latency responses were coming through the lateral geniculate or could they come over some other pathways, such as some of the "unspecific" nuclei of the thalamus ?

R. W. Doty: There are in the cat many non-striate areas from which photic responses can be elicited (6, 11, 20, 28, 51). In some of these areas and under some conditions the latency can be the same as that to the striate area, as it was in the supra-sylvian and ectosylvian areas in cat NDEH — 59; but in many instances it is much longer. Borenstein, Bruner and Buser[1] have shown that the pulvinar and nucleus lateralis posterior probably relay the photic response to the middle surprasylvian gyrus, but believe the mesencephalic reticular formation may also play some role here. Ingvar and Hunter[2], of course, have also shown an extensive distribution of photically elicited responses in the brain stem which is altered and augmented by cortical ablation.

W. A. Beresford: You said that after ablation of the non-striate cortex lying laterally in the lateral gyrus you could find no retrograde cell degeneration in the lateral geniculate body. Where in the thalamus could you find such degeneration ?

After removal of the striate cortices in newborn kittens you found a severe atrophy of the lateral geniculate body. Did this include the *pars ventralis* ?

Your animals could still discriminate form and a different cortical area to that in normal cats showed evoked potentials to light stimulus. You seem to interpret this as a new or better developed visual pathway via the thalamus to the cortex. Have you ablated the cortical area showing the abnormally increased response to light stimuli to attempt to find by retrograde cell degeneration which thalamic nucleus is projecting to this cortex ?

R. W. Doty: Extirpation of the "high amplitude strip" in the middle of the marginal gyrus did not produce any readily apparent degeneration in the thalamus beyond that attributable to slight inadvertent invasion of the optic radiation. This also holds for small extirpations of the posterior suprasylvian gyrus; i. e. an extensive cortical loss seems necessary to produce degeneration in regions such as the pulvinar.

There is no obvious degeneration in the ventral nucleus of the lateral geniculate body in any of my animals with neonatal extirpations. However, for a sound anatomical statement on this point I would prefer to have some unilateral extirpations for definitive comparisons.

D. Whitteridge: I have explored the extent of the visual area in about half-a-dozen cats using long steel needles to record from the medial surface of the hemisphere. I should like to support Talbot's (1942)[3] conclusions that a comparatively small amount of visual area I is exposed on the posterolateral surface of the cortex, that the lower field is represented anteriorly and the upper field on the deep aspect of the posterior pole, with the horizontal meridian running downwards and backwards in the direction of the posterior tip of the gyrus splenialis. It is easy to obtain well localised responsive areas not more than 10° diameter situated 30° to 60° from the optic axis by leading from the medial surface.

I think that Talbot is also right that there is a visual area II, but so far it can only be identified in relation to visual area I. I think that early responses appearing in the cortex after 30—40 msecs are well localised, but that late responses beginning after 70 msecs can be set up from points widely separated in the visual field and even in the ipsilateral visual field.[4]

[1] Borenstein, P., J. Bruner et P. Buser: Etude du système thalamocortical d'association visuelle et auditive chez le chat sous chloralose. Contrôle réticulaire des systèmes associatifs. J. Physiol. (Paris) 50, 166—170 (1958).

[2] Ingvar, D. H., and J. Hunter: Influence of visual cortex on light impulses in the brain stem of the unanesthetized cat. Acta physiol. scand. 33, 194—218 (1955).

[3] Talbot, S. A.: A lateral localization in the cat's visual cortex. Fed. Proc. 1, 84 (1942).

[4] Subsequently Dr. Doty has visited Edinburgh and we have both seen in cats under chloralose anaesthesia well localised early responses from visual area I. We agree that the late responses show much less localisation. It is difficult, however, to describe visual area I completely until visual area II can be identified with certainty wherever one meets with it.

R. W. Doty: Dr. Whitteridge and I obviously held rather different opinions concerning the degree of localization of the cortical response to a localized photic stimulus. He generously proposed that en route home I might stop in Edinburgh where in his laboratory we could jointly ask nature itself to resolve our differences. This we did, and in two thoroughly pleasant and busy days asked two cats where the potentials appeared in their cerebral cortex when a spot of light of 10′ to 1°40′ diameter was flashed on a perimeter arm before their eye.

I think Dr. Whitteridge definitely scored the best in our argument. His system of projecting the light flash on a surface in front of the animal appears to give much less light-scattering effect than did that which I used projecting the light directly into the animal's eye. Chloralose anesthesia may also offer some advantages over Nembutal for this type of work. From the experience in his laboratories it appears that when that retinal area is photically excited which is appropriate to the cortex from which one is recording, the latency of the potential at the cortex will be essentially the same as that to full-field stimulation of comparable intensity. It is the latency rather than amplitude which is the reliable criterion of the point to point relationship and one can state almost categorically that unless the latency of the cortical response is less than 50 msec one is not stimulating the appropriate retinal point. Thus in my Fig. 11[11 (1958)] the latency of 43 msec indicates this point was correctly localized, whereas the much longer latencies of 70—100 msec observed in the search for the horizontal meridian (Figs. 12, 13, 14, 15 etc. ref. 11; 1958) clearly indicate the appropriate retinal locus was not found. I am still puzzled as to why my exploration never quite managed to find these points, but Whitteridge's demonstration convinces me that the situation exists very much like Talbot and Marshall (52) described it.

The problem of "on-off reciprocity"(11) may have been explained in these meetings by Sickel's report of the existence of this phenomenon in the isolated retina.

Nevertheless there is still much to be said about the later, often larger responses which even with Whitteridge's apparatus can be triggered at a cortical point by stimulation far removed from the retinal locus giving the earliest evoked potentials. It seems my work dealt mostly with these later responses. Some of these responses can be attributed to light-scattering. However, the latencies may actually be too long to fit this explanation since a 1000 fold decrease in light stimulus intensity which reduces the cortical potential to the vanishing point causes only a change from 31 to 43 msec in latency (e. g. Fig. 11, in 11). This fact plus the data from electrical stimulation of the retina (12) thus prompts me still to maintain my opinion that a localized retinal stimulus can produce a widespread cortical effect. There may then, conceivably, exist two processes, one which rapidly affects the cortex in a topographically organized manner and a second slower, possibly intraretinal process which elaborates the stimulus over a much wider area.

Fibre Degeneration Following Lesions of the Visual Cortex of the Cat*

By

W. A. Beresford

With 5 Figures

Introduction

Previous workers Probst (12), Polyak (11), and Barris, Ingram and Ranson (1) made lesions in the cat's visual cortex and traced the resulting fibre degeneration into subcortical areas of the brain with the Marchi method. My experiments are a repetition of their work with the substitution of the silver staining

---

* From the University Laboratory of Physiology, Oxford.

16a

method of NAUTA and GYGAX for the Marchi method. As the silver stain, also used by SZENTÁGOTHAI (*13*) in similar experiments, reveals the degeneration of finer fibres than are shown by the method of Marchi based on myelin degeneration products, more details of the efferents of the visual cortex can be given.

Experimental procedure

In the cortex of adult cats under anaesthesia three types of unilateral lesions were made:
1. Undercuts of the posterior part of the lateral gyrus via the posterior suprasylvian gyrus.

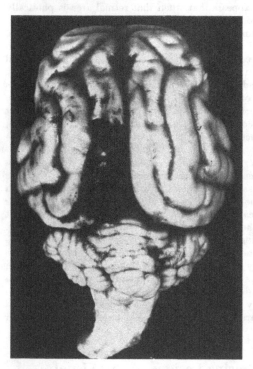

Fig. 1. A lesion of type 2. Parts of the left lateral and posterolateral gyri were ablated (C/VCL/13)

2. The ablation of part of the lateral and postlateral gyri with some damage to the suprasylvian gyrus.

3. Small lesions of the posterior part of the lateral gyrus made through a burr hole over the gyrus.

These lesions all resulted in the same distribution of subcortical degeneration. These lesions will be described as lesions of the visual cortex as they involved the posterior lateral gyrus and medial posterolateral gyrus. These gyri contain cortical area 17 and part of area 18, and the surrounding cortex, which was injured partially in the lesions of types 1 and 2, contains areas 5 and 19. The restricted lesions penetrated the white matter of the lateral gyrus so the possibility of damage to fibres leaving parastriate cortex cannot be excluded for lesions of type 3.

The animals were allowed to survive 5 to 8 days before being anaesthetised with Nembutal and killed by perfusion via the aorta of 0.9% saline followed by 10% formalin in 0.9% saline. Frozen sections of 25 micron's thickness were cut in the transverse plane of the WINKLER and POTTER (*14*) atlas or in the sagittal plane. The sections were stained according to the method of NAUTA and GYGAX (*9*) with some modification in the details.

Criteria of degeneration

A degenerating fibre was taken to be one that appears as a series of darkly stained fragments differing from one another slightly in both size and shape. The problems in recognising the products of degeneration in sections stained by their methods are discussed in detail by GLEES and NAUTA (*5*). A variable proportion of normal fibres show artifacts such as varicosities and intermittent impregnation that can easily be mistaken for the distortions and disintegration of fibres undergoing degeneration. Although it is possible to distinguish fibres undergoing degeneration from normal fibres with these artifacts, it is of great help to know the extent and the type of artifact that the staining solutions are inducing in a normal control specimen of the brain structure under investigation, e. g. the lateral geniculate body. The sections cut transversely contained both the ipsi- and the contralateral thalamus or colliculus so both received the same treatment. To give the sections cut sagittally similar treatments, corresponding ipsilateral and contralateral sections were taken together through the same staining solutions. Except for the callosal projection to the contralateral cortex only very rarely could a "degenerating" fibre be seen in the side of the brain contralateral to the lesion. It is assumed from this and from the Marchi findings (1) that no degeneration from the visual cortical lesion crossed the midline subcortically, that the contralateral structures are providing the control that the degeneration within the ipsilateral structures is a result of the cortical lesion. NAUTA and WHITLOCK (10) report that with survival times of up to ten days the Nauta method impregnates axons undergoing Wallerian degeneration, but not axons degenerating retrogradely. As survival times were no longer than eight days in this work it has been assumed that the degeneration seen has been Wallerian.

Description of the degeneration

It has been customary for experimenters using the Nauta method to distinguish between degenerating fibres of passage and the more haphazardly orientated degenerating terminal or preterminal fibres within an area defined by their presence as a site of "terminal degeneration". But the Nauta stain shows only randomly orientated fine degenerating fibres around and over a nerve cell. It is inferred from a study of the picture of *synapsing* fibres given by other silver stains and by the electron microscope that the fine degenerating fibres in the Nauta picture are, or will soon give rise to, fibres that terminate on that or adjacent cells. However in some areas e.g. the pulvinar in this experiment, the fine degenerating fibres seen to be distributed around the cells may have branched off from the fibres of passage and in order to *pass by* the cells and fibre bundles to reach an adjacent nucleus e.g. the posterior nucleus, must pursue an apparently haphazard and meandering course. If the method showed axons terminating on cells it would be possible to say that the fine fibre degeneration was of terminals or of a not very obvious kind of fibre of passage. As the method reveals only degenerating fibres it would seem safer to choose a term that describes the appearance of the degeneration rather than a term that infers an unseen relationship between fibre and cell. It is suggested that "directed" might be applied to fibres orientated through or towards a particular structure and "undirected" to fibres having no particular orientation. Within a nucleus the degeneration will be described as dense, medium or mild. The individual degenerating fibres will be described, by their thickness, in three categories large, medium, and fine. The largest pyramidal fibres are "large" and no fibres of this size leave the visual cortex.

The limits and nomenclature of the nuclei in which degeneration has been found are based on INGRAM, HANNETT and RANSON's (6) atlas of the diencephalon of the cat.

Results

Directed fibre degeneration. Disintegrating fibres run from the lateral gyrus to the neighbouring posterior suprasylvian gyrus and via the corpus callosum to the lateral gyrus of the other hemisphere. Subcortically fibres go from the internal capsule into the thalamic radiations, passing in both branches of the optic tract around and through the lateral geniculate body (dorsal part), and traverse the pulvinar, pulvinar pars posterior, posterior nucleus, and lateral posterior nucleus to enter the superior colliculus as part of the mesencephalic branch of the optic tract.

A tract of degenerating fibres maintained a ventrally directed path in the internal capsule and did not turn medially into the thalamus. In transverse sections of the posterior thalamus and of the colliculi some degenerating fibres were visible in the cerebral peduncle and pons ipsilateral to the lesion.

Undirected fibre degeneration. *1. Superior colliculus.* Dense degeneration was found in the lateral two thirds of the superior colliculus. Disintegrating fibres of medium and fine diameters were present in the superficial part of the stratum griseum intermedium. The most ventral extent of this degeneration was marked by the giant cells situated in the deeper part of the s.g.i. These cells did not have

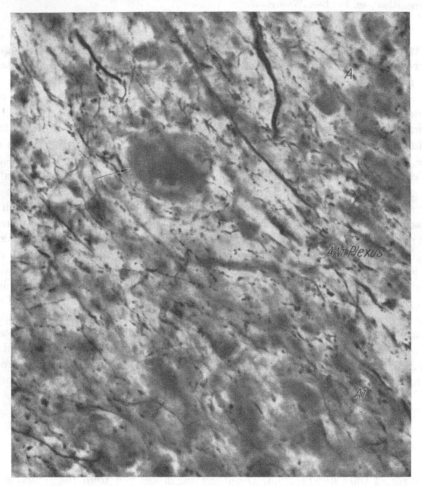

Fig. 2. A large cell (arrowed) in the AAl interlaminar plexus of the left ipsilateral LGBd. Degenerating fibres are visible in A, Al and AAl (C/VCL/12)

fine degenerating fibres around them and probably do not receive direct afferents from the visual cortex, but they do serve as a convenient reference feature.

The stratum griseum superficiale showed undirected fine fibre degeneration and some degenerating fibres traversed this stratum and then ran in the superficial stratum zonale.

2. Posterior nucleus. Dense undirected degeneration was evident in this nucleus which lies just medially to the medial interlaminar part of the lateral geniculate body (dorsal part). In the dorsal area of the nucleus considerable directed degeneration is present.

3a. Lateral geniculate body (dorsal part). Degenerating fibres of medium and fine thickness are to be found in the dorsolateral branch of the optic tract where it enfolds the lateral geniculate body and in the posterior part of the ventromedial branch. Fibres of the dorsolateral branch give two distinct kinds of degeneration within the lateral geniculate body.

i) Medium and a few thinner fibres run in fasciculi through the dorsal part of the lateral geniculate body in a lateral to medial direction. It is inferred from their size that they are myelinated and would produce the directed degeneration on which BARRIS et al. (*1*)

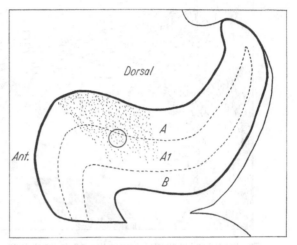

with the Marchi technique have commented, "a few degenerated fibres passed through the dorsal nucleus of the lateral geniculate body, but none seemed to terminate there".

ii) A medium undirected degeneration of fine fibres. Fine degenerating fibres pass from the optic tract into lamina A and can be seen in lamina Al and the AAl interlaminar plexus. The number of fibres in A appeared to be more than twice the number in lamina Al. No degenerating fibres

Fig. 3. A diagram of a sagittal section of the LGB showing the position at which figure 2 was taken (circle) and the distribution of degeneration (dotted), following a small anterior visual cortex lesion (C/VCL/12)

were seen to pass from the ventromedial branch of the optic tract into the lateral geniculate body. Although the occasional fibre could be found in lamina B, it was straight and somewhat larger than the fine fibres found in laminae A and Al. Degeneration was absent from the most posterior part of the lateral geniculate body, but this may be because the lesions did not involve the whole visual cortex.

3b. Lateral geniculate body (ventral part). A mild undirected degeneration was present in the central part of the LGBv. The fibres were of medium and fine sizes.

4a. Pulvinar, pulvinar pars posterior and lateral posterior nucleus. All these structures contain fasciculi of degenerated fibres. Between the fasciculi there are a considerable number of fine fibres running in an undirected manner. The density of both the directed and the undirected degeneration within these structures increases with proximity to the posterior nucleus.

4b. The reticular nucleus of the thalamus. Part of this nucleus is represented by a few scattered large cells lying just dorsally to the LGB and laterally to the pulvinar. They are surrounded by directed and undirected degenerating fibres.

5. The nucleus of the optic tract and pretectal region. The nucleus of the optic tract consists of large cells between the fibre bundles of the mesencephalic branch of the optic tract. The bundles contain directed disintegrating medium and fine fibres and between the bundles are many medium and fine degenerating fibres running more randomly. The lateral portion of the pretectal area that lies ventrally to the optic tract contained a number of bundles of degenerating fibres but very little undirected degeneration.

6. *The ipsilateral suprasylvian gyrus and contralateral lateral gyrus* have medium undirected degeneration in layers V and VI and a few disintegrating fibres running radially or obliquely decreasing in number from layers IV to II.

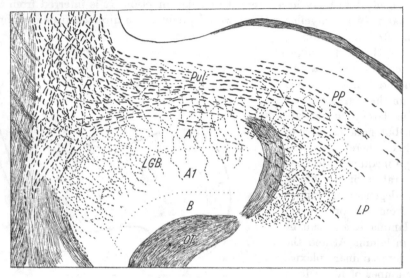

Fig. 4. The directed and undirected degeneration seen in the thalamus is shown schematically in its relationship to the nuclei

Conclusions

1. As degenerated fibres run from the visual cortex to the brain structures listed in the section of results all these structures *may* receive a visual cortical projection. Previous authors have moreover found myelin degeneration running in the transverse peduncular tract and into the anterior pons after lesions of the cat's visual cortex. Some degeneration was found in the cerebral peduncle in this experiment. But the peduncular site in which the degeneration is to be expected from the Marchi work is at the edge of the section and contains a number of stained normal fibres cut almost in cross section. Both factors result in an increase in artifacts making it very difficult to distinguish degenerating fibres. In this situation the Marchi method gives a clearer picture than the Nauta of the course of the myelinated fibre projection.

2. The structures in which the cortical efferents terminate are assumed to be those containing undirected disintegrating fibres surrounding the nerve cells. In the lateral geniculate body, posterior nucleus, nucleus of the optic tract and superior colliculus the undirected degeneration is limited to the nuclei and does not lie between the degenerated fibres coming from the cortex and another structure containing undirected fibre degeneration. The reticular nucleus, pulvinar and lateral posterior nucleus contain directed degenerating fibres and an undirected fibre component that might

a) terminate within the nucleus,

b) pass through the nucleus to the adjacent LGBd in the case of the reticular nucleus or to the posterior nucleus in the case of the pulvinar,

c) terminate within and outside the nucleus.

These three possibilities are shown in a diagram.

From these results it is concluded that the cat's visual cortex projects to the ipsilateral parastriate cortex, superior colliculus, nucleus of the optic tract, posterior nucleus and lateral geniculate body, and to the contralateral visual

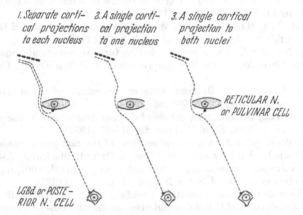

Fig. 5. In the confusion of degenerating fibres around the cells of the pulvinar and reticular nuclei three possible patterns of cortical projection are illustrated

cortex. It is intended to examine the pontine projections in more detail, to look for more conclusive evidence of corticofugal terminations with the Glees technique and to attempt lesions limited to specific cortical areas within the visual cortex.

Summary

Experimental lesions made in the visual cortex (striate and the surrounding parastriate) resulted in a degeneration of the efferent fibres whose path to and within other areas of the brain was revealed by the Nauta and Gygax silver impregnation method. Within a nucleus this method shows fibres of small diameter curving around cells in a manner suggestive of a terminal plexus. Such degeneration is usually described as "terminal" but it is suggested that "terminal" is misleading as it is an inferred conclusion used as a descriptive term. The degenerating fibres are described as "directed" or "undirected" according to whether or not they have a definite linear orientation through a structure. Degeneration is seen in the visual cortex (a) of both sides of the brain, and in the ipsilateral superior colliculus (b), nucleus of the optic tract (c), posterior nucleus (d), lateral geniculate body (e), reticular nucleus of the thalamus (f), pulvinar and lateral posterior nucleus (g), pons (h). In the reticular nucleus and pulvinar the undirected degeneration might consist of fibres that had turned out of the main bundles and were themselves directed for another nucleus e.g. LGBd or P. Only for the structures (a) to (e) was it concluded from their undirected degeneration and its relationship to the fibres coming from the cortex and to the degeneration in neighbouring structures, that they received a visual cortical projection.

References

1. BARRIS, R. W., W. R. INGRAM and S. W. RANSON: Optic connections of the diencephalon and midbrain. J. comp. Neurol. **62**, 117—153 (1935).
2. BOWSHER, D., A. BRODAL and F. WALBERG: The relative values of the Marchi method and some silver impregnation techniques. Brain **83**, 150—160 (1960).
3. CHANG, H. T.: Cortical response to activity of callosal fibres. J. Neurophysiol. **16**, 117—132 (1953).
4. CURTIS, H. J.: Intercortical connections of corpus callosum as indicated by evoked potentials. J. Neurophysiol. **3**, 407—413 (1940).
5. GLEES, P., and W. J. H. NAUTA: A critical review of studies on axonal and terminal degeneration. Mschr. Psychiat. Neurol. **129**, 74—91 (1955).
6. INGRAM, W. R., F. I. HANNETT and S. W. RANSON: The topography of the nuclei of the diencephalon of the cat. J. comp. Neurol. **55**, 333—394 (1932).
7. LORENTE DE NO, R.: Cerebral cortex: architecture, intracortical connections, motor projections. In: Physiology of the Nervous System by J. Fulton (Oxford University Press) 1943.
8. NAUTA, W. J. H., and V. M. BUCHER: Efferent connections of the striate cortex in the albino rat. J. comp. Neurol. **100**, 257—286 (1954).
9. — and P. A. GYGAX: Silver impregnation of degenerating axons in the central nervous system: a modified technic. Stain Technol. **29**, 91—93 (1954).
10. — and D. G. WHITLOCK: An anatomical analysis of the nonspecific thalamic projection system. In: Brain Mechanisms and Consciousness. Oxford: Blackwell 1954.
11. POLYAK, S.: An experimental study of the association, callosal, and projection fibres of the cerebral cortex of the cat. J. comp. Neurol. **44**, 197—258 (1927).
12. PROBST, M.: Über den Verlauf der zentralen Sehfasern (Rinden-Sehhügelfasern) und deren Endigung im Zwischen- und Mittelhirn und über die Assoziations- und Commissurenfasern der Sehsphäre. Arch. Psychiat. Nervenkr. **35**, 22—43 (1902).
13. SZENTÁGOTHAI, J.: Die zentrale Innervation der Augenbewegungen. Arch. Psychiat. Nervenkr. **116**, 721—760 (1943).
14. WINKLER, C., and A. POTTER: An anatomical guide to experimental researches on the cat's brain. Amsterdam: Versluys 1914.

Acknowledgement

The author is grateful for the advice and criticisms of Dr. P. GLEES and Dr. MARIANNE FILLENZ and for the photographic assistance of Miss F. GREENE. The award of a Medical Research Council scholarship is gratefully acknowledged.

Discussion

P. GLEES: The likelihood of a callosal connexion of area 17 deserves attention as neurophysiological methods e.g. CURTIS (4) showed this connexion in the cat but not in the monkey.

W. A. BERESFORD: The Nauta method shows that, in the cat, after lateral gyrus lesions degenerating fibres pass via the corpus callosum into the contralateral lateral gyrus and invade area 17. As these fibres pass into the gyrus presumably they terminate there as there is no more distant structure to which they could continue.

2. The cortical layers in which the majority of the callosal fibres terminate can be still considered controversial. NAUTA and BUCHER (8) stressed that the majority of the visual cortical callosal fibres in the rat ran in an undirected manner in layers VI and V with only a few radial and oblique fibres in layers III and II. The distribution of visual callosal afferents revealed by NAUTA's technique in the cat is similar to that described by him for the rat.

LORENTE DE NO (7) and CHANG (3) using Golgi preparations of the rat both describe callosal fibres as running to the supragranular layers. The infragranular layers of the cortex have more fibres than the supragranular layers, so even with the selection of the Golgi method whatever criteria the two authors were using to decide the source of a fibre may have been of no help there. They say that few callosal fibres terminate in the deeper layers. The Nauta method shows that supragranular part of the picture given by the Golgi method and suggests that the main callosal projection is to the deepest cortical layers. As it is suspected that the Nauta method does not show the degeneration of the finest fibres, BROWSHER, BRODAL and WALBERG (2), it might be objected that the disintegrating fibres seen in V and VI branched, becoming too thin to be seen, and proceeded more superficially. To check this possibility one might cut thin sections and stain with a more completely impregnating silver stain such as the GLEES.

A. ARDUINI: It is remarked that the transcallosal pathways are not easily activated even when a synchronized volley arrives at the striate cortex through the optic radiations.

W. A. BERESFORD: I think there are several questions worth asking when the physiologist finds it difficult to activate the visual callosal pathway in the cat. 1. Is there anatomical evidence for a connection, and of what kind of fibres does it consist? 2. Is the "activating" stimulus the one most likely to fire the cells giving rise to callosal fibres? 3. Is the recording being taken under the most favourable conditions of location, anaesthesia etc.? 4. Is there evidence that the small activity of this pathway assists the cat in its use of vision?

In answer to:

1. NAUTA treated sections show fine and medium sized fibres passing from the visual cortex to the area 17 of the other hemisphere. POLYAK (11) showed with the Marchi method that this projection contained myelinated fibres.

2. If the striate cortex contains excitatory and inhibitory synapses, shocking the optic radiations to fire synchronously the afferents (and efferents) to the cortex may result in the inhibitory effects upon cells neutralising the excitatory. Functional evidence, 4. below, suggests that a small light stimulus should induce callosal activity.

3. As the callosal fibres appear to terminate in the deepest layers, if the recording is taken from the surface of the cortex the activity in the fibres may seem to be less than it is.

4. MYERS[1] has performed a series of visual discrimination experiments using cats with the optic chiasma cut through in the midline. His experiments show that the cat can use the connection between the two visual cortical areas to convey information concerning the *difference* between two stimuli e. g. ☐ versus 0 from an eye to the opposite cortex. In the intact animal such information could be carried more directly to the opposite cortex by the optic fibres that cross in the chiasma. In the normal animal I feel that the corpus callosum is more likely to convey information about *where* on the retina of the other eye the image of a stimulus is falling. When will this information not be able to reach the cortex from its own ipsilateral lateral geniculate body? The cat is said to have 130° of binocular overlap in its visual fields. So in a central sector of the unfixated visual field (180°—130°) the image will fall on the temporal quadrants of each eye, and from work on other species the temporal quadrants are believed to project to the ipsilateral lateral geniculate body.

M. VERZEANO: Did you find any descending fibres which might go to the caudal part of the n. reticularis of the thalamus or to other "unspecific" nuclei?

W. A. BERESFORD: No degenerating fibres could be traced to the midline thalamic nuclei. The most medial incursion of degeneration in the thalamus was into the lateral posterior nucleus. The reticular nucleus of the thalamus could receive a visual cortical projection as fibres go to and through it.

R. W. DOTY: Do the ipsilateral cortico-cortical connections appear to be diffuse, or is there perhaps some grouping of fibres passing to the ipsilateral suprasylvian and ectosylvian areas?

W. A. BERESFORD: Degenerating fibres run from a lesion of the posterior lateral gyrus into the ipsilateral suprasylvian gyrus, only a few fibres pass just into the ectosylvian gyrus. The degeneration was quite widespread in the posterior suprasylvian gyrus, but I would rather not describe the projection as "diffuse" until some quantitative meaning can be given to the term. If the lesion was confined to the grey matter of one cortical area one might say that a lesion of area x produced degeneration of a certain intensity in an area of extent y.

---

[1] MYERS, R. E., and R. W. SPERRY: Interhemispheric communication through the corpus callosum. Arch. Neurol. Psychiatr. (Chicago) 80, 298—303 (1958).

Neuere Beobachtungen über Sehstrahlung und Sehrinde*

Von

Hans-Lukas Teuber

Mit 5 Abbildungen

Der Bericht, den ich Ihnen geben möchte, bedarf der Rechtfertigung, und zwar in zweierlei Hinsicht: Ich spreche von einer Gattung, von der wir in diesem Symposion wenig gehört haben — dem Menschen — und fasse zusammen, was ich zum Teil schon an anderen Stellen (besonders in einer bald erscheinenden Monographie, *69*) im einzelnen beschrieben habe.

Doch gehören Beobachtungen über das zentrale Sehsystem des Menschen in den Rahmen des Symposions; denn fast alle Tierversuche an der Sehrinde sind durch klinische oder experimentelle Erfahrungen am Menschen angeregt worden. Vielleicht lohnt es sich zu sehen, wie weit diese Erfahrungen beim Menschen gekommen sind und wie sie zu den experimentellen Befunden an höheren Tieren passen. Es mag auch nützlich sein, hier mit einigen neuen Zusätzen kurz zusammenzufassen, was ausführlicher englisch veröffentlicht ist: die Zusammenfassung verschärft die Betonung, macht die Lücken in den eigenen Beobachtungen deutlicher, und zeigt vielleicht, in welcher Hinsicht auch die Tierexperimente etwas Vorläufiges haben.

Fragestellung. Wir können die Übersicht über unsere Ergebnisse beim Menschen in zwei Fragen ordnen: die erste gilt der *Form* der Sehfelddefekte nach fokalen Verletzungen der zentralen Sehbahn; die zweite gilt dem *Wesen* der Sehleistungen im Restfeld. Um das Wichtigste vorauszunehmen, die Messung der Sehfelddefekte bestätigt (mit einigen Einschränkungen) das klassische Prinzip der retinotopen Projektion, wie es uns Whitteridge so klar in seinen eigenen Versuchsberichten dargestellt hat (*85*). Der zentrale Abschnitt der Sehbahn repräsentiert demnach in seiner räumlichen Anordnung die entsprechende Anordnung der Netzhaut und des Gesichtsfeldes; denn den Lücken im Gewebe entsprechen ganz spezifische Lücken im perimetrischen Feld. Aber diese mosaikartige Entsprechung gilt nur für die Defekte, die erworbenen Lücken. Sobald wir uns mit den überlebenden Sehleistungen im Restfeld befassen, wird es deutlich, daß noch andere Prinzipien im Spiele sind: Die Leistungen des Restfeldes sind nämlich in ganz bestimmter Art verändert.

Diese Veränderungen, die nicht fokal, sondern diffus sind (d. h. über das ganze erhaltene Sehfeld verteilt), erinnern eher an die radikalen Dinge, die Dotys neuere Tierexperimente uns nahelegen (*17*): Wechselwirkungen zwischen weit getrennten Teilen der Sehrinde, selbst von einer Hemisphäre zur andern, und Abhängigkeit der höheren Sehleistungen von Hirnregionen, die deutlich außerhalb des klassischen Projektionsgebietes zu liegen kommen.

* Aus dem Psychophysiologischen Laboratorium New York University-Bellevue Medical Center, New York, N. Y., USA. Unterstützt vom öffentlichen Gesundheitsdienst der Vereinigten Staaten (USPHS Grant M-3347).

Art der Fälle. Bevor ich von den Ergebnissen spreche, möchte ich nur kurz etwas über unsere Fälle und Arbeitsmethoden mitteilen: Die meisten unserer Berichte beruhen auf Untersuchungen an einer Gruppe von 232 Patienten, gewöhnlich im frühen und mittleren Mannesalter, deren Zustand wir seit mehr als zehn Jahren beobachten. Alle diese Patienten haben Schußverletzungen des Gehirns, meistens aus dem zweiten Weltkrieg; sie werden in unserem Laboratorium geprüft, weil sie die Verletzung haben, und nicht, weil irgendwelche klinischen Nachfolgen der Verletzung auftreten (67). Die Fälle unterscheiden sich also von denen die sonst untersucht werden: nicht nur Verletzte mit Komplikationen wurden geprüft, sondern auch solche, die nichts als die durchdringende Verletzung aufweisen und sonst völlig unauffällig sind. Gedeckte Schädelverletzungen wurden ausgeschlossen; nur solche mit nachweislichen Verlusten an Hirnsubstanz, als Folge von Geschossen, die durch die Hirnhäute ins Gewebe eindrangen, wurden in die Versuchsgruppe aufgenommen. Außerdem haben wir 118 Leute mit Schußverletzungen des peripheren Nervensystems (aber nicht des Gehirns), die uns als Kontrollfälle dienen. Von den 232 Hirnverletzten haben sich 203 ausführlichen und oft wiederholten Sehfeldprüfungen und anderen Studien ihrer posttraumatischen Sehleistungen unterzogen. Unter diesen 203 Fällen finden sich 46 mit Sehfelddefekten aller Art, von denen wir hier besonders sprechen werden (s. a. 69).

Methoden. Die Sehfeldprüfungen werden alle unter gleichförmigen Bedingungen, an einem Brombachschen Perimeter und Kampimeter unter 7 Fußkerzen-Beleuchtung, mit weißen, roten und grünen Marken von 1° und $^1/_2$° Durchmesser, ausgeführt (69). Neuerdings haben wir auch eine zusätzliche Methode, die Latenzperimetrie, eingeführt. Diese Methode, die von zwei unserer Mitarbeiter, STEPHAN CHOROVER und RITA RUDEL, ausgearbeitet wird, ist in mancher Hinsicht komplementär zu der von BAY (6, 15) geforderten Messung der lokalen „Verschwindezeiten". Wir messen die Zeit vom objektiven Erscheinen eines Lichtpunktes (in den verschiedensten, ausgewählten Stellen des Sehfeldes) bis zum Anschlagen einer Taste durch den Patienten, also eine regionale Reaktionszeit. Diese Methode verspricht eine bessere Bestimmung der amblyopen Gesichtsfeldbezirke, die hier als Regionen mit verlangsamter Reaktionszeit erscheinen. Es ist bezeichnend für unsere Fälle von fokalen Schußverletzungen des Gehirns, daß wir nur selten Allgemeinverlängerungen der Reaktionszeiten antreffen, ganz im Gegensatz zu Fällen von Hirntumoren oder Blutungen, bei denen die große Ermüdbarkeit unsere Art von Prüfungen überhaupt sehr erschwert. In der Zukunft hoffen wir übrigens auch die Apparatur von HARMS (27) zur weiteren Untersuchung unserer Fälle mittels einer dynamischen Perimetrie zu verwenden.

Ein weiterer Punkt zur Methode: bei gewöhnlicher Perimetrie und bei den zusätzlichen Prüfungen (s. u.) benutzen wir regelmäßig zur Fixationskontrolle den blinden Fleck (solange dieser nicht in einem erworbenen Skotom verborgen liegt). Ein Tupfen Leuchtfarbe wird auf Perimeter (und Campimeter) dort aufgetragen, wo die Projektion des blinden Flecks des jeweiligen Patienten fällt. Sobald der Patient seine Sehrichtung ändert, wird dieser Leuchtpunkt für ihn sichtbar, so daß wir eine (wenigstens subjektive) Kontrolle für seine Fixation gewinnen (70, 75). Zugleich gestattet dieser Kunstgriff aber eine Abschätzung (nach Richtung und Sehwinkelgraden) für die Verlagerung des Fixierpunktes in den häufigen Fällen, in denen sich eine Pseudofovea gebildet hat (69).

Unsere ergänzenden Methoden, die andernorts im einzelnen beschrieben wurden (66, 69, 71—74), sind vor allem dazu bestimmt, ein Bild von den Leistungen im überlebenden Rest des Gesichtsfelds zu verschaffen. Diese Methoden zeigen vielfach, daß solche Restgebiete, die im üblichen Perimeter- und Kampimeterversuch völlig unversehrt zu sein scheinen, eben doch ganz charakteristische Veränderungen aufweisen. So prüfen wir die Hell- und Dunkeladaptation, für ausgewählte Stellen des Sehfelds, außerdem Flimmerverschmelzung an vielen Stellen, d. h. Flimmerperimetrie (3, 4, 70, 71, s. u.) und auch obere und untere Schwellen für wahre und scheinbare Bewegung (72—74). Andere Methoden, einschließlich Tachistoskopie, gelten der Untersuchung der Farbwahrnehmung, den Nachbildern und gewissen „höheren" Sehleistungen, wie z. B. der Entdeckung von versteckten Figuren (76).

Mit Hilfe dieser beiden Methoden — der Messung von erworbenen Skotomen einerseits und der Prüfung der überlebenden Sehleistungen andererseits, wird es nun möglich, die beiden Fragen zu stellen, mit denen wir diese Diskussion begonnen haben: *Die Frage nach der Form der erworbenen Defekte*, und *die Frage nach dem Wesen der veränderten Sehleistungen im Rest des Feldes*.

Form der Sehfelddefekte

Die Prinzipien der retinotopen Projektion. *Lateraler Projektionstypus.* Einsichten in die räumliche Organisation der zentralen Sehbahn begannen vor mehr als hundert Jahren mit der Entdeckung des Prinzips der lateralen Projektion (z. B. PANIZZA, 1855, *53*), wonach die homonymen linken Hälften des Sehfeldes in der rechten Sehstrahlung und -rinde vertreten sind, und dem entsprechend die rechte Hälfte des Sehfeldes in der linken. Dieser Projektionstypus genügte zum Verständnis der rechts- und linksseitigen Hemianopsien.

Vertikaler Projektionstypus. Etwas später kam man zum analogen Prinzip der vertikalen Projektion, wonach die obere Hälfte des Sehfelds in die untere Calcarina-Furche gelangt, und umgekehrt für die untere Hälfte des Feldes. Dieser vertikale Typus wurde besonders durch HENSCHEN (*30*) und dann durch HOLMES (*32, 33*) und MARIE und CHATELIN (*49*) auf Grund der Fülle von Occipitalhirnverletzungen im ersten Weltkriege erforscht. Das vertikale Prinzip hilft zum Verständnis der horizontalen Sehfelddefekte: Verlust der unteren Teile des Sehfelds nach Zerstörung der oberen Anteile der Calcarina-Region und entsprechend für die oberen Teile des Sehfelds; solche Verluste, die durch Verletzung der *unteren* Anteile der Calcarina-Furche verursacht sind, traten bedeutend seltener auf (*11*), und zwar nicht nur im ersten (*56, 65, 78, 86*), sondern auch im zweiten Weltkrieg (*18, 69*). Dies hängt zweifellos damit zusammen, daß die untere Hälfte der Sehrinde doch näher als die obere Hälfte an lebenswichtige Hinterhirnregionen grenzt. Schußverletzungen dieser unteren Sehrindenanteile verlaufen deshalb weit häufiger tödlich, so daß die Seltenheit ausgedehnter Defekte in der oberen Hälfte des Sehfelds verständlich wird.

Der fronto-caudale Projektionstypus. Im Gegensatz zur Projektion nach Breite und Höhe — dem lateralen und vertikalen Prinzip, die recht früh angenommen wurden, dauerte es lange, bevor sich Einigkeit über die Vertretung der konzentrischen Zonen ergab, d. h. der Sehfeldgebiete von der Fovea auswärts bis zur äußersten Peripherie. Es war wiederum besonders HOLMES, der darauf hinwies, daß der foveale Bezirk wohl doch am weitesten nach hinten zu liegen kommt, im caudalen Teil der Sehrinde, also besonders auf den Lippen der Calcarina, während die mehr peripheren Anteile entsprechend weiter vorn, in der Tiefe der Calcarina-Furche, ihre Vertretung finden (*33, 34*). Solch eine frontocaudale Gliederung innerhalb der Sehrinde würde dann zur Folge haben, daß eine Verletzung nahe am Occipitalpol die zentrale Region des Sehfeldes selektiv zerstören könnte, wie man es an einem unserer eigenen Fälle (in Abb. 1, oben) gut sehen kann. Umgekehrt sollte man dann auch Verluste der Peripherie des Sehfeldes antreffen, bei denen der caudale Anteil, also die Lippen der Calcarina und damit der Foveal-Bezirk, erhalten sein könnten, wie man das tatsächlich in einem andern unserer Fälle (in Abb. 1, unten) zu sehen bekommt. Solche röhrenförmigen Gesichtsfelder auf Grund von Verletzungen unterscheiden sich vom hysterischen Tunnelfeld, indem sie sich ausweiten, wenn man den Abstand von der Fläche vergrößert, auf der das ausgesparte Sehfeld vermessen wird (*69*).

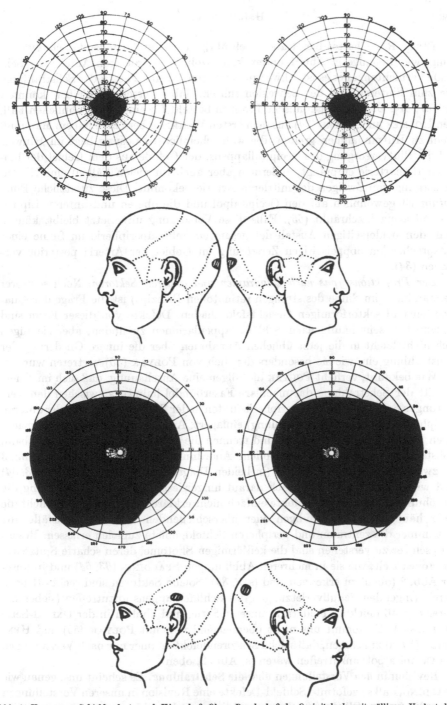

Abb. 1. *Homonyme Sehfeldverluste nach Hirnschuß. Oben: Durchschuß des Occipitalpols*, mit völligem Verlust der Zentralregion im Sehfeld (schwarz), mit Schwellenänderung im Randbezirk (um das Skotom herum, getüpfelt). Der gestrichelte Bezirk rechts über dem Skotom deutet eine Region an, in der dieser Patient Farbmarken (1°, rot, blau und grün) unterschied. In dieser Gegend hatte der Patient eine Pseudofovea gebildet. Der Patient nahm sein inselförmiges Skotom als solches nicht wahr, wußte aber, daß er Einzelheiten unterhalb seines Fixierpunktes (d. h. unterhalb der neuen Fovea) nicht erkennen konnte. Große Figuren, die dem Skotom umschrieben wurden, konnte er gut unterscheiden. — *Unten: Durchschuß parietal mit Läsion des linken parieto-temporalen und rechten parietalen Gebietes:* völliger Verlust des peripheren Feldes, und Aussparung der Zentralregion. Trotz dieser radikalen Einengung seines Gesichtsfeldes konnte dieser Patient lesen und sich räumlich gut orientieren; er betätigte sich als Sortierer im Postamt. Dunkeladaptation im Restfeld war deutlich gestört: die Adaptationskurve zeigte keine zweite Senkung (im Gegensatz zum Normalen), und blieb hinter der normalen Kurve um $4^{1}/_{2}$ logarithmische Einheiten zurück. (Für Einzelheiten über beide Fälle siehe *69*.)

17*

Etwas Rätselhaftes bleibt aber doch übrig: eine durchdringende Schußverletzung, wie diejenige in Abb. 1 unten, kann wohl die vordersten Anteile der Sehrinde vernichten, aber es ist schwer zu verstehen, wie die Fasern der Sehstrahlung,
die zum hinteren Teil der Sehregion führen, dabei verschont bleiben konnten
(12, 37, 57). Dasselbe anatomische Problem besteht für einen ganz ähnlichen Fall,
den Holmes und Lister (34) aus dem ersten Weltkrieg berichtet haben. Man muß
wohl zu Hilfsannahmen greifen: die wahrscheinlichste Lösung liegt im Hinweis
auf die Blutversorgung des Occipitallappens, der Gefäße aus dem Gebiet der hinteren Hirnarterie empfängt, außerdem aber auch (in vielen Fällen) eine Neben-
versorgung von Zweigen der mittleren Arterie bekommt. Diese zusätzliche Blut-
zufuhr ist gewöhnlich auf den Occipitalpol und die oberen und unteren Lippen
der Calcarina beschränkt (55). Falls diese Versorgung unverletzt bleibt, könnte
man den beiderseitigen Ausfall der gesamten Sehfeldperipherie im Sinne einer
entsprechenden doppelseitigen Zerstörung im Gebiet der Arteria posterior verstehen (34).

Der Projektionstypus nach Quadranten und anderen Sektoren. Noch schwerer
verständlich (im Sinne des strengen retinotopen Prinzips) ist die Frage der Quadranten und sektorförmigen Gesichtsfeldschäden. Defekte von dieser Form sind
bekanntlich sehr häufig nach Schläfenlappenläsionen zu finden, aber sie fügen
sich nicht leicht in die jetzt üblichen Annahmen über die innere Gliederung der
Sehstrahlung ein, wie sie besonders deutlich von Polyak (55) vertreten wurden.

Wie bekannt, verficht Polyak die allgemeine Anschauung, daß sich im Querschnitt der Sehstrahlung das maculäre Faserbündel halbwegs zwischen den Vertretungen der oberen Sehfeldperipherie (unten in der Sehstrahlung) und der unteren
Peripherie (oben in der Sehstrahlung) einlagert. Auf diese Weise liegen die macu-
lären Fasern dann mehr lateral, und trennen die peripheren Anteile der Sehbahn
vollständig voneinander. Diese übliche Anordnung (s. a. 51) erscheint in Abb. 3
im zweiten Diagramm von links (in beiden Diagrammreihen). Spalding (63, 64)
und wir (67, 69) haben mehrfach darauf hingewiesen, daß diese Anordnung die
gewöhnlichen Quadrantendefekte einfach nicht erklären kann, vor allem nicht die
(sehr häufigen) unvollständigen oder überschießenden Quadrantenausfälle, die
fast immer die zentralen und peripheren Sehfeldgebiete zugleich erfassen. Besonders schwer zu verstehen sind die keilförmigen Skotome, deren scharfe Spitze auf
die Fovea zielt, wie sie in mehreren Abbildungen Spaldings (63, 64) und in unserer Abb. 2 (oben) zu erkennen sind (s. a. 80). Solche Sektoren sind recht oft nach
durchdringenden Schußverletzungen des Schläfenlappens anzutreffen (siebenmal
unter den 46 defekten Feldern in unserer Serie, und ähnlich in der Oxford-Serie
Spaldings). Es kommt uns nicht überzeugend vor, mit Polyak (55) und Henschen (30) anzunehmen, daß solche Sektorendefekte immer nur nach Verletzungen
des Occipitalpols anzutreffen wären (s. Abb. 2, oben).

Revision in den Vorstellungen über die Sehstrahlung. Es scheint uns, genau wie
Spalding, daß so geformte Sehfeld-Defekte eine Revision in unseren Vorstellungen
über die innere Gliederung der menschlichen Sehstrahlung erzwingen — mindestens jedenfalls für den vorderen Verlauf der Sehstrahlung, wie dies in Abb. 3
(im dritten Diagramm von links) schematisch angedeutet ist.

Wie das Schema zeigt, nehmen wir an, daß die Vertretung der zentralsten
Teile des Sehfeldes sich im vorderen Verlauf der Sehstrahlung fächerförmig an

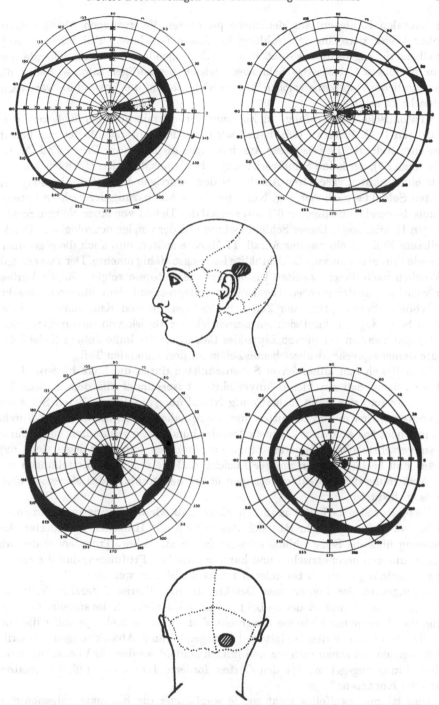

Abb. 2. *Homonyme Sehfeldverluste nach Hirnschuß. Oben:* Keilförmiges Skotom (schwarz = blind, getüpfelt = amblyopisch), nach Verletzung der Hirnsubstanz, durch Einschuß gerade oberhalb und hinter der linken Ohrmuschel. *Unten:* Unregelmäßig geformtes, parazentrales Skotom nach Schußverletzung der rechten Occipitalregion. Man beachte die Inkongruenz der beiden monocularen Felder, besonders die zipfelförmige Erstreckung am oberen Ende des Skotoms für das rechte Auge, und das Fehlen dieses Zipfels für das linke Auge. (Für weitere Einzelheiten siehe *69*.)

der lateralen Kante entlang den mehr peripheren Vertretungen überlagert. In solcher Weise wäre die Sehstrahlung in diesem (vorderen) Teil ihres Verlaufs lamellenartig angeordnet, so daß eine durchdringende Verletzung zentrale und mehr periphere Gebiete des Sehfeldes zugleich beschädigen könnte. Selbst die eigentümliche Abspitzung solcher Sektorendefekte, auf die Fovea hin, wäre dann vielleicht zu erklären.

Anatomische Nachprüfung. In Zusammenarbeit mit unserem Kollegen, dem Anatomen P. J. Harman (*26*), haben wir einen Fall untersucht, der uns beinah zum unmittelbaren Beweis dieser Anschauungen dienen kann. Dieser Fall (M. R., siehe auch *69*), der keine Schußverletzung, aber langwährenden Hochdruck hatte, erlitt einen akuten vasculären Anfall, der den sofortigen Verlust des homonymen rechten Sehfeldes nach sich zog. Nur eine kleine Aussparung der rechten unteren Macula-Gegend (von ungefähr 6°) unterschied den Defekt von einer völligen rechtsseitigen Hemianopsie. Dieser Sehfeld-Befund war der einzige neurologische Defekt in diesem Fall, bis ein zweiter Anfall, 17 Monate später, nun auch die gegenüberliegende (linke) homonyme Sehfeldhälfte leistungsunfähig machte. Der Tod erfolgte 7 Wochen nach diesem zweiten Insult, und die Autopsie zeigte völligen Verlust der Sehrinde in der rechten Hemisphäre, entsprechend dem jüngeren Infarkt, mit völliger Schrumpfung der Zellen im rechten äußeren Kniehöcker. Auf der linken Seite dagegen fand sich ein umschriebener Bezirk von unversehrter Sehrinde, und zwar an der oberen Lippe der Calcarina; der linke äußere Kniehöcker zeigte dementsprechend überlebende Zellen im dorsocaudalen Teil.

Es ließ sich nun anhand von Serienschnitten durch die linke hintere Hemisphäre zeigen, daß ein kleines unversehrtes Faserbündel aus dem Kniehöcker ausstrahlte und sich dann fächerförmig lateral über die degenerierten Sehfasern verbreiterte. Erst in den Schnitten, die der Annäherung an die Calcarina-Furche entsprachen, zog sich diese „Lamelle" wieder bündelartig zusammen, um dann in die unversehrte obere Calcarina-Lippe einzumünden (zur Histologie siehe *69*). Dieser Fall bestärkt uns in unserer Ansicht, daß die üblichen Vorstellungen von der Anordnung der Sehfeldvertretungen in der Sehstrahlung des Menschen einer Revision bedürfen.

Diese Revision bedeutet natürlich nicht, daß wir das retinotope Prinzip als solches ablehnen; vielmehr läßt sich das Prinzip mit Hilfe der veränderten Anschauung über die Sehstrahlung schärfer fassen als bisher. Trotzdem finden wir aber in unseren perimetrischen und kampimetrischen Prüfungen, daß die retinotope Anordnung in einem besonderen Punkt modifiziert werden muß.

Inkongruenz der homonymen Defekte. In der älteren Literatur (z. B. bei Henschen *30, 31*, und wiederum bei Polyak, *55*) findet sich die schroffe Behauptung, daß homonyme Skotome kongruent sind — um so mehr, je näher die entsprechende Läsion an den Occipitalpol zu liegen kommt. Abweichungen von strikter Kongruenz zwischen rechtem und linkem Sehfeld werden für Verletzungen der Sehstrahlung zugegeben; für den Cortex forderte Henschen (*30, 31*) „mathematische Kongruenz".

Dies ist nun zweifellos nicht so; je sorgfältiger die Skotome aufgenommen werden, um so deutlicher werden die kleinen, aber statistisch zuverlässigen Unterschiede zwischen den beiden Sehfeldern, wie das z. B. in Abb. 2 unten zu erkennen ist.

Solche regelmäßigen Abweichungen von strenger Kongruenz weisen darauf hin, daß die Vertretungen der monocularen Felder sich eben doch nicht so genau im Cortex zusammenordnen, wie man oft angenommen hat (69). Vielleicht enden die ipsi- und kontralateralen Fasern eben doch in verschiedenen Tiefen der Rinde, wie es (u. a.) KLEIST vorgeschlagen hat (39, s. a. 2). Auf jeden Fall können unsere Beobachtungen nicht zur Auflösung der scheinbaren Widersprüche zwischen den Ergebnissen von HUBEL (35, 36) und GRÜSSER und GRÜSSER (25) über den relativen Anteil der monocularen und binocularen Zellen in der Sehrinde beitragen;

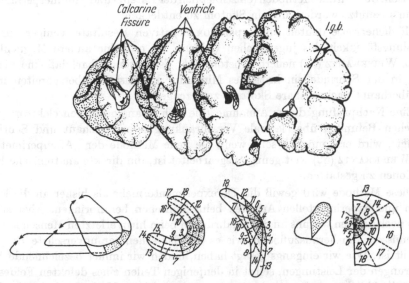

Abb. 3. *Vorschlag zur Gliederung der Sehstrahlung. Oben:* Verlauf der linken Sehstrahlung (grob schematisch), vom linken äußeren Kniehöcker (l. g. b., ganz rechts) bis zum Eintritt in die Calcarina-Furche (links). *Unten:* Diagramme zur Darstellung der Projektion der rechten Sehfeldhälfte (ganz rechts) in (von rechts nach links): Kniehöcker. vorderem Verlauf der Sehstrahlung und beginnende Einmündung in die Calcarina-Furche. Die Querschnitte durch die Sehstrahlung (in der oberen und unteren Diagramm-Serie) sollen andeuten, wie die (getüpfelte) Vertretung des zentralen Feldbezirks sich zunächst fächerförmig an der lateralen Kante der Sehstrahlung verbreitet, um sich dann erst nahe der Calcarina-Furche in ein konzentriertes Bündel zusammenzuziehen. (Für weitere Einzelheiten siehe Text, und SPALDING, 63—64, HARMAN und TEUBER, 26, 69.)

aber die von uns beobachtete Inkongruenz der homonymen Skotome zeigt doch, daß hier ein wichtiges ungelöstes Problem liegt. Das gleiche läßt sich ja über das überraschend kleine Ausmaß der binocularen Summation sagen, die man bei getrenntäugiger Reizung mit Flimmerlicht vorfindet (38, 62, 68, 77).

Ausblick: Stand der Frage nach dem retinotopen Prinzip. Zusammenfassend können wir sagen, daß die retinotopischen Grundsätze sich zweifellos auf die Form der Sehfeld-Defekte anwenden lassen: den Gewebslücken scheinen die Skotome nach Lage und Umriß gut zu entsprechen, vorausgesetzt, a) daß man die Vorstellungen über den Verlauf der Sehstrahlung abändert, wie wir es hier vorgeschlagen haben, und b) daß man sich der Inkongruenz der Sehfelder bewußt bleibt: homonyme Defekte, selbst nach Verletzungen des Occipitalpols, sind geometrisch ähnlich, wenn man die beiden monocularen Felder miteinander vergleicht, aber die Defekte sind nicht superponierbar, sie sind also nicht geometrisch identisch.

Mit diesen Einschränkungen gilt das retinotope Prinzip für unser Material genauso wie für die vielen klassischen Studien auf diesem Gebiet (32, 46, 49, 56).

Es bleibt nur offen, wie weit man von solchen Beobachtungen an jungen Erwachsenen auf die Situation bei Neugeborenen schließen kann. Doty selbst hat uns gewarnt (17), seine Resultate, die er an Carnivoren erhalten hat, unbesehen auf Primaten auszudehnen (s. aber 16, 41). Aber wir haben einen ganz eigentümlichen Fall, J. H., der als einjähriges Kind eine zufällige Schußverletzung erlitt. In diesem Fall (der Mann ist jetzt über 30 Jahre alt) ist die Kugel, die durch den rechten Parietallappen eindrang, immer noch im Röntgenbild in der rechten Calcarina-Gegend zu sehen. Trotzdem ist es uns nicht gelungen, einen Sehfelddefekt nachzuweisen, obwohl alle Methoden (einschließlich der Latenz- und Flimmerperimetrie) von uns benutzt wurden, um ein Skotom zu entdecken.

Möglicherweise deuten solche paradox negativen Resultate weniger auf die Erholungsfähigkeit des jugendlichen Gehirns, als auf eine andere Möglichkeit, die L. Weiskrantz (81) neuerlich betont hat: Es ist vorstellbar, daß eine Verletzung in der Sehrinde ein kritisches Minimum an Ausmaß überschreiten muß, um überhaupt nachweisbare Skotome zu erzeugen.

Eine Nachprüfung dieser Annahme (die sich zwanglos zu den elektrophysiologischen Befunden über laterale Verschränkungen in Netzhaut und Sehrinde einfügt), wird erst möglich sein, wenn die neue Methode der „Affenperimetrie" von Weiskrantz (82) weit genug ausgearbeitet ist, um direkte anatomische Korrelationen zu gestatten.

Diese Methode wird gewiß die Tierexperimente mehr als bisher an die klinischen und experimentellen Arbeiten beim Menschen heranbringen. Aber selbst dann noch werden wir uns an die Erfahrungen beim hirnverletzten Menschen wenden müssen, um herauszufinden, wie es um das scheinbar unversehrte Restfeld bestellt ist. Wie wir eingangs gesagt haben, finden wir immer bezeichnende Veränderungen der Leistungen, selbst in denjenigen Teilen eines defekten Feldes, in denen die üblichen perimetrischen und campimetrischen Methoden keine Ausfälle nachweisen. Zu diesen eigentümlichen Leistungsänderungen wollen wir uns nun wenden.

Wesen der Sehleistungen im Restfeld

Es ist seit langem bekannt, daß das erlebte Sehfeld für den Patienten sehr anders „aussieht" als das Gesichtsfeld, das wir mit dem Perimeter erhalten (19—21, 40, 56, 69, 73). Viele der Phänomene, die das erlebte Gesichtsfeld bestimmen, lassen sich ganz offensichtlich in keiner Weise aus dem retinotopen Prinzip ableiten.

Ergänzungserscheinungen. Poppelreuter (56) war wohl der erste, der auf diese eigentümlichen Phänomene hinwies: Gestalten, von denen ein Teil in das Gebiet eines erworbenen Skotoms hineinragt, werden vom Patienten ergänzt, d. h. die Figur wird als Ganzes gesehen (20, 23, 56, 68).

Konturergänzung. Solche „totalisierende Gestaltergänzung", wie sie Poppelreuter nannte, betrifft vor allem einfache und bilateral- oder sonst mehrfachsymmetrische Figuren (Fuchs, 20), ist aber doch anders als eine bloße Einfüllung von wirklichen Lücken aufzufassen, wie sie im gewöhnlichen Wahrnehmen der Normalen, besonders bei niedriger Beleuchtung oder kurzer Belichtung (z. B. im Tachistoskop), auftritt (7, 10).

Tatsächlich schließt sich das erlebte Sehfeld für einen Patienten wie den in Abb. 1 (oben) ohne weiteres zur Einheit: er sieht das zentrale Skotom in keiner Weise, wohl aber empfindet er eine diffuse Herabsetzung in seiner Sehschärfe. Auch alle die anderen Patienten (mit Einschluß von denen, deren Sehfelder hier abgebildet sind) sehen die Umrisse ihrer Skotome gerade so wenig, wie wir Normalsichtigen die äußere Grenze unserer Sehfelder als solche wahrzunehmen vermögen. Die Ergänzungsprozesse, die bei solchen „negativen" Skotomen am Werk sind, müssen nicht mit der bekannten Nichtwahrnehmung einer schweren Rindenblindheit (57, 58) gleichgesetzt werden: solche Verleugnung hat sich zu keiner Zeit in irgendeinem unserer 46 Fälle von Hirnschuß nachweisen lassen, obwohl sieben dieser Leute ursprünglich völlig blind waren und erst nach Minuten, Stunden und (in einem Fall) mehreren Tagen das Sehvermögen in Teilen des defekten Feldes wiedergewannen. Offenbar bedarf es vielfacher oder weitausgebreiteter Herde, bevor man das klassische Anton-Syndrom (Ableugnung der Blindheit, 1) beobachten kann.

Farbergänzung. In eigentümlicher Weise kann sich das Ergänzungsphänomen auf Farbprozesse erstrecken. So beklagt sich ein Mann mit akuter rechtsseitiger Hemianopsie, daß die Buchseite nach rechts hin weiß und leer aussähe, während die linke Hälfte mit gewöhnlichen Buchstaben bedeckt sei. Noch seltsamer (und seltener) sind Fälle von Farbkontrast in kleinen Skotomen, besonders den eigenartigen krallenförmigen Ausbuchtungen unregelmäßiger Felddefekte, die nahe an die Fovea reichen.

Solche Skotome bilden eine Ausnahme vom allgemeinen Ergänzungsprinzip, da sie sich den Sehdingen oft als schattenhafte Linien überlagern, also doch positive und nicht negative Skotome darstellen. Diese kleinen Skotome können bei Fixation auf eine helle grüne (bzw. rote) Fläche in der Kontrastfarbe (also rot bzw. grün) erscheinen. Läßt man den Patienten danach sein Nachbild beschreiben, das auf einer grauen Fläche dann eben rot (bzw. grün) erscheint, so berichtet er, daß in diesem Nachbild ein schattenhaftes Gebilde in der Gegenfarbe erscheint, also grün auf rot (bzw. umgekehrt). Diese seltsamen Phänomene, die sich natürlich ganz besonders schwer mit dem retinotopen Prinzip vereinbaren lassen, wurden unseres Wissens zuerst von BRÜCKNER im ersten Weltkrieg beobachtet (13, s. a. 69).

Ergänzung für Bewegung. Von besonderer Wichtigkeit für die Psychophysiologie des Sehens sind schließlich diejenigen Ergänzungsphänomene, die das Bewegungssehen betreffen. Wir haben uns besonders mit der sog. scheinbaren Bewegung beschäftigt, die ja das *experimentum crucis* in der frühen Gestaltpsychologie geliefert hat (42, 83). Im einfachsten Fall werden zwei Lichtpunkte abwechselnd auf einem Schirm geboten. Falls die Punkte am selben Ort erscheinen, bekommt man Flimmern, und mit steigender Frequenz Verschmelzung; falls aber ein räumlicher Abstand zwischen den beiden Lichtpunkten, A und B, eingeführt wird, bekommt man erst sukzessives Auf- und Ableuchten von zwei deutlich getrennten Lichtern, dann teilweise oder schattenhafte Bewegung von A zu B, und, mit schnellerem Alternieren, eine überzeugende Bewegungswahrnehmung, in der ein einziger Lichtpunkt hin- und herhuscht. Wird das Alternieren noch weiter beschleunigt, so zerfällt der Bewegungsprozeß wieder, um schließlich in getrenntes Flimmern der getrennt gesehenen Lichtpunkte A und B einzumünden; noch schnelleres Pulsieren führt dann zur Verschmelzung in A sowohl als B.

Diese Staffelung der Phänomene wurde von uns bei den Hirnverletzten, mit und ohne Gesichtsfelddefekten, und bei den normalen Kontrollpersonen (Peripheralnerven-Verletzten) untersucht. Der Abstand zwischen den Leuchtpunkten, ihre Lage im Sehfeld, und die Pausen zwischen den 20 mikrosekunden-langen Lichtblitzen wurden alle systematisch variiert (*69, 72, 74*). Das wesentliche Ergebnis war in defekten Feldern eine charakteristische Herabsetzung in der Variationsbreite der Pausen, die mit optimalen Bewegungseindrücken verträglich waren, so daß kleine Änderungen der Pausenlänge bei Normalen den Bewegungseindruck noch nicht zerstörten, wohl aber bei Fällen von Sehfelddefekten, obgleich die Prüfung in den scheinbar intakten Teilen des Feldes vorgenommen wurde. Außerdem aber war die nötige Geschwindigkeit des Alternierens bei den Sehfeldgestörten (aber nicht bei den anderen Hirnverletzten) erhöht, so daß optimale Bewegung erst bei schnellerem Alternieren entstand. Dies führte dann dazu, daß in manchen Teilen eines defekten Feldes keine Scheinbewegung auftrat, da die Sukzessiv-Stadien dort unmittelbar in das getrennte Flimmern (das Simultan-Stadium) übergingen. In den gleichen Feldbezirken war übrigens auch die Verschmelzungsfrequenz für Flimmerlicht bedeutend herabgesetzt (s. u., und Abb. 5), ein Zeichen für die enge physiologische Beziehung zwischen Flimmer- und Bewegungssehen.

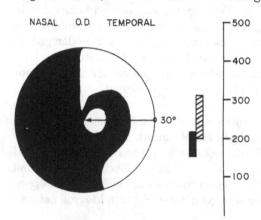

Abb. 4. *„Ergänzung" von scheinbarer Bewegung. Links:* Ausschnitt aus dem perimetrischen Sehfeld für das rechte Auge, in einem Fall von homonymer linksseitiger Hemianopsie (nach Schußverletzung der rechten Occipitalregion), mit halbringförmigem Defekt in der rechten Sehfeldhälfte. Ein Leuchtpunkt wurde im Fixierpunkt geboten (Pfeilspitze), ein zweiter Leuchtpunkt 30° rechts davon, auf dem horizontalen Meridian (Ende des Pfeils). Abwechselndes Aufleuchten der Punkte erzeugte scheinbare Bewegung über die vom Pfeil angedeutete Strecke, also quer durch das halbringförmige Skotom hindurch. Die Ordinate (rechts), in Mikrosekunden, gibt die Zeitintervalle zwischen den beiden Lichtblitzen, für die Bewegungswahrnehmungen erhalten wurden (schwarz für den Patienten, schraffiert für eine normale Kontrollperson). Man beachte die kürzeren Intervalle, und die Einengung der Schwellenwerte für den Patienten. (Für weitere Einzelheiten siehe Text.)

Am eigentümlichsten aber war die Anwendung dieser Bewegungsprüfungen auf das Studium der Ergänzungsphänomene (s. Abb. 4). Man konnte nämlich die beiden Leuchtpunkte so verteilen, daß sie zu beiden Seiten eines Skotoms fielen: in dieser Weise mußte dann die wahrgenommene Bewegung den Bezirk der erworbenen Blindheit durchqueren, was in allen Fällen ohne weiteres geschah. Wie die Abbildung (Abb. 4) zeigt, gelang dies sogar in Fällen, wo sich ein Skotom als Halbring um den Fovealbezirk herum an eine Hemianopsie anschmiegte, so daß gar keine „Öffnung" zwischen dem zentralen und peripheren Feld bestand. Auch hier vollzog sich die Bewegungswahrnehmung wie beim Normalen, nur daß der Schwellenbereich für optimale Bewegung im angedeuteten Sinn begrenzt und verschoben war (siehe die Ordinate in Abb. 4). Solche „Ergänzung" von Scheinbewegung (das gleiche gilt für wirkliche Bewegung von Sehdingen über ein Skotom hinweg) zwingt uns, über die physischen Grundlagen des Bewegungssehens anders zu denken, als es der ursprüngliche Isomorphismus (*42*) uns nahegelegt hatte.

„Auslöschung". Ergänzungsphänomene lassen das defekte Sehfeld sozusagen größer erscheinen als es „wirklich" (d. h., perimetrisch) ist. Umgekehrt aber gibt es vielerlei Erscheinungen, die das Sehfeld mehr einschränken als bloße perimetrische Vermessung von Skotomen uns erwarten läßt. Seit LOEBS Versuchen mit bilateraler Doppelreizung im Sehfeld (47), im Straßburger Laboratorium von GOLTZ, ist es bekannt, daß in gewissen Sehfeldern nach Hirnläsion ein Reiz, der allein auftritt, wohl gesehen und beschrieben wird; führt man nun aber einen zweiten Reiz anderswo ins Sehfeld ein, so behauptet der Patient, daß der Eindruck des ersten Reizes schwächer wird oder ganz erlischt (Auslöschung, "extinction", s. auch 7, 14, 52, 56). Dieses Auslöschungsphänomen spricht für eine starke Interferenz zwischen gleichzeitigen Ereignissen in weitgetrennten Bezirken des gestörten Sehsystems.

Leider bleiben hier immer noch viele unbeantwortete Fragen. Die Auslöschung ist nämlich nicht obligat; wir wissen nicht, warum dieses Phänomen bei manchen Patienten zu finden ist, aber nicht bei anderen mit ganz ähnlichen Sehfeldern, und ganz ähnlichen Verletzungen. Bedarf es eines besonderen Zustandes im verletzten Substrat, oder einer besonderen Kombination von Verletzungen? Hier vor allem wären Tierversuche nützlich, aber bisher ist es nicht gelungen, dieses so augenfällige menschliche Symptom durch gezielte Abtragung von Hirnteilen beim Tier zu erzeugen.

Andere Anzeichen der Leistungsänderung im Sehfeld. Ergänzung und Auslöschung sind positive und negative Zeichen für die beträchtliche räumliche Wechselwirkung im Sehfeld, und somit Zeichen für eine Wirkungsweise, die vom bloßen retinotopen Prinzip her nicht verständlich wäre. Ebenso kennzeichnend aber für defekte Sehfelder sind die Veränderungen im zeitlichen Ablauf der Wahrnehmung.

Adaptationsstörungen. So ist der Verlauf der Hell- und Dunkeladaptation verlangsamt, und beide sind in ihrem Ausmaß eingeengt (69, 79). Ebenso finden wir (s. o.), daß die Bewegungswahrnehmung, einschließlich der Scheinbewegung, typische Schwellenänderungen zeigt, die sich nicht nur in der Nähe von Skotomen, sondern auch in den scheinbar unversehrten Teilen eines geschädigten Sehfeldes feststellen lassen.

Flimmerverschmelzung. Besonders deutlich zeigt sich die Leistungsänderung im Restfeld mit Hilfe der Flimmerperimetrie (3, 4, 10, 69, 70—73). Wie unsere zusammenfassenden Kurven (Abb. 5) deutlich machen, findet man eine systematische Herabsetzung der Verschmelzungsfrequenz für Flimmerlicht, selbst in der scheinbar intakten Hälfte des Sehfeldes, bei unseren Hemianopikern. Die Erniedrigung der Schwellen ist zwar nicht groß, ist aber statistisch zuverlässig: Es sieht so aus, als ob die Unversehrtheit der anderen (hier beschädigten) Hemisphäre nötig wäre, um optimale zeitliche Auflösung von Reizfolgen in der scheinbar unverletzten Hemisphäre zu ermöglichen. Daß kein ganz allgemeiner Defekt vorliegt, zeigen die Stirnhirnverletzten (s. Abb. 5), bei denen keine Herabsetzung der Verschmelzungsfrequenzen zu finden war. Leider fehlen uns vorläufig noch die nötigen Messungen bei Scheitel- und Schläfenlappenverletzungen (mit unversehrten Gesichtsfeldern). Ohne diese zusätzlichen Gruppen können wir ja nicht entscheiden, ob Sehfeldverluste nicht nur hinreichend, sondern auch notwendig sind, um bleibende Schwellenänderungen hervorzubringen.

Ergänzende Beobachtungen mit Doppelreizen, die kurz nacheinander an derselben Netzhautstelle geboten werden, sind kürzlich von Battersby und Wagman mitgeteilt worden (5). In defekten Feldern fand sich, daß die Schwelle für den ersten der beiden Lichtblitze normal sein konnte, obwohl der zweite Reiz abnorm erhöht werden mußte, um vom Patienten wahrgenommen zu werden. Auch hier wäre also mit einer Störung im zeitlichen Ablauf der Empfindung zu rechnen, und zwar in Bezirken, für die perimetrische Prüfungen gar keine Schäden nachgewiesen hatten.

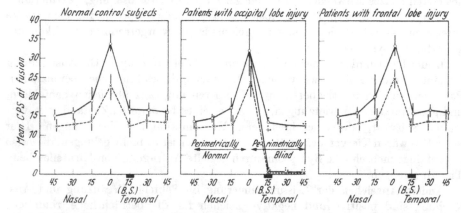

Abb. 5. *Ergebnisse der Flimmerperimetrie bei zehn normalen Kontrollpersonen* (links), *zehn Stirnhirnverletzten* (rechts) *und zehn Occipitalverletzten mit hemianopischen Felddefekten* (in der Mitte). Die Kurven verbinden Durchschnittswerte für subjektive Verschmelzung (in Lichtblitzen pro Sekunde auf der Ordinate), für ausgewählte Sehfeldstellen (Abszisse), im Zentrum (0°) und 15°, 30° und 45° rechts und links vom Fixierpunkt, auf dem horizontalen Meridian. Die vertikalen Querstriche geben die Streuung der Schwellenwerte über und unter dem Durchschnitt. Die ausgezogenen Kurven beruhen auf Versuchen mit weißen Lichtern von 2° Durchmesser, die unterbrochenen Kurven geben die Werte für solche mit 0,5° Durchmesser. Die Stirnhirnverletzten unterscheiden sich nicht von den Normalen. Die Occipitalverletzten zeigen eine kleine, aber statistisch zuverlässige Herabsetzung der Schwellenwerte im scheinbar intakten Halbfeld; auf der deutlich geschädigten Seite zeigten fünf der Fälle gar keine Reaktion auf das Flimmerlicht, während bei den anderen fünf Schwellen für das größere (2°) Licht erhalten wurden. (Für weitere Einzelheiten, auch zur Methodik, siehe Teuber und Bender, *70—73*; Battersby, *3*; Battersby et al., *4*; Teuber et al., *69*.)

Verlagerungserscheinungen. Zeitliche und räumliche Faktoren kombinieren sich in der Erzeugung von Verlagerungserscheinungen und Verzerrungen im Restfeld. Je länger die Fixation anhält, um so mehr treten diese Erscheinungen auf: gesehene Konturen verschieben sich, oft vom Fixierpunkt fort (*8, 9*), erscheinen verzerrt (*7*) oder vervielfältigt (*73*). Diese Phänomene treten häufig im akuten Zustand kurz nach einer Occipitalhirnverletzung auf, klingen dann ab, aber kehren oft nach Jahren anfallsweise wieder zurück (*69*). Diese eigenartigen Raumstörungen sind viel häufiger nach rechtshirnigen als nach linkshirnigen Verletzungen zu finden (*69*, s. a. *28, 48, 50, 54*, und besonders Hécaen und Badaraco, *29*, die ähnliche Resultate haben, ohne besonders darauf hinzuweisen).

Manche von diesen Verlagerungserscheinungen im Restfeld ähneln den sog. figuralen Nach-Effekten bei Normalen, wie das W. Köhler betont hat (*43*, in der Diskussion im Hixon Symposion, s. a. *44, 45*). Diese Phänomene deuten darauf hin, daß die räumliche Projektion im Sehsystem wohl kaum genügt, um die räumliche Ordnung der Sehdinge zu gewährleisten; andere aktive Leistungen des Substrats, die uns eben noch ganz verborgen sind, müssen hier mit im Spiele sein.

Unspezifische Veränderungen: Beeinträchtigung der optischen Analyse. Man kann das bisher Gesagte so zusammenfassen, daß wir zwei Arten von Sehfeldveränderungen gefunden haben: solche, die als umschriebene *Skotome* den *fokalen* Verletzungen im Substrat entsprechen, und solche, die *außerhalb der Skotome, und im ganzen Restfeld,* zu finden sind. Beide Arten von Sehveränderungen sind aber doch spezifisch in dem Sinne, daß sie an eine Läsion im cerebralen Sehsystem gebunden sind.

Es gibt nun aber auch Veränderungen in gewissen „höheren" Sehleistungen, die über diese spezifischen Symptome hinausgehen, da sie bei allen Untergruppen von Hirnverletzten auftreten, gleichgültig, ob Felddefekte vorhanden sind oder nicht, und ganz unabhängig von der Lage der Verletzung im Großhirn. Ein besonders überraschendes „unspezifisches" Symptom dieser Art stellte sich heraus, als wir unsere Verletzten mit „verborgenen Figuren" prüften (*76*), d. h., mit geometrischen Figuren, deren Konturen in andere, größere Gestalten so eingebettet waren, daß eine Tarnwirkung entstand (*24, 42, 60, 84*).

Die Fähigkeit, solche versteckten Liniengebilde optisch „auszuwickeln", ist beim Durchschnitt der Hinterhauptverletzten (mit Felddefekt) deutlich gegenüber den Kontrollpersonen herabgesetzt, aber dieselbe Herabsetzung fand sich bei hirnverletzten Gruppen *ohne* Sehfeldverluste (*76*). Läsionen im Stirnhirn, im Scheitel- oder Schläfenlappen, in der rechten oder linken Hemisphäre — alle waren durchschnittlich gerade so stark behindert wie die Occipitalverletzten; keine der Untergruppen bei den Hirnverletzten konnte in dieser Hinsicht von einer oder mehreren von den anderen Gruppen unterschieden werden (*67*).

Wir haben also hier *ein visuelles „Allgemeinsymptom"*, das sich, als nicht fokal, von den spezifischen Änderungen unterscheidet. Es scheint also so, wie wir andernorts gesagt haben (*67, 68, 76*), daß Verletzungen von der Art der hier beschriebenen zweierlei Symptome erzeugen, *spezifische und unspezifische,* und daß diese beiden Typen von Symptomen in notwendiger Verknüpfung nebeneinander stehen. Dies könnte entweder bedeuten, daß die Verletzungen zugleich fokal und diffus sind, oder daß die Sehleistungen selbst fokal und diffus vertreten sind. Unsere Fälle können die Frage nicht entscheiden, aber sie können diese Frage entschiedener stellen, als die widersprechenden Tierversuche dies bisher getan haben.

Wahrscheinlich ist es doch so, daß Verletzungen der Sehstrahlung und Sehrinde des Menschen zweierlei Folgen haben — solche die dem retinotopen Prinzip (mit gewissen Revisionen) entsprechen, und solche die im Gegenteil sich nur so verstehen lassen, daß wir für die höheren Sehleistungen weiterzerstreute Prozesse als physiologische Korrelate annehmen müssen, die sich über viele Teile des Sehrinde, und über die Sehrinde hinaus auf andere Hirnteile erstrecken.

Summary

This report describes alterations in the visual field of man following gunshot wounds of optic radiation and cortex. The validity of the principle of retinotopic projection was assessed in 46 cases of field defect (among 203 cases of penetrating brain injury). We found that the principle of retinotopic projection could predict the shape of areas of acquired blindness in a given visual field but not the nature of altered visual performance in the remainder of that field.

The scotomas corresponded in position and outline to the gaps in the substrate; this correspondence was in accord with currently accepted notions about the representation of different parts of the field in visual radiation and visual cortex. Our observations differed from current conceptions in only two points: 1. The accepted views regarding the course of the macular fibers within the optic radiation have to be revised. A cross-section through the anterior portion of the optic radiation discloses the macular fibers, not as a concentrated bundle, but as an extended band which overlaps the peripheral fibers laterally. 2. Homonymous scotomas in corresponding parts of monocular fields are similar but not congruent. Apparently, even at the level of the visual cortex, there is no perfect alignment of representations of the two monocular fields. The principle of retinotopic projection is valid, with these two qualifications, as far as the shape of scotomas is concerned.

By contrast, examinations of visual function in seemingly intact areas of a defective field led to results which cannot be derived from the principle of retinotopic projection. Perceived contours, colors and movements are "completed", across scotomas; the visual process creates a functioning field which extends well beyond the field determined by perimetry. Conversely, the functioning field is limited by altered adaptation, displacements of contours, and other changes which implicate those regions that appeared to be intact on perimetric testing. Thresholds for flicker fusion are reduced, even in the seemingly normal half of fields with hemianopia, suggesting that the integrity of both occipital lobes is a prerequisite for optimal stimulus utilization in either half of the visual field. An analogous result was obtained on tests of somatic sensation after injuries of parietal structures: abnormal sensory thresholds of one hand were accompanied by subtle but significant alterations in tactile discrimination in both hands (22, 61). Finally, certain higher visual achievements (such as the detection of "hidden figures") were found to be impaired in all of our groups with brain injury, regardless of presence or absence of otherwise demonstrable field defects.

Alterations in perception thus ranged from circumscribed gaps (in perimetrically determined fields) to subtle but systematic threshold changes and other abnormalities in the remaining parts of the field, and thence to nonspecific alterations in performance which appeared, irrespective of the state of the visual field, and with lesions in any cerebral lobe.

These results could mean that the lesions are both focal and diffuse, or that the functions have specific as well as general representation. Our observations cannot decide between these two alternatives, but we believe that the second of the two may eventually turn out to be correct. Accordingly, normal visual performance may depend in some respects on the integrity of narrowly circumscribed structures which conform to the retinotopic principle in lateral geniculate, optic radiation and cortex. At the same time, however, there is evidence that normal performance requires complex lateral interaction within the optic structures, at all levels of the visual pathways. Beyond this, normal performance appears to involve additional regions of the CNS which lie outside the classical retino-geniculo-calcarine structures.

Literatur

1. Anton, G.: Über Herderkrankungen des Gehirns, welche vom Patienten selbst nicht wahrgenommen werden. Wien. klin. Wschr. 11, 227—229 (1898).
2. Bárány, R.: La bipartition de la couche interne des grains, est-elle l'expression anatomique de la réprésentation isolée des champs visuels monoculaires dans l'écorce cérébrale? Trab. Lab. Invest. biol. Univ. Madr. 22, 359—368 (1924).
3. Battersby, W. S.: The regional gradient of critical flicker frequency after frontal or occipital injury. J. exp. Psychol. 42, 59—68 (1951).
4. — M. B. Bender and H.-L. Teuber: Effects of total light flux on critical flicker frequency after frontal lobe lesion. J. exp. Psychol. 42, 135—142 (1951).
5. — and I. H. Wagman: Alterations of visual excitability in patients with lesions of the central optic pathways. Trans. Amer. neurol. Ass. 84, 156—159 (1959).
6. Bay, E.: Agnosie und Funktionswandel; eine hirnpathologische Studie. Berlin: Springer 1950.
7. Bender, M. B., and H.-L. Teuber: Phenomena of fluctuation, extinction, and completion in visual perception. Arch. Neurol. Psychiat. (Chicago) 55, 627—658 (1946).
8. — — Spatial organization of visual perception following injury to the brain. Arch. Neurol. Psychiat. (Chicago) 58, 721—739 (1947).
9. — — Spatial organization of visual perception following injury to the brain. Arch. Neurol. Psychiat. (Chicago) 59, 39—62 (1948).
10. — — Psychopathology of vision. Chap. 8, pp. 163—192, in: Progress in Neurology and Psychiatry, vol. IV (ed. E. A. Spiegel). New York: Grune & Stratton 1949.
11. Best, F.: Ergebnisse der Kriegsjahre für die Kenntnis der Sehbahnen und Sehzentren. Zbl. ges. Ophthal. 3, 193—207, 241—254 (1920).
12. Brouwer, B.: Über die Projektion der Macula auf die Area striata des Menschen. J. Psychol. Neurol. (Lpz.) 40, 147—159 (1930).
13. Brückner, A.: Zur Frage der Lokalisation des Kontrastes und verwandter Erscheinungen in der Sehsinnsubstanz. Z. Augenheilk. 38, 1—14 (1917).
14. Bruns, L.: Ein Beitrag zur einseitigen Wahrnehmung doppelseitiger Reize bei Herden einer Großhirnhemisphäre. Neurol. Cbl. (Lpz.) 5, 198—199 (1886).
15. Cibis, P., u. H. Müller: Lokaladaptometrische Untersuchungen am Projektionsperimeter nach Maggiore. Albrecht v. Graefes Arch. Ophthal. 148, 468—489 (1948).
16. Denny-Brown, D., and R. W. Chambers: Visuo-motor function in the cerebral cortex. J. nerv. ment. Dis. 121, 288—289 (1955).
17. Doty, R. W.: Functional significance of the topographical aspects of the retino-cortical projection. Dieses Symposion, pp. 228—245, 1961.
18. Faust, C.: Die cerebralen Herdstörungen bei Interhauptsverletzungen und ihre Beurteilung (Arbeit und Gesundheit, n. S., no. 57). Stuttgart: Thieme 1955.
19. Fuchs, W.: Untersuchungen über das Sehen der Hemianopiker und Hemiamblyopiker: I. Verlagerungserscheinungen. Z. Psychol. 84, 67—169 (1920).
20. — Untersuchungen über das Sehen der Hemianopiker und Hemiamblyopiker: II. Die totalisierende Gestaltauffassung. Z. Psychol. 86, 1—143 (1921).
21. Gelb, A., u. K. Goldstein: Psychologische Analysen hirnpathologischer Fälle. Leipzig: Barth 1920.
22. Ghent, L., J. Semmes, S. Weinstein and H.-L. Teuber: Tactile discrimination after unilateral brain injury in man. Amer. Psychologist 10, 408 (1955).
23. Goldstein, K.: Die Lokalisation in der Großhirnrinde. In: Handb. norm. pathol. Physiol. (ed. A. Bethe et al.) 10, 600—842. Berlin: Springer 1927.
24. Gottschaldt, K.: Über den Einfluß der Erfahrung auf die Wahrnehmung von Figuren. Psychol. Forsch. 8, 261—317 (1926).
25. Grüsser-Cornehls, U., u. O. J. Grüsser: Reaktionsmuster der Neurone im zentralen visuellen System von Fischen, Kaninchen und Katzen auf monoculare und binoculare Lichtreize. Dieses Symposion, pp. 275—287, 1961.
26. Harman, P. J., and H.-L. Teuber: The geniculo-calcarine system of M. R.; a case of cortical blindness. Paper read at Spring mtg. of Amer. Anatomists, Seattle, Wash. 1959.
27. Harms, H.: Persönliche Mitteilung (1958).

28. Hebb, D. O.: Intelligence in man after large removals of cerebral tissue: defects following right temporal lobectomy. J. gen. Psychol. 21, 437—446 (1939).
29. Hécaen, H., et J. G. Badaraco: Séméiologie des hallucinations visuelles en clinique neurologique. Acta neurol. lat.-amer. 2, 23—57 (1956).
30. Henschen, S. E.: Die zentralen Sehstörungen. In: Handbuch der Neurologie (ed. M. Lewandowsky) 1, 891—918. Berlin: Springer 1910.
31. — Die Vertretung der beiden Augen in der Sehbahn und in der Sehrinde. Albrecht v. Graefes Arch. Ophthal. 117, 419—459 (1926).
32. Holmes, G.: Disturbances of vision by cerebral lesions. Brit. J. Ophthal. 2, 353—384 (1918).
33. — The organization of the visual cortex in man (Ferrier Lecture, delivered May 18, 1944). Proc. roy. Soc. B 132, 348—361 (1945).
34. — and W. T. Lister: Disturbances of vision from cerebral lesions, with special reference to the cortical representation of the macula. Brain 39, 34—73 (1916).
35. Hubel, D. H.: Cortical unit responses to visual stimuli in unanesthetized cats. Amer. J. Ophthal. 46, 110—112 (1959).
36. — and T. H. Wiesel: Receptive fields of single neurones in the cat's striate cortex. J. Physiol. (Lond.) 148, 574—591 (1959).
37. Inouye, T.: Die Sehstörungen nach Schußverletzungen der corticalen Sehsphäre, nach Beobachtungen an Verwundeten der letzten japanischen Kriege. Leipzig: Engelmann 1909.
38. Ireland, F. H.: A comparison of critical flicker frequencies under conditions of monocular and binocular stimulation. J. exp. Psychol. 40, 282—286 (1950).
39. Kleist, K.: Die einzeläugigen Gesichtsfelder und ihre Vertretung in den beiden Lagern der verdoppelten inneren Körnerschicht der Sehrinde. Klin. Wschr. 5, 3—10 (1926).
40. Klüver, H.: Visual disturbances after cerebral lesions. Psychol. Bull. 24, 316—358 (1927).
41. — Certain effects of lesions of the occipital lobes in macaques. J. Psychol. (Provincetown) 4, 383—401 (1937).
42. Köhler, W.: Gestalt Psychology. New York: Liveright 1947.
43. — Diskussion, p. 200 in: Cerebral Mechanisms in Behavior (ed. L. A. Jeffress). New York: Wiley 1951.
44. — and J. Fishback: The destruction of the Müller-Lyer illusion in repeated trials. 1, 2. J. exp. Psychol. 40, 267—281, 398—410 (1950).
45. — and H. Wallach: Figural after-effects; an investigation of visual processes. Proc. Amer. phil. Soc. 88, 269—357 (1944).
46. Lenz, G.: Die Kriegsverletzungen der cerebralen Sehbahn. In: Handbuch der Neurologie (ed. O. Bumke und O. Foerster). Erg.bd. 1, 668—729. Berlin: Springer 1924.
47. Loeb, J.: Die Sehstörungen nach Verletzung der Großhirnrinde. Pflügers Arch. ges. Physiol. 34, 67—172 (1884).
48. Luria, A. R.: Disorders of "simultaneous perception" in a case of bilateral occipito-parietal brain-injury. Brain 82, 437—449 (1959).
49. Marie, P., et C. Chatelin: Les troubles visuels dûs aux lésions des voies optiques intra-cérébrales et de la sphère visuelle corticale dans les blessures du crâne par coup de feu. Rev. neurol. 28, 882—925 (1915).
50. Milner, B.: Psychological defects produced by temporal lobe excision. Res. Publ. Ass. nerv. ment. Dis. 36, 244—257 (1958).
51. Monbrun, A.: Les hémianopsies en quadrant et le centre cortical de la vision. Presse méd. 25, 607—609 (1917).
52. Oppenheim, H.: Über eine durch eine klinisch bisher nicht verwerthete Untersuchungs-methode ermittelte Form der Sensibilitätsstörung bei einseitigen Erkrankungen des Groß-hirns. Neurol. Cbl. (Lpz.) 4, 529—533 (1885).
53. Panizza, B.: Osservazioni sul nervo ottico. G. I. R. Ist. Lombardo 7, 237—252 (1855).
54. Paterson, A., and O. L. Zangwill: Disorders of visual space perception associated with lesions of the right cerebral hemisphere. Brain 67, 331—358 (1944).
55. Polyak, S.: The vertebrate visual system (ed. H. Klüver). Chicago: Univ. Chicago Press 1957.
56. Poppelreuter, W.: Die psychischen Schädigungen durch Kopfschuß im Kriege 1914—16; die Störungen der niederen und höheren Sehleistungen durch Verletzung des Occipitalhirns, vol. I. Leipzig: Voss 1917.

57. REDLICH, E., u. G. BONVICINI: Über das Fehlen der Wahrnehmung der eigenen Blindheit bei Hirnkrankheiten. Jb. Psychiat. Neurol. **29**, 1—133 (1908).

58. REDLICH, R. C., and J. F. DORSEY: Denial of blindness by patients with cerebral disease. Arch. Neurol. Psychiat. (Chicago) *53*, 407—417 (1945).

59. RØNNE, H.: Über doppelseitige Hemianopsie mit erhaltener Macula. Klin. Mbl. Augenheilk. **53**, 470—487 (1914).

60. RUPP, H.: Über optische Analyse. Psychol. Forsch. **4**, 262—300 (1923).

61. SEMMES, J., S. WEINSTEIN, L. GHENT and H.-L. TEUBER: Somatosensory changes after penetrating brain wounds in man. Cambridge, Mass. (USA): Harvard Univ. Press 1960.

62. SHERRINGTON, C. S.: The integrative action of the nervous system. New Haven: Yale Univ. Press 1906 (Neugedruckt: London: Cambridge Univ. Press 1947).

63. SPALDING, J. M. K.: Wounds of the visual pathway: I. The visual radiation. J. Neurol. Neurosurg. Psychiat. **15**, 99—109 (1952).

64. — Wounds of the visual pathway: II. The striate cortex. J. Neurol. Neurosurg. Psychiat. **15**, 169—183 (1952).

65. SZILY, A. VON: Atlas der Kriegsaugenheilkunde, samt begleitendem Text (Sammlung der kriegsophthalmologischen Beobachtungen und Erfahrungen aus der Universitäts-Augenklinik in Freiburg i. Br.), vol. I. Siehe Kap. III: Kriegshemianopsien, pp. 78—132. Stuttgart: Enke 1918.

66. TEUBER, H.-L.: Neuropsychology. Amer. Lecture Series (no. 81, 30—52). Springfield, Ill.: Thomas 1950.

67. — Some alterations in behavior after cerebral lesions in man. Pp. 157—194 in: Evolution of Nervous Control. Washington, D. C.: Amer. Assoc. Adv. Sci. 1959.

68. — Perception. Chap. LXV, pp. 1595—1668 in: Handbook of Physiology-Neurophysiology III. Washington, D. C.: Amer. Physiol. Soc. 1960.

69. — W. S. BATTERSBY and M. B. BENDER: Visual field defects after penetrating missile wounds of the brain. Cambridge, Mass. (USA): Harvard Univ. Press 1960.

70. — and M. B. BENDER: Flicker-perimeter (demonstration). Trans. Amer. neurol. Ass. **73**, 174—175 (1948).

71. — — Critical flicker frequency in defective fields of vision. Fed. Proc. **7**, 123—124 (1948).

72. — — Changes in visual perception of flicker, apparent motion, and real motion after cerebral lesions. Amer. Psychologist **3**, 246—247 (1948).

73. — — Alterations in pattern vision following trauma of occipital lobes in man. J. gen. Psychol. **40**, 37—57 (1949).

74. — — Perception of apparent movement across acquired scotomata in the visual field. Amer. Psychologist **5**, 271 (1950).

75. — — Neuro-ophthalmology; the oculomotor system. Chap. 8, pp. 148—178 in: Progress in Neurology and Psychiatry, vol. VI (ed. E. A. SPIEGEL). New York: Grune & Stratton 1951.

76. — and S. WEINSTEIN: Ability to discover hidden figures after cerebral lesions. Arch. Neurol. Psychiat. (Chicago) **76**, 369—379 (1956).

77. THOMAS, G. J.: A comparison of uniocular and binocular critical flicker frequencies: Simultaneous and alternate flashes. Amer. J. Psychol. **68**, 37—53 (1955).

78. UHTHOFF, W.: Die Verletzungen der zentralen Bahnen und des Sehzentrums bei Schädelschüssen, speziell Hinterhauptschüssen. Pp. 303—320 in: Handb. d. ärztl. Erfahrungen im Weltkriege 1914—18 (ed. O. v. SCHJERNING), vol. V: Augenheilkunde (ed. T. AXENFELD). Leipzig: Barth 1922.

79. ULLRICH, N.: Adaptationsstörungen bei Sehhirnverletzten. Dtsch. Z. Nervenheilk. **155**, 1—31 (1943).

80. VAN BUREN, J. M., and M. BALDWIN: The architecture of the optic radiation in the temporal lobe of man. Brain **81**, 15—40 (1958).

81. WEISKRANTZ, L.: Encephalization and the scotoma. Unpublished manuscript, Psychol. Laboratory, Cambridge Univ. (1958).

82. — Persönliche Mitteilung (1960).

83. Wertheimer, M.: Experimentelle Studien über das Sehen von Bewegung. Z. Psychol. 61, 161—265 (1912).
84. — Untersuchungen zur Lehre von der Gestalt. Psychol. Forsch. 4, 301—350 (1923).
85. Whitteridge, D., and P. M. Daniel: The representation of the visual field on the calcarine cortex. (Dieses Symposion, pp. 222—228, 1961.)
86. Wilbrand, H., u. A. Saenger: Die Verletzungen der Sehbahnen des Gehirns mit besonderer Berücksichtigung der Kriegsverletzungen. Wiesbaden: Bergmann 1918.

Diskussion

M. Monjé: Ich möchte auf die perimetrischen Methoden hinweisen, an besonders interessierenden Stellen der Netzhaut die Empfindlichkeit zu messen. Die Methoden wurden zunächst in Amerika von Sloan, dann in Deutschland von Harms und Monjé eingeführt. Harms spricht von quantitativer Perimetrie, Monjé von Lichtsinnperimetrie. Der einfachste Weg, die Empfindlichkeit zu messen, ist der, daß man mit einem kleinen Projektor, z. B. einem Kampimeter, auf eine große, als Adaptationsfläche dienende Wand Marken projiziert. Mit Hilfe von Graufiltern und einer Irisblende kann man die Intensität des Prüfreizes solange verändern, bis der Untersuchte den Prüfreiz gerade bemerkt. Der Prüfreiz wird stets an dieselbe Stelle der Wand projiziert, verändert wird die Stelle, an der die Versuchsperson zu fixieren hat. Es handelt sich also um eine echte Perimetrie, nicht um eine Kampimetrie. Mit Hilfe dieser Methode konnten wir z. B. bei einem Patienten mit einer Schußverletzung am Hinterkopf feststellen, daß die Empfindlichkeit im rechten oberen Quadranten des Restgesichtsfeldes wesentlich herabgemindert war. Frühere Beobachter hatten diese Tatsache übersehen. Die angeführte Methode hat eine Reihe von großen Vorteilen; z. B. lassen sich Refraktionsanomalien ausgleichen, ohne daß das Gesichtsfeld durch das Brillengestell eingeengt wird oder der Astigmatismus schräg einfallende Strahlen stört.

H. Kornhuber: Der Befund von Prof. Teuber, daß homonyme *Quadrantenanopsien* durch Läsionen im *vordersten* Teil der Sehstrahlung entstehen können, wird durch unsere Erfahrungen bestätigt. Bei cerebralen Gefäßinsulten, die Quadrantenanopsien machen, entstehen oft zugleich *Thalamussyndrome*. Und im Gegensatz zu Läsionen in den mittleren und hinteren Abschnitten der Sehstrahlung mit ziemlich vollständiger Hemianopsie finden sich bei Insulten mit Quadrantenanopsien seltener *Störungen des optokinetischen Nystagmus*, offenbar weil im vordersten Abschnitt der Sehstrahlung die cortico-fugalen optisch-motorischen Fasern schon von der sensorischen Sehstrahlung getrennt sind.

H.-L. Teuber (zu Monjé): Es ist zweifellos besser, bei der Perimetrie Prüfmarken zu verwenden, deren Helligkeit sich stetig verändern läßt. Die Methoden von Harms und Monjé sind besonders günstig, weil sie sich mit kleinen Zusätzen mit der Flimmerperimetrie verbinden lassen. Außerdem kann man leicht den Kunstgriff zur Fixationskontrolle hinzufügen, den ich oben beschrieben habe, und zwar Lichtpunkte in der Gegend der blinden Flecks, die die Versuchsperson nicht sieht, solange sie richtig fixiert.

Zu Kornhuber: Die wichtige Frage nach dem Stand der okulomotorischen Leistungen haben wir hier nicht behandeln können. Die Symptomverbindungen, die Herr Dr. Kornhuber beschreibt, sind bei Gefäßinsulten sicher sehr häufig anzutreffen, obwohl sie bei durchdringenden Hirnverletzungen, wie den von uns beschriebenen, doch wohl nicht obligat sind. Ich möchte übrigens auch darauf hinweisen, daß willkürliche Spähbewegungen der Augen („optisches Suchen") von frontalen und parieto-occipitalen Stellen aus gestört werden können. An unseren Fällen kann man das mit einer Variation der Poppelreuterschen Suchfeldmethode (56) deutlich zeigen (10, 66), und zwar noch viele Jahre nach der Verletzung.

Reaktionsmuster der Neurone im zentralen visuellen System von Fischen, Kaninchen und Katzen auf monoculare und binoculare Lichtreize*

Von

URSULA GRÜSSER-CORNEHLS** und O.-J. GRÜSSER**

Mit 5 Abbildungen

In den meisten früheren Untersuchungen (*2, 3, 12, 13, 15, 21*) über die Lichtreaktionen corticaler Neurone wurden monoculare und binoculare Lichtreize nicht unterschieden oder monoculare Lichtreize angewandt. Einen ersten Anhalt für das Zusammenwirken der Afferenzen aus beiden Augen ergaben Untersuchungen, bei denen der Nervus opticus des einen Auges elektrisch gereizt wurde, während das andere Auge physiologisch erregt wurde (*16, 17a*). Für die Katze wurden inzwischen auch die ersten Ergebnisse bei binocularer Lichtreizung im Geniculatum [COHN (*8*), ERULKAR u. FILLENZ (*10*), GRÜSSER u. SAUR (*16a*)] und im visuellen Cortex [HUBEL u. WIESEL (*18*), CORNEHLS u. GRÜSSER (*9, 14*) und BURNS, HERON u. GRAFSTEIN (*7*)] mitgeteilt.

Die folgende Mitteilung ist ein Zwischenbericht über die Resultate mit binocularen Lichtreizen von 87 Neuronen im Geniculatum laterale und 185 Neuronen im visuellen Cortex, die bis jetzt von über 400 registrierten Neuronen aus dem zentralen Sehsystem der Katze quantitativ ausgewertet wurden. Da zu erwarten war, daß mit der phylogenetischen Entwicklung des Binocularsehens in der Wirbeltierreihe andersartige Verschaltungen im zentralen visuellen System auftreten, haben wir vergleichend zur Katze noch Tiere untersucht, deren Augen zur Seite schauen, und die keinen bzw. nur einen spärlichen binocularen Sehraum haben. 35 Neurone wurden aus dem Tectum opticum von Fischen [Hechte *(Esox lucius)* und Schleien *(Tinca vulgaris)*], 45 visuelle Neurone aus der Sehrinde des Kaninchens registriert.

Methodik

45 Katzen in encephale isolé-Präparation nach BREMER, zusätzlich Curarin, künstliche Beatmung, Rotlichtbestrahlung, Blutdruckregulation mit Effortil. 10 Kaninchen curarisiert und künstlich beatmet. 18 Fische curarisiert, in einem speziellen Halter fixiert und mit kontinuierlichem Frischwasserstrom „beatmet". Alle Tiere waren helladaptiert.

Elektroden: Mikropipetten, unter 1 μ Spitzendurchmesser, 3 n-KCl- oder 4 n-NaCl-Füllung. Registrierung über imperative Eingangsstufe mit Kathodenfolgeschaltung nach TÖNNIES, übliche CW-Verstärkung, Mehrfachoszillograph, Recordine-Kamera von Dr. J. F. TÖNNIES.

Lichtreizung mit einem elektrisch gesteuerten binocularen Lichtreizgerät (*9*), das eine strenge Trennung der Strahlengänge für beide Augen hatte. Die beiden Augen wurden durch Spiegel und ein optisches System von der gleichen Wolframbandlampe getrennt belichtet. Die Beleuchtungsstärke der Mattscheibe vor jedem Auge konnte durch Filter und Graukeile reduziert werden (0,01—650 Lux). Der Lichtreiz wurde durch je einen elektronisch gesteuerten, elektromagnetischen Verschluß im Brennpunkt der beiden Strahlengänge ein- und ausgeschaltet. Die Frequenz der weißen Lichtreize war bis zu 70 pro sec beliebig regelbar (Hell-Dunkel-Verhältnis 1:1). Die Belichtung des rechten und linken Auges war mit gleicher oder verschiedener Frequenz und in jeder beliebigen Phasenverschiebung möglich.

* Aus der Abteilung für klinische Neurophysiologie der Universität Freiburg i. Br.
** Nervenklinik der Universität Göttingen. Mit Unterstützung der Deutschen Forschungsgemeinschaft.

Ergebnisse

1. Tectum opticum (Fisch). Sämtliche registrierten Neurone reagierten nur auf Belichtung des *contralateralen* Auges. Die Reaktionsmuster (on-, off-, on-off-Neurone) wurden durch gleichzeitige synchrone oder phasenverschobene Belichtung des ipsilateralen Auges nicht beeinflußt (Abb. 1). Die kritische Flimmerfusionsfrequenz (CFF) war ebenfalls durch das contralaterale Auge bestimmt und wurde

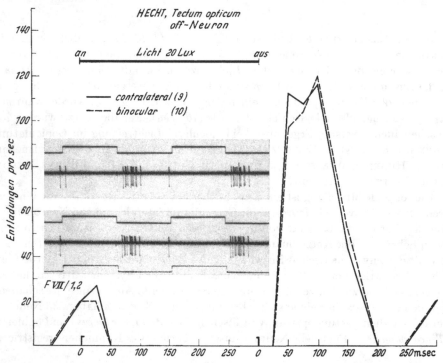

Abb. 1. *Off-Neuron* im Tectum opticum vom Hecht *(Esox lucius)*. Reaktion auf contralaterale und synchrone binoculare Lichtreize (jeweils 20 Lux, weißes Licht) ergibt keine Differenz. Auf den ipsilateralen Lichtreiz erfolgte keine Reaktion

binocular nicht modifiziert. Auch die Reaktion des von der Tectum-Oberfläche abgeleiteten *Elektrocorticogramms* (ECG) auf Belichtung des contralateralen Auges wurde ebenfalls durch Belichtung des ipsilateralen Auges nicht modifiziert. Wie bei den einzelnen Neuronen ergab im ECG die Belichtung des ipsilateralen Auges auch bei hohen Beleuchtungsstärken keine ECG-Reaktion.

Auffallend war an den Neuronen im Tectum die sehr niedrige spontane Entladungsfrequenz (um 1—2/sec). Die Reaktionstypen waren denen im visuellen Cortex der Katze bei monocularer Belichtung ähnlich. Ein registriertes on-off-Neuron hatte vor der on- und der off-Aktivierung jeweils eine kurze Hemmphase.

2. Visueller Cortex des Kaninchens. Registriert wurde aus dem von Korn-müller *(23)* mit Hilfe von Oberflächenableitungen abgegrenzten Hirnrindenfeld (visuelle Area I). Nur etwa ein Drittel der Neurone ließ sich durch Licht- oder Dunkelreize aktivieren. Jeweils etwa die Hälfte gehörten dem on- oder dem off-System (off-Neurone und on-off-Neurone) an. *Sämtliche Neurone reagierten nur* auf Belichtung des *contralateralen* Auges. Ihre Reaktionsmuster wurden nicht durch gleichzeitige Belichtung des ipsilateralen Auges modifiziert. Das Fehlen von ipsilateral aktivierten Neuronen ist wahrscheinlich durch die geringe Anzahl der registrierten licht- oder dunkelaktivierten Neurone (45) zu erklären.

3. Geniculatum laterale der Katze. Zusammen mit SAUR wurden 87 Neurone im Geniculatum laterale registriert. Die Ergebnisse wurden ausführlich an anderer Stelle dargestellt (*16a*). 31 Neurone (19 on-, 12 off-) reagierten auf Belichtung des ipsilateralen Auges, 53 Neurone (29 on-, 22 off-, 2 Z-) auf Belichtung des contralateralen Auges. 3 Neurone reagierten weder auf das ipsi- noch auf das contralaterale Auge. 8 Neurone hatten eine statistisch signifikante Verminderung der Entladungsfrequenz in den Aktivierungsphasen bei synchroner binocularer Belichtung im Vergleich zur monocularen Belichtung des dominanten Auges. Diese binoculare Verminderung weist darauf hin, daß gewisse binoculare Koordinationsvorgänge schon auf der Ebene des Geniculatum laterale der Katze eintreten.

Die *CFF war rein monocular determiniert*; binoculare Flimmerbelichtung, synchron oder in Phasenverschiebung, ergab bei gleichen Beleuchtungsstärken keine signifikante Differenz im Vergleich zur Flimmerbelichtung des dominanten Auges.

2 Neurone wurden sowohl bei Belichtung als auch bei Verdunklung gehemmt (Z-Neurone).

Die Neuronentladungen wurden als postsynaptische Nervenzellentladungen durch 2 Komponenten des extracellulär positiven spike ($\alpha\beta$-spike) identifiziert. Diese Selektion erfaßte, wie in einer anderen Arbeit (*17*) gezeigt wurde, Nervenzellen, die von rasch leitenden und solche, die von langsamer leitenden Opticusfasern aktiviert wurden.

4. Primärer visueller Cortex der Katze. Über 300 Neurone wurden über längere Zeit photographisch registriert, 185 davon bis jetzt quantitativ ausgewertet.

a) Als „*monocular dominant*" werden die Neurone bezeichnet, deren Entladungsmuster bei binocularer synchroner und gleich heller Belichtung von *einem* Auge bestimmt werden, d. h. ihr binoculares Entladungsmuster unterscheidet sich nicht oder nur quantitativ von dem monocularen Entladungsmuster bei Belichtung des „dominanten Auges".

80% der 185 Neurone waren monocular dominant. Für etwa 40% dieser Neurone war das ipsilaterale Auge, für etwa 60% das contralaterale Auge dominant.

Unter diesen Neuronen mit monocularer Dominanz waren zwei Gruppen zu unterscheiden. Etwa die Hälfte (etwa 40% der 185 ausgewerteten Neurone) reagierte nur bei Belichtung des dominanten Auges, während die *Belichtung des nicht dominanten Auges keine Änderung* der spontanen Entladungsfrequenz auslöste. Binoculare Belichtung (synchron oder phasenverschoben) ergab das gleiche Reaktionsmuster wie die Belichtung des dominanten Auges. Auch verschiedene Beleuchtungsstärken der Mattscheiben vor beiden Augen änderten an dieser rein monocularen Bestimmtheit nichts.

Für die andere Hälfte der monocular dominanten Neurone war *die Entladungsfrequenz* in den on- oder off-Aktivierungsphasen *bei binocularer Belichtung* im Vergleich zur Belichtung des dominanten Auges *signifikant vermindert*. Diese binoculare Verminderung lag zwischen 10 und 30%. Ein großer Teil dieser binocular beeinflußten Neurone reagierte auf Belichtung des nicht dominanten Auges nach dem C-Typ (*12, 22*) mit einer variablen Hemmung bei „Licht an" und „Licht aus".

Die monocular dominanten Neurone umfassen die seither beschriebenen corticalen Reaktionstypen: Die Neurone des on-Systems (B-Neurone) verhalten sich zu den Neuronen des off-Systems (D- und E-Neurone) im ausgewerteten Neuronenkollektiv zahlenmäßig etwa wie 4 zu 3.

Die Untersuchungen haben ergeben, daß Entladungsmuster nach dem C-Typ zum großen Teil durch Belichtung des *nicht dominanten* Auges zustande kommen.

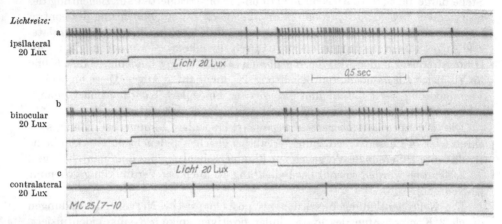

Abb. 2 a—c. *Off-Neuron* (D-Typ) im primären visuellen Cortex der Katze. a Reaktion auf ipsilateralen Lichtreiz (20 Lux, diffuses weißes Licht); b Reaktion auf synchrone binoculare Lichtreize jeweils 20 Lux ergibt eine deutliche Verminderung der off-Aktivierung im Vergleich zur Belichtung des dominanten ipsilateralen Auges. c Reaktion auf den contralateralen Lichtreiz nach Typ C mit schwacher Spätaktivierung nach „Licht an" und „Licht aus", jeweils nach vorausgehender Hemmung. Empfindlichkeit der Verstärkung im Vergleich zu a und b reduziert

b) 18 Neurone (etwa 10%) reagierten sowohl auf monoculare Belichtung des ipsilateralen als auch auf Belichtung des contralateralen Auges. Die Entladungsmuster waren im Vergleich zu den Neuronen mit monocularer Dominanz meist weniger frequent und für das linke und rechte Auge verschieden.

Die statistische Auswertung eines solchen Neurons ist in Abb. 3 dargestellt. Es reagierte auf das contralaterale Auge mit einer gruppierten on-Reaktion, auf das ipsilaterale mit einer on-off-Reaktion. Wurden beide Augen synchron belichtet, so war das Neuron fast vollständig gehemmt, wurden beide Augen alternierend belichtet, so ergab sich wiederum eine verstärkte on-off-Aktivierung. Die binocularen Entladungsmuster lassen sich aus den monocularen Reaktionen ableiten, wenn man annimmt, daß die Hemmungsvorgänge sich durchsetzen. Wurde das linke und das rechte Auge synchron, aber mit verschieden hellen Lichtreizen beleuchtet, so änderten sich mit den monocularen Erregungs- und Hemmungsvorgängen die binocularen Entladungsmuster.

c) Etwa 5% der ausgewerteten Neurone reagierten wie das in Abb. 4 gezeigte. Belichtung des ipsi- oder contralateralen Auges ergab bei diesen Neuronen keine oder nur eine außerordentlich geringfügige Reaktion. Auffallend war bei diesen Neuronen die niedrige spontane Entladungsfrequenz. Wurden beide Augen synchron belichtet, so trat eine regelmäßige, jedoch immer kurze und relativ frequente on- und off-Reaktion auf. Der Grad dieser binocularen Bahnung war von der Phasenlage der ipsi- und contralateralen Lichtreize abhängig. Bei synchroner Belichtung war die binoculare Summation am stärksten und bei binocularer Belichtung in Gegentaktfolge am schwächsten (Abb. 4e). Diese Neurone vermitteln in ihrem Informationsgehalt ebenfalls echte binoculare Effekte. Da ihre Entladungsfrequenz von der zeitlichen Verschiebung der afferenten Impulse aus beiden Augen abhängt, könnte man sich vorstellen, daß sie binoculare Latenzzeitdifferenzen messen.

d) Nur etwa 5% der registrierten Neurone reagierten weder auf monoculare Belichtung jedes Auges noch auf binoculare Belichtung. Diese Neurone waren also echte A-Neurone im Sinne der ersten Nomenklatur von JUNG, VON BAUMGARTEN und BAUMGARTNER (19, 21, 22).

Die überwiegende Mehrheit der registrierten Neurone (etwa 80%) konnte in ihrer Entladungsform als $\alpha\beta$-spike und damit als postsynaptisch in der Hirnrinde identifiziert werden. In seltenen Fällen waren intracelluläre Ableitungen möglich (Potentialhöhe bis — 50 mV). Die Neurone, die extracellulär einen $\alpha\beta$-spike hatten, zeigten dann einen typischen IS-SD-spike nach ECCLES u. Mitarb.

e) *Flimmerbelichtung.* Die kritische Flimmerfusionsfrequenz (CFF) der echten binocularen Neurone (Gruppe b und c) war unter gleichen Reizbedingungen weit niedriger als die CFF der Neurone mit monocularer Dominanz. Es kann noch nicht gesagt werden, ob die CFF der binocularen Neurone ebenso wie die CFF der monocular dominanten Neurone in gesetzmäßiger Weise von der Beleuchtungsstärke abhängig ist.

Bei den meisten untersuchten monocular dominanten Neuronen unterschied sich die binoculare CFF bei sonst gleichen Lichtbedingungen nicht von der monocularen CFF. Dann hatte auch eine Phasenverschiebung der Lichtreize oder eine alternierende Belichtung der beiden Augen keinen Einfluß auf die CFF.

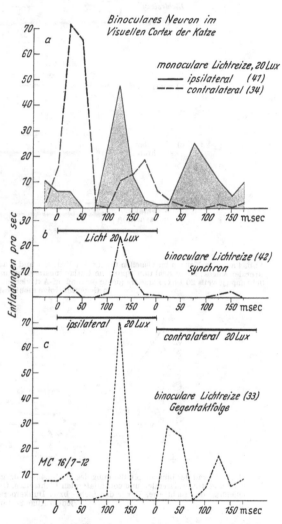

Abb. 3 a—c. a Statistische Auswertung der Reaktionen eines echten *binocularen Neurons* im visuellen Cortex der Katze auf monoculare Lichtreize. Auf den contralateralen Lichtreiz gruppierte *on-Aktivierung*, auf den ipsilateralen Lichtreiz *on-off-Aktivierung*. Beleuchtungsstärke jeweils 20 Lux. b *Synchrone binoculare Lichtreize* (jeweils 20 Lux) ergeben nur eine sehr geringfügige späte on-Aktivierung. c *Binoculare Lichtreize in Gegentaktfolge* (jeweils 20 Lux), jetzt wieder gruppierte Reaktionen, die sich als Summierung der on- und off-Reaktionen auf den ipsi- bzw. contralateralen Lichtreiz ableiten lassen (siehe Text). Abszisse: Jeweils Zeit in msec, Ordinate: Entladungsfrequenz (pro sec)

Eine Minderheit der monocular dominanten Neurone ließ jedoch einen solchen Einfluß erkennen. Bei einigen Neuronen erhöhte sich die CFF bei synchroner binocularer Belichtung im Vergleich zur monocularen oder alternierenden binocularen

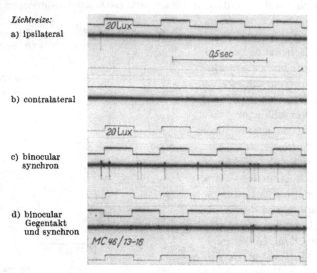

Abb. 4 a—d. a Neuron im visuellen Cortex der Katze. a und b auf monoculare Belichtung des ipsi- oder contralateralen Auges: keine Reaktion. Spontane Entladungsfrequenz unter 2 pro sec. c Bei synchroner binocularer Belichtung (jeweils 20 Lux) kurze frequente on- und off-Aktivierung. d Diese binoculare Bahnung ist bei Belichtung in Gegentaktfolge nicht festzustellen

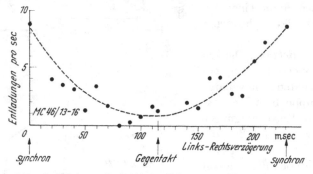

Abb. 4e. Der Grad der binocularen Bahnung des in Abb.4a—d dargestellten Neurons ist abhängig von der zeitlichen Verschiebung des ipsilateralen und contralateralen Lichtreizes. Ordinate: Entladungsfrequenz, Abszisse: zeitliche Verschiebung der Lichtreize, Dauer der Licht- bzw. Dunkelperioden jeweils 115 msec, Beleuchtungsstärke auf jedem Auge 20 Lux

Belichtung, bei einem anderen Teil jedoch trat das Gegenteil ein. In Abb. 5 ist ein Neuron dargestellt, das bei synchroner binocularer Belichtung eine höhere CFF hatte als bei alternierender Belichtung. Insgesamt kann jedoch gesagt werden, *daß für das gesamte corticale Neuronenkollektiv die CFF weitgehend monocular determiniert war und nur unwesentlich binocular beeinflußt wurde.*

Besprechung der Ergebnisse

Aus den mitgeteilten Resultaten geht hervor, daß die binocularen Koordinationsvorgänge an den Nervenzellen des zentralen visuellen Systems im Laufe der phylogenetischen Entwicklung des Sehens mit dem Auftreten eines binocularen

Sehraumes sich wandeln. Bei den Fischen und beim Kaninchen, die keinen oder nur einen geringfügigen binocularen Sehraum haben (das Kaninchen z. B. nach PORTMANN nur hinter seinem Kopf, besteht eine unioculare Projektion zur contralateralen Sehrinde. Die Lichtreaktionen der visuellen Neurone werden jeweils nur vom einen Auge bestimmt und sind vom anderen nicht beeinflußt.

Dieses Prinzip wird in Form der monocularen Dominanz auch dann für einen großen Teil der Neurone des zentralen Sehsystems in der phylogenetischen Entwicklung aufrecht erhalten, wenn durch das Zusammenrücken der beiden Augen ein ausgedehnter binocularer Sehraum entstanden ist. Parallel mit der Größe des binocularen Sehraumes erhöht sich die Zahl der nicht gekreuzten Sehnervenfasern und damit der Grad der räumlichen Vermischung der afferenten Systeme aus beiden Augen. Ein Teil der Neurone der monocularen Systeme erhält einen Erregungszufluß aus dem jeweils nicht dominanten Auge, so daß bei binocularer Belichtung zwar die monoculare Dominanz erhalten bleibt, jedoch eine Modifikation der Entladungsmuster durch die Afferenzen vom nicht dominanten Auge eintritt.

Neben dieser *binocularen Modifikation* der Entladungsmuster, die als Ausdruck einer Lockerung des Prinzips der monocularen Dominanz aufgefaßt werden kann,

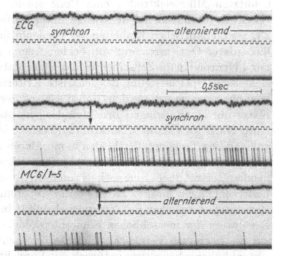

Abb. 5. *On-Neuron* (B-Typ) im primären visuellen Cortex der Katze. Flimmerlichtreaktionen auf binoculare Belichtung. Die Lichtreize werden abwechselnd binocular synchron und binocular alternierend geschaltet. Bei synchroner Belichtung erfolgt eine regelmäßige Neuronreaktion, bei alternierender Belichtung fehlt diese. Flimmerfrequenz 36 Lichtreize pro sec. Das contralaterale Auge ist dominant. Eine solche Erhöhung der CFF bei binocularer synchroner Belichtung konnte nur bei einem kleinen Prozentsatz der untersuchten Neurone festgestellt werden. Im Elektrocorticogramm der Area 17 (ECG) ebenfalls deutliche Bahnung der Flimmerlichtreaktion bei synchroner Belichtung. Es ist nur die Photozelle für das contralaterale Auge abgebildet. Wechsel der Phasenbeziehung durch Pfeil markiert

tritt bei der Katze ein zweites Neuronensystem auf, welches echte binoculare Effekte vermittelt. Unter der Voraussetzung, daß mit der angewandten Mikroelektrodentechnik keine Selektion der Neurone vorgenommen wurde, kann angenommen werden, daß dieses binoculare System in der primären Sehrinde durch weniger Neurone vertreten ist als die dem ipsi- und contralateralen Auge zugeordneten Systeme mit monocularer Dominanz.

Soweit man von den Entladungsmustern der Neurone auf den Informationsinhalt schließen kann, vermitteln die Neurone der vorwiegend monocularen Systeme Hell- (on-System) und Dunkelinformationen (off-System) einschließlich der monocularen Simultan- und Sukzessivkontraste (*3, 4, 5, 12, 15, 19, 22*). Der hemmende Einfluß des nicht dominanten Auges auf etwa die Hälfte dieser Neurone steht vielleicht mit der binocularen Rivalität beider Augen und der sinnesphysiologisch eindrucksvollen wechselseitigen Suppression in Zusammenhang.

Die Neurone des echten binocularen Systems vermitteln wahrscheinlich verschiedene Informationsgehalte, wobei man einmal an binoculare Kontrastphänomene (z. B. Neuron der Abb. 3), aber auch an stereoskopische Informationen denken muß. Eine solche Beziehung zum stereoskopischen Sehen liegt vor allem bei jenen Neuronen nahe, die Latenzzeitdifferenzen der afferenten Erregungen aus beiden Augen messen (Abb. 4e).

Für die Existenz echter binocularer Neurone im Geniculatum laterale ergaben sich gewisse Widersprüche der verschiedenen Untersucher, wobei für den Unterschied teilweise die Versuchsbedingungen (Narkose, Adaptation) und die Größe der benützten Mikroelektroden eine Rolle spielt. P. O. Bishop, Burke, Davis u. Hayhow (6) haben bei der Katze unter Anwendung strenger Kriterien unter 230 postsynaptischen Einheiten der Geniculatumregion nur 19 gefunden, die bei binocularer Opticusreizung von beiden Augen aktivierbar waren. Davon waren nur 4 Neurone in die Zellschichten des Geniculatum laterale zu lokalisieren. Da die elektrische Opticusreizung das schärfste Kriterium einer binocularen Interaktion erlaubt, kann gesagt werden, daß diese auf der Ebene des Geniculatum bei der Katze nur einen geringen Bruchteil der synaptischen Übertragungsvorgänge betrifft. Nach de Valois u. Mitarb. (25) besteht im Affengeniculatum offenbar eine vollständige Trennung der beiden monocularen Systeme.

Beziehungen zu subjektiv sinnesphysiologischen Erscheinungen. Wie im abschließenden Referat dieses Symposions von Prof. Jung (20, 22) berichtet wird, waren die Untersuchungen unseres Labors unter anderem auch dahingehend ausgerichtet, Beziehungen zwischen der Neuronenaktivität im Sehsystem und den subjektiven Resultaten der menschlichen Sinnesphysiologie herzustellen. Dieser im Hinblick auf die begrenzte Vergleichbarkeit des menschlichen Sehsystems mit dem Sehsystem höherer Säugetiere natürlich mit Vorsicht anzustellende Vergleich hat zwei Hypothesen zur Voraussetzung. Einmal muß angenommen werden, daß das on-System den Informationsinhalt „heller" und das off-System den Informationsinhalt „dunkler" vermittelt. Zum anderen wird vorausgesetzt, daß der Grad der subjektiven Hell- oder Dunkelwahrnehmung dem Grad der Aktivierung der Neurone des on- bzw. off-Systems parallel geht. Für die Richtigkeit beider Hypothesen lassen sich hinreichend wahrscheinliche Argumente bringen.

Unter diesen Voraussetzungen lassen sich auch Parallelen zwischen subjektiven Phänomenen bei der binocularen Wahrnehmung und den oben mitgeteilten Befunden an Katzen erheben.

1. Die *binoculare Rivalität* („Wettstreit der Sehfelder") zeigt sich in dem hemmenden Einfluß des nicht dominanten Auges, zum anderen aber auch bei einigen echten binocularen Neuronen. Der hemmende Einfluß des nicht dominanten Auges ist bei Flimmerlicht stärker als bei langdauernden Lichtreizen. Dies entspricht der binocularen Dominanz einer Kontur über eine nicht konturierte Fläche, da in Folge der unwillkürlichen Augenbewegungen an der Kontur ständige „Flimmererregungen" zustande kommen.

2. Unter günstigen Bedingungen sieht man bei verschiedenen Eindrücken auf beide Augen nicht den einen oder den anderen, noch beide zusammen verschmolzen zu einem einheitlichen Gebilde, sondern den einen *und* den anderen. Ein solches Experiment läßt sich z. B. anstellen, wenn man mit dem einen Auge eine Briefmarke mit dem anderen ein 10-Pfennig-Stück auf korrespondierenden Netzhautstellen unter tachistoskopischen Bedingungen anschaut. Dann sieht man nicht einen „Briefmarkenpfennig" sondern beide Gegenstände, d. h. der Informationsgehalt

entspricht näherungsweise der Summe der einzelnen Informationen durch jedes Auge. Bei längerer binocularer Fixierung tritt dann die langsame Periodik der wechselseitigen binocularen Hemmung auf, man sieht *entweder* eine Briefmarke *oder* ein 10-Pfennig-Stück. Ein solches Verhalten ist zu erwarten, wenn monocular dominante Systeme in Funktion treten, nicht jedoch, wenn nur Neurone aktiviert würden, die eine echte binoculare Konvergenz zeigen.

3. Der *Fechnersche Paradoxeffekt* (*11*) läßt sich auf die einfache Formel bringen, daß näherungsweise die subjektive binoculare Helligkeit dem arithmetischen Mittel aus den beiden monocularen Helligkeiten entspricht. Nimmt man an, daß bei diffuser Belichtung die subjektive Helligkeit mit dem mittleren Erregungsniveau der on-Neurone im visuellen Cortex parallel geht (Hypothese 1 u. 2), so läßt sich in der binocularen Verminderung der Entladungsfrequenz eine gewisse Analogie zum Fechnerschen Paradoxeffekt finden: Bei monocularer Belichtung werden im Vergleich zur binocularen Belichtung weniger Neurone, dafür aber stärker aktiviert. Die binoculare Belichtung erhöht die Zahl der aktivierten Neurone, vermindert jedoch ihre Entladungsfrequenz, so daß das mittlere corticale Erregungsniveau nur wenig ansteigt. In den untersuchten Helligkeitsbereichen nimmt bei Verdoppelung der Beleuchtungsstärke die Entladungsfrequenz der Neurone des on-Systems um 10—30% zu. Dies entspricht etwa der Zunahme der monocularen Aktivierung im Vergleich zur binocularen Aktivierung bei gleicher Beleuchtungsstärke. Die beiden dominanten Systeme reagieren bei binocularer Belichtung näherungsweise so, als ob monocular jedes Auge mit der halben Beleuchtungsstärke belichtet würde. Für die Neuronreaktionen bei verschiedenen Beleuchtungsstärken des linken und rechten Auges gilt Analoges.

4. SHERRINGTON (*24*) hat in seiner berühmten Untersuchung gezeigt, daß sich die *binoculare Flimmerfusionsfrequenz* nur geringfügig von der monocularen unterscheidet, wobei auch die Phasenverschiebung zwischen dem linken und rechten Auge nur eine geringfügige Rolle spielt. BAKER (*1*) hat seine Resultate kürzlich bestätigt und durch die Beobachtung ergänzt, daß der binoculare Einfluß zwar sehr geringfügig (höhere CFF bei synchroner Belichtung), jedoch konstant ist.

SHERRINGTON schloß aus seinen Resultaten, daß die für die CFF und die Wahrnehmung von Flimmerlicht verantwortlichen Neuronensysteme im zentralen Sehsystem eine weitgehende Trennung in ihrer Zuordnung zum linken und rechten Auge haben.

Diese weitgehende Trennung ist in den Neuronensystemen mit monocularer Dominanz gegeben. Betrachtet man die CFF als einen statistischen Vorgang im zentralen Neuronensystem, so korrespondieren die hier mitgeteilten Resultate über die CFF corticaler Neurone mit den subjektiven Resultaten SHERRINGTONs.

Herrn H. KAPP, dem Techniker der Abt. f. Klinische Neurophysiologie, sei auch an dieser Stelle für seine Hilfe gedankt.

Summary

1. The results of microelectrode recordings of the central visual system of 45 cats (encephale isolé, curarization), 10 rabbits (curarization) and 10 fishes (Esox lucius and Tinca vulgaris) were described. The responses of 185 neurons of cats, 45 of rabbits and 35 of fishes to monocular and binocular light stimuli applied with a special electronic binocular stimulator were quantitatively analysed.

2. The neurons in the optic tectum of fishes responded only to contralateral light stimuli. No binocular interaction was found. The same was true for the primary visual cortex of the rabbit, but it is assumed, that according to a small EEG-evoked-potential a small number of neurons also show reactions to ipsilateral light stimuli.

3. The spontaneous discharge frequency of central visual neurons of fishes was very low (1—2 per sec); in rabbits it was significantly lower (4—7 per sec) than in cats (6—15 per sec).

4. In the lateral geniculate body of cats (87 neurons), 31 neurons were activated by light or dark stimuli to the ipsilateral eye, 53 by stimulation of the contralateral, 3 showed no response. No neuron could be found which responded to the stimulation of either eye. Ten percent of the geniculate neurons showed a significant diminution of discharge frequency during the activation period with binocular stimuli compared with monocular stimulation of the dominant eye. The CFF was determined by the dominant eye. The neuronal discharges were identified as postsynaptic nerve cell spikes by the two components of their extracellular potential ($\alpha\beta$-spike).

5. 80 percent of the neurons in the primary visual cortex of cats were monocularly dominant (ca. 35 percent ipsilateral and 45 percent contralateral). One half of these neurons showed no alteration of discharge patterns to binocular light stimuli in comparison with the stimulation of the dominant eye. The other half had a significant binocular diminution, which was dependent upon the phase lag between the stimuli to the two eyes. Most of the neurons of this type responded to light or dark stimuli of the non dominant eye with a moderate inhibition (type C).

6. Ten percent of the neurons in the primary visual cortex responded to monocular stimuli of both eyes and had no monocular dominance. With binocular stimuli phenomena of inhibitory interaction and of occlusion were observed.

7. A fourth group of 5 percent of the analysed cortical neurons responded only to binocular stimuli and not to monocular stimulation of either eye. The binocular summation was most evident with synchronous light stimuli and only small if both stimuli were in alternating phases.

8. The last group (ca. 5 percent) consisted of neurons which responded neither to monocular nor to binocular light stimuli (so-called A-neurons).

9. The percentage values are preliminary. It is possible that the quantitative analysis of all recorded neurons in the visual cortex (ca. 300) may reveal slightly different percentages.

10. The CFF of the binocular activated neurons was, as a rule, in lower range of frequencies and not always dependent upon light intensity. The CFF of monocular dominant neurons depended on light intensity roughly corresponding to Porter's law. The CFF of most of these neurons showed no binocular influence; some had a small decrease, some a small, but significant increase of CFF with binocular light stimuli. The increase was highest with synchronous binocular light stimuli.

11. The results are compared with psycho-physiological findings (binocular summation and rivalry, binocular CFF).

Literatur

1. BAKER, C. H.: The dependence of binocular fusion on timing of peripheral stimuli and on central process. I. Symmetrical flicker. Canad. J. Psychol. 6, 1—10 (1952).
2. BAUMGARTEN, R. VON, and R. JUNG: Microelectrode studies on the visual cortex. Rev. neurol. 87, 151—155 (1952).
3. BAUMGARTNER, G.: Reaktionen einzelner Neurone im optischen Cortex der Katze nach Lichtblitzen. Pflügers Arch. ges. Physiol. 261, 457—469 (1955).
4. — u. P. HAKAS: Reaktionen einzelner Opticusneurone und corticaler Nervenzellen der Katze im Hell-Dunkel-Grenzfeld (Simultankontrast). Pflügers Arch. ges. Physiol. 270, 29 (1959).
5. — Die Reaktionen der Neurone des zentralen visuellen Systems im simultanen Helligkeits-kontrast. In diesem Symposion, S. 296—313.
6. BISHOP, P. O., W. BURKE, R. DAVIS and W. R. HAYHOW: Binocular interaction in the lateral geniculate nucleus — a general review. Trans. ophthal. Soc. Aust. 18, 15—34 (1958).
7. BURNS, B. D., W. HERON and B. GRAFSTEIN: Responses of cerebral cortex to diffuse mon-ocular and binocular stimulation. Amer. J. Physiol. 198, 200—204 (1960).
8. COHN, R.: Laminar electrical responses in lateral geniculate body of cat. J. Neurophysiol. 19, 317—324 (1956).
9. CORNEHLS, U., u. O.-J. GRÜSSER: Ein elektronisch gesteuertes Doppellichtreizgerät. Pflügers Arch. ges. Physiol. 270, 78 (1959).
10. ERULKAR, S. D., and M. FILLENZ: Pattern of discharge of single units of the lateral geni-culate body of the cat in response to binocular stimulation. J. Physiol. (Lond.) 140, 6—7 P (1958).
11. FECHNER, G. TH.: Über einige Verhältnisse des binocularen Sehens. Abh. Kgl. Sächs. Ges. Wiss. 5, 337—564 (1861).
12. GRÜSSER, O.-J.: Reaktionen einzelner corticaler und retinaler Neurone der Katze auf Flimmerlicht und ihre Beziehungen zur subjektiven Sinnesphysiologie. Med. Diss. Frei-burg 1956.
13. — u. O. CREUTZFELDT: Eine neurophysiologische Grundlage des Brücke-Bartley-Effektes: Maxima der Impulsfrequenz retinaler und corticaler Neurone bei Flimmerlicht mittlerer Frequenzen. Pflügers Arch. ges. Physiol. 263, 668—681 (1957).
14. — u. U. GRÜSSER-CORNEHLS: Entladungsmuster der Neurone des visuellen Cortex bei monocularer und binocularer Belichtung. (26. Tagg. Dtsch. Physiol. Ges.) Pflügers Arch. ges. Physiol. 272, 51 (1960).
15. — u. A. GRÜTZNER: Neurophysiologische Grundlagen der periodischen Nachbildphasen nach Lichtblitzen. Albrecht v. Graefes Arch. Ophthal. 160, 65—93 (1958).
16. — — Reaktionen einzelner Neurone des optischen Cortex der Katze nach elektrischen Reizserien des Nervus opticus. Arch. Psychiat. Nervenkr. 197, 405—432 (1958).
16a. — u. G. SAUR: Mikroelektrodenuntersuchungen am Geniculatum laterale der Katze: Mono- und binoculare Lichtreize. Pflügers Arch. ges. Physiol. 271, 595—612 (1960).
17. GRÜSSER-CORNEHLS, U., u. O.-J. GRÜSSER: Mikroelektrodenuntersuchungen am Genicula-tum laterale der Katze. Nervenzell- und Axonentladungen nach elektrischer Opticus-reizung. Pflügers Arch. ges. Physiol. 271, 50—63 (1960).
17a. GRÜTZNER, A., O.-J. GRÜSSER u. G. BAUMGARTNER: Reaktionen einzelner Neurone im optischen Cortex der Katze nach elektrischer Reizung des Nervus opticus. Arch. Psychiat. Nervenkr. 197, 377—404 (1958).
18. HUBEL, D. H., u. T. N. WIESEL: Receptive fields of single neurones in the cat's striate cortex. J. Physiol. (Lond.) 148, 574—591 (1959).
19. JUNG, R.: Neuronal discharge. EEG. Clin. Neurophysiol. Suppl. 4, 57—71 (1953).
20. — Korrelationen von Neuronentätigkeit und Sehen. Dieses Symposion S. 410 ff.
21. — R. VON BAUMGARTEN u. G. BAUMGARTNER: Mikroableitungen von einzelnen Nerven-zellen im optischen Cortex der Katze: Die lichtaktivierten B-Neurone. Arch. Psychiat. Nervenkr. 189, 521—539 (1952).
22. — O. CREUTZFELDT u. O.-J. GRÜSSER: Die Mikrophysiologie corticaler Neurone und ihre Bedeutung für die Sinnes- und Hirnfunktionen. Dtsch. med. Wschr. 82, 1050—1054 (1957).

23. Kornmüller, A. E.: Architektonische Lokalisation bioelektrischer Erscheinungen auf der Großhirnrinde. I. Untersuchungen am Kaninchen bei Augenbelichtung. Z. Psychol. Neurol. **44**, 447—459 (1932).
24. Sherrington, C. S.: On binocular flicker and the correlation of activity of "corresponding" retinal points. Brit. J. Psychol. **1**, 26—60 (1904).
25. Valois, R. L. de, C. J. Smith, A. J. Karoly and S. T. Kitai: Eelectrical responses of primate visual system. II. Recordings from single on-cells of macaque lateral geniculate nucleus. J. comp. physiol. Psychol. **52**, 635—641 (1959).

Diskussion

Mit 1 Abbildung

R. L. de Valois: Have you any evidence which would indicate that these various types of cells are located in different regions of the cortex or at different depths?

H.-L. Teuber: The change in fusion-frequency when intermittent stimulation of one eye is added to intermittent stimulation of the other is not „unwesentlich" (insignificant). Sherrington[3] had concluded that there was practically no difference between binocular flicker-fusion values in man when the flashes to one eye were in phase with those to the other, and when the two trains of flashes were out of phase. However, the more recent work of Ireland[1] and of Thomas[2] has shown clearly that there are small but significant differences between fusion thresholds under these different conditions, so that there must be some central interaction between the two monocular processes. As you may recall, Sherrington concluded from his seeming failure to find interaction that binocular vision was "psychic" rather than physiologic. The recent work, fortunately, suggests that Sherrington's conclusion was not inescapable.

U. Grüsser-Cornehls (zu de Valois): Wir haben die Area 17 von occipital nach frontal in etwa 3 gleich große Felder eingeteilt und im einzelnen Versuch notiert, aus welchen Feldern registriert wurde. Soweit bisher zu übersehen ist, besteht keine Differenz in der Verteilung der binocularen Reaktionstypen im Hinblick auf diese Felder. Allerdings wurden die Resultate noch nicht mit der χ^2-Methode berechnet, da wir bisher erst knapp die Hälfte der registrierten Neurone quantitativ ausgewertet haben.

In bezug auf die Tiefe hatten wir den Eindruck, daß die rein monocularen Neurone aus tieferen Schichten stammen, jedoch ist diese Beobachtung nur mit großer Einschränkung verwertbar, da man nahe an der Mantelkante in verschiedenen Tiefen aus gleichen Zellschichten registrieren kann.

(Zu Teuber) Mit „unwesentlich" war geringfügig und nicht insignifikant gemeint. Sherrington hat diese geringfügige Differenz zwischen monocularer und binocularer CFF ja schon beschrieben, und neuere Autoren (Baker, Bott u. a.) haben eine Differenz beschrieben, die bis zu 10% der CFF beträgt. Uns erscheint wichtig, daß jedoch eine erhebliche Änderung der CFF nicht eintritt, wie sie zu erwarten wäre, wenn die Afferenzen von beiden Augen an den für die CFF „zuständigen" Neuronen konvergieren würden.

Die sinnesphysiologischen Resultate lassen sich aus den mitgeteilten neurophysiologischen Resultaten begründen, wenn man bedenkt, daß die subjektive CFF statistisch gesehen ein Grenzprozeß ist, wofür auch die subjektive Wahrnehmung der Inkonstanz des Flimmerns knapp unterhalb der CFF spricht.

Befindet sich auch nur eine kleine Minderheit von Neuronen in der Hirnrinde, bei denen die binoculare CFF höher als die monoculare CFF ist bzw. die binocular synchrone CFF höher als die binocular alternierende, so wird der Grenzwert für das gesamte Kollektiv ansteigen. Aber

[1] Ireland, F. H.: A comparison of critical flicker frequencies under conditions of monocular and binocular stimulation. J. exp. Psychol. **40**, 282—286 (1950).

[2] Thomas, G. J.: A comparison of uniocular and binocular critical flicker frequencies: Simultaneous and alternate flashes. Amer. J. Psychol. **68**, 37—53 (1955).

[3] Sherrington, C. S.: The integrative action of the nervous system. New Haven: Yale Univ. Press 1906.

selbst wenn solche Neurone (Abb. 5) nicht vorhanden wären, könnte eine Erhöhung der binocularen CFF begründet werden, da oberhalb der definierten neuronalen CFF unregelmäßig
einzelne Entladungen immer noch in Abhängigkeit von der Flimmerfrequenz stehen. Dies läßt
sich beweisen durch Analyse von Entladungsintervallen relativ zum Flimmerintervall: Es
treten Maxima der Entladungsintervalle um ganzzahlig vielfache Werte der Flimmerlicht-
intervalle auf. Damit ist die subjektive CFF neurophysiologisch direkt als statististischer Grenzprozeß begründet. Da nun bei binocularer Flimmerbelichtung etwa doppelt soviel Neurone in
der Sehrinde aktiviert werden, erfolgt notwendigerweise eine Erhöhung der binocularen CFF
für das ganze Kollektiv, wenn man annimmt, daß beide Augen statistisch weitgehend unabhän-
gige Prozesse auslösen. Es tritt also ein ähnlicher Fall auf, wie bei der Erhöhung der binocularen absoluten Schwelle im Vergleich zur monocularen, die ebenfalls als statistischer Vorgang
durch die Addierung der Meldungen aus zwei stochastischen Informationssystemen erklärt
werden kann.

L. WIDÉN: With your experimental technique, Dr. GRÜSSER, it is hardly possible to determine whether a spike recorded in the visual cortex is a presynaptic impulse in an optic
radiation fibre or a postsynaptic response from a cortical unit, since you stimulate the optic
nerve — and not the optic radiation — and consequently the LGD synapses would lie between
the stimulating and the recording electrodes. All recorded spikes would thus have "post-
synaptic" characteristics. When studying a unit in the visual cortex with your technique there
is, in our experience, no way of discriminating between phenomena due to LGD synapses and
those due to cortical synapses since spikes recorded from both these foci following stimulation
of the optic tract or nerve may show equally long latencies and, in double shock experiments,
equally long periods of unresponsiveness.

O.-J. GRÜSSER: Die Frage war für unsere Untersuchungen
natürlich von Wichtigkeit. Wir haben daher versucht, physiologische Kriterien für die postsynaptische Natur einer Entladung
zu finden, d. h. für die Ableitung von Nervenzellen. Ein solches
Kriterium gibt es: Alle Neuronentladungen, die konstant im extracellulären positiven Aktionspotential zwei Komponenten aufzeigen
($\alpha\beta$-spike), können als postsynaptische Registrierungen von Nervenzellen angesehen werden. Da ein $\alpha\beta$-spike auch noch als Registrierung an einer Axonaufzweigung interpretiert werden könnte,
möchte ich die beiden Beobachtungen mitteilen, die vielleicht beweisend sind, daß ein $\alpha\beta$-spike eine Registrierung von der Nervenzelle darstellt:

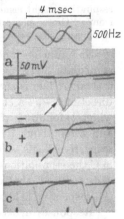

1. Bei intracellulärer Ableitung haben Neurone, die extracellulär einen $\alpha\beta$-spike aufwiesen, die typischen IS-SD-Potentiale von
ECCLES u. Mitarb. (Abb. 6).
2. Reizt man den Nervus opticus mit hochfrequenten elektrischen Doppelreizen unter 2—3 msec Intervall, so findet man
bei Neuronen mit $\alpha\beta$-spike in der Regel Intervalle, bei denen
der erste elektrische Reiz mit einem kompletten $\alpha\beta$-spike, der
zweite jedoch nur mit einem α-spike beantwortet wird. Der α-
spike scheint ein präsynaptisches, der β-spike ein postsynap-
tisches Potential zu sein[1].

Abb. 6. *Intracelluläre Ableitung einer Nervenzelle des
visuellen Cortex der Katze.*
IS-SD-spike (Pfeil). Nach
Verletzung der Membran in
c) Zerfall des IS- und SD-
spike. DC-Registrierung

---

[1] *Anmerkung bei der Korrektur:* Dieses Kriterium bewährt sich auch bei elektrischer
Radiatioreizung, wie neuere Versuche mit K. HELLNER ergeben haben. Die maximale
Reizfolgefrequenz des α-spikes corticaler Neurone liegt signifikant weit über der maxi-
malen Reizfolgefrequenz des β-spikes.

Recordings with Multiple Microelectrodes from the Lateral Geniculate and the Visual Cortex of the Cat[1,2]

By

K. Negishi[3] and M. Verzeano

With 8 Figures

Previous studies, based on the use of single and multiple microelectrodes, have indicated that neuronal activity propagates in cortical and thalamic networks. Such propagation may take place spontaneously (13, 14, 15, 16, 17) or may be triggered by sensory stimulation (9, 12, 16). In the latter case it may, within certain limits, be "driven" at the frequency of stimulation (9, 16).

This report deals with the study of such phenomena in the lateral geniculate body, the nucleus reticularis of the thalamus and the visual cortex of the cat, and with their relations to visual stimulation.

The type of microelectrodes, the experimental techniques and the electronic devices used in this study are the same as those used in previous studies and have been described elsewhere (13, 16, 17). The animals were paralyzed with flaxedil and maintained with artificial respiration. Light nembutal anesthesia was used in a few experiments. Brief flashes of light from a "Grass" photostimulator were used for contralateral visual stimulation. The location of the recording points in the brain was checked histologically (fig. 1).

Spontaneous and evoked propagation of neuronal activity in the lateral geniculate body, recorded with four microelectrodes (a, b, c, d) displayed along a straight line is shown in Fig. 2. In A propagation occurs spontaneously in the direction c−b−a at 1, 2, 3 and 5, 6, 7; in B it is triggered by a single stimulus which is followed, after about 30 msec, by a first volley of impulses (at 1, 2, 3, 4) and after about 70 msec by a second volley of impulses which appear in the respective fields of the microelectrodes in the order b−a−c−d (at 5, 6, 7, 8); in C the stimulation is repetitive, the latency of the first volley of impulses (1, 2, 3 4) is reduced, that of the second volley is increased and its impulses appear in the respective fields of the microelectrodes in the changed order a−d−b (5, 6, 7).

Responses evoked in the visual cortex by single and repetitive stimulation, recorded with three mircoelectrodes (a, b, c) displayed in such a way as to form a triangle, are shown in Fig. 3. Early (1, 2, 3, 4) and late (5, 6) responses are seen in A, B and C. As the frequency of stimulation is increased from 1 to 3 flashes/second the order in which impulses appear in the respective fields of the microelectrodes changes: in the late response, from c−a−b− (in A: 5, 6, 7) it changes to a−c−b (in B: 5, 6, 7), then again to c−a−b (in C: 5, 6, 7), while the intervals 5 to 6 and 6 to 7 become shorter; in the early response the order changes from c−b−a (in B: 1, 2, 3) to c−a−b (in C: 1, 2, 3). As the frequency of stimulation is further increased (in D) the order of appearance of the impulses in the fields of the microelectrodes continues to change.

---

[1] From the Department of Biophysics and Nuclear Medicine University of California, Los Angeles.

[2] Aided by grant B-649 from the USPH Service.

[3] Visiting Investigator, University of Kanazawa, Japan.

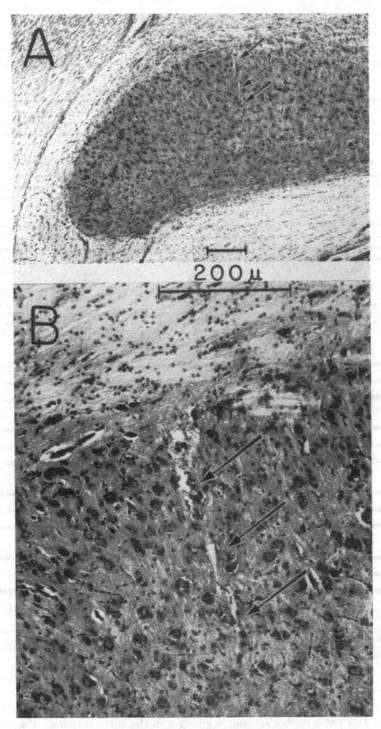

Fig. 1. Microphotographs showing, at two different magnifications (*A* and *B*), tracks (indicated by arrows) of triple microelectrodes penetrating into the lateral geniculate body

Similar phenomena occur in response to visual stimuli in the caudal part
(Fig. 4) of the nucleus reticularis of the thalamus. Fig. 5 shows responses evoked,
in this nucleus, by single and repetitive stimulation, recorded with three microelectrodes displayed along a straight line. In A, an early response is seen at 1, 2, 3

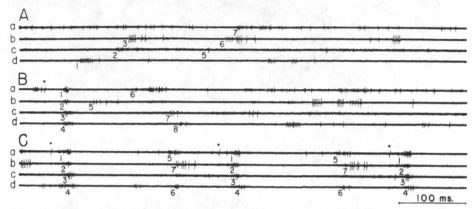

Fig. 2. *Spontaneous and evoked neuronal activity in the lateral geniculate, recorded with four microelectrodes* (*a, b, c, d*)
displayed along a straight line. A: spontaneous activity. B: activity evoked by a single flash of light. C: activit*y*
evoked by repetitive flashes. Microelectrode tip diameters: $a = 5\ \mu$; $b = 2\ \mu$; $c = 3\ \mu$; $d = 4\ \mu$. Distances between
tips: a to $b = 156\ \mu$; b to $c = 160\ \mu$; c to $d = 156\ \mu$. Recordings obtained 1 hour and 20 minutes after the administration of 6 mg of nembutal/kg. In this and all other pictures the numerals (1, 2, 3, etc.) indicate the order in which
neuronal activity appears in the respective fields of the microelectrodes. Stimuli are indicated by black dots.

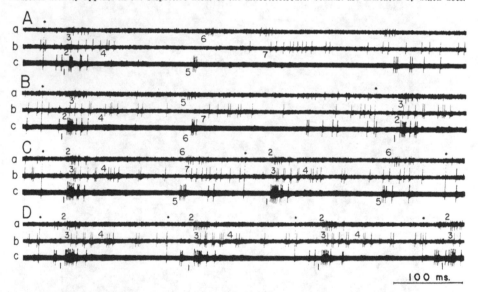

Fig. 3. *Evoked neuronal activity in the visual cortex recorded with three microelectrodes* (*a, b, c*) whose tips were displayed
in such a way as to form a triangle. *A*: single flash. *B, C, D*: low frequency stimulation. Microelectrode tips:
$a = 3\ \mu$; $b = 3\ \mu$; $c = 2\ \mu$. Distances between tips: a to $b = 120\ \mu$; b to $c = 200\ \mu$; a to $c = 235\ \mu$.

and two late responses at 4, 5, 6 and 7, 8, 9. As the frequency of stimulation is
increased, the order of appearance of neuronal activity in the respective fields
of the microelectrodes changes: in B, at 1.5 flashes/second, it changes in the late
response. In C, at 6 flashes/second, it changes in the early response. Fig. 6 shows
responses evoked in the same nucleus by repetitive stimulation at increasing

frequencies and recorded with four mircoelectrodes displayed along a straight line. Each flash of light triggers a response in the vicinity of electrode tips a and b while, at the same time, it causes extinction of the activity of the neuron recorded by tip c. The latency of the response at tips a and b and that of the extinction at

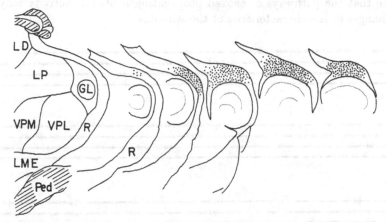

Fig. 4. Diagrammatic representation of transverse serial sections of thalamus of cat, indicating (black dots) location, in the nucleus reticularis, of the points from which neuronal activity can be recorded in response to visual stimulation.

tip c, as well as the number and grouping of spikes generated by the neurons recorded at a, b and c, vary with the frequency of stimulation, but the coupling of triggered activity at a and b with extinction of activity at c remains unchanged.

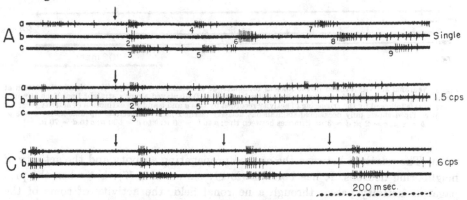

Fig. 5. Neuronal activity evoked in the nucleus reticularis of the thalamus by visual stimulation recorded with three microelectrodes displayed along a straight line. A: single flash; B: 1.5 flashes/sec.; C: 6 flashes/sec. Microelectrode tips: $a = 3\ \mu$; $b = 2\ \mu$; $c = 2\ \mu$; Distances between tips: a to $b = 250\ \mu$; b to $c = 500\ \mu$.

When the latencies of the responses in the nucleus reticularis are compared with those in the lateral geniculate body, it is found that, most frequently, the latency of the early response in the nucleus reticularis is longer than the one in the lateral geniculate (Fig. 7).

The significance of these findings in connection with central visual mechanisms may be sought in:

a) The relations between the frequency of the visual stimuli and the order in which neurons in the networks of the lateral geniculate, the nucleus reticularis, or the visual cortex become active after a stimulus. The changes which occur in the order of activation as a consequence of changes in the frequency of stimulation indicate that the pathways of evoked propagating neuronal activity may vary with changes in the characteristics of the stimulus.

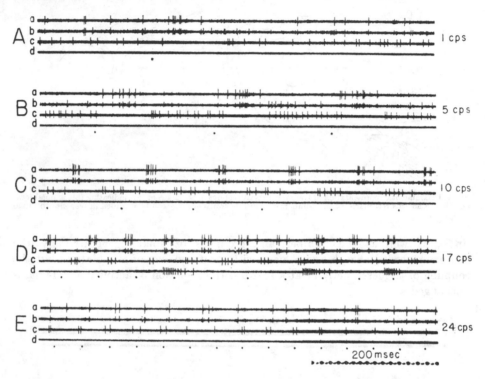

Fig. 6. Neuronal activity evoked in the nucleus reticularis of the thalamus, by repetitive visual stimulation at various frequencies, recorded with four microelectrodes (a, b, c, d) displayed along a straight line. Each stimulus (black dot) is followed by the triggering of activity recorded by tips a and b and the extinction of activity recorded by tip c. Tip d shows only occasional spontaneous activity (strip D). Microelectrode tip diamaters: $a = 3\ \mu$; $b = 2\ \mu$; $c = 2\ \mu$; $d = 3\ \mu$; distances between tips: a to $b = 60\ \mu$; b to $c = 500\ \mu$; c to $d = 70\ \mu$.

b) The relations between the evoked propagating activity and the activity of neighboring neurons. It has been previously shown (16, 17) that when the propagating activity passes through a neuronal field, the activity of some of the neighboring neurons may be extinguished. In this series of investigations it has been found that, when the propagated activity is triggered by visual stimulation, this effect on neighboring neurons may change with the frequency of stimulation (Fig. 8). This indicates, again, that the pathways of evoked propagating neuronal activity may vary with changes in the characteristics of the stimulus and suggests, in addition, that excitatory and inhibitory actions associated with it, may also vary with changes in the characteristics of the stimulus.

c) The relations between the activity of the nonspecific nuclei of the thalamus and that of the visual cortex or the lateral geniculate body.

Anatomical evidence indicating that relations may exist between the nucleus reticularis and other thalamic nuclei has been brought forth by ROSE and WOOL-SEY (*11*), ROSE (*10*), and by AKIMOTO, NEGISHI and YAMADA (*4*). Electrophysiological evidence indicating that sensory information arrives in nonspecific nuclei of the thalamus has been brought forth by FRENCH, VERZEANO and MAGOUN (*7*) and more recently by ALBE-FESSARD et al. (*1, 2*). JUNG and his collaborators (*3, 5, 6, 8*) have demonstrated that the activity of some of the nonspecific nuclei of the thalamus may influence that of neurons in the visual cortex. All these studies, thus, converge to suggest that the activity of the nonspecific nuclei of the thalamus may be related to or have an influence upon sensory mechanisms. The findings presented here indicate that visual stimulation evokes neuronal responses in the nucleus reticularis and triggers the propagation of neuronal activity through the neuronal networks of this nucleus. They further indicate that temporal and spatial relations between these neuronal responses are similar

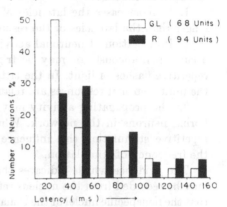

Fig. 7. Frequency distributions of latencies of neuronal responses evoked, by visual stimulation, in the lateral geniculate and the nucleus reticularis of the thalamus.

to those which occur, under similar conditions, in the lateral geniculate body or the visual cortex. Additional evidence is thus provided which suggests that sensory information arrives in nonspecific nuclei of the thalamus and that the activity of these nuclei may be implicated in central visual mechanisms.

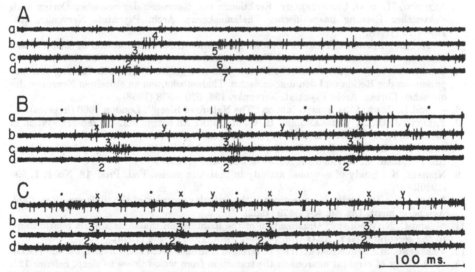

Fig. 8. Relations between propagating activity and neighboring neurons in lateral geniculate, studied with four microelectrodes (*a, b, c, d*) displayed along a straight line. *A*: spontaneous activity showing propagation at 1, 2, 3, 4; *B*: stimulation with flashes of light at low frequency; following each flash, neuronal activity appears in the order *a—d—c* (at 1, 2, 3), while the activity of the neurons recorded by *b* is extinguished (*x — y*). *C*: stimulation at an increased frequency; following each flash, activity appears in the order *d—c—b* (at 1, 2, 3) while the activity of the neurons recorded by *a* is extinguished (*x — y*). Microelectrode tips and distances as in fig. 2.

Summary

The neuronal responses evoked by visual stimulation with brief flashes of light, in the visual cortex, the lateral geniculate body and the nucleus reticularis thalami have been studied by means of recordings with multiple microelectrodes, in cats immobilized with flaxedil and maintained with artificial respiration. It has been found that:

1. In most cases the latencies of the responses in the nucleus reticularis are longer than the latencies of the responses in the lateral geniculate body.

2. Propagation of neuronal activity through the networks of these structures occurs spontaneously or may be triggered by visual stimulation with single or repetitive flashes of light. In the latter case the temporal and spatial patterns of the multineuronal responses are related to the frequency of stimulation.

3. The propagating activity may have an influence on the activity of neighboring neurons in the network. When the propagating activity is triggered by repetitive stimulation this influence on neighboring neurons may change with the frequency of stimulation.

The evidence which indicates that neuronal responses to visual stimulation may be recorded from the nucleus reticularis gives additional support to the view that the nonspecific nuclei of the thalamus may be implicated in visual mechanisms.

References

1. Albe-Fessard, D., C. Rocha-Miranda et E. Oswaldo-Cruz: Activités d'origine somesthésique évoquées au niveau du cortex non-spécifique et du centre médian du thalamus chez le singe anasthésié au chloralose. EEG clin. Neurophysiol. 11, 777—787 (1959).
2. — et A. Rougeul: Activités d'origine somesthésique evoquées sur le cortex non spécifique du chat anesthésié au chloralose: rôle du centre médian du thalamus. EEG clin. Neurophysiol. 10, 131—152 (1958).
3. Akimoto, H., u. O. Creutzfeldt: Reaktionen von Neuronen des optischen Cortex nach elektrischer Reizung unspezifischer Thalamuskerne. Arch. Psychiat. Nervenkr. 196, 494—519 (1958).
4. — K. Negishi and K. Yamada: Studies on thalamo-cortical connection in cat by means of retrograde degeneration method. Folia psychiat neurol. jap. 10, 39—82 (1956).
5. Creutzfeldt, O., u. H. Akimoto: Konvergenz und gegenseitige Beeinflussung von Impulsen aus der Retina und den unspezifischen Thalamuskernen an einzelnen Neuronen des optischen Cortex. Arch. Psychiat. Nervenkr. 196, 520—538 (1958).
6. — and R. Jung: Ciba Symposium on "The Nature of Sleep", London 1960 (in press).
7. French, J. D., M. Verzeano and H. W. Magoun: An extralemniscal sensory system in the brain. A. M. A. Arch. Neurol. Psychiat. 69, 505—518 (1953).
8. Jung, R.: Microphysiology of cortical neurons and its significance for psychophysiology. An. Fac. med. Montevideo 44, No. 3—4, 323—332 (1959).
9. Negishi, K.: Study of neuronal activity in thalamic nuclei. Fed. Proc. 19, No. 1, 1, 300 (1960).
10. Rose, J. E.: The cortical connections of the reticular complex of the thalamus. Res. Publ. Ass. nerv. ment. Dis. 30, 454—479 (1952).
11. — and C. N. Woolsey: Organization of the mammalian thalamus and its relationships to the cerebral cortex. EEG clin. Neurophysiol. 1, 391—404 (1949).
12. Verzeano, M.: Sequential activity of cerebral neurons. Arch. int. Physiol. 63, 458 (1955).
13. — Activity of cerebral neurons in the transition from wakefulness to sleep. Science 124, 366 (1956).
14. — and I. Calma: Unit-activity in spindle bursts. J. Neurophysiol. 17, 417 (1954).
15. — R. Naquet and E. E. King: Action of barbiturates and convulsants on the unit-activity of the diffusely projecting nuclei of the thalamus. J. Neurophysiol. 18, 502 (1955).

16. VERZEANO, M. and K. NEGISHI: Neuronal activity in cortical and thalamic networks. J. gen. Physiol. Suppl. *43*, 177—195 (1960).

17. — — Neuronal activity in wakefulness and in sleep. Ciba Symposium on "The Nature of Sleep". London, 1960 (in press).

Discussion

R. JUNG: Dr. VERZEANO's findings, indicating the existence of spontaneously circulating neuronal activity in the geniculate and visual cortex, may be of psychophysiological importance. I believe that *I, myself, can see, entoptically, visual correlates of these neuronal activities:* Watching my visual field, in complete darkness, after bleaching of all after images, I see in my „Eigengrau" small patches of lighter greyness with internal movements, sometimes circling around, sometimes expanding and shrinking. Most of these circles have diameters of a few degrees and show oscillations at 1 to 10 per second. Sometimes larger fields of cloud like forms appear, with slow circular movements over several quadrants of the paracentral visual field. If you accept my suggestion that the visual „Eigengrau" corresponds to the resting activity of B- and D-neurons, signalling brightness and darkness respectively, the moving images could be explained by the relative preponderance of B- or D-neurons in the pathways of this circulating activity. Furthermore, we may assume that these neuronal impulses have some relation to spatial distribution within the visual field.

When a *flickering light* is projected on closed eyes these circular images are enhanced and enlarged in the peripheral field to *huge concentric rings shrinking or expanding around a brighter center in the foveal area.* This may correspond to changes in the pathways of the circulating neuronal activity, similar to those suggested by the results obtained in the experiments with flickering light, conducted by NEGISHI and VERZEANO. I must add, that I am aneidetic and that I am unable to see spontaneously arising complex visual images with closed eyes, except the classical after images.

R. L. DE VALOIS: Recording from the retina one finds cells which fire with different latencies or with different patterns of response to light stimuli. Is it possible that some of what you have presented as evidence for waves of activity spreading through the geniculate and thalamus could just be simultaneous recordings from these different types of cells?

O.-J. GRÜSSER: Die beschriebenen rhythmischen Aktivierungsphasen der Geniculatumneurone nach kurzen Lichtreizen lassen sich auch schon im retinalen Neuronensystem finden. Es ist daher sehr schwer zu beurteilen, was bei Registrierungen aus dem Geniculatum als retinaler Effekt vorhanden ist und was neu an Geniculatumneuronen auftritt. Vergleichende Messungen der Latenzzeiten der sekundären und tertiären Aktivierungsphasen der on-Neurone in der Retina und im Geniculatum laterale haben ergeben, daß nicht nur die Primäraktivierungen, sondern auch die späteren Aktivierungsphasen weitgehend durch retinale Vorgänge bedingt sind.

M. VERZEANO: Professor JUNG's suggestions are very pertinent and very stimulating. It seems to me that it is quite possible that there may be some relations between the spontaneous or evoked circulating neuronal activity and the phenomena described by Professor JUNG. More particularly so, in the case of the flicker experiment. When the circulating neuronal activity was "driven" with repetitive flashes of light we found that, at a given frequency, the spatial and temporal interneuronal relations remain fairly much stationary, suggesting that the network territory over which the neuronal activity circulates remains fairly much the same. This might explain the enhancement of the circles mentioned by Professor JUNG in relation to his flicker experiment on closed eyes.

(To O.-J. GRÜSSER and R. L. DE VALOIS) I think that it is, indeed, possible that some of the spatial and temporal characteristics of the circulating neuronal activity observed in the geniculate may be directly related to phenomena which occur in the neuronal networks of the retina, as Dr. GRÜSSER suggests. It seems to me that it should be very interesting to investigate the interneuronal relations in the complex networks of the retina.

II. Corticale Mechanismen des Kontrast- und Bewegungssehens. Receptive Felder

Die Reaktionen der Neurone des zentralen visuellen Systems der Katze im simultanen Helligkeitskontrast*

Von

Günter Baumgartner

Mit 7 Abbildungen

Um die zentrale Verarbeitung der visuellen Afferenz zu studieren, haben wir in Fortsetzung der Kontrastlichtuntersuchungen an Fasern des Tractus opticus (s. S. 45) mit gleicher Methode auch Neurone des *Corpus geniculatum laterale* und des *optischen Cortex (Area 17)* der Katze (encéphale isolé) registriert. Auch vom Genicula- tum wurde nach Freilegung und nicht stereotaktisch abgeleitet. Die Bestimmung der horizontalen Durchmesser der Feldzentren er- folgte in der gleichen Weise wie bei den Tractusfasern (vgl. S. 47). Kurze Mitteilungen dieser Unter- suchungen erfolgten 1959 (*4*) und 1960 (*5*).

Ergebnisse. Die corticalen Neu- rone zeigen eine geringere Ent- ladungsfrequenz bei ihrer Licht- oder Dunkelaktivierung als die Neurone des Corp. genic. lat., die bei diffuser Belichtung wie Trac- tusfasern reagieren. Wie die on- Fasern des Tr. opt. werden auch die on-Zentrum-Neurone des Corp. genic. lat. durch Kontrastreiz

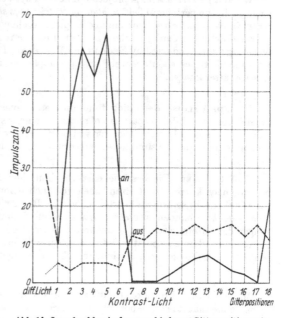

Abb. 1b. Impulszahlen in den verschiedenen Gitterpositionen in den ersten 500 msec nach Belichtung (—) und Verdunkelung (· · ·)

deutlich stärker aktiviert als durch diffuses Licht. Ebenso wie dort findet sich die *maximale Aktivierung im Grenzgebiet am Übergang vom Hell- zum Dunkelfeld.* Die Aktivierungskurve bei breiten Hellfeldern verläuft wiederum M-förmig. Bei schmalen Hellfeldern kommt es entsprechend nur noch zu einer verstärkten Aktivierungsspitze. Das gleiche gilt für die corticalen on-Zentrum-Neurone (B-Neurone).

---

* Aus der Abteilung für Klinische Neurophysiologie der Universität Freiburg im Breisgau.

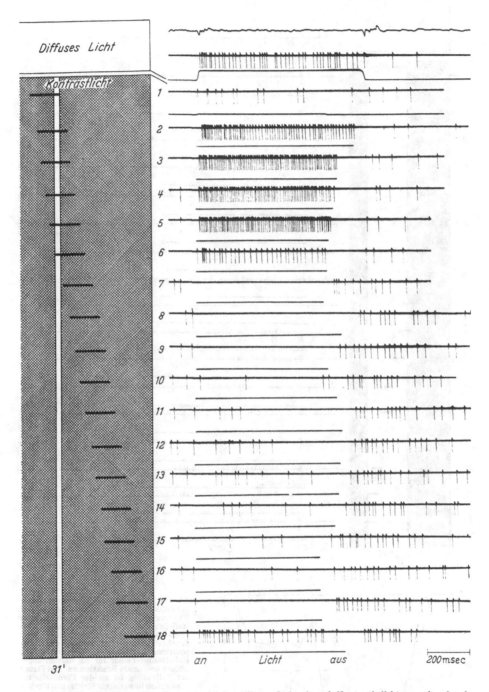

Abb. 1a. *On-Zentrum-Neuron des Corp. gen. lat.* bei diffusem Lichtreiz und Kontrastbelichtung mit schmalem Hellfeld (31′) und breitem Dunkelfeld (schraffiert). Die schwarzen Balken entsprechen größen- und lagerichtig dem Horizontaldurchmesser des Feldzentrums innerhalb des Kontrastfeldes in den verschiedenen Gitterpositionen. Bei der Registrierung der diffusen Belichtung ist als erste Kurve das EEG mit abgebildet. Die Photozelle ist nur in den zwei obersten Registrierungen dargestellt, danach durch einen Strich markiert

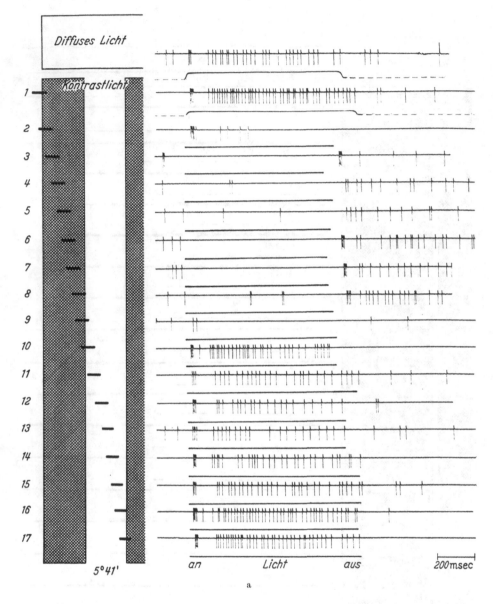

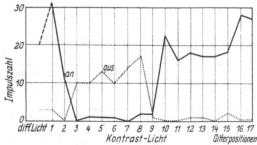

a

b

Abb. 2a. *On-Zentrum-B-Neuron des Cortex* bei diffuser und Kontrast-Belichtung. Der Kontrastreiz besteht hier aus gleich breiten Hell- (weiß) und Dunkelfeldern (schraffiert) von 5° 41'. Der schwarze Balken gibt wieder den horizontalen Durchmesser des Feldzentrums und dessen Lage innerhalb der Hell-Dunkel-Felder für die danach abgebildete neuronale Reaktion an. Die Dauer der Belichtung ist an der Photozelle ersichtlich bzw. durch Striche markiert

Abb. 2b. Impulszahlen in verschiedenen Gitterpositionen der Abb. 2a für die ersten 500 msec nach Belichtung (—) und nach Verdunkelung (...)

Abb. 1 zeigt ein *on-Zentrum-Neuron des Corp. genic. lat.*, welches bei diffusem Licht und mit einem schmalen Hellfeld getestet wurde. Vor den neuronalen Reaktionen ist die Ausleuchtung des receptiven Feldzentrums im Kontrast (s. S. 47) schematisch angegeben. Man sieht, daß die Aktivierung auf Belichtung im Kontrast erheblich stärker ist als bei diffuser Belichtung. Die Lichtaktivierung des Neurons erfolgt nur, wenn ein Teil des receptiven Feldzentrums im Hellfeld liegt. Befindet sich das receptive Feldzentrum jedoch im Kontrastschatten, so kommt es nach Belichtung zu einer Hemmung des Neurons (Pos. 7, 8, 9, 16 und 17) und nach Verdunkelung zur Aktivierung. Die Lichthemmung ist dann am deutlichsten, wenn sich das receptive Feldzentrum im Randbereich des Dunkelfeldes befindet. Sie nimmt ab, wenn es in die Mitte des Dunkelfeldes gerät.

Das *corticale on-Zentrum-Neuron (B-Neuron)* der Abb. 2a, welches mit breitem Hellfeld (5° 41') getestet wurde, zeigt eine maximale Aktivierung, wenn das receptive Feldzentrum an der Kontrastgrenze im Hellfeld liegt (Pos. 1, 10, 16 und 17) und eine Umkehr der Reaktion, d. h. eine Hemmung bei Belichtung und eine Aktivierung bei Verdunkelung im Dunkelfeld (Pos. 3—8). Dabei ist der Aktivierungsverlauf sowohl auf Belichtung wie auf Verdunkelung je nach der Lage der Kontrastgrenze zum Feldzentrum etwas verschieden (Abb. 2b). Dies zeigt, daß die Wirkung der antagonistischen Randzone auf das Neuron in bezug auf die senkrechte Kontrastgrenze nicht symmetrisch ist. Das vom Betrachter aus rechts des Feldzentrums gelegene Umfeld hat eine deutlich stärkere inhibitorische Wirkung als das links gelegene. Infolgedessen kommt es bei Beschattung der rechten Umfeldzone in Pos. 1 und 16 zu einer stärkeren Aktivierung bei Belichtung als in Pos. 10. Umgekehrt ist entsprechend die Aktivierung auf Verdunkelung dann am stärksten, wenn sie nach Belichtung der rechts gelegenen Randzone auftritt (Pos. 8).

Auch bei der Aktivierung nach Verdunkelung behält das Neuron das charakteristische Verhalten eines on-Zentrum-Neurons bei. Es zeigt also nach kurzer Latenz eine Primärerregung mit anschließend postexcitatorischer Hemmung und langsam abklingender Nacherregung.

Auf Abb. 3a ist ein mit schmalem Hellfeld getestetes off-Zentrum-Neuron des Geniculatum dargestellt. Befindet sich das receptive Feldzentrum dieses Neurons völlig im Dunkelfeld (Pos. 1, 9—17), so reagiert das Neuron auf Belichtung mit einer on-Aktivierung. Diese Aktivierung zeigt allerdings im Gegensatz zur Lichtaktivierung des reinen on-Zentrum-Neurons die typisch langsam abklingende Aktivierung der off-Zentrum-Neurone. Der Aktivierung kann auch eine kurze präexcitatorische Hemmung vorausgehen. Bei Verdunkelung kommt es in diesen Positionen nur zu einer geringen Aktivierung, manche Neurone werden auch kurz gehemmt. Wird das Feldzentrum belichtet, so verhält sich das Neuron wie bei diffuser Belichtung, d. h. es kommt zu einer Lichthemmung.

Die Kurve der Abb. 3b zeigt die Impulszahl in verschiedenen Gitterpositionen für die ersten 500 msec nach Belichtung (an) und Verdunkelung (aus). Dabei ergibt sich auch bei den off-Zentrum-Neuronen ein M-förmiger Aktivierungsverlauf der on-Reaktion. Die Aktivierungsmaxima liegen bei ihnen jedoch im Dunkelfeld an der Grenze zum Hellfeld und nicht im Hellfeld an der Grenze zum Dunkelfeld wie bei den on-Zentrum-Neuronen. Auch die off-Reaktion zeigt hier

Aktivierungsspitzen an der Kontrastgrenze. Diese Maxima sind aber gegen die der on-Aktivierungen des Neurons in das Hellfeld verschoben.

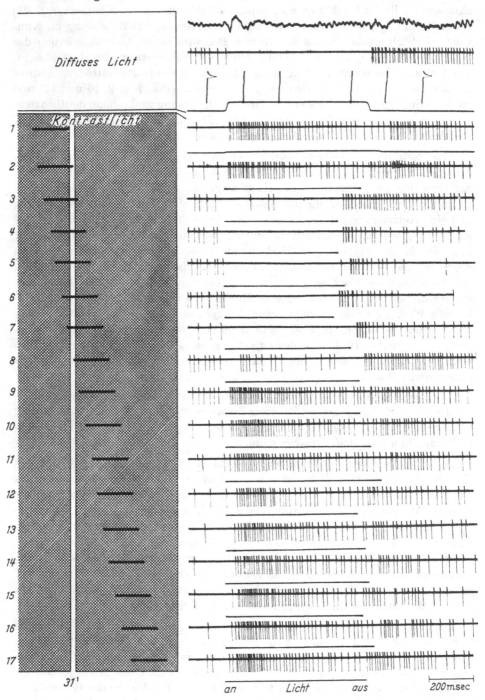

Abb. 3a. *Off-Zentrum-Neuron des Corp. gen. lat.* bei diffuser Belichtung und Kontrastlichtreizen mit schmalem Hellfeld (31'). (Legende s. Abb. 1 und 2 und Text)

Die folgende Abb. 4 zeigt ein entsprechendes Beispiel eines *corticalen off-Zentrum-Neurons (D-Neuron)*, das mit einer Hellfeldbreite von 2° 4′ untersucht wurde. Wie zu erwarten, ergeben auch die corticalen off-Zentrum-Neurone eine Reaktionsumkehr bei Belichtung, wenn das receptive Feldzentrum im Kontrastschatten liegt. Die maximale Aktivierung tritt wieder am Übergang zum Hellfeld auf. Die Impulszahlen in den verschiedenen Gitterpositionen sind bei diesem Neuron wie bei dem Beispiel des on-Zentrum-Neurons des Tr. opt. (s. S. 47) für verschiedene Intervalle nach Belichtung getrennt ausgezählt. Auch hier ist ersichtlich, daß sich erst nach den ersten 100 msec nach Belichtung die kontrastabhängigen Aktivierungsunterschiede entwickeln. Die off-Aktivierung dieses Neurons verhält sich uncharakteristisch und wurde deshalb nicht gezeichnet.

Auf Abb. 5 sind noch einmal die Aktivierungskurven eines corticalen on-Zentrum-Neurons bei breitem (5° 41′) und schmalem Hellfeld (2° 50′) abgebildet. Die gestrichelte Linie zeigt die Kontrolle bei Rückbewegung des Kontrastgitters. Die Verschmälerung des Hellfeldes führt also auch bei corticalen Neuronen zu einer deutlichen Zunahme der Aktivierung.

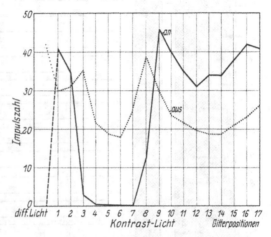

Abb. 3b. Impulszahlen des Neurons in verschiedenen Gitterpositionen 500 msec nach Belichtung (—) und Verdunkelung (...)

An dem Beispiel der on-off-Tractusfasern (s. S. 50) wurde gezeigt, daß die on-off-Neurone, welche bei Belichtung präexcitatorisch gehemmt werden, ein off-Zentrum besitzen. Diese on-off-Neurone verhalten sich im Kontrast genau wie die reinen off-Neurone. Bei Annäherung an die Dunkelgrenze wird im Hellfeld die präexcitatorische Hemmung zu einer Dauerhemmung, d. h. die Neurone reagieren dann wie reine off-Neurone. Im Dunkelfeld selbst kommt es zur üblichen Reaktionsumkehr mit maximaler Aktivierung an der Kontrastgrenze.

Die präexcitatorisch gehemmten on-off-Neurone unterscheiden sich danach von den reinen off-Neuronen durch eine intensivere Wirkung des antagonistischen Umfeldes. Dies zeigt sich daran, daß die off-Hemmung bei diffuser Belichtung durch die antagonistische on-Erregung der Randzone durchbrochen wird und diese Hemmung verstärkt werden kann, wenn man einen Teil des Umfeldes beschattet. Die stärkere Umfeldwirkung führt bei asymmetrischer Anordnung des receptiven Feldes bei den präexcitatorisch gehemmten on-off-Neuronen zu außergewöhnlichen asymmetrischen Aktivierungsverläufen im Kontrast. Ein solches Beispiel zeigt die Abb. 6. Es sind dort die Impulszahlen eines präexcitatorisch gehemmten on-off-Neurons, welches mit verschiedenen Hellfeldbreiten (5° 41′ und 1° 31′) untersucht wurde, in verschiedenen Gitterpositionen dargestellt.

Der mittlere horizontale Durchmesser der Feldzentren von 8 on-Zentrum-Neuronen des Corp. genic. lat. betrug 0,85 mm (0,63—0,97 mm). Die entsprechen-

302 G. BAUMGARTNER:

den Werte von 17 corticalen on-Zentrum-Neuronen waren 0,42 mm (0,18–0,68 mm).
4 off-Zentrum-Neurone des Corp. genic. lat. ergaben einen mittleren Durchmesser
von 0,73 mm (0,48–1,07 mm), 8 off-Zentrum-Neurone des Cortex 0,61 mm (0,27
bis 0,86 mm) (s. S. 47 und 49).

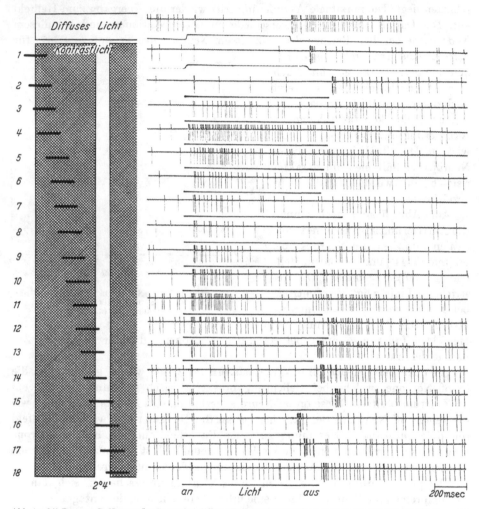

Abb. 4a. *Off-Zentrum-D-Neuron des Cortex* bei diffuser Belichtung und Kontrastlichtreiz (Hellfeld 2°4'). (Legende
s. Abb. 1 und 2 und Text)

Besprechung. Wie schon aus Untersuchungen von HUBEL (1960) (*13*) hervorgeht, sind die Tractusfasern und die Neurone des Corp. gen. lat. auf Lichtreize
stärker aktivierbar als die Neurone der Area 17. In dieser Versuchsserie wurden die
Geniculatum-Neurone nicht differenziert. Es kann sich bei ihnen deshalb zum
Teil auch um noch unverschaltete Tractusfasern gehandelt haben. Kontrollab-
leitungen der Radiatio optica ergaben aber keine Unterschiede.

Grundsätzlich verschieden verhalten sich in sämtlichen optischen Zentren
die on- und off-Zentrum-Neurone. Sie reagieren im Kontrast genauso entgegengesetzt wie bei diffuser Belichtung.

Ein weiterer Unterschied zwischen on-Zentrum-Neuronen des Cortex und denen des Tr. opt. und des Corp. genic. lat. ist die Größe der horizontalen Durchmesser ihrer receptiven Feldzentren, soweit sie durch die Kontrastmessung erfaßt werden. Wie oben berichtet, liegen die Durchmesserwerte des Cortex unter denen des Corp. genic. lat. und des Tractus. Unter der Voraussetzung, daß keine Faserselektion erfolgte, ergibt sich nach der *t*-Verteilung eine signifikante Differenz ($p < 0,01$) zwischen den Neuronen des Corp. genic. lat. und Cortex und des Tr. opt. und Cortex, während der Unterschied zwischen den Neuronen des Corp. genic. lat. und Tr. opt. danach zufällig ist (s. Tab. 1). Inwieweit auch bei den off-Zentrum-Neuronen eine Veränderung der Feldzentrum-

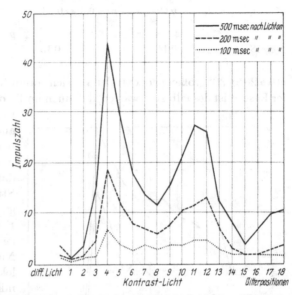

Abb. 4 b. Impulszahlen des Neurons in verschiedenen Gitterpositionen in den ersten 100, 200 und 500 msec nach Belichtung

Durchmesser erfolgt, muß auf Grund der bisherigen Messungen noch offenbleiben.

Die Größe der Feldzentren ist bekanntermaßen von der Lage der receptiven Feldzentren im Gesichtsfeld abhängig und nimmt nach zentral ab. Da die receptiven Felder der getesteten Neurone im Gesichtsfeld verschieden lokalisiert sind, ist es denkbar, daß wir cortical bevorzugt zentral gelegene Neurone und im Tr. opt. und Corp. genic. lat. peripherer repräsentierte Neurone registriert haben. Die Signifikanz der Tab. 1 ist deshalb noch nicht gesichert, da sie nur gilt, wenn keine Selektion erfolgte. Es ist jedoch wahrscheinlich, daß ihr ein echter Unterschied entspricht, da das gesamte ausgeleuchtete Gesichtsfeldgebiet nur 30° × 50° betrug und die untersuchten Neurone aus einem

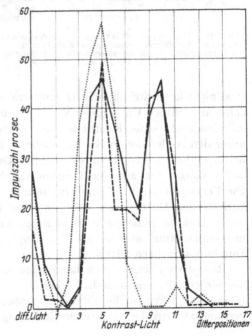

Abb. 5. *Kontrastaktivierung eines B-Neurons im visuellen Cortex:* Impulszahlen des corticalen on-Zentrum-Neurons in verschiedenen Gitterpositionen bei Kontrastbelichtungen mit breitem (5° 41′) und schmalem (2° 50′) Hellfeld. Die Impulszahlen sind jeweils über 500 msec nach Belichtung ausgezählt worden. Die gestrichelte Kurve zeigt die Kontrolle bei Rückbewegung des Kontrastgitters (-- = 5° 41′, … = 2° 50′)

Tabelle 1

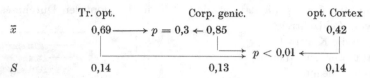

	Tr. opt.	Corp. genic.	opt. Cortex
$\bar{x}$	0,69 ⟶ $p = 0,3$ ⟵ 0,85		0,42
	⌞_____ ⌟ ⟶ $p < 0,01$ ⟵ ⌞		
S	0,14	0,13	0,14

etwa 20° × 30° großen perizentralen Bereich stammten. Bei dem Überwiegen zentraler Fasern ist deshalb zu erwarten, daß auch im Tr. opt. gelegentlich zentralere Neurone abgeleitet und umgekehrt auch corticale Neurone des mehr peripher gelegenen Gesichtsfeldes mit erfaßt wurden. Dafür spricht, daß wir auch cortical öfter durch Streulicht aktivierte Neurone registriert haben, deren receptive Felder sicher außerhalb des ausgeleuchteten Gesichtsfeldes lagen. Nicht auszuschließen ist eine Selektion nach Fasergröße. Es ist mir aber nicht bekannt, ob die Fasergröße mit der Feldgröße korreliert, d.h. ob ein statistischer Fehler in diesem Falle überhaupt möglich ist.

Unabhängig davon ist die Verkleinerung der Durchmesser der corticalen Feldzentren jedoch auf die jeweils kontrastaktiven Felder einzuschränken. Hubel und Wiesel (14) (1959) fanden nämlich die receptiven Felder cortical nicht konzentrisch, sondern längsoval mit beliebiger Orientierung der Längsachse angeordnet. Unter dieser Voraussetzung ist bei der Messung der Feldzentren mit einer senkrechten Kontrastgrenze eine *Selektion* von Neuronen zu erwarten, die unter den so definierten Kontrastbedingungen besonders deutlich reagieren. Das heißt, wir haben vermutlich bevorzugt die Durchmesser von Feldzentren gemessen, deren Längsachse mit der Richtung der Kontrastgrenze übereingestimmt hat. Die Verkleinerung der Feldzentrumsdurchmesser gilt also zunächst nur für den horizontalen Durchmesser von receptiven Feldern, deren Längsachse senkrecht angeordnet ist. Diese methodische Beschränkung ist aber auch für die Messungen im Geniculatum laterale und Tract. opt. anzunehmen, was den Vergleich der Durchmessergrößen erlaubt.

Receptive Felder, deren Längsachse mit der Richtung der Kontrastgrenze übereinstimmt, zeigen deshalb eine besonders starke Kontrastaktivierung, weil bei ihnen im Kontrast die Wirkung der antagonistischen Randzone am intensivsten vermindert wird. Da die laterale Hemmung und die laterale Aktivierung mit der

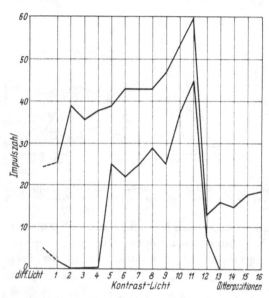

Abb. 6. Impulszahlen eines off-Zentrum-Neurons des Corp. gen. lat., welches bei diffuser Belichtung on-off-Reaktionen zeigt, bei Kontrastbelichtungen mit unterschiedlicher Hellfeldbreite (5°41′ und 1°31′; s. Text)

Entfernung abnehmen, können sie sich bei einem längsovalen receptiven Feld senkrecht zur Längsachse stärker auswirken. Es sind daher dann die größten Aktivierungsunterschiede zwischen Kontrast- und diffusen Lichtreizen zu erwarten, wenn die Richtung der Kontrastgrenze mit der Längsachse des receptiven Feldes übereinstimmt. Eine Verkleinerung des Zentrumdurchmessers, auch wenn sie nur funktionell ist, bedeutet eine Zunahme des antagonistischen Randzonenfeldes, was wiederum die Aktivierung im Kontrast gegenüber der Aktivierung bei diffuser Belichtung hervorhebt. Unter diesen Umständen muß aber auch die maximale Aktivierung an der Kontrastgrenze mit zunehmender Entfernung von der Kontrastgrenze steiler abfallen als bei den größeren und konzentrisch angeordneten Feldzentren des Tr. optic. und des Corp. genic. lat. Wie Abb. 7 zeigt, ist dies auch der Fall. In dieser Abbildung ist die Aktivität von 5 Tractusfasern, 6 Geniculatumneuronen und 7 corticalen Elementen in verschiedenen, aber unter sich gleichen Abständen von der Kontrastgrenze aufgezeichnet. Der Nullpunkt der Abszisse stimmt mit der Kontrastgrenze überein. Die Kontrastgrenze selbst ist willkürlich auf Grund der maximalen Aktivierung des Neurons festgelegt. Die Aktivierung in verschiedenen Abständen (Gitterpositionen) von der Kontrastgrenze ist in % der Maximalaktivität angegeben. Man sieht hier, daß der Abfall der Kontrastaktivierung bei corticalen Neuronen deutlich steiler ist als bei den Neuronen des Tr. opt. und des Corp. genic. lat.

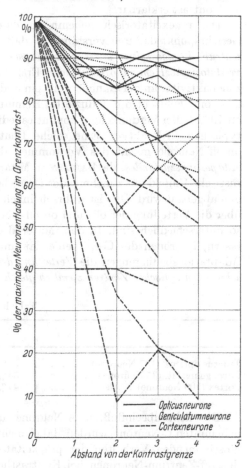

Ab. 7. Entladungszahlen von 5 on-Zentrum-Neuronen des Tractus opticus, 6 on-Zentrum-Neuronen des Corp. gen. lat. und 7 on-Zentrum-Neuronen des Cortex (Area 17) in verschiedenem Abstand von der Kontrastgrenze. Die maximale Entladungszahl in den ersten 500 msec nach Kontrastbelichtung wurde für das jeweilige Neuron als 100% gesetzt und darauf die Verminderung der Impulszahlen nach Verschiebung des Kontrastes bezogen. Die Einheit der Abszisse entspricht einer Verschiebung der Kontrastgrenze um 41'

Wir haben bisher meistens nur die horizontalen Durchmesser der receptiven Feldzentren untersucht und keine Gesamtfeldbestimmung vorgenommen, wie dies HUBEL (13) und WIESEL (14) für corticale Neurone und für Neurone des Corp. genic. lat. und Tractusfasern getan haben. Die von HUBEL und WIESEL (14) nachgewiesene Feldasymmetrie kommt aber auch dabei gut zum Ausdruck, sofern sie in bezug auf die senkrechte Kontrastgrenze auftritt. Bei präexcitatorisch gehemmten on-off-Neuronen wird dies besonders gut sichtbar.

Off-Feldzentren wurden bisher nicht ausreichend untersucht. Wir haben aber den Eindruck, daß die off-Feldzentren der präexcitatorisch gehemmten on-off-Neurone im Verhältnis zur antagonistischen Randzone kleiner sind als die Zentren der reinen off-Neurone. Damit wären das Überwiegen der Randzonenaktivität bei diesen Neuronen und die häufigen starken Asymmetrien des Aktivierungsverlaufes im Kontrast erklärbar.

Die präexcitatorisch gehemmten *on-off-Reaktionen* werden unter diesem Gesichtspunkt dadurch verständlich, daß sich bei diffuser Belichtung das *Feldzentrum infolge seines kürzeren Synapsenweges zunächst durchsetzt und die präexcitatorische Hemmung verursacht*. Erst danach trifft die antagonistische Randzonenaktivität an der Ganglienzelle ein und durchbricht infolge ihres Überwiegens die vom Feldzentrum induzierte Hemmung, d. h. sie verursacht den späten on-Effekt. Bei Verdunkelung kommt es lediglich zu der vom Zentrum gesteuerten typischen off-Reaktion. Eine solche Deutung der präexcitatorisch gehemmten on-off-Neurone macht das Vorkommen dieser Neurone zu einer *Funktion des Adaptationszustandes*, da BARLOW u. Mitarb. (*1*) gezeigt haben, daß das antagonistische Umfeld mit zunehmender Dunkeladaptation bis zum völligen Verschwinden abgebaut wird. Dies ist wahrscheinlich einer der Gründe, weshalb die Angaben über die Verteilung der off- und on-off-Neurone von Untersucher zu Untersucher so unterschiedlich sind. In dem Material dieser Versuchsserie war bei Opticusfasern, Neuronen des Corp. genic. lat. und corticalen Neuronen unter gleichen Adaptationsbedingungen die *Verteilung der lichtbeeinflußten Neurone in den verschiedenen optischen Zentren ziemlich gleich*.

Tabelle 2.

	on	off	präexcitat. gehemmte on-off
Tractus opticus (127 Neurone)	52%	15%	33%
Corp. genic. lat. (35 Neurone)	54%	17%	29%
Cortex (109 Neurone)	47% (B)	24% (D)	29% (E)

Die lichtunbeeinflußten A-Neurone und die seltenen licht- und dunkelgehemmten C-Neurone wurden dabei nicht berücksichtigt. Aus dem völlig übereinstimmenden Verhalten der präexcitatorisch gehemmten on-off-Neurone mit den off-Zentrum-Neuronen bei Kontrastlichtreizen geht hervor, daß es sich bei diesem Typ der on-off-Neurone um off-Zentrum-Neurone handelt. Wir nehmen deshalb an, daß die Informationsleistung der off-Zentrum-on-off-Neurone mit der der off-Zentrum-Neurone (D-Neurone) identisch ist. Ich bezeichne sie deshalb auch als *on-off-D-Neurone* entsprechend den dunkelmeldenden corticalen D-Neuronen. Ob ihnen zusätzlich eine Funktion bei der Wahrnehmung der Bewegungsrichtung zukommt, wozu sie besonders wegen ihrer starken, oft asymmetrischen Umfeldwirkung geeignet sind, wird zunächst offengelassen.

Die Diskriminationsleistung des Sehens für schwarze und weiße Objekte ist etwa die gleiche. Man muß deshalb für das on- und off-System vergleichbare informative Voraussetzungen fordern. Addiert man präexcitatorisch gehemmte on-off- und reine off-Zentrum-Neurone, so ergeben sich zwei weitgehend ausgeglichene Systeme von ungefähr je 50% die Information „heller" und 50% die

Information „dunkler" übertragenden Neuronen. Die Zuordnung der on-off-D-Neurone zum off-System scheint daher auch unter diesem Gesichtspunkt gerechtfertigt.

Gibt es aber off-Zentrum-Neurone, die bei relativem Überwiegen der Umfeldaktivität als on-off-D-Neurone reagieren, so sind auch on-Zentrum-Neurone zu erwarten, bei denen die Aktivität der Randzone überwiegt. Auch diese Neurone müssen on-off-Reaktionen zeigen. In diesem Falle darf es jedoch zu keiner präexcitatorischen Hemmung, sondern es muß nach kurzer Latenz durch die direkt durchgeschaltete on-Erregung des Zentrums zu einer Aktivierung und zu einer späten Hemmung bei Belichtung infolge der inhibitorischen Randzonenaktivität kommen. Die off-Aktivierung dagegen kann erst mit langer Latenz auftreten. Solche *on-off-B-Neurone* existieren, sie sind aber sehr selten (<1% im Tr. opt. und Cortex bei den von uns verwandten Lichtintensitäten), weshalb sie die Symmetrie des Systems nicht stören (s. S. 379). Wahrscheinlich sind sie eine Untergruppe der B-Neurone mit on-Zentrum und melden Helligkeit (B = brightness).

Die Interpretation der obigen Befunde geschah unter der Voraussetzung, daß die Katze farbenblind ist (MEYER, MILES, RATOOSH 1954) (*17*). Sofern das Farbensehen mit erwogen werden muß, werden die Verhältnisse entsprechend komplizierter. Doch ist die Diskriminationsleistung des Farbsehens nicht wesentlich von der des Hell-Dunkel-Sehens verschieden, und die Helligkeitskontrastphänomene sind auf die Farbenkontraste transponierbar. Es ist deshalb zu erwarten, daß auch im Bereich des Farbsehens Feldorganisationen analoger Art mit entsprechenden Farbpaaren (Gelb-Blau, Rot-Grün) existieren, was nach DE VALOIS' Untersuchungen (s. S. 182) wahrscheinlich ist.

Der hier verwandte Reizparameter war ein senkrechter simultaner Helligkeitskontrast. Es ist durchaus denkbar, daß durch kompliziertere Reizanordnungen funktionell anders integrierende Systeme gefunden werden, die von uns gar nicht erfaßt wurden.

Ferner können wir noch nicht ausreichend beurteilen, inwieweit die Veränderung des Intensitätsniveaus neue Gesichtspunkte ergibt. Da keine strenge Trennung der antagonistischen Bereiche innerhalb einer Feldorganisation anzunehmen ist, sondern diese als überlappend gedacht werden müssen (*1*), sind bei intensitätsgekoppelten Empfindlichkeitsverschiebungen Reaktionsveränderungen denkbar.

Auch im Geniculatum und im Cortex entsprechen die Aktivierungsmaxima der lichtaktivierten on-Zentrum-Neurone den Orten subjektiv maximaler *Kontrastaufhellung*. Entsprechend stimmen die Maxima der off-Zentrum-Neurone bei Belichtung mit den Orten subjektiv stärkster *Kontrastverdunkelung* überein. Es ist lange bekannt, daß die subjektive Kontrastinduktion vom Verhältnis der Lichtintensität der kontrastierenden Felder abhängt (*7, 12*). Auch diese Abhängigkeit ist neuronal zu erwarten. Obwohl wir bisher keine Versuche mit helligkeitsvariierten Kontrastfeldern gemacht haben, ist mit ziemlicher Sicherheit vorauszusagen, daß bei nicht völliger Abdunkelung bei Kontrastlichtreizen durch die nur partielle Reduktion der Randzonenaktivität im Dunkelfeldbereich Aktivierungsveränderungen auftreten, wie sie den subjektiven Erfahrungen entsprechen.

Die Reduktion der lateralen Hemmung der on-Zentrum-Neurone bzw. der lateralen Aktivierung der off-Zentrum-Neurone mit der Entfernung macht die Distanzabhängigkeit des Kontrastes verständlich (*9, 18*). Ferner entspricht, wie schon erwähnt, das relativ späte Auftreten der Kontrastempfindung dem Verhalten der Neurone (s. Abb. 1b, S. 47, und Abb. 4b). Das Zeitverhalten der neuronalen Kontrastverarbeitung vermag auch zu erklären, weshalb es trotz der subjektiven Aufhellung eines Lichtreizes gleicher Intensität bei intermittierender Applikation (brightness enhancement) zu keiner Verbesserung, sondern zu einer Verschlechterung der Diskriminationsleistung (8) kommt. Wenn, und das ist kaum zu bezweifeln, das optische Auflösungsvermögen von der Kontrastverschärfung mit abhängig ist, muß es schlechter sein, wenn die zeitliche Voraussetzung zur Entwicklung der Kontrastverschärfung nicht vorhanden ist.

1958 beschrieb Diamond (6) die Umkehrung des Pulfrich-Effektes durch Kontrastverdunkelung.

Die von Fertsch und Pulfrich beschriebene Vortäuschung (19) einer ellipsoiden bis kreisförmigen Bahn durch ein in einer Ebene parallel vor den Augen schwindendes Pendel, das gleichzeitig mit dem einen Auge direkt und mit dem anderen Auge durch ein neutrales Filter beobachtet wird, wird durch die verlängerte Empfindungszeit auf dem abgefilterten Auge erklärt. Dadurch wird der Erregungsablauf an den homonyme Gesichtsfeldstellen vertretenden Neuronen verändert, was eine Querdisparation mit entsprechender Bewegungstäuschung hervorruft.

Diamond (6) hat das bewegte Objekt vor dem einen Auge nicht durch Filter, sondern durch Kontrast verdunkelt und fand eine Umkehrung der Bewegungsrichtung. Das heißt, wenn eine Bewegung von links nach rechts bei einem Filter vor dem linken Auge eine Entfernung des Objektes verursacht, erscheint die gleiche Bewegung bei Kontrastverdunkelung als Annäherung.

Diamond hat daraus geschlossen, daß die Helligkeitsreduktion durch Kontrast und durch Intensitätsverminderung auf zwei prinzipiell verschiedene Mechanismen zurückzuführen ist. Dies wird durch das Kontrastverhalten der Neurone bestätigt. Gleichzeitig läßt sich dadurch diese Umkehrung einfach erklären. Verwendet man ein Filter vor einem Auge, so werden die Latenzen sämtlicher neuronalen Erregungen auf dem einen Auge verlängert. Bei der Verdunkelung durch Kontrast kommt es dagegen durch die Kontrastaktivierung zu einer Verkürzung sowohl der on- wie der off-Reaktionen, was die Umkehrung einfach erklärt und die oben angeführte übliche Deutung des Pulfrich-Effektes indirekt wahrscheinlich macht.

Das Verhalten der Neurone des visuellen Systems der Katze im Kontrast entspricht also einer Reihe von subjektiv sinnesphysiologischen Erfahrungen direkt, und die Parallelität ist so zwingend, daß man vermuten kann, daß ähnliche Mechanismen auch im visuellen Apparat des Menschen wirksam sind. Auch Schuberts (20) Nachweis der Kontrastbildung als einer Funktion des photopischen Sehens, die bei zunehmender Dunkeladaptation verlorengeht, spricht in dieser Richtung. Er stimmt mit dem von Barlow u. Mitarb. (1) nachgewiesenen Abbau der antagonistischen Randzone bei zunehmender Dunkeladaptation überein und unterstützt die Auffassung, daß der Feldantagonismus dem Simultankontrast zugrunde liegt. Es ist deshalb anzunehmen, daß der Mechanismus der Kontrastbildung auf die seit Hartline 1949 (10) am Limulus bekannte laterale Hemmung und die von Kuffler (15, 16) an der Katze zusätzlich beschriebene laterale Aktivierung zurückzuführen ist. Wie die Kontrastversuche zeigen, ist die laterale Hemmung des on-Systems allein für die Erklärung des Effektes nicht ausreichend. Für die Kontrastverdunkelung ist die laterale Aktivierung des off-Systems entscheidend.

Überträgt man die Ergebnisse dieser Untersuchungen auf das menschliche Sehen, dann erlaubt die „Hermannsche Gittertäuschung" (11) eine direkte Bestimmung der Durchmesser der Feldzentren beim Menschen (*2, 3*). Im Hermannschen Gitter sieht man eine *Verdunkelung* an den *Kreuzungsstellen eines weißen Gitters auf schwarzem Untergrund* und eine *Aufhellung der Kreuzungen eines dunklen Gitters* auf *hellem Grund*. Dieser Effekt *fehlt* bei mittlerem Objekt-Augenabstand im Bereich des *fovealen Sehens*. Die Verdunkelung an den Kreuzungsstellen der Hellbalken läßt sich neuronal dadurch erklären, daß in diesem Bereich die lichtaktivierten on-Elemente aus den Umfeldern vermehrt inhibitorische Impulse erhalten, da die Umfelder im Bereich der Kreuzungsstellen weniger beschattet werden. Die Aktivierung an den Kreuzungsstellen muß also geringer sein, das heißt die Kreuzungsstellen müssen als graue Punkte erscheinen. Die Aufhellung der Dunkelfelder ergibt sich umgekehrt durch die verminderte Aktivierung der off-Zentrum-Neurone an den Kreuzungsstellen infolge der dort ausgedehnteren Beschattung der aktivierenden Randzone. Dadurch wird bei Belichtung die on-Reaktion der off-Zentrum-Neurone weniger intensiv, das heißt die Kreuzungsstellen erscheinen weniger dunkel als die übrigen Schwarzbalkenbereiche.

Es ist bekannt, daß beim Betrachten des Hermannschen Gitters die Dunkelpunkte verschwinden, wenn man sie fixiert und daß sie um so deutlicher auftreten, je weiter im peripheren Gesichtsfeld sie gesehen werden. *Vergrößert man aber den Objektabstand, so tritt* in einer für verschiedene Versuchspersonen ziemlich definierten, von der Balkenbreite abhängigen Entfernung die *Verdunkelung auch im Fixierpunkt auf*. Sind unsere Voraussetzungen richtig, so besagt dies, daß die antagonistische Feldorganisation auch für die Fovea gilt, daß dort die receptiven Felder aber wesentlich *kleiner* sind als in den peripheren Gesichtsfeldbereichen. Denn es ist einleuchtend, daß dann eine Kreuzung keine Informationsänderungen hervorrufen kann, wenn die receptiven Felder im Verhältnis zu den Kreuzungspunkten so klein sind, daß für sie eine zusätzliche Umfeldhemmung keine Rolle spielt. *Aus der Balkenbreite und dem Objektabstand, bei dem* für einen bestimmten Gesichtsfeldbereich eine *Verdunkelung oder Aufhellung eintritt, läßt sich so die Größe der receptiven Felder in der Fovea bestimmen*. Dabei ist von der Voraussetzung auszugehen, daß die maximale Verdunkelung dann auftritt, wenn das zentral aktivierende Feld bei Hellneuronen der Balkenbreite entspricht und damit die Umfeldhemmung in der Kreuzung im Verhältnis zu der Hemmung im Balkenbereich ein Maximum erreicht. Sie muß bei weiterer Entfernung wieder abfallen, was sich auch subjektiv zeigen läßt. Die subjektive Verdunkelung an der Kreuzung beginnt schon früher, da eine verstärkte Umfeldhemmung schon bei geringerer Entfernung wirksam wird. Zur Bestimmung der Feldgröße ist jedoch nur die Entfernung bei maximaler Verdunkelung des Kreuzungspunktes verwendbar. Bestimmt man auf diese Weise die Sehwinkelgrößen der Kreuzungspunkte bei maximaler Verdunkelung im fovealen Bereich, so ergeben sich *Sehwinkelgrößen von 4—5'. Der Durchmesser eines fovealen Feldzentrums beträgt also etwa 20 μ.*

Dieses Beispiel zeigt, daß die Ergebnisse neuronaler Kontrastuntersuchungen auch auf die subjektive Sinnesphysiologie beim Menschen anwendbar sind.

Summary

1. Neurons of the lateral geniculate body and of the primary visual cortex were examined by the same contrast illumination method as previously used for retinal ganglion cells (v. p. 45) and the horizontal diameter of their receptive field center was determined by this method.

2. All visual neurons located in the geniculate and cortex responded in a similar way as did retinal ganglions cells. However, the activation frequency was markedly lower in cortical neurons than in neurons of the optic tract and of the lateral geniculate body. Further, on-field center diameters were considerably smaller in the horizontal plane for cortical B-neurons than for on-neurons of the optic tract and of the lateral geniculate body.

3. This smaller diameter of on-field centers in the cortex may indicate an additional *contrast sharpening effect at cortical neurons* if compared with HUBEL's results (same order of magnitude of the entire receptive field). Apparently lateral inhibition by the surrounding field may be more effective in cortical neurons, possibly by the elongated form of their receptive field (HUBEL u. WIESEL).

4. On-off-responding-neurons of the E-type with preexcitatory inhibition at light-on (called *on-off-D-neurons*) respond to light-off with shorter latency of activation and have always *off-center fields*. Their response under contrast conditions shows no essential difference to true or off-D-neurons. Those rare *on-off-B-neurons*, responding to light stimuli by on-activation of short latency always show a delayed off-activation. They probably have on-field centers. The type of response to diffuse illumination (on-, off-, or on-off) depends upon the preponderant excitation of its surrounding.

5. Amongst the population of visual neurons examined by contrast (127 optic tract fibers, 35 geniculate neurons and 109 cortical neurons) were approximately *50% on-center neurons and 50% off-center neurons*.

6. The neuronal mechanism of simultaneous brightness contrast can readily be explained by *lateral inhibition within the on-system*, and *lateral activation within the off-system*.

7. In the visual centers, as in the optic tract, the response of on- and off-center neurons under contrast stimulation conditions *corresponded exactly to the subjective perception of simultaneous contrast*, if activation of on-center neurons correlates with the information "brighter", activation of off-center neurons with "darker" in their receptive field centers.

8. By application of these rules to human vision the diameter of the receptive field center of visual neurons can be measured in man. For foveal vision in the human eye a diameter of 20 μ (4–5') was found.

Literatur

1. BARLOW, H. B., R. FITZHUGH and S. W. KUFFLER: Change of organization in the receptive fields of the cat's retina during dark adaptation. J. Physiol. (Lond.) 137, 338—354 (1957).
2. BAUMGARTNER, G.: Die neuronale Aktivität des visuellen Systems der Katze und ihre Beziehungen zur subjektiven Sinnesphysiologie. Habilitationsschrift Freiburg i. Br. 1960.
3. — Indirekte Größenbestimmung der receptiven Felder der Retina beim Menschen mittels der Hermannschen Gittertäuschung. Pflügers Arch. ges. Physiol. 272, 21 (1960).
4. — u. P. HAKAS: Reaktionen einzelner Opticusneurone und corticaler Nervenzellen der Katze im Hell-Dunkel-Grenzfeld (Simultankontrast). Pflügers Arch. ges. Physiol. 270, 29 (1959).
5. — — Vergleich der receptiven Felder einzelner On-Neurone des N. optic., des Corp. geniculat. lat. und des optischen Cortex der Katze. Zbl. ges. Neurol. Psychiat. 155, 243—244 (1960).
6. DIAMOND, A. L.: Simultaneous brightness contrast and the Pulfrich phenomenon. J. opt. Soc. Amer. 48, 887—890 (1958).

7. EBBINGHAUS, H.: Die Gesetzmäßigkeiten des Helligkeitskontrastes. S.-B. Akad. Wiss., Berlin 1887/2, 995—1009 (1887).
8. GERATHEWOHL, S. J., and W. F. TAYLOR: Effect of intermittent light on the readability of printed matter under condition of decreasing contrast. J. exp. Psychol. 46, 278—282 (1953).
9. HARMS, H., u. E. AULHORN: Studien über den Grenzkontrast. I. Ein neues Grenzphänomen. Albrecht v. Graefes Arch. Ophthal. 157, 400—415 (1955).
10. HARTLINE, H. K.: Inhibition of visual receptors by illuminating in the limulus eye. Fed. Proc. 8, 69 (1949).
11. HERMANN, L.: Eine Erscheinung des simultanen Kontrastes. Pflügers Arch. ges. Physiol. 3, 13—15 (1870).
12. HESS, C., u. H. PRETORI: Messende Untersuchungen über die Gesetzmäßigkeiten des simultanen Helligkeitskontrastes. Albrecht v. Graefes Arch. Ophthal. 40, IV, 1—24 (1894).
13. HUBEL, D. H.: Single unit activity on laterale geniculate body and optic tract of unrestrained cats. J. Physiol. (Lond.) 150, 91—104 (1960).
14. — and T. B. WIESEL: Receptive field of single neurons in the cats striate cortex. J. Physiol. (Lond.) 148, 574—591 (1959).
15. KUFFLER, S. W.: Neurons in the retina: organization, inhibition and excitation problems. Cold Spring Harbor Symposion on quantitative Biology 17, 281—292 (1952).
16. — Discharge patterns and functional organization of mammalian retina. J. Neurophysiol. 16, 37—69 (1953).
17. MEYER, D. R., R. C. MILES and PH. RATOOSH: Absence of color vision in cat. J. Neurophysiol. 17, 289—294 (1954).
18. MONJÉ, M.: Über die Lichtempfindlichkeit im Bereich des Rand- und des Binnenkontrastes. Pflügers Arch. ges. Physiol. 262, 92—106 (1955).
19. PULFRICH, C.: Die Stereoskopie im Dienste der isochromen und heterochromen Photometrie. Naturwissenschaften 10, 553—564 (1922).
20. SCHUBERT, G.: Foveale Helligkeitsschwelle und Simultankontrast. Albrecht v. Graefes Arch. Ophthal. 159, 60—65 (1957).

Diskussion

L. M. HURVICH: I think these are beautiful experiments. As I followed your analysis of the records along with the diagram of the position of the receptive field in relation to the black and white striped pattern I expected the impulse decrement to become greatest in the middle position because presumably there would now be interactive effects coming from both white stripes. This didn't materialize. However it seems to me that you have an ideal technique for evaluating the contrast effects of both the spatial and intensity parameters with your set-up.

W. SICKEL: Eine Verbesserung des Auflösungsvermögens für Tonhöhenunterschiede auf zentralen Stationen wird in Einklang mit den Mikroelektrodenbefunden KATSUKIs durch die Koincidenz-Siebschaltung (Zusammenfassung direkter und verzögerterInformation—TEUBNER, Tübingen) befriedigend nachgebildet. Anfrage, inwieweit dieses Modell eine brauchbare Vorstellung für die hier gezeigten Befunde liefert.

R. JUNG: KATSUKI[1] hat im akustischen System gefunden, daß die Einengung und Verschärfung zwar auf den unteren Stationen bis zum Tectum auftritt, aber *nicht im Cortex*, wo die akustischen receptiven Felder wieder breiter werden. Das ist ein prinzipieller Unterschied zwischen BAUMGARTNERs Befunden im optischen System und KATSUKIs im akustischen. Im sensiblen System hat MOUNTCASTLE[2] wiederum ähnliche Befunde mit lateraler Hemmung im Thalamus und Cortex festgestellt.

1. KATSUKI, Y., J. SUMI, H. UCHIYAMA and T. WATANABE: Electric responses of auditory neurons in cat to sound stimulation. J. Neurophysiol. 21, 569—588 (1958).
2 MOUNTCASTLE, V. B., and T. P. S. POWELL: Neural mechanisms subserving cutaneous sensibility, with special reference to the role of afferent inhibition in sensory perception and discrimination. Bull. Johns Hopk. Hosp. 105, 201—232 (1959).

Fast alle funktionellen Charakteristiken des visuellen Systems sind durch zwei einfache Prinzipien zu erklären: 1. Die laterale Hemmung synergistischer Neurone, die zur Bildverschärfung und zum Simultankontrast führt, und 2. die reziproke Hemmung antagonistischer Neurone, des B- und D-Systems. B bedeutet Belichtung oder Helligkeit, D Dunkelheit und beide hemmen sich gegenseitig offenbar auf allen Stationen von der Retina über das Geniculatum bis zum Cortex. Ich halte es für möglich, daß auch die von BAUMGARTNER gefundene Verkleinerung der corticalen Feldzentren *durch laterale Hemmung im Cortex* entsteht, die in den beiden reziproken Neuronensystemen B und D zur Wirkung kommt. Dadurch wird eine weitere Kontrastverschärfung im Cortex erreicht, wie schon TSCHERMAK 1903 postuliert hat.

H. BARLOW: I would like to ask a question about these very interesting results and also to make a comment about Professor JUNG's interpretation. First, if I have understood correctly, you find that the central zone of the receptive field is considerably smaller in the cortical neurons than it is when recording from optic nerve or geniculate neurons. Can you really be sure that you are recording from comparable regions from the visual field ? I can imagine great difficulties in being sure on this point, and there are other possible sources of error. For instance when isolating a nerve fibre you might tend to pick a big one connecting to a big receptive field, or when penetrating the cortex you might first encounter cells which connect ultimately to small retinal ganglion cells.

My comment on the interpretation of your results is this. Professor JUNG suggests that they can be explained by further lateral inhibition occurring in the cortex. The trouble with this explanation is that if you repeat the transformation effected by lateral inhibition you do not get more and better lateral inhibition, but some very strange things happen instead. Imagine a border separating black and white areas and consider the impulse frequencies in a row of "on" centre units crossing from black to white. Their discharge frequencies will be medium (spontaneous), low (inhibition), high (excited), medium (excited and inhibited). After a repeat of the transformation a similar row would be medium, high, low, high, low, medium. So you would get multiple fringes at borders, not enhanced contrast. There is something here that needs further thought.

F. BREMER: Has Dr. BAUMGARTNER any idea of the respective importance of the retinal, subcortical and cortical seats of the inhibitory mechanisms involved in the beautiful contrasted effects he has shown us. As he knows, the direct evidence for active inhibitory effects at the cortical level, especially the demonstration of neurone hyperpolarization, is still rather scanty.

The complexity which the visual contrast effects may show has been revealed by LETTVIN's neurophysiological experiments on the frog's optic lobe. There, the effect of a curvilinear lightshadow contrast on the retina was striking, while a rectilinear contrast was without effect! My colleague JUNG and I could see this surprising phenomenon when we visited McCULLOCH's and LETTVIN's laboratory last year, in Boston.

G. BAUMGARTNER (zu BARLOW): Wir konnten bisher keine korrespondierenden Neurone von Retina, Geniculatum und Cortex vergleichen. Die receptiven Felder der in diesen Versuchen ausgewerteten Neurone des Tract. opt. des Geniculatum und des Cortex lagen aber innerhalb eines perizentralen Gesichtsfeldbereiches von $20° \times 30°$. Bei dem Überwiegen perizentraler Fasern sollte man deshalb erwarten, daß auch an Neuronen des Tract. opt. oder des Geniculatum für manche Felder kleine Durchmesser festzustellen sind. Dies war nicht der Fall.

Es ist nicht bekannt, ob die Größe der rezeptiven Felder mit den Durchmessern der entsprechenden Opticusfasern positiv korreliert. Vom zentralen zum peripheren Gesichtsfeld vergrößert sich der Felddurchmesser ziemlich kontinuierlich. Dagegen gruppiert sich die Leitungsgeschwindigkeit der Opticusfasern um drei deutlich differente Maxima. Es ist deshalb nicht möglich, den Faserdurchmesser einfach mit der Feldgröße in Beziehung zu setzen.

Allein durch eine verstärkte laterale Hemmung im Cortex ist, wie Dr. BARLOW feststellt, eine Verbesserung des Grenzkontrastes nicht zu erklären. Doch ist zu berücksichtigen, daß 1. cortical eine Umorganisation der konzentrischen peripheren Felder in *längsovale rezeptive* Felder erfolgt, wie HUBEL und WIESEL gezeigt haben und daß 2. die laterale Hemmung distanzabhängig ist. Infolge der Distanzabhängigkeit der lateralen Hemmung ist ein exponentieller Anstieg der Aktivierung der on-Zentrum-Neurone bei Annäherung an die Kontrastgrenze zu erwarten. Das gilt in ähnlicher Weise schon für die Retina. Die corticalen Felder werden aber durch ihre längsovale Anordnung für Kontrastgrenzen, die senkrecht zur Längsachse ihrer rezeptiven Felder verlaufen, zusätzlich besonders kontrastaktiv. Denn bei ihnen kommt es im Grenzkontrast zur Beschattung einer maximal großen, dem Feldzentrum dicht benachbarten Hemmungsfläche. Der Anstieg des Aktivierungsverlaufes bei Annäherung an die Kontrastgrenze muß daher steiler werden. Das läßt sich experimentell zeigen.

Gegenüber den Feldvermessungen mit Lichtpunkten kann die Kontrastmethode eine funktionelle Verkleinerung der Feldzentrumsdurchmesser ergeben. Denn bei breitem Hellfeld, welches zur Messung der Felder meist verwendet wurde (s. Abb. 2a), wird die laterale Hemmung im Grenzkontrast nur an *einer* Seite des rezeptiven Feldes durch Beschattung aufgehoben. An der anderen Seite bleibt das hemmende Umfeld belichtet. Dadurch könnte eine stärkere Verkleinerung der corticalen Felddurchmesser gegenüber denen der Retina bzw. des Geniculatum verursacht werden, da die laterale Hemmung parallel zur Längsachse der receptiven Felder cortical ein Maximum erreicht. Dies kann die Unterschiede zwischen den Befunden von HUBEL und WIESEL und unseren Messungen erklären. Für die normale Kontrastbildung sind aber Flächenkontraste wie die von mir verwendeten wichtiger als Punktlichtreize.

(Zu BREMER): Obwohl ein direkter Nachweis einer zentralen Hemmung, wie Prof. BREMER betont, noch fehlt, ist am Vorkommen zentraler Hemmungsmechanismen meines Erachtens kaum zu zweifeln. Ohne eine zentrale Hemmung wäre beispielsweise nicht zu verstehen, wie ein durch unspezifische Reizung im Dunkeln aktiviertes Neuron durch Licht gehemmt werden kann. Es ist in diesem Falle nicht anzunehmen, daß die Aktivierung sekundär über spezifische Afferenzen erfolgt, die durch Licht blockiert werden. Außerdem kann man häufiger beobachten, daß lokal ausgelöste Verletzungsentladungen von corticalen off-(D-) Neuronen durch Licht gehemmt werden. Auch dies ist nur durch die Existenz einer corticalen Hemmung verständlich, da nicht einzusehen ist, weshalb eine lokal ausgelöste hochfrequente Entladung durch Wegfall einer geringen aus der Peripherie ankommenden spontanen Aktivierung blockiert werden sollte.

(Zu SICKEL): Es ist wahrscheinlich, daß für die visuelle Information nicht nur Ortswerte, sondern auch Zeitwerte von Bedeutung sind und die Zusammenfassung von direkter und verzögerter Information eine große Rolle spielt. Wie dies geschieht, weiß ich nicht. Ich kann deshalb auch nicht sagen, inwieweit das Teubner-Modell brauchbaren Modellcharakter hat.

(Zu HURVICH): Den von Dr. HURVICH postulierten Effekt verminderten Mittelkontrasts bei größerer Spaltbreite im Vergleich zu schmalen Streifen zeigt die Abb. 5.

Reaktionsmuster einzelner Neurone in Geniculatum laterale und visuellen Cortex der Katze bei Reizung mit optokinetischen Streifenmustern*

Von

O.-J. GRÜSSER** und URSULA GRÜSSER-CORNEHLS**

Mit 5 Abbildungen

Wird ein ruhender Lichtreiz bewegt, so treten in der Wahrnehmung zwei neue Qualitäten auf: die Richtung und die Geschwindigkeit der Bewegung. Aus den bisher bekannten Daten über die Funktion der Neurone des visuellen Systems kann man sich zunächst 3 Möglichkeiten für die Informationsvermittlung dieser beiden neuen Größen in der Wahrnehmung denken:

* Aus der Abteilung für klinische Neurophysiologie der Universität Freiburg i. Br.
** Nervenklinik der Universität Göttingen. Mit Unterstützung der Deutschen Forschungsgemeinschaft.

1. Der Bewegungseindruck ergibt sich durch die zeitliche Folge der Aktivierung verschiedener Neurone, die verschiedenen Gesichtsfeldpunkten zugeordnet sind.

2. Die Bewegungsrichtung und die Geschwindigkeit äußern sich im Entladungsmuster der visuellen Neurone.

3. Es gibt spezifische „Bewegungsneurone", die auf unbewegte Licht- und Dunkelreize nicht reagieren.

Doty (4) und Whitteridge (11) haben in diesem Symposion gezeigt, daß eine relativ strenge retino-corticale Punkt-zu-Punkt-Projektion besteht. Daraus kann geschlossen werden, daß das in der Hypothese 1 Ausgesagte eine Rolle spielt, da Bewegungseindrücke subjektiv schon zustande kommen, wenn zwei unbewegte kurze Lichtreize kurz nacheinander auf verschiedenen Netzhautstellen wahrgenommen werden (Phi-Phänomen von Wertheimer).

Um die Hypothesen 1—3 zu prüfen, wurden 30 Neurone im Geniculatum laterale und 75 Neurone im visuellen Cortex registriert und ihr Verhalten auf *bewegte Hell-Dunkel-Streifenmuster* geprüft. Wie bei den Reizen zur Auslösung eines optokinetischen Nystagmus beim Menschen (9) wechselten Hell- und Dunkelstreifen in kontinuierlicher Folge ab.

Methodik

11 Katzen in encephale isolé-Präparation nach Bremer, zusätzlich Curarin zur Unterdrückung von Augenbewegungen, künstliche Beatmung, Rotlichtbestrahlung, Effortil zur Blutdruckregulation. Horizontale Lagerung.

Registrierung mit Mikropipetten unter 1 μ Spitzendurchmesser, 3-m-KCl- oder 4-n-NaCl-Lösung, imperative Eingangsstufe nach Tönnies, übliche CW-Verstärkung, Mehrfachkathodenstrahloszillograph, Recordine-Kamera.

Lichtreizung: Um eine Wolframfadenlampe rotierte eine doppelte Zylindertrommel mit streifenförmigen Öffnungen. Projektion dieser Zylindertrommelstreifen auf eine 30 cm vor den Augen angebrachte Mattscheibe, die 60 Grad breit und etwa 50 Grad hoch war. Die Geschwindigkeit der auf diese Mattscheibe projizierten Hell-Dunkel-Streifen konnte durch ein Getriebe am Motor der Zylindertrommel in 3 Stufen reguliert werden. Das Hell-Dunkel-Verhältnis des Streifenmusters war durch Verdrehen der beiden Zylindertrommeln gegeneinander zwischen 1:2 und 2:1 beliebig regelbar. Die Beleuchtungsstärke konnte durch einen, der Wolframfadenlampe vorgeschalteten Widerstand reguliert werden, jedoch wurde davon nur wenig Gebrauch gemacht, da sich dadurch die spektrale Zusammensetzung änderte.

Zwei Arten der Lichtreizung wurden benützt: Bei einem Drittel der Neurone wurden die bewegten Hell-Dunkel-Muster auf die ganze Mattscheibe projiziert. Bei den übrigen Neuronen wurde, um Symmetriebedingungen zu erreichen, folgendes Verfahren angewandt: Zunächst wurde mit Hilfe von vertikalen und horizontalen verschiebbaren Blenden das receptive „Feldzentrum" (on- oder off-Aktivierung) bestimmt. Eine Maske, die einen kreisrunden Ausschnitt von 21 Winkelgraden hatte, wurde dann so auf der Mattscheibe angebracht, daß das Feldzentrum des registrierten Neurons in der Mitte des runden Ausschnittes lag. Die Genauigkeit der Bestimmung des Feldzentrums und der „Zentrierung" des runden Reizfeldes (Maskenausschnitt) relativ zum Feldzentrum war mit einer Fehlerbreite von $\pm$ 2 Grad möglich. Senkrecht zur Bewegungsrichtung waren am Rand des runden Reizfeldes 2 etwa 2 mm breite Photodioden angebracht, die den Ein- und Austritt der Hell- bzw. Dunkelstreifen ins Reizfeld anzeigten. Beide Photozellen wurden getrennt registriert, so daß aus ihren Ausschlägen ermittelt werden konnte, wann der Licht- oder Dunkelreiz die Mitte des Reizfeldes erreicht hatte, wie groß die Winkelgeschwindigkeit der Streifenmuster und das Hell-Dunkel-Verhältnis sowie die Winkelbreite der Streifen (jeweils gemessen in Relation zum Katzenauge) war.

8 verschiedene Bewegungsrichtungen konnten durch Kippung des rotierenden Zylinders untersucht werden: Oben, unten, links und rechts horizontal, links und rechts schräg nach oben,

links und rechts schräg nach unten, jeweils um 45 Grad gegen die vertikale bzw. horizontale Bewegungsrichtung geneigt.

Die registrierten Neuronenreaktionen wurden quantitativ ausgewertet, indem die mittlere Entladungsfrequenz aus 10—20 Reizantworten bestimmt wurde. Soweit erforderlich wurden unterschiedliche Reaktionen bei verschiedenen Bewegungsrichtungen statistisch auf Signifikanz geprüft.

Bei den meisten registrierten Neuronen wurde der Reaktionstyp auf unbewegte Lichtreize geprüft. Es wurde dazu ein Strahlengang des an anderer Stelle beschriebenen binocularen Lichtreizgerätes (3) auf das Reizfeld projiziert. Zur Bestimmung des Reaktionstyps wurden Lichtreize von 0,5—1 sec Dauer angewandt. Die Leuchtdichte betrug etwa 600 asb.

Ergebnisse

1. Spezifische „Bewegungsneurone"? Zur Prüfung der Frage, ob spezifische „Bewegungsneurone" registriert werden können, muß die Art und Weise, wie die Neurone im Versuch ausgewählt wurden, berücksichtigt werden. Die Feldzentren sämtlicher untersuchten Neurone lagen innerhalb eines Radius von etwa 15 Winkelgraden um das foveale Gebiet. Dies bedeutet eine erhebliche Selektion der Neurone und damit eine Einschränkung der Gültigkeit der Resultate für das foveale und parafoveale Sehen.

Die überwiegende Mehrheit wurde in den einzelnen Experimenten bei gleichzeitiger Reizung beider Augen mit bewegten Streifenmustern durch Bewegungen der Mikroelektrode mit Hilfe eines Mikromanipulators gesucht. Durch Abdecken des linken oder des rechten Auges mit einer Metallblende wurde festgestellt, von welchem Auge her die „dominante Aktivierung" erfolgte. Das nicht dominante Auge blieb dann mit der Blende abgedeckt; die weitere Untersuchung erfolgte monocular über das dominante Auge. Alle Neurone, die in dieser Arbeit verwertet wurden, gehörten den, dem ipsi- oder kontralateralen Auge zugeordneten, „dominanten Neuronensystemen" mit keinen oder nur schwachen binocularen Effekten (s. GRÜSSER-CORNEHLS u. GRÜSSER) an. Binocular aktivierte Neurone wurden in dieser Serie nicht untersucht.

Nachdem im Versuch das dominante Auge ermittelt wurde, erfolgte die Bestimmung der Lage des Zentrums des receptiven Feldes und die Bestimmung des Reaktionstyps auf unbewegte Lichtreize.

Sämtliche Neurone, die auf bewegte Streifenmuster reagierten, konnten auch durch unbewegte Hell-Dunkel-Reize aktiviert werden.

Eine Minderheit der Neurone wurde während langsamer Flimmerbelichtung (1—3 pro sec) der Mattscheibe gesucht. Diese Neurone wurden anschließend mit bewegten Hell-Dunkel-Streifen getestet. *Sämtliche Neurone waren auch in dieser Folge durch beide Reizarten zu aktivieren.*

Unter den angegebenen Reizbedingungen (encephale isolé-Präparationen, Helladaptation, photopische Beleuchtungsstärken, foveale und parafoveale Gesichtsfeldausschnitte) konnten also *keine spezifischen Bewegungsneurone* im Geniculatum oder visuellen Cortex gefunden werden.

2. Das Entladungsmuster auf bewegte und unbewegte Lichtreize. Die Neurone *des on-Systems* (on-Neurone bzw. B-Neurone) im Geniculatum und im visuellen Cortex reagierten auf den unbewegten Lichtreiz mit einer initial meist frequenten Aktivierung, die mit längerer Dauer des Lichtreizes abnahm (*10*). Bei „Licht aus" folgte eine Hemmung, an die sich bei einem Teil der Neurone eine Nachaktivierung anschloß. Durch bewegte Hell-Dunkel-Streifen wurden die on-(B-) Neurone aktiviert, wenn das Feldzentrum erhellt, gehemmt, wenn es dunkel war. Die Dauer der Aktivierung entsprach der Breite der Hellstreifen. Während der Zeit, in welcher der Dunkelstreifen das receptive Feld bedeckte, wurden die Neurone gehemmt. Einige on-Neurone hatten nach der initialen Dunkelhemmung während der Dunkelphase eine Nachaktivierung.

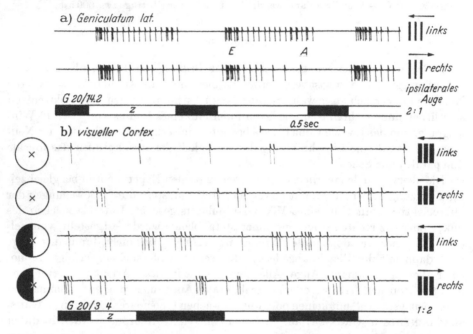

Abb. 1a. *On-Neuron* im Geniculatum laterale (G 20/14,2). Hell-Dunkel-Verhältnis 2:1, rundes Reizfeld 21° Durchmesser. Streifengeschwindigkeit 26° 16′ sec⁻¹. Dauer der Hell-Dunkel-Periode: 0,8 sec = 23°. Die Streifenbewegung nach links ergibt eine geringere „Eintrittsaktivierung" (E) als die Streifenbewegung nach rechts. Beim Austritt des Lichtreizes aus dem receptiven Feld folgt bei Bewegung nach links ein erneuter Anstieg der Entladungsfrequenz (A), der bei der Bewegung nach rechts fehlt. Die Hell-Dunkel-Streifen sind wie in sämtlichen anderen Abbildungen so eingezeichnet, daß sie die Belichtungsverhältnisse im *Zentrum des Reizfeldes*, also auch etwa im Zentrum des receptiven Feldes des registrierten Neurons wiedergeben

Abb. 1b. *On-off-Neuron (E-Typ)* im visuellen Cortex. Hell-Dunkel-Verhältnis 1:2, Streifengeschwindigkeit 26° 16′sec⁻¹, Periodendauer 0,8 sec = 23°, Reizfelddurchmesser 21°. Werden die Streifenmuster auf das ganze Reizfeld projiziert, so erfolgt bei Bewegung nach horizontal links oder rechts nur eine schwache Reaktion. Jedoch deutlicher Unterschied bei den verschiedenen Bewegungsrichtungen. Wird das linke Halbfeld abgedeckt, das Feldzentrum des Neurons also in eine Kontrastsituation gebracht, so erfolgt auf die bewegten Hell-Dunkel-Reize eine stärkere Aktivierung, die jedoch wiederum eine deutliche Differenz zwischen links und rechts ergibt

Die Entladungsfrequenz der Hellaktivierung verminderte sich mit der Dauer der Belichtung des receptiven Feldes, jedoch löste der Austritt des Hellstreifens aus dem receptiven Feld bei einem Teil der on-Neurone eine zweite Aktivierungsphase aus. Diese sei „Austrittsaktivierung" genannt. Die Entladungsfrequenz der Austrittsaktivierung war immer geringer als die Entladungsfrequenz der „Eintrittsaktivierung" (s. Abb. 1a und 2a).

Das Auftreten einer Austrittsaktivierung war nach den Resultaten von Baumgartner (1, 2) über Simultankontrasterregung mit unbewegten Streifenmustern an den visuellen Neuronen zu erwarten.

Die Neurone des *off-Systems* (on-off- und off-Neurone bzw. D- und E-Neurone) wurden durch die bewegten Streifenmuster ebenfalls analog zu ihren Reaktionsmustern auf unbewegte Licht- oder Dunkelreize aktiviert. Ein reines off-Neuron wurde in der Regel dann aktiviert, wenn der Dunkelreiz das receptive Feldzentrum bedeckte und gehemmt, wenn der Lichtreiz sich über das Feldzentrum bewegte. Einige Neurone, die auf den unbewegten Lichtreiz mit einer reinen off-Aktivierung und einer Hemmung während des Lichtreizes antworteten, reagierten auf die bewegten Streifenmuster mit einer on-off-Aktivierung. Die Entladungsmuster dieser Neurone waren dann in der Regel richtungsabhängig.

3. **Der Einfluß des Hell-Dunkel-Verhältnisses der bewegten Streifenmuster.** Das Hell-Dunkel-Verhältnis der optokinetischen Reize konnte zwischen 1:2 und 2:1 variiert werden. Die Winkelgröße der Hell-Dunkel-Periode lag zwischen 18° und 26°. Das Hell-Dunkel-Verhältnis beeinflußte die Entladungsmuster der Neurone bei sonst gleichen Reizbedingungen (Bewegungsrichtung und Geschwindigkeit). Die Stärke der Eintritts- und Austrittsaktivierung war vom Hell-Dunkel-Verhältnis abhängig. Die Eintrittsaktivierung war in der Regel um so stärker, je länger die Dunkelphase relativ zur Hellphase (Abb. 2a) war. Die Austrittsaktivierung verhielt sich bei einigen Neuronen umgekehrt und war um so frequenter, je mehr die Dauer der Lichtperiode relativ zur Dunkel-Periode erhöht wurde.

Bei den Neuronen des off-Systems beeinflußte das Hell-Dunkel-Verhältnis die off-Aktivierung und die postinhibitorische on-Aktivierung. Der Einfluß der Änderung des Hell-Dunkel-Verhältnisses waren jedoch von Neuron zu Neuron verschieden. Bis jetzt konnte noch keine allgemeine Regel für den Einfluß des Hell-Dunkel-Verhältnisses auf die Aktivierung der Neurone des off-Systems gefunden werden.

4. **Die Geschwindigkeit der bewegten Streifenmuster.** Diese wurde zwischen 7° sec^{-1} und 32° sec^{-1} variiert. Sie beeinflußte ebenfalls das Entladungsmuster der untersuchten Neurone. Bei der Mehrheit der Neurone des on- und off-Systems erhöhte sich die Entladungsfrequenz in den Aktivierungsphasen mit Zunahme der Streifengeschwindigkeit. Einzelne Neurone zeigten jedoch das gegenteilige Verhalten vor allem in den initialen Aktivierungsphasen.

5. **Die Bewegungsrichtung.** 8 verschiedene Bewegungsrichtungen (s. Methodik) konnten untersucht werden, jedoch wurden nur bei einem kleinen Teil der Neurone alle Bewegungsrichtungen geprüft.

Die Neurone des *on-Systems* (Abb. 1a) einschließlich der corticalen B-Neurone (Abb. 2a) wurden in der Regel in ihren Entladungsmustern nur wenig von der Änderung der Bewegungsrichtung beeinflußt. Die Entladungsfrequenz der Eintritts- oder der Austrittsaktivierung variierte meist nur wenig mit dem Wechsel der Bewegungsrichtung. Die Austrittsaktivierung einiger Neurone war jedoch von der Bewegungsrichtung abhängig. Das in Abb. 1a gezeigte Neuron hatte z. B. bei horizontaler Bewegung der Streifenmuster nach links eine deutliche Austrittsaktivierung, die bei der Bewegung horizontal nach rechts fehlte. In dieser Richtung war jedoch die Eintrittsaktivierung dafür stärker ausgeprägt. Solche Differenzen ließen sich statistisch sichern.

In einzelnen Fällen war die Nachaktivierung der on-Neurone während der Dunkelperiode von der Bewegungsrichtung zu beeinflussen und trat dann nicht bei allen untersuchten Bewegungsrichtungen auf. Dies war vor allem der Fall, wenn das Hell-Dunkel-Verhältnis 1:2 betrug.

Insgesamt kann jedoch gesagt werden, daß die Entladungsmuster der Neurone des on-Systems im Geniculatum und visuellen Cortex eine relativ hohe Richtungsunabhängigkeit hatten.

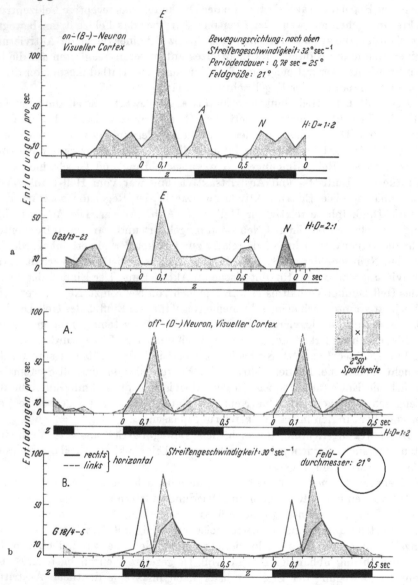

Abb. 2a. Abhängigkeit der Entladungsfrequenz eines *on-(B)-Neurons* im visuellen Cortex der Katze vom Hell-Dunkel-Verhältnis der bewegten Streifenmuster. Abszisse: Zeit in sec, Ordinate: Entladungsfrequenz (pro sec), Bewegungsrichtung vertikal nach oben. Streifengeschwindigkeit 32° sec⁻¹. Periodendauer 0,78 sec = 25°, Feldgröße 21°. Die „Eintrittsaktivierung", wenn ein Lichtreiz das receptorische Feld erreicht hat, ist bei relativ längerer Dunkelphase größer. Deutliche „Austrittsaktivierung".

Abb. 2b. *Off-Neuron (D-Typ)* im visuellen Cortex (G 18/4—5). Horizontale Bewegung nach links und rechts, Hell-Dunkel-Verhältnis 1:2, Streifengeschwindigkeit 30° sec⁻¹. Dauer der Hell-Dunkel-Periode 0,75 sec = 22° 30'. Wird das Reizfeld auf einen Spalt von 2° 50' verengt (A), so ergeben sich bei Bewegungen nach rechts und nach links keine differenten Reaktionen. Wird das übliche Reizfeld von 21° Durchmesser benützt, so unterscheidet sich die Reaktion bei der Bewegung der Streifenmuster nach links und nach rechts (B). Ordinate: Entladungsfrequenz, Abszisse: Zeit in sec

Die Neurone des *off-Systems* (off- und on-off- bzw. D- und E-Neurone) unter-schieden sich von den Neuronen des on-Systems hinsichtlich der Abhängigkeit der Entladungsmuster von der Bewegungsrichtung der Hell-Dunkel-Streifen. Nur ein kleiner Teil der Neurone des off-Systems war im Entladungsmuster relativ

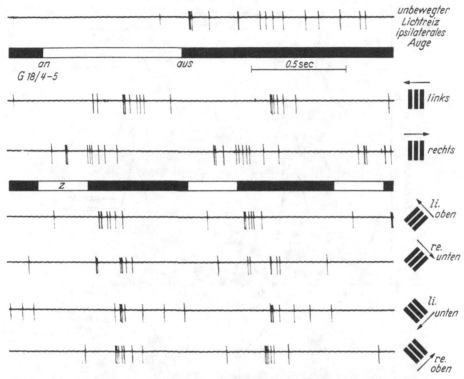

Abb. 3. *Off-Neuron (D-Typ)* im visuellen Cortex (G 18/4—5). Reizfeldgröße 21°. Auf unbewegten Lichtreiz reine off-Aktivierung. Bewegte Hell-Dunkel-Streifen (Geschwindigkeit 30° sec⁻¹, Periodendauer 0,86 sec = 26°) lösen je nach Bewegungsrichtung verschieden gruppierte off-Reaktionen aus. Anmerkung b. d. Korrektur: Die 3. Reihe (Bewegung nach rechts) wurde irrtümlich falsch abgebildet. Die Reihe muß um 7,5 mm nach rechts verschoben gedacht werden.

richtungskonstant. Diese Neurone waren dann meist „reine" off-Neurone (D-Neurone), die sowohl auf unbewegte Lichtreize mit einer on-Hemmung und off-Aktivierung reagierten, als auch auf Bewegungsreize nur dann aktiviert wurden, wenn sich der Dunkelstreifen durch das receptive Feldzentrum bewegte.

Die Mehrheit der Neurone des off-Systems war jedoch im Entladungsmuster auf optokinetische Reize „richtungslabil", wobei in der Regel sich der Einfluß der Bewegungsrichtung außer in der off-Aktivierung auch in einer Änderung der Dauer der on-Hemmung und der postinhibitorischen on-Aktivierung äußerte. Beispiele für solche Neurone sind in Abb. 4 und 5 gezeigt. Das Verhältnis der on- zur off-Aktivierung sowie die Gruppierung der Entladung und die Dauer der Aktivierungs-phasen waren bei diesen Neuronen richtungsabhängig.

Neurone, die auf unbewegte Lichtreize nach dem on-off-Typ (E-Neurone) re-agierten, waren bevorzugt richtungslabil. Jedoch ergab sich auch bei Neuronen mit „reiner" off-Reaktion auf unbewegte Lichtreize eine Abhängigkeit der Entladungs-muster von der Bewegungsrichtung

Vergleicht man das Verhalten der Neurone des on- und des off-Systems miteinander, so ergab sich aus unseren Befunden der Eindruck, daß die Neurone des off-Systems in ihren Entladungsmustern deutlich mehr von der Richtung der bewegten Hell-Dunkel-Reize abhängig waren als die Neurone des on-Systems.

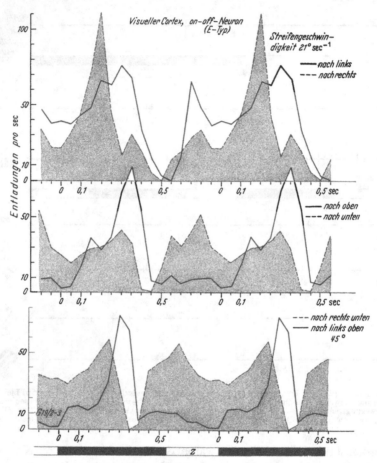

Abb. 4. Quantitative Auswertung (Mittelwerte aus jeweils 15 Reaktionen) der Entladungsmuster eines *on-off-* *(E)-Neurons* im visuellen Cortex. Hell-Dunkel-Verhältnis des Streifenmusters 1:2. Streifengeschwindigkeit 21° sec⁻¹. Periodendauer 0,8 sec = 17°. Ordinate: jeweils Entladungsfrequenz (pro sec), Abszisse: Zeit in Sekunden. Dieses Neuron läßt eine deutlicheDifferenz der Entladungsmuster bei verschiedenen Bewegungsrichtungen erkennen

6. Reaktionsmuster bei unvollständiger Belichtung des receptiven Feldes. Der Einfluß des receptiven Feldes auf die Entladungsmuster der visuellen Neurone bei bewegtem Hell-Dunkel-Reiz wurde mit 2 Methoden geprüft:

a) Hatte ein Neuron „richtungslabile" Entladungsmuster, so konnten diese in „richtungsstabile" umgewandelt werden, wenn das Reizfeld auf das Feldzentrum eingeengt wurde (Abb. 2b). Dies ist ein Hinweis dafür, daß die Verschiedenheit der Entladungsmuster bei Richtungsänderung durch den Einfluß der (hemmenden) Randzone des receptiven Feldes bedingt ist.

b) Durch Abdecken einer Hälfte des Reizfeldes mit einer Blende wurde das receptive Feldzentrum in eine *Kontrastsituation* gebracht (Abb. 1b). Dadurch

änderte sich ebenfalls das Entladungsmuster der Neurone auf die bewegten Lichtreize, wobei Richtungsdifferenzen in der Regel verstärkt wurden. Wie nach den
Ergebnissen BAUMGARTNERs (1, 2) mit unbewegten Lichtreizen zu erwarten war,
war die Aktivierung in dieser Kontrastsituation höher als bei Belichtung des
ganzen Reizfeldes.

**7. Unterschiede zwischen Geniculatum-Neuronen und Neuronen im visuellen
Cortex.** Um signifikante Aussagen über Differenzen der Beeinflussung der neuronalen Entladungsmuster durch Richtungsänderung der optokinetischen Reize auf
den beiden Stufen des zentralen visuellen Systems machen zu können, ist das vorliegende Material noch zu klein. Auffallend war jedoch, daß richtungslabile Neurone im visuellen Cortex relativ häufiger waren als im Geniculatum laterale. Auch
die Neurone des off-Systems waren im Geniculatum laterale vorwiegend richtungs-
stabil und änderten ihre Entladungsmuster beim Wechsel der Bewegungsrichtung
der Hell-Dunkel-Streifen nur wenig.

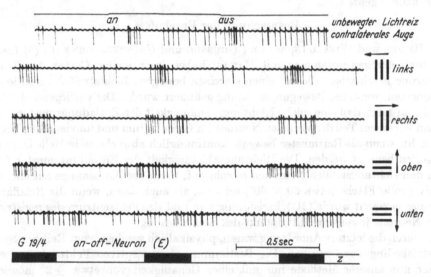

Abb. 5. *On-off-(E-) Neuron* im visuellen Cortex. Belichtung des contralateralen Auges (G 19/4). In der obersten
Reihe Reaktion auf unbewegten Lichtreiz, darunter Reaktionen auf bewegte Streifenmuster; Hell-Dunkel-Verhältnis 2:1, Streifengeschwindigkeit 23° 20′ sec⁻¹, Periodendauer 0,8 sec = 18° 20′, Reizfeldgröße 21°. Die Entladungsmuster (off- oder on-off-Aktivierung) sind abhängig von der Bewegungsrichtung

**8. Beeinflussung der Neurone des visuellen Cortex durch Reizung des frontalen
Augenfeldes.** Elektrische Reizung (Thyratron, 16—50 pro sec) bestimmter Areale
des motorischen Cortex bewirkt an der encéphale-isolé-Katze eine konjugierte
Augenbewegung nach kontralateral und unten. In 2 orientierenden Versuchen
wurde der Einfluß einer solchen Reizung auf die spontanen und durch Bewegungsreize ausgelösten Entladungsmuster der Neurone in der Sehrinde untersucht. Dabei
ergab sich, daß das spontane Entladungsmuster der visuellen Neurone durch Reizung des frontalen Augenfeldes beeinflußt werden kann. Beobachtet wurden in der
Regel nach variablen Latenzzeiten zwischen 80 und 200 msec nicht-rhythmische
Aktivierungen, die die Reizung oft um mehrere Sekunden überdauerten. In den
Versuchen konnten die Tiere keine wirklichen Augenbewegungen ausführen, da

sie nach der Bestimmung der elektrischen Reizschwelle für die vom frontalen Augenfeld ausgelösten Augenbewegungen curarisiert wurden.

Wurde die optische Reizung mit Streifenmustern mit der elektrischen Reizung des frontalen Augenfeldes kombiniert, so traten deutliche Veränderungen der durch die visuellen Reize ausgelösten Entladungsmuster auf.

Diese Beobachtung weist darauf hin, daß das primäre corticale Sehzentrum Afferenzen aus Strukturen erhält, welche die Augenbewegungen steuern. Diese Verbindung könnte der neurophysiologische Ausdruck für die ,,Efferenzkopie" von v. HOLST und MITTELSTAEDT sein. Mit dem sehr groben elektrischen Reiz lassen sich natürlich keine genaueren Daten über das Zusammenspiel von Motorik und Sensorik im zentralen visuellen System ermitteln.

Über den Weg der Impulse innerhalb der Afferenzen aus dem frontalen Augenfeld kann nichts Näheres ausgesagt werden; die lange Latenzzeit der Aktivierung spricht für eine komplexe Verschaltung, die möglicherweise über subcorticale Strukturen geht.

Besprechung der Ergebnisse

HUBEL und WIESEL (8, 8a) und GRÜSSER und GRÜSSER-CORNEHLS (5) (nach Untersuchungen zusammen mit HAKAS) haben im visuellen Cortex der Katze Neurone beschrieben, die auf einen *einzelnen* bewegten Lichtstreifen verschieden reagierten, wenn die Bewegungsrichtung geändert wurde. Die vorliegende Untersuchung zeigt, daß eine solche Richtungsabhängigkeit der Entladungsmuster auch dann bei einem Teil der visuellen Neurone im Geniculatum und im visuellen Cortex besteht, wenn als Reizmuster bewegte kontinuierlich abwechselnde Hell- Dunkel-Streifen benutzt werden. Die Richtungsabhängigkeit der Entladungsmuster trat bei den richtungslabilen Neuronen sowohl auf, wenn das Katzenauge auf eine relativ große Fläche (etwa $50 \times 60°$) schaute, als auch dann, wenn die Reizfläche kleiner gemacht wurde ($21°$), kreisförmig war und das Feldzentrum des registrierten Neurons jeweils im Mittelpunkt des Reizfeldes lag.

Durch die letztere Anordnung waren, physikalisch gesehen, vom Reiz her Symmetriebedingungen gegeben. Die Bestimmung des receptiven Feldzentrums war zwar mit unserer Methode nur mit einer Genauigkeit von etwa $\pm 2°$ möglich, jedoch lag auch bei nicht genauer Zentrierung das ganze receptive Feld (maximal $12°$ Ausdehnung) (8a) innerhalb des runden Reizfeldes. Bei der Bestimmung des rezeptiven Feldzentrums, von dem die registrierten Neurone aktiviert werden konnten, war oft auffallend, daß es außerordentlich klein war ($2—4°$).

Die in der Einleitung erwähnten drei Möglichkeiten für die Informationsvermittlung von Bewegungsrichtung und Geschwindigkeit eines optokinetischen Reizes ließen sich mit der angewandten Technik relativ sicher prüfen. Es kann gesagt werden, daß die *Bewegungsrichtung und Geschwindigkeit durch die zeitliche Folge der Aktivierung der Neurone*, die den verschiedenen Punkten im Gesichtsfeld zugeordnet sind, gemeldet wird. Zum anderen *beeinflussen beide Bewegungsgrößen die Entladungsmuster eines Teils der Neurone*, vor allem jene des off-Systems. Spezifische Bewegungsneurone, die nicht auf unbewegte Lichtreize reagieren, konnten im Geniculatum und im Cortex im Bereich der Projektionsgebiete der fovealen und parafovealen Retina nicht gefunden werden. Der Unterschied zu den andersartigen Resultaten von HUBEL und WIESEL (8), die über spezifische Bewegungsneurone berichteten, mag in den Versuchsbedingungen (Narkose und kleine Lichtstreifen) begründet sein.

Der Grund für die Abhängigkeit der Entladungsmuster von der Bewegungsrichtung ist wahrscheinlich in der Asymmetrie der receptiven Felder (BAUMGARTNER, *1, 2*; HUBEL u. WIESEL, *8a*; KUFFLER, *11*) zu sehen. Es ist anzunehmen, daß die Richtungslabilität der Entladungsmuster auf optokinetische Reize um so mehr zunimmt, je mehr die Peripherie des receptiven Feldes das Entladungsmuster bestimmt. Diese Annahme läßt sich prüfen durch Einengen des Reizfeldes. Wird dadurch nur noch das Feldzentrum durch die bewegten Lichtreize erregt, so wandeln sich richtungslabile Entladungsmuster in richtungsstabile Entladungsmuster um.

Dem Techniker der Abt. für Klin. Neurophysiologie, Herrn H. KAPP, danken wir für seine Hilfe und Überwachung der benutzten elektronischen Geräte.

Summary

1. Single neurons in the primary visual cortex and the lateral geniculate body of cats (encephale isolé, curarization) were recorded from by means of micropipettes (tip diameter below 1 μ). The neuronal reactions to diffuse light stimuli and to *moving* light-dark stripes, which were projected to a screen of 30 cm distance from the eye, were quantitatively analysed. Eight different movement directions were tested.

2. The receptive field centers of all recorded neurons were located within an area of 15 degrees around the central region of the retina.

3. No neuron specialized for the reception of moving patterns could be found; all neurons which responded to moving light-dark stripes were also activated by stationary light-dark stimuli and vice versa.

4. The neurons of the *on-system* (B) responded to moving light-dark stripes with an activation during the illumination of the receptive field center. Darkening of the field center elicited an inhibition. Some neurons had an afteractivation ("after image") following a short inhibitory period during darkening of receptive field. The discharge patterns depended upon velocity of stripe movement, width, brightness and light-dark ratio of the stripes and in some neurons also on the direction of movement.

5. The discharge frequency of the *on*-neurons, as a rule, had a maximum with entrance of a bright stripe into the receptive field center and partly a second maximum when the light stripe left it („Eintritts- und Austrittsaktivierung"). This observation corresponded to BAUMGARTNER's results that neuronal activation by an stationary light-dark grid reaches maximal values if the receptive field is in a contrast situation.

6. The neurons of the *off-system* (so-called off- and on-off-neurons, D, E) showed a similar dependance upon the different mentioned factors of the moving light stimuli as the on-neurons. The most effective stimulus for neuronal activation was darkening of the receptive field. In many of these neurons, contrary to the on-system, the discharge patterns were highly influenced by alteration of the movement direction.

7. The influence of direction was higher in cortical neurons than in the neurons of the lateral geniculate body. However, the number of analysed geniculate neurons was too small for measuring the statistical significance of this observation.

8. Electrical stimulation of the cortical eye field in encephale isolé cats elicited contraversive and downward eye movements. The same electrical stimulation influenced the spontaneous discharge patterns of cortical visual neurons and also modified their reactions to moving light-dark stripes. This was also observed after supression of eye movements by curarization. Thus the primary visual cortex receives impulses from the optomotor field and this may correspond to the ,,Efferenzkopie", postulated in the ,,Reafferenzprinzip" of v. Holst and Mittelstaedt.

Literatur

1. Baumgartner, G.: Die Reaktionen der Neurone des zentralen visuellen Systems der Katze im simultanen Helligkeitskontrast. Dieses Symposion. 296—313.
2. — u. P. Hakas: Reaktionen einzelner Opticusneurone und corticaler Nervenzellen der Katze im Hell-Dunkel-Grenzfeld (Simultankontrast). Pflügers Arch. ges. Physiol. 270, 29 (1960).
3. Cornehls, U., u. O.-J. Grüsser: Ein elektronisch gesteuertes Doppellichtreizgerät. Pflügers Arch. ges. Physiol. 270, 78—79 (1959).
4. Doty, R. W.: Functional significance of the topographical aspects of the retino-cortical projection. Dieses Symposion. 228—247.
5. Grüsser, O.-J., u. U. Grüsser-Cornehls: Mikroelektrodenuntersuchungen zur Konvergenz verstibulärer und retinaler Afferenzen an einzelnen Neuronen des optischen Cortex der Katze. Pflügers Arch. ges. Physiol. 270, 227—238 (1960).
6. Grüsser-Cornehls, U., u. O.-J. Grüsser: Reaktionsmuster einzelner Neurone im zentralen visuellen System von Fischen, Kaninchen und Katzen auf monoculare und binoculare Lichtreize. Dieses Symposion. 275—287.
7. Holst, E. v., u. H. Mittelstaedt: Das Reafferenzprinzip. Naturwissenschaften 37, 256—272 (1950).
8. Hubel, D. H.: Cortical unit responses to visual stimuli in non anesthetized cats. Amer. J. Ophthal. 46, 110—122 (1958).
8a. — and T. N. Wiesel: Receptive fields of single neurones in the cats striate cortex. J. Physiol. (Lond.) 148, 574—591 (1959).
9. Jung, R.: Nystagmographie: Zur Physiologie und Pathologie des optisch-vestibulären Systems beim Menschen. Handb. der Inneren Medizin. 4. Aufl. Band V, 1, 1206—1402. Berlin-Göttingen-Heidelberg: Springer 1953.
10. — R. v. Baumgarten u. G. Baumgartner: Mikroableitungen von einzelnen Nervenzellen im optischen Cortex der Katze: Die lichtaktivierten B-Neurone. Arch. Psychiat. Nervenkr. 189, 521—539 (1952).
11. Kuffler, S. W.: Discharge patterns and functional organization of mammalian retina. J. Neurophysiol. 16, 37—68 (1953).
12. Whitteridge, D. and P. M. Daniel: The representation of the visual field on the calcarine cortex. Dieses Symposion. 222—228.

Diskussion

P. Glees: Mir erscheint unwahrscheinlich, daß elektrische Reizung des frontalen Augenfeldes den Neuronen der Sehrinde ein sinnvolles Erregungsmuster zutragen kann, da elektrische Reizung durch Erfassung aller Rindenelemente wahrscheinlich chaotische Meldungen überträgt. Eine Interaktion zwischen retinaler und frontaler Reizung ist ja zu sehen, aber sie könnte unspezifisch sein.

F. Bremer: A cortico-reticular influence followed by an unspecific activation of the visual cortex seems also to me a more plausible explanation than a direct cortico-cortical regulation effect. In extensive recent researches, Fangel and Kaada found that the frontal oculo-motor field is characterized by a great density of cortico-reticular fibers.

R. L. DE VALOIS: I believe that many of the differential responses which you were giving as evidence for movement perception would have been produced if the receptive field of the cell were not accurately located in the center of your stimulating area. This is particularly true for latency differences. For instance if the cell's receptive field were to the left of center then it would have fired sooner to movement from the left than from the right. Are you sure that this possibility has been well controlled for?

H. SCHOBER: Die Abhängigkeit der Reaktion der corticalen oder Geniculatum-Neurone von der Bewegungsrichtung der Streifenmuster im Gesichtsfeld kann auch weitgehend physikalisch bedingt sein. Die Objektsymmetrie besteht nämlich nur außerhalb des Auges und die vom Autor benutzten Photozellen messen auch nur diese Objektsymmetrie. Die physikalische Lichtverteilung auf der Netzhaut ist aber niemals symmetrisch, sie wird durch die Eigenart der Beugungsfigur (Rechteckmuster gegen runde Pupille) weitgehend modifiziert. Eine bewegte asymmetrische Objektfigur muß aber in jeder Richtung zu anderen Reaktionen führen und muß daher schon rein physikalisch viele der hier beschriebenen Vorgänge verursachen.

G. BAUMGARTNER: Für die Meldung von Bewegungsreizen sind *Neurone mit off-Zentrum* dann gut geeignet, wenn die Wirkung des Umfeldes im Vergleich zu der des Zentrums relativ intensiv ist wie bei den präexcitatorisch gehemmten on-off- oder E-Neuronen. Ist das receptive Feld nämlich hinsichtlich eines bewegten Kontrastreizes asymmetrisch eingeordnet, so muß es je nach Richtung der Hell-Dunkel-Folge zu unterschiedlichen Aktivierungen kommen. Wie GRÜSSER ausführt, macht dies eine richtungsspezifische Information über einzelne Neurone denkbar. Ich habe im Tractus opticus bisher keine solchen richtungsmeldenden Neurone gesehen und HUBEL fand sie auch nicht im Geniculatum. Der Nachweis richtungsspezifischer Reaktionen im Geniculatum ist für diese Auffassung deshalb von Wichtigkeit. Auch die von HUBEL publizierten richtungsspezifischen Cortexneurone sind off-Zentrum-Neurone. Dies spricht dafür, daß die off-Zentrum-Neurone, und zwar die mit starker Umfeldaktivität, für die Bewegungswahrnehmung eine besondere Bedeutung haben.

R. JUNG: Ergibt sich aus diesen übereinstimmenden Ergebnissen von BAUMGARTNER, HUBEL und GRÜSSER, daß die *Neurone der on-off- oder E-Gruppe* eine für Bewegungsreize spezialisierte Gruppe der dunkelaktivierten Neurone sind? In diesem Fall müßten solche richtungsspezifischen Effekte auch an den on-off-Neuronen der Retina und des Geniculatum nachweisbar sein. Wenn im Geniculatum oder der Retina richtungsspezifische Neurone vorkommen, müßten solche Neurone im Geniculatum, wenn sie sinnvolle Informationen melden sollen, auch vestibulär beeinflußt sein. Hier hat Dr. GRÜSSER jedoch keine vestibuläre Afferenz gefunden. Sie wäre aber nur in der Retina entbehrlich, da die Augenbewegungen vestibulär reguliert sind.

O.-J. GRÜSSER (zu GLEES): Ich glaube auch nicht, daß durch elektrische Reizung ein physiologisches Erregungsmuster zustande kommt; an den Neuronen der Sehrinde ist wenigstens nur eine diffuse Aktivierung zu beobachten. Ob diese „spezifisch" oder „unspezifisch" ist, kann man an der Aktivierung selbst nicht erkennen. Eine diffuse Aktivierung allein weist zwar mehr in die Richtung des „Unspezifischen", jedoch läßt sich auch solches Entladungsmuster auch durch spezifische Reize erzeugen (z. B. durch statistisch verteilte mittelfrequente elektrische Opticusreize oder durch in der Frequenz um die CFF zufällig schwankende Lichtblitze). Es ist noch nicht systematisch untersucht, von welchen Rindenpunkten eine Aktivierung der visuellen Neurone zu erreichen ist. Durch elektrische Reizung der akustischen Rinde kann man z. B. keinen Effekt an den visuellen Neuronen sehen, obwohl diese Reizung sicher auch eine unspezifische "arousal reaction" bewirkt.

(zu BREMER): Die relativ langen Latenzzeiten sprechen für eine polysynaptische Verschaltung des afferenten Zuflusses zur Sehrinde aus dem frontalen Augenfeld. Daß dieser Zufluß über subcorticale Strukturen erfolgt, ist denkbar. Vielleicht sind dabei die gleichen Strukturen beteiligt, die auch Meldungen aus dem vestibulären System zur Sehrinde vermitteln.

(zu DE VALOIS): Die Bestimmungen des Feldzentrums war etwa mit einer Genauigkeit von ± 2 Grad möglich. Damit können auch Differenzen der Latenzzeiten bei verschiedener Streifenrichtung auftreten. Da das runde Reizfeld eine Größe von 21 Grad hatte und die größten rezeptiven Felder corticaler Neurone in ihrer längsten Ausdehnung wohl nicht mehr als 15 Grad betragen, ist es unwahrscheinlich, daß eine durch die Methodik bedingte ungenaue Zentrierung von Reizfeld und rezeptivem Feld auch die verschiedenen Entladungsmuster bei verschiedenen Bewegungsrichtungen bedingt. Für diese Meinung spricht auch, daß richtungsvariable Entladungsmuster auch bei großer Reizfläche (etwa 60 Grad) auftreten. Schließlich sei auf die Ergebnisse von HUBEL und WIESEL hingewiesen, die mit einzelnen Lichtstreifen, die genau projiziert wurden, ebenfalls richtungsabhängige Reaktionen an corticalen Neuronen gefunden haben.

(zu SCHOBER): Dieser Einwand ist physikalisch als Ursache einer Richtungsabhängigkeit der Entladungsmuster denkbar. Würde er physiologisch eine wesentliche Rolle spielen, so müßte man erwarten, daß Neurone, deren retinale receptive Felder etwa im gleichen Abstand und etwa gleicher Richtung vom optischen Abbildungszentrum des Auges liegen, sich ähnlich verhalten. Dies ist nicht der Fall. Es gibt Neurone (vor allem des on-Systems) die richtungsunabhängig immer die gleichen Reaktionen auf die Streifenmuster zeigten. Daher ist anzunehmen, daß doch ein physiologischer Faktor, der in der asymmetrischen Organisation der rezeptiven Felder gesehen werden kann, eine Rolle spielt.

(zu JUNG und BAUMGARTNER): Die Neurone des off-Systems waren zum Teil deutlich stärker im Entladungsmuster von der Bewegungsrichtung abhängig als die on-Neurone. Daraus läßt sich jedoch nicht eine Spezialisierung der Informationsübertragung dieser Neurone für Bewegungsreize ableiten, da diese Neurone ja auch auf unbewegte Lichtreize reagieren. Die stärkere Richtungsabhängigkeit corticaler Neurone im Vergleich zu Geniculatumneuronen war auffallend, jedoch ließen sich auch an den letzteren Einflüsse der Bewegungsrichtung auf das Entladungsmuster feststellen (Abb. 1). Zur statistischen Sicherung der Differenz zwischen Geniculatum- und Cortexneuronen war die Zahl der registrierten Geniculatum-Neurone zu klein.

III. Koordination spezifischer und unspezifischer Afferenzen in Area 17

The Cortex as a Sensory Analyser[1,2]

By

GEORGE H. BISHOP

With 3 Figures

1. The sensory systems. The vertebrate brain has acquired seriatim in its phylogeny a sequence of brains, central structures employing afferent information for control of behavior. Each of these central brains has developed out of one or another afferent level; a medullary level related to cranial and spinal nerves; the cerebellum from Vth and VIIIth nerve nuclei; the vestibular apparatus from another division of the VIIIth, the thalamus from the IInd; and cortex from the olfactory apparatus. Each center secondarily acquires connections not only from its own level, but from all levels of the body. For instance the eye is a diencephalic

[1] Washington University School of Medicine, St. Louis, Missouri.

[2] This work was conducted in part under contract between Washington University and the Office of Naval Research, and in part under a grant from the Supreme Council, Thirty-third Degree Scottish Rite, Northern Jurisdiction, USA, through the National Association for Mental Health.

structure, but the "optic" thalamus also receives auditory and somaesthetic paths. From the primitive pallium, starting as a facilitator of olfactory function (HERRICK, 1948) and still so operating as the pyriform lobe of mammals, a general cortex developed which made secondary connections with other levels; not directly, but only through the sensory centers of the thalamus. This relation is exemplified in the reptilian brain. Not until the mammal, however, were added the more direct and specific relays of the main sensory systems of audition, vision and body sense, through thalamic relay to projection cortex.

That this direct relay is a highly specialized relation is indicated by the fact that only a portion of the largest afferent fibers of any modality projects thus directly to cortex (BISHOP, 1959). In the cat optic nerve where the maximal fiber size is 12 μ, only the fibers from 12 to 6 μ in diameter producing a first spike in the optic tract relay in the lateral geniculate and activate the visual area of cortex (BISHOP and CLARE, 1955). Medium sized fibers activate other thalamic nuclei, and the smallest fibers pass to brainstem structures, the pretectal area and colliculus. Analogously in the somaesthetic system only the large sensory fibers of the beta group ascend the dorsal column where they synapse to form the medial lemniscus. This relays again in the ventral nucleus of thalamus to activate somaesthetic cortex. The medium sized gamma-delta path ascending the lateral column in the spinal lemniscus passes initially to the intralaminar thalamic region, though in the ascending scale of the mammals an increasing number of fibers joins the medial lemniscus to reach the ventral nucleus and cortex. The smallest fibers relay to the medullary reticular substance, and relay again to medial thalamus. The somaesthetic system thus parallels the visual system, and from the form and conditions of the cortical response, the auditory system appears to have a similar configuration, though the details have not been worked out.

One difference is noteworthy; when the visual cortex of man is destroyed, all visual sense is lost, but when the somaesthetic area is destroyed pain and temperature and crude touch persist. Those sensations are lost in either system which are mediated by the larger fiber group, but the smaller and unmyelinated groups of the somaesthetic system still mediate characteristic sensations. This indicates that the small-fiber paths must finally be relayed to cortex, which appears to be essential for sensory perception in the mammal. But they are not projected primarily to the somaesthetic area. The projection area of cortex must not be the locus of the subjective awareness of these sensations. It is rather an analyser contributing to fine discrimination in spatial contacts via a special group of tactile and proprioceptive endings, mediated by way of the dorsal cord columns. From this point of view all of our visual sensations are similarly devoted to the fine discrimination of information from *distance* receptors, comparable to those so acutely discriminating *contact* sensations mediated by way of the medial lemniscus system. The optic system in man has lost, if it ever acquired, a sensory correlate of the afferent activity presented to structures below cortex, however this activity may contribute to behavioral reactions to light stimuli. Correspondingly no path is known from colliculus to cortex, although a path from cortex to colliculus is present in the cat.

In spite of this difference, all of the main afferent systems are laid out on so similar a pattern that information about one should be useful in understanding the functioning of the others. Some recent work on the somaesthetic system has furnished data that may have general significance for all cortical sensory functioning. (Further details and references will be found in BISHOP, 1959). This work deals with the analysis of paths to higher levels of the somaesthetic system, and with the functioning of these centers themselves. Here one can trace the development in phylogeny of these structures, and evaluate their contribution to behavior.

2. The somaesthetic afferent paths.

In the vertebrates below mammals no dorsal column–medial lemniscus–ventral nucleus path is present. The main afferent

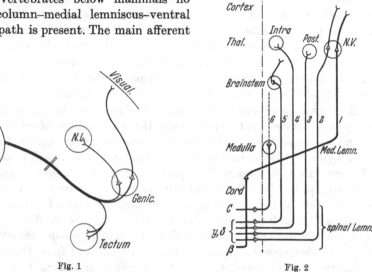

Fig. 1   Fig. 2

Fig. 1. Distribution of fibers of the optic tract. Visual, optic cortex; Genic., dorsal nucleus of the lateral geniculate; N. L., nucleus lateralis; and Tectum, superior colliculus and pretectal area. Of size ranges in the optic tract, the largest, approximately 5 to 12 mμ in diameter, terminate chiefly in the A layer of the dorsal nucleus of the geniculate, and relay to optic cortex. The smaller relay in the B layer to other thalamic nuclei. The smallest fibers terminate without relay in colliculus and pretectal areas. Two other tracts, the anterior and posterior accessory, are present in some animals presumably as relics of a more primitive stage of development. The size distribution in the optic tract is essentially like that of white matter below cortex generally, see fig. 3

Fig. 2. Somaesthetic afferent paths. Six afferent paths, at least four of them presumably sensory, can be designated; 1, medial lemniscus, large fibers of the dorsal cord column. 2 to 6, spinal lemniscus, smaller myelinated and unmyelinated fibers ascending the lateral column after synapse. 2, 3, 4, three spinothalamic paths to ventral nucleus, posterior nuclei and intralaminar region respectively. 5, path to brainstem relaying to thalamus. 6, unmyelinated fiber path relaying in the medulla to higher centers, presumably medial thalamus. In addition many fibers from the cord terminate along the reticular formation of medulla and brainstem, of unknown sensory implication

paths rising from the lateral column constitute the *spinal lemniscus* of the comparative anatomists (HERRICK, 1948). In mammals this comprises those fibers postsynaptic to the smaller myelinated and unmyelinated fibers of peripheral nerves. Different components of this lemniscus bundle can be traced to various loci of termination. It has long been presumed, because of the prominence of the spinothalamic tract in man and other primates, that the chief destination of the anterolateral cord bundle was the ventrolateral nucleus of the thalamus. However a majority of the fibers (75% in the human) of the bundle arising from the lateral cord column terminate not in this nucleus but below the thalamus, in the reticular formation of medulla and brainstem. In addition, the premammalian vertebrates had a more primitive spinothalamic tract, which is presumably the precursor of the "pain" path recently investigated by the Nauta degeneration technique (MEHLER, 1957; MEHLER, FEFERMAN and NAUTA, 1960). Fibers from cells in the spinal cord pass without synapse to certain of the intralaminar nuclei and presumably mediate pain and temperature senses.

This medial bundle is the most prominent spinothalamic connection in the lower mammals, but increasing numbers of fibers are found to take a more lateral course in the classical spinothalamic tract as one ascends the scale of mammalian evolution toward the primates and man Thus two spinothalamic components arise from the spinal lemniscus. The lateral of these, like the dorsal column-medial lemniscus terminating in the same region of thalamus, is not present below the mammals.

A third component of the spinal lemniscus bundle terminates in the upper brainstem medial and anterior to the red nucleus, and their postsynaptic responses occur in the region around the *centrum medianum* of the thalamus (COLLINS and O'LEARY, 1954). Responses here to peripheral nerve stimulation occur after section of the dorsal column of the cord, but not after section of the lateral column. This path thus constitutes a brainstem relay parallel to the medial spinothalamic tract investigated by MEHLER, and its synapses are peculiarly sensitive to anaesthetics, appropriate to the early loss of pain in progressive general anaesthesia.

Still a fourth component of the spinal lemniscus, the *unmyelinated fiber group*, has been traced to a still lower level of the reticular formation in the medulla (COLLINS and RANDT, 1959). Here it is relayed upward through reticulothalamic connections again to the medial region of thalamus. Since stimulation of unmyelinated fibers induces sensations of pain and temperature, this afferent path is specifically a sensory one, and is presumably relayed to cortex by some route at present unknown.

A fifth group of spinal lemniscus fibers constitutes a third spinothalamic path, whose course and functioning have been recently studied (POGGIO and MOUNTCASTLE, 1960). These fibers accompany the classical spinothalamic bundle, but do not terminate in the ventral nucleus. Rather they pass to the posterior thalamic group of nuclei, a region between the ventral nucleus and the intralaminar nuclei. Their projections to cortex can be inferred from cortical degeneration experiments (ROSE and WOOLSEY, 1958). When the secondary somatic area of cortex is detroyed, or when all cortex except this is destroyed, slight retrograde degeneration of the posterior thalamic region is observed, but when destruction of surrounding cortex is added to destruction of somatic sensory area II, degeneration occurs. The cells of these nuclei thus appear to have rather widespread terminations in cortex, which include sensory II. Their failure to degenerate after removal of any one region of cortex has led ROSE to term their projections *sustaining* projections, in contrast to the *essential* projections to regions of cortex whose destruction causes degeneration in the thalamus.

While certain direct correlations are possible to be made between these somaesthetic paths and those of the visual system, not all the components that can be differentiated in the former are at present known in the latter. However comparable distributions cannot be excluded. Auditory and visual stimuli activate cells in the posterior nuclei, and in the brainstem reticular substance. In certain animals posterior and anterior accessory optic tracts are demonstrable, presumably as relics of a more primitive stage of development and many fibers from the spinal cord distribute to the reticular substance of the brainstem, again a persistence of a primitive condition.

3. The activation of cortex from the periphery; sensory vs. afferent functions. The idea of a generalized brainstem center capable of being activated by more than one modality is supported by the study of individual cell responses in the posterior thalamic nuclei following sensory stimulation at the periphery of the body (Poggio and Mountcastle, 1960). Here single cells may be found which respond to stimuli applied at widely different loci, to stimuli which should arouse different types of sensation, and even to auditory as well as somatosensory activation. This thalamic region, in contrast to the ventral nucleus, is neither space nor modality specific and is interpreted as a polysensory integrative apparatus. It thus appears to transmit to cortex, including the secondary somatic area and adjacent regions, aspects of sensation quite different from those presumably analytic in character assignable to the primary projection area. The auditory cortex and thalamus show similar complications. Concerning the *visual system*, information on subcortical structures other than the lateral geniculate is limited. It may be suggested that the visual *sensory* function is more narrowly limited to its large fiber projection to cortex than is the case for somaesthetic sensory function, but paths from the retina to brainstem and thalamic structures may still mediate some contribution to responses to light, if not to visual sensations.

What does the cortex do with these various components of afferent information that reach it eventually by such different routes? Is there any sharp line to be drawn between sensory and afferent, or do what we call *afferent but nonsensory paths* modulate or otherwise contribute to the sensations mediated more specifically? It has been emphasized by Herrick that both analysis and integration are involved in cortical processes, and that the more primitive neuropil net of lower animals tended to serve rather nonspecific integrative functions. In this primitive neuropil, differentiation occurred by crystallization out of the diffuse network of more definitive paths connecting specific loci. The differentiation of definitive paths to separate loci is illustrated in the extreme by the approximately point to point relations between periphery and cortex for visual and somaesthetic systems. This design affords the highest degree of analytic functioning. The polyvalent regions of the posterior nuclei of thalamus with their more diffuse projections to relatively nonspecific cortical areas are appropriate to integrative functioning. The medial spinothalamic tract to the intralaminar nuclei may represent a third type of afferent, less specifically projected than is the medial lemniscus component but more specific in terms of sensation than is the parallel path to the posterior nuclei. Still other paths innervating a generalized and nonspecific brainstem region may exert a more diffuse effect as a modulation of the more specific cortical activity, that mediated over more obviously sensory paths. The final integration of all afferent activity contributory to sensory experience must be still more diffusely represented in cortex than are its various constituent elements.

The work all too briefly summarized here indicates that not all of the differentiation of sensory information is performed by cortex. Throughout their courses each of the afferent systems is differentiated into qualitatively different components, each component handling its own input to cortex according to its nature. The sensory picture presented to cortex from any peripheral source must be a corresponding composite. The roots of this complex innervation lie in the phylogenetic development of the vertebrates, and one of the differential criteria of these multiple paths corresponding to their evolutionary origin appears to be the *fiber size* range characteristic of each.

4. The significance of fiber size in central functioning. In relation to the mammalian acquisition of the medial lemniscus path to cortex and of the larger fiber component of the optic tract, activating a visual projection area, the cortex itself has acquired a corresponding large fiber system in other areas as well as in those of sensory projection.

The fiber size distribution in the white matter below cortex has been studied by means of the electron microscope (unpublished work). The lateral and suprasylvian areas of the cat, the cat corpus callosum, various areas in the more primitive mole cortex, tissues from biopsies at frontal lobotomy in the human, and the cat optic nerve and tract all show a common pattern. Practically all of the fibers are myelinated, but many lose their myelin as they ascend through cortex. The smallest fibers are less than 0.5 μ in diameter, some as

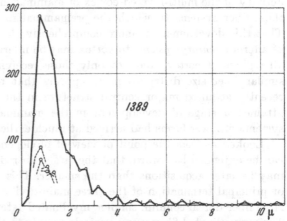

Fig. 3. Plot of 1389 fibers counted in five photographs from the electron microscope at magnification of 3.75 mm per μ, in white matter below the cortical visual area of the cat. Addition of further counts fails to change the picture significantly other than to smooth the curve, although an occasional fiber of 12 and 13 μ diameter has been found. The peaks of distribution in the five photographs as counted separately are indicated in dotted curves. This size distribution prevails in other areas of cortex, both sensory and association, also in the corpus callosum and in the optic tract of the cat

small as 0.2 μ, the largest, 12 to 14 μ. The peak in a plot of numbers against diameters lies at 0.8 μ; the major elevation of *fibers up to 3 or 4 μ* in diameter which includes this peak constitutes over *80% of the fibers present.*

The fibers of this size in the optic chiefly innervate the *superior colliculus and pretectal area* of the brainstem. From 3 to 5 or 6 μ the number of fibers per size decreases, including 12 to 15% of the total. This range accounts for the second spike in the cat optic nerve record after conduction. These fibers terminate in the lateral geniculate nucleus, and their stimulation is followed by a response in the lateral nucleus of the thalamus (BISHOP and CLARE, 1955). The largest 2 or 3% of the total relay in the geniculate to cortex and correspond to the first spike in the optic nerve record. Comparing these size ranges with those of the sensory fibers of peripheral nerves, the smallest in cortex, though all myelinated, correspond in size to the unmyelinated C group, plus the small myelinated fiber range included conventionally in the late part of the delta wave of peripheral nerves. The middle range corresponds in fiber diameter to the gamma-delta range of peripheral nerves, synapsing in the cord to form the spinal lemnicus and the three spinothalamic paths included in it. The large fiber range corresponds to the dorsal column beta group relaying at the medial lemnicsus to the ventral nucleus and somaesthetic cortex.

In the turtle brain, most of the fibers are unmyelinated, and all are small. The total seems to correspond to not more than the smallest size range of the mammal. The turtle and frog, however, have in their peripheral nerves fibers as large as are found in mammalian nerves. In a sense then one may say that the mammalian cortex, as compared to the turtle, has acquired an overlay of larger fiber components as an extension to cortex of the distribution already present peripherally in the premammalian vertebrates. The relatively small number of larger fibers present even in the higher mammals suggests that most of the cortical activity of the multi-layered cortex of mammals must be performed by means of those fiber systems to which the premammalian singlelayered cortex is limited. That this development is more comprehensive however than a simple extension of afferent *sensory systems* to cortex may be inferred from the circumstance that all regions of cortex, and not only those receiving sensory radiations, show a similar fiber size distribution. It appears that the cortex, which is the most recently acquired major central structure in the evolving nervous system, has attained a stage of development in the mammal that the peripheral nervous systems of lower forms had arrived at much earlier.

Looked at from the point of view of phylogenetic development, this concept can be extended backward, that the larger fibered systems *of the spinal cord* also may be later acquisitions than the smaller. This is also consistent with the loci of principal termination of the three main divisions of the sensory systems, the large fiber dorsal column, smaller myelinated lateral column, and unmyelinated. The unmyelinated fiber group projects mainly to the medulla in the somaesthetic system, and to the brainstem in the visual system, both very old regions and early developed, and still serving what must be subcortical functions in the mammal. The smaller myelinated lateral column component projects to the thalamus, but only diffusely to cortex, and did so in the premammalian land vertebrates. Only the large fiber dorsal column component projects conspicuously to a specialized area of cortex in all the main sensory systems. The alpha group of sensory fibers does not project at all to cortex, but synapses in CLARK's column (LLOYD and McINTYRE, 1950) to give rise to the dorsal or neospinocerebellar tract, a path again not present below mammals.

What advantages the cortex, and in fact the older parts of the nervous system derive from a large fiber path as compared to a smaller, it is at present impossible to say. It has been suggested that the high speed of conduction associated with large diameter should offer an obvious advantage. Another possibility is that a larger fiber might support greater numbers of, or more powerful synaptic endings. Both these ideas meet with exceptions and objections, and seem not to offer a sufficient advantage to call for such an extensive phylogenetic addition to the more primitive apparatus. A cue may be available in the fact that, at least in the sensory systems, the large fiber component appears to be employed in a new set of paths and central interconnections affording a more acute discrimination of fine detail than appears to have been available by the use of more primitive arrangements.

Aside from arguments which must at present be teleological, the recognition of the arrangement of nervous structures in relation to fiber size offers an approach to their further analysis. The fact that there are three fiber systems, phylogenetically successive and functionally each an addition to rather than a replacement of previously developed apparatus, offers a significant scheme of sensory pattern that should be worthy of further study.

Summary

We make a distinction between sensory and afferent paths, but the distinction is not a sharp one and we do not know where it lies. We know of three sensory paths of increasing discriminatory functioning in the somaesthetic system, and corresponding paths in the visual system, only one of which is predominent in sensory functioning. Even less is known about the fiber size relations in the auditory system. Fiber size relationships are a convenient means of designating these paths, and correlations with identifiable phylogenetic stages of central nervous system development offer a rationale of the differences in their relations to cortex. It appears that any afferent path, projecting immediately to any lower level, may be extended by relay upwards to have its appropriate influence on cortex itself, and hence (somehow) potentially on subjective phenomena such as sensory perception. However not all such paths have been demonstrated to have such a central effect, and the different sensory systems may differ in the comprehensiveness with which their cortical levels are affected by one afferent path or another. The significance is still unknown of the fact that a large-fiber range correlates with the more discriminating functioning of a more sophisticated projection area of cortex.

References

BISHOP, G. H.: The relation between nerve fiber size and sensory modality; phylogenetic implications of the afferent innervation of cortex. J. nerv. ment. Dis. 128, 89—114 (1959).
— and MARGARET H. CLARE: Organization and distribution of fibers in the optic nerve of the cat. J. comp. Neurol. 103, 269—304 (1955).
COLLINS, WM. F., and J. L. O'LEARY: Study of a somatic evoked response in midbrain reticular substance. E. E. G. Clin. Neurophysiol. 6, 619—628 (1954).
— and C. RANDT: Evoked central nervous system activity relating to peripheral unmyelinated or C fibers in cat. J. Neurophysiol. 21, 343—352 (1958).
HERRICK, C. J.: The brain of the tiger salamander. Chicago: Univ. of Chicago Press 1948.
LLOYD, D. P. C., and A. K. McINTYRE: Dorsal column conduction of group I muscle afferent impulses and their relay through CLARK's column. J. Neurophysiol. 13, 39—54 (1950).
MEHLER, WM. R.: The mammalian "pain" tract in phylogeny. Anat. Rec. 127, 332 (1957).
— M. E. FEFERMAN and W. J. H. NAUTA: Ascending axonal degeneration following anterolateral cordotomy. An experimental study in the monkey. Brain 83, in press (1960).
POGGIO, G. F., and V. B. MOUNTCASTLE: A study of the functional contributions of the lemniscal and spinothalamic systems to somatic sensibility. Bull. Johns Hopk. Hosp. 106, 266—316 (1960).
ROSE, J. E., and C. N. WOOLSEY: Cortical connections and functional organization of the thalamic auditory system of the cat. In Biological and Biochemical Bases of Behavior. H. F. HARLOW and C. N. WOOLSEY ed. Univ. of Wisconsin Press 1958.

Discussion

P. GLEES: 1. If I understand Prof. BISHOP's paper correctly he assumes that the phylogenetic older systems are characterized by thin or very thin fibres. He finds support for this view in HERRICK's classical teaching. However a study of the pyramidal system of lower mammals and primates has convinced me that the primates have many more fine fibres in the pyramidal tract than lower mammals and also more smaller cells in the sensory-motor cortex.

2. Assuming BISHOP's assertion that 80% of all afferent fibres to the cortex are unmyelinated is correct, is it possible that the electron-microscopical pictures dissolve the fibrilles of single conduction into a wealth of smaller elements which in itself do not conduct individually. How does the electron microscopist discriminate between the very fine glial fibres, dendrites and branching axons?

R. JUNG: BISHOPs Beitrag ist eine gute Einleitung und allgemeine morphologische Grundlage zur Konvergenz spezifischer und unspezifischer Afferenzen. Die Afferenz dünner Fasern ist zweifellos eine vernachlässigte Dimension, die jetzt durch die Elektronenmikroskopie aktuell geworden ist. BISHOPs vergleichende und phylogenetische Aspekte und das somato-sensorische System können wir hier nicht diskutieren und wir werden uns auf Fragen des visuellen Systems beschränken:

Die physiologischen Korrelationen spezifischer Afferenzen der Sehrinde durch dünne Opticusfasern sind noch ungenügend bekannt. Neuronale Korrelate im Cortex sind die B-Neurone langer Latenz (B$_2$-Entladung 50—150 msec nach Lichtreizen) und der Typus 3 nach Opticusreiz (25—150 msec Latenz nach GRÜTZNER, GRÜSSER u. BAUMGARTNER). Ob sie durch solche dünnen Fasern mit vielen Zwischenneuronen und das unspezifische System aktiviert werden, wissen wir allerdings noch nicht sicher.

Für BISHOPs Vorstellung, daß dünne Fasern und Kollateralen mit dem unspezifischen System zur visuellen Information beitragen, gibt es auch morphologische Grundlagen: SZENTÁGOTHAI (persönliche Mitteilung) hat viele direkte Endigungen von Opticusfasern im Mesencephalon der Katze gefunden: in der homo- und kontralateralen F. reticularis, prätectal und im Tectum, dagegen nicht im Prägeniculatum und im medialen Thalamus. Es ist wahrscheinlich, daß diese Opticus-Reticularis-Verbindungen nicht nur unspezifische Aktivierungen auslösen, sondern auch *spezifische Funktionen* für die optisch-vestibuläre Koordination und damit auch für die optische Information haben (vgl. Schema S. 423). Da SZENTÁGOTHAIs Untersuchungen mit der Nauta-Methode durchgeführt wurden, konnte er auch dünne markarme und marklose Fasern darstellen. Sind diese direkten extrageniculären Opticusverbindungen nach BISHOPs Meinung ein Homologon der „unspezifischen" Reticularis-Kollateralen des Lemniscus medialis oder des spinothalamischen Systems?

Ich glaube auch, daß die unspezifischen Verbindungen und dünnen Fasern zur Information, Modulation und Integration der Sinnesafferenzen beitragen. Aber der Beweis ist schwierig. Dafür sprechen vielleicht Narkoseversuche mit erhaltenem evoked potential im Cortex, aber gestörter reticulärer Nebenleitung und entsprechend gestörter Wahrnehmung. Von den neuronalen Einzelmechanismen wissen wir noch zu wenig und elektrische Reizversuche, die in den folgenden Beiträgen diskutiert werden, sind nicht ohne weiteres mit physiologischen Bedingungen gleichzusetzen.

G. H. BISHOP (to R. JUNG): It is obvious that the limited measurements made so far are more appropriate to speculations than to conclusions; and I am glad to hear of other work in progress. It may be of interest here that the optic system, like the somatic, has had very primitive connections, for instance the socalled anterior and posterior accessory tracts, barely recognizable in only some mammals. In addition, in all the afferent systems there must be many fibers, particularly demonstrable from the spinal ascending tracts, terminating along the reticular system and presumably not strictly sensory. They might however, by relays, condition ("activate"?) the thalamus and cortex to more strictly sensory reception. In fact for an understanding of the neurophysiology of the central nervous system as a whole we may be giving too much emphasis to the distinction between "sensory" and "afferent". The action of the nervous system is to organize behavior, both subjective and objective, and who at present can draw a physiological line between these two aspects of central function?

(To P. GLEES): 1. My statements applied to the afferent paths up to the thalamic level; we have not yet examined the motor paths. The pyramidal tract I understand to include fibers from other than the motor projection area. It would indeed be desirable to have data on more different representatives of the mammals, pending which any inferences I would propose are properly taken with due skepticism. 2. The statement concerning 80% of fibers counted applies to those measured in white matter below cortex, and to myelinated fibers only, including naturally both afferent and efferent. The number of unmyelinated fibers we found here was so small that they were ignored, and they may well have been glial fibers. It is indeed difficult to differentiate unmyelinated components, especially within the cortex, unless they can be actually traced for instance to glial cells, although in many places their distribution and relations to other structures are probably significant. Many of the small fibers at least lose their myelin as they pass upward through cortex, and in general within cortex it appears to be impossible to make fiber counts that would be conclusive.

Le potentiel évoqué de l'aire visuelle corticale*

Par

Frederic Bremer

Avec 6 Figures

I. Introduction

La réponse du cortex visuel des mammifères supérieurs provoquée par une volée d'influx synchrones est caractérisée par une succession d'oscillations électriques, les unes — les plus précoces — de signe positif, les autres de signe négatif.

La configuration oscillographique de ce potentiel évoqué avait paru posséder un caractère spécifique que des recherches récentes n'ont pas confirmé. En réalité, les différences d'avec les potentiels évoqués des autres aires corticales de réception des mammifères sont plutôt d'ordre quantitatif que qualitatif (14). Cette remarque n'est évidemment plus valable lorsqu'il s'agit de réponses à des stimuli physiologiques. Les influx suscités par un bref éclair représentent en réalité les décharges efférentes très complexes, déjà hautement organisées, du «petit cerveau qui est derrière les bâtonnets et les cônes» (Granit, 37). Aussi la réponse de l'aire visuelle à un stimulus photique diffère-t-elle fortement, par sa latence, sa durée et la complexité de sa phase surface-négative, des réponses suscitées par un choc électrique appliqué sur le nerf optique, le corps genouillé latéral ou les radiations optiques.

Une autre remarque préalable doit encore être faite. Un potentiel évoqué cortical dérivé par une macroélectrode représente déjà un processus d'*averaging*, ainsi que l'a souligné justement Rosenblith (53). Cette qualité lui confère la valeur d'une donnée statistique, dont l'empirisme expérimental a su largement profiter. Mais elle implique aussi les incertitudes interprétatives qui s'attachent à des tracés oscillographiques enregistrant simultanément les réponses intégrées de myriades d'éléments nerveux dont la seule homogénéité fonctionnelle est leur appartenance à un même système de projection sensorielle.

II. La réponse de l'aire visuelle à un stimulus «central»

1. **Configuration oscillographique du potentiel évoqué.** Le terme «central», qui n'a de signification que topographique, trouve sa justification dans l'analogie frappante des réponses suscitées par un bref stimulus électrique appliqué en n'importe quel point de la voie visuelle, depuis le nerf jusqu'aux radiations optiques. La description et l'analyse qui vont suivre s'appliquent au potentiel évoqué recueilli, en dérivation monopolaire de surface, en un point quelconque de l'*area striata* du chat.

* Laboratoire de Pathologie Générale, Université de Bruxelles.

Le potentiel évoqué de l'aire visuelle (fig. 1) est constitué par le groupement de trois pointes positives initiales et de trois potentiels plus lents, successivement positif, négatif, positif. La latence de la pointe 1 dépend du point d'application du stimulus. Elle est suivie d'une petite déflexion surface-positive, numérotée 2, que l'on serait tenté de négliger n'était sa remarquable constance. La pointe positive 3 s'inscrit généralement sur le tracé du potentiel 4. Celui-ci, nettement plus lent que les pointes initiales, est lui aussi surface-positif. Le potentiel 5, négatif, qui lui fait suite, est de latence et d'amplitude variable et plus lent que la phase 4. Un potentiel tardif positif inconstant, de plus longue durée encore, de faible voltage et de signification incertaine, termine cette réponse primaire à laquelle peut faire suite une post-décharge, rapide ou lente selon l'état fonctionnel du cerveau. De petites oscillations brèves surnuméraires peuvent surcharger le tracé des ondes lentes (*5, 13, 14*). Elles résultant vraisemblablement de l'irradiation à l'écorce de la post-décharge rapide du corps genouillé décrite par P. O. Bishop et ses collaborateurs (*7*).

L'interprétation de cette séquence d'oscillations se base sur la théorie du volume conducteur et sur l'action de différents facteurs de modification (paramètres et point d'application du stimulus, réfractorité post-réactionnelle, processus de facilitations, effets d'agents pharmacologiques appliqués localement, excision de la substance grise). Les controverses ont porté principalement sur l'interprétation des composantes brèves initiales de la réponse.

L'accord est fait actuellement en ce qui concerne la constitution de la pointe 1 et des potentiels 4 et 5. La première représente le potentiel d'action sommé des radiations optiques. Il peut être précédé d'une très petite oscillation traduisant la diffusion physique des potentiels d'action des segments initiaux de la voie optique[1]. La pointe 1 est le seul élément du potentiel évoqué qui subsiste clairement après une excision corticale suffisamment large et faite correctement (fig. 2, A et B). Son voltage est directement fonction, jusqu'à un maximum, de l'intensité du stimulus, c'est à dire du nombre de fibres afférentes activées simultanément.

Les potentiels 4 et 5 ne sont pas formellement différents du complexe positif-négatif qui caractérise les potentiels évoqués de toutes les aires de réception de l'isocortex et dont l'analyse microphysiologique (voir *44*) a montré qu'il représente vraisemblablement l'activation synaptique successive des somas des neurones de couches corticales immédiatement voisines de la couche granulaire réceptrice puis des dendrites superficiels de ces mêmes cellules pyramidales. Leurs propriétés permettent d'homologuer ces potentiels lents à des potentiels post-synaptiques d'excitation, donc à des dépolarisations neuroniques membranaires, auxquelles est associée ou non l'émission d'un ou plusieurs spikes. Une incertitude persiste encore en ce qui concerne le processus du passage de l'activation axo-somatique à la dépolarisation dendritique. Parmi les auteurs qui se sont préoccupés de ce problème, les uns ont admis une propagation antidromique de la dépolarisation somatique post-synaptique le long du tronc dendritique des cellules pyramidales vers les arborisations dendritiques de la couche moléculaire. D'autres expérimentateurs, dont la conclusion est basée sur l'analyse des modifications que subit la réponse d'une aire corticale réceptrice lorsqu'elle est enregistrée à des profondeurs

---

[1] Chang et Kaada (1950) avaient assigné à cet accident inconstant le numéro 1. Cette numérotation n'a pas été adoptée par la majorité des auteurs.

différentes de l'écorce, ainsi que sur des arguments pharmacologiques indiquant l'indépendance réactionnelle des deux phases de la réponse, ont conçu le passage de la phase positive à la phase négative comme étant le résultat d'une succession de transmissions interneuroniques ascendantes. Les arguments indirects sont sans doute les plus convaincants. La possibilité d'augmenter électivement et considérablement le voltage de la phase négative à la suite d'une application locale de strychnine ne paraît pas con-
ciliable avec l'hypothèse que ce potentiel résulterait de la propagation antidromique, sans relais synaptiques, de la dépolari-sation des somas neuroniques vers les

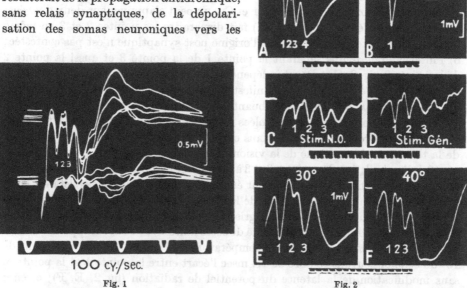

Fig. 1   Fig. 2

Fig. 1. *Réponses de l'aire visuelle primaire à un stimulus « nerf optique »*. Chat, encéphale isolé; dérivations mono-polaires de surface de l'aire visuelle (tracé supérieur) et du gyrus suprasylvien adjacent (négativité réactionnelle vers le haut); cinq balayages cathodiques superposés; temps en intervalles de 10 msec. Remarquer le contraste de la constance d'amplitude des pointes initiales 1, 2 et 3 de la réponse de l'aire visuelle avec la variabilité spontanée des potentiels post-synaptiques 4 et 5; noter aussi l'inconstance et le retard de la réponse du gyrus suprasylvien

Fig. 2. *Analyse du potentiel évoqué de l'aire visuelle suscité par un stimulus « genouillé »*. Chats, encéphale isolé; réponses enregistrées comme celle de la figure 1. *A* et *B*, réponses dérivées de la surface cérébrale avant et après l'excision de l'écorce visuelle; stimulus « genouillé »; *C* et *D*, constance de l'espacement des pointes 1, 2 et 3 dans les réponses au stimulus « nerf optique » (C) et au stimulus genouillé (D); *E* et *F*, rapprochement des pointes 1, 2 et 3 déterminé par l'élévation locale de la température de l'écorce; remarquer la constance de la latence de la pointe 1
Partout le temps est en msec. (d'après BREMER et STOUPEL, 1956, 1957)

dendrites superficiels. Au surplus, VON EULER, GREEN et RICCI (*56*) n'ont pu se convaincre de l'existence d'une propagation antidromique somato-dendritique dans le cas des cellules pyramidales de l'archicortex hippocampien.

L'opinion de PURPURA et GRUNDFEST (*52*) qui voient dans le potentiel surface-positif lent (l'onde 4 du potentiel évoqué de l'aire visuelle) un potentiel d'inhibition, homologue au potentiel postsynaptique d'inhibition, mis en évidence par ECCLES et ses collaborateurs (voir *33*) dans leurs enregistrements intracellulaires de la réponse des motoneurones spinaux à une volée d'influx inhibiteurs, ne semble pas avoir recueilli beaucoup de créance.

La signification de la pointe 3, et accessoirement aussi celle de la pointe 2, est celle qui comporte encore le plus d'incertitude. Dans une analyse, basée en particulier sur des enregistrements différentiels en profondeur, BISHOP et CLARE

(*5*, *6*), étaient arrivés à la conclusion que ces deux oscillations révélaient des activations synaptiques interneuroniques ascendantes, précédant celles des cellules pyramidales dont le complexe positif-négatif est l'expression. Cette interprétation, si elle avait pu être étayée de preuves définitives, aurait établi la notion qu'il était possible de suivre dans l'intimité de l'écorce, par une simple dérivation macroélectrodique, la succession des processus réactionnels s'échelonnant depuis l'arrivée des influx corticipètes jusqu'à la réaction des dendrites superficiels. Cette considération justifie l'intérêt que les expérimentateurs ont porté à ces deux oscillations du tracé de la réponse de l'aire visuelle à une volée d'influx afférents synchrones. La conception de Bishop et Clare peut s'appuyer sur deux données: a) l'excision de l'écorce (fig. 2, A ,B) fait disparaitre les pointes 2 et 3 en même temps que les potentiels 4 et 5 dont l'origine post-synaptique n'est pas contestée; b) l'intervalle de temps séparant la pointe 1 de la pointe 3 et aussi la pointe 2 de la pointe 3 (fig. 2, C et D) est indépendant de la distance du point d'application du stimulus de l'écorce, donnée manifestement incompatible avec l'interprétation de Chang et Kaada (1950) attribuant l'échelonnement des trois pointes à la dispersion spatio-temporelle de volées rétino-corticales d'influx de vitesses de conduction différentes, et voyant dans cette hétérogénéité un argument à l'appui de la théorie trichromatique de la vision des couleurs.

Mais l'assimilation des pointes 2 et 3 à des potentiels post-synaptiques successifs, rencontre des difficultés que l'on peut énumérer comme suit: a) persistance de la brieveté des potentiels et de la fixité de leur espacement dans les conditions de dépression fonctionnelle de la substance grise corticale ainsi que dans la dynamogenèse réticulaire (fig. 4, A et B); b) contraste de cette fixité avec l'effet frappant qu'exercent les modifications locales de la température de l'écorce, un réchauffement de 10° de celle-ci pouvant réduire de 1,4 msec l'écart entre la pointe 1 et la pointe 3, sans modification de la latence du potentiel de radiation (fig. 2, E, F); c) effet faible ou même nul sur l'amplitude de la pointe 3 (la seule susceptible de mesures précises) des modifications fonctionnelles de l'écorce du moment qu'elles ne comportent pas de changement d'amplitude du potentiel de radiation; cette faible réactivité de la pointe 3, qui contraste avec la facilité avec laquelle les mêmes modifications influencent le voltage des phases 4 et 5, a été observée au cours de la strychnisation, de la narcose et de l'anoxie locales de l'écorce (*23*, *13*, *39* bis). Dans la potentiation réticulaire, le fait que le voltage de la pointe 3 est habituellement un peu plus augmenté que celui de la pointe 1 (fig. 4) peut s'expliquer par un effet d'addition de ce potentiel avec un potentiel 4 très amplifié et débutant précocement.

Ces données diverses nous ont fait proposer (*13*, *14*) l'hypothèse d'après laquelle les pointes 2 et 3, si étroitement jumelées, seraient produites par un ralentissement très marqué des influx corticipètes dans les terminaisons amyéliniques intracorticales des fibres afférentes. L'existence d'une composante présynaptique dans la constitution de la pointe 3 ressort également d'observations microphysiologiques de Widén et Ajmone Marsan (*58*) montrant que les éléments générateurs du *spike* correspondant à cette oscillation du potentiel évoqué de surface pouvaient présenter une période réfractaire absolue à peu près aussi brève que celle des fibres de radiation produisant le pointe 1 et que cette brieveté, que montre la fig. 3, Bet C, contrastait avec la longue dépression postréactionnelle des potentiels 4 et 5, évènements post-synaptiques. Pour mettre en évidence ce contraste il était évidemment nécessaire d'appliquer les deux stimuli sur les radiations optiques et d'éliminer ainsi la dépression postréactionnelle résultant d'une stimulation faite présynaptiquement par rapport au relais genouillé.

Cependant, il nous parait plausible d'admettre (cf. également 58) la possibilité d'une contribution post-synaptique précoce à la constitution de la pointe 3. Cette opinion peut se baser notamment sur les cas exceptionnels où une strychnisation locale de l'écorce a renforcé une pointe 3 bien dissociée du potentiel 4 et sur l'étude comparative des dépressions postréactionnelles des trois pointes et des potentiels 4 et 5 (*34, 54*).

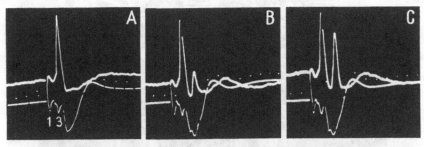

Fig. 3. *Relation des oscillations du potentiel évoqué de surface avec des potentiels d'action unitaires intracorticaux.* Chat légèrement endormi au pentobarbital. *A—C, spikes* unitaires (tracés supérieurs) correspondant à la pointe 3 des tracés de surface (tracés inférieurs); stimulus appliqué sur les radiations optiques (en B et C, paires de stimuli); remarquer en B la brieveté de la période réfractaires du processus responsable de la pointe 3; échelle de temps: 2 msec (d'après WIDÉN et AJMONE MARSAN, 1960)

2. Modifications fonctionnelles de la réponse. Certaines de ces modifications ont déjà été évoquées lors de l'analyse de la configuration oscillographique de la réponse. Dans ce qui va suivre, nous étudierons surtout les changements réversibles de l'amplitude du potentiel de radiation et des phases lentes, positive et négative de la réponse. Les facteurs suivants seront examinés en raison de l'intérêt particulier qui s'attache au déterminisme de leurs effects physiologiques: réfractorité post-réactionnelle; facilitation post-tétanique; facilitation par sommation temporelle; potentiation par illumination rétinienne (effet CHANG, *22*); facilitation par stimulation réticulaire d'éveil.

A priori, toute modification du potentiel de l'aire visuelle évoqué par un stimulus invariable appliqué en amont du corps genouillé ou directement sur ce dernier peut dépendre, soit d'une variation des propriétés fonctionnelles du noyau de relais (excitabilité directe ou transmissibilité synaptique selon le cas), soit de facteurs intracorticaux, soit des deux groupes de facteurs simultanément. La variation d'excitabilité ou de transmissibilité du corps genouillé est mise en évidence par une modification d'amplitude du potentiel de radiation (pointe 1) ainsi que — cas d'un stimulus infragéniculé — d'une modification de la réponse du noyau thalamique enregistré en même temps que la réponse corticale.

Le cycle de restauration postréactionnelle de la réponse de l'aire visuelle du Chat a été réétudié récemment par SCHOOLMAN et EVARTS (*54*) appliquant deux brefs stimuli successifs sur les radiations optiques. Cette méthode qui vise à éliminer la variable thalamique a mis en évidence le parallélisme général des courbes de restauration des potentiels 3, 4 et 5 et l'existence, chez l'animal non narcotisé, d'un retard de l'apparition de la dépression postréactionnelle de la réponse, retard s'expliquant par un processus de facilitation initial et le recrutement de neurones non activés par le premier stimulus. Cette facilitation, qui se manifeste malgré la dépression post-réactionnelle, est abolie par la narcose barbiturique.

La dépression postréactionnelle, dans la courbe de restauration étudiée chez des chats porteurs d'électrodes implantées en expériences chroniques, s'est révélée être paradoxalement plus profonde et plus longue chez l'animal éveillé que chez le même animal endormi (35).

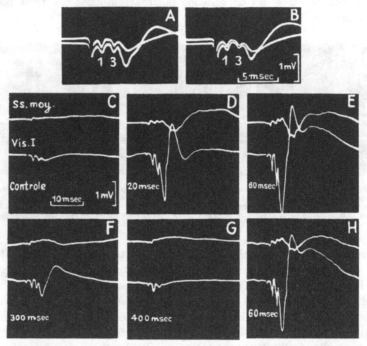

Fig. 4. *Potentiation de la réponse de l'aire visuelle à un choc «genouillé» sous l'effet d'un stimulus réticulaire conditionnant.* Chats, encéphale isolé; *A* et *B*, paires de réponses à un choc «genouillé»; la plus ample de chaque paire est la réponse potentiée par une brève stimulation réticulaire répétitive, faite immédiatement avant l'enregistrement; remarquer l'invariance des pointes 1 et 3 et de leur espacement; *C—H*, stimulus conditionnant constitué par un tétanos de 5 impulsions rectangulaires, de durée 0,3 msec, à la fréquence de 500/sec, appliqué sur la formation réticulaire mésencéphalique; intervalles entre stimulus conditionnant et stimulus «genouillé» testant indiqués en msec sous les différents tracés, qui sont reproduits dans l'ordre de leur enregistrement (d'après BREMER et STOUPEL, 1959)

La facilitation post-tétanique de la réponse du corps genouillé, et secondairement de la réponse de l'aire visuelle, a été étudiée par HUGHES, EVARTS et MARSHALL (*40*). De même que dans le cas de la facilitation post-tétanique au niveau spinal, l'augmentation de voltage du potentiel d'action des fibres présynaptiques ne semble pas constituer un facteur déterminant essentiel de l'effet. Une hypothèse plausible tend à rattacher le phénomène à une modification transitoire du processus chimique de la transmission synaptique (cf. *33*).

Deux autres phénomènes de facilitation se signalent particulièrement à l'attention en raison de la puissance de la dynamogenèse dont ils sont l'expression et de l'intérêt physiologique qui s'attache à l'élucidation de leurs mécanismes. Ce sont la facilitation «réticulaire» de la réponse à un choc «nerf optique» ou à un choc

« genouillé » (fig. 4) et la facilitation de la réponse à ce même stimulus thalamique que détermine l'illumination de la rétine.

La facilitation réticulaire des potentiels évoqués corticaux, dont celle de la réponse de l'aire visuelle n'est qu'un cas particulier (*15, 16, 29, 32*), se manifeste dans: a) l'interaction dynamogénique des influx spécifiques et des influx suscités par la stimulation électrique de la formation réticulaire mésencéphalique ou thalamique, un bref stimulus conditionnant pouvant être efficace (fig. 4); b) l'éveil thalamo-cortical provoqué par des stimulations sensorielles; c) l'éveil faisant suite à l'injection d'amphétamine.

Les données dont on dispose pour déterminer le mécanisme du phénomène sont les suivantes: a) les influx réticulaires ascendants produisent, quand ils sont répétitifs, une activation manifeste de l'isocortex, démontrée par la fois par des enregistrements macro- et microélectrodiques, dont ceux qui ont été obtenus dans le laboratoire de Freiburg (*27, 28*) sont les plus significatifs ici puisqu'ils concernent l'air visuelle; b) les réactions corticales aux influx réticulaires d'origine mésencéphalique ou thalamique sont nettement différentes par leur latence et leur morphologie des réponses suscitées par des influx spécifiques et l'on peut admettre que ces différences s'expliquent par l'interposition de relais interneuroniques plus ou moins nombreux sur la voie des influx non spécifiques; c) l'évail réticulaire et les éveils physiologiques s'accompagnent de l'apparition d'une négativité électrique (*negative shift*) de la surface corticale (*8, 18, 21*), qu'il est plausible de rapporter à une dépolarisation réactionnelle inégale des somas et des dendrites des cellules pyramidales; d) l'enregistrement microphysiologique des potentiels unitaires de l'aire visuelle a mis en évidence, dans une proportion élevée de ces enregistrements (environ 80%), les convergences d'influx visuels spécifiques et non spécifiques sur les mêmes cellules de l'aire visuelle (*27, 28*); cette convergence neuronique s'est manifetée le plus souvent par la facilitation de la réponse de l'aire visuelle à des stimulations rétiniennes physiologiques; e) le processus de dynamogenèse peut affecter directement l'écorce: la facilitation de la transmission dans le noyau thalamique (démontrée par l'augmentation de la réponse du corps genouillé latéral à un choc nerf optique) ne suffit apparemment pas à rendre compte des potentiations spectaculaires de la réponse corticale et peut d'ailleurs faire défaut (*15*).

A la lumière de l'ensemble de ces données, il parait légitime d'expliquer la facilitation réticulaire de la réponse de l'aire visuelle et celle des réponses «secondaires» qui l'accompagnet dans les aires associatives (fig. 4) par la convergence hétérosynaptique des influx réticulaires ascendants et des influx spécifiques sur les neurones thalamiques spécifiques et sur les interneurones corticaux conduisant aux esthésioneurones des aires de réception sensorielles ou aux cellules pyramidales qui sont leurs homologues dans les aires associatives. L'organisation synaptique corticale des projections réticulaires et spécifiques rendrait compte du fait que les influx d'éveil, tout en facilitant puissamment les réponses sensorielles primaires et «secondaires» de l'écorce ne réalisent pas les configurations réactionnelles qui sont la condition de la sensation et de ses manifestations comportementales (*17*).

La combinaison de facilitations ressortissant à des mécanismes différents, en particulier à celui de la sommation temporelle, et de la facilitation réticulaire, a mis clairement en évidence leur dépendance commune de la frange sous-liminaire de la réponse au stimulus conditonnant (*17*). Dans ces expériences où le stimulus était appliqué sur le corps genouillé, il s'est révélé en effet que l'existence préalable de l'une des facilitations empêchait la manifestation de l'autre. Cette non-additivité s'explique par la limitation des disponibilités de la frange sous-liminaire. Par contraste, l'effet d'une potentiation strychnique de la réponse peut être encore augmenté fortement par une stimulation réticulaire (*15, 17*), comme si l'action du poison avait comme effet d'élargir la frange sous-liminaire et de permettre ainsi l'addition d'un recrutement neuronique à celui qui est déjà manifeste dans la réponse de contrôle.

La potentiation de la réponse de l'aire visuelle à un choc «genouillé» que détermine l'illumination rétinienne, avait paru à Chang (*22*) résulter de la sensibilisation facilitatrice du corps genouillé et de l'écorce par les influx issus de l'activation rétinienne photique. Cette interprétation, qui avait été admise implicitement par les auteurs (*13, 46*) qui confirmèrent les observations de Chang n'était pas toutefois sans rencontrer des difficultés, dont la plus sérieuse est le délai relativement considérable qui peut s'écouler entre le début de la stimulation lumineuse rétinienne continue et celui de la potentiation de la réponse. Les recherches de Arduini et Hirao (*1*), dont notre collègue Arduini nous fait part à ce Symposium, les ont conduits à reconsidérer le problème et les ont amenés à la conclusion inattendue que l'effet de l'éclairement rétinien sur le potentiel évoqué cortical résulterait de l'abolition de l'activité rétinienne spontanée et de la suppression corrélative d'une décharge d'influx corticipètes, d'effet inhibiteur sur le corps genouillé et sur l'écorce et transmis bilatéralement à partir de chaque oeil par des fibres corticipètes spéciales. Posternak, Fleming et Evarts (*51*) avaient déjà été amenés à postuler, eux aussi, une influence inhibitrice tonique s'exerçant à partir de la rétine sur la réactivité de l'*area striata*, à la suite d'expériences leur ayant montré une augmentation de la réponse du cortex visuel à un choc appliqué sur la radiation optique, après la section du nerf optique ou la destruction du corps genouillé.

L'effet Chang représenterait donc, dans cette hypothèse, la libération du corps genouillé et de l'écorce d'une inhibition tonique d'origine rétinienne. Arduini et Hirao ne se dissimulent pas les difficultés que rencontre cette interprétation dans des conditions expérimentales, comme celles des observations de Chang, où en raison d'une narcose barbiturique profonde, l'existence d'une activité rétinienne spontanée est problématique.

III. Le potentiel de l'aire visuelle évoqué par un stimulus photique

L'intérêt qui s'attache à cette réponse ressortit plus spécialement à la physiologie visuelle. Car, entre le stimulus photique si simple qu'il soit et la volée d'influx enregistrée dans le nerf optique s'interpose l'enchevêtrement infiniment complexe des processus de l'excitation photochimique de récepteurs répartis en des catégories multiples, puis de l'activation synaptique et de l'inhibition associée de deux couches neuroniques successives.

Il n'est donc pas surprenant, dans ces conditions, que les différences morphologiques entre les potentiels évoqués de l'aire visuelle suscités par des stimuli «périphériques» et «centraux» soient bien plus marquées que celles qui s'observent entre, par exemple, les réponses de l'aire auditive corticale à un «clic» et à un choc électrique appliqué sur le corps genouillé médian. Dans les deux cas, la différence de latence des deux réponses est plus grande que celle qui résulterait simplement de l'inégalité de distance des points d'application des stimuli. Mais la phase surface-négative de la réponse de l'aire visuelle à un bref stimulus photique (fig. 5, A) est accidentée d'indentations profondes qui ne s'observent pas dans le cas des potentiles évoqués des autres aires de réception et dont le déterminisme est certainement intrarétinien car elles existent déjà dans le potentiel évoqué de la bandelette optique (50).

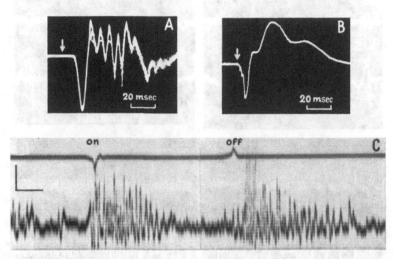

Fig. 5. *Réponse de l'aire visuelle du chat au stimulus photique. A* et *B*, chats narcotisés; *A*, réponse à un éclair bref appliqué sur l'oeil contralatéral; tracés superposés; *B*, pour comparaison, réponse (enregistrée à la même vitesse) à un stimulus «nerf optique » (d'après BUSER, 1957); *C*, encéphale isolé; adaptation partielle à l'obscurité; réponse à l'illumination de l'oeil contralatéral; barre de temps: 0.2 sec; remarquer l'intensité de la postdécharge rapide dans les effets *on* et *off* (d'après BREMER, 1949)

En raison de sa constitution même, le potentiel évoqué cortical suscité par un stimulus photique ne peut fournir, lui aussi, que des informations statistiques, compliquées par l'incidence de facteurs extrarétiniens, en particulier intracorticaux. Cette considération vaut pour les réponses *on* et *off* (fig. 5, C) à une illumination rétinienne plus ou moins prolongée, pour le rôle de l'adaptation à l'obscurité et à la lumière (24) et pour l'interférence de l'activité corticale spontanée avec la réponse enregistrée chez l'animal non anesthésié. Cette activité tend à brouiller les réponses au point de les rendre parfois presque indiscernables et de nécessiter, pour les dégager du bruit de fond de l'activité corticale autochtone, la dépression de celle-ci par une narcose corticale locale (24) ou générale, en particulier chloralosique (9, 10, 19, 20), ou bien encore une transsection mésencéphalique (11).

Chez l'homme, où le problème de l'enregistrement des réponses est rendu très difficile par la réduction de voltage des potentiels réactionnels résultant de leur dérivation transcranienne, la difficulté a été tournée par le recours à des techniques compliquées d'intégration électronique (2, 25, 53). Les tracés recueillis au moyen de ces méthodes ont permis de préciser la situation de la projection cranienne de la réponse de l'aire visuelle chez l'Homme, la latence exacte de cette réponse, sa configuration, sa relation temporelle avec l'ERG (49).

L'étude de la relation de l'activité rythmique corticale provoquée par les
stimulations photiques (exemple de post-décharge lente) a été reprise au moyen
de la combinaison de la technique d'intégration avec l'analyse par la méthode de
l'autocorrélation de l'activité rythmique dominante de l'EEG. Cette étude a
amené BARLOW (2) à admettre, en accord avec la conclusion qu'avait déjà déduite
BARTLEY (4) de ses expériences sur l'animal anesthésié, qu'il existe une relation

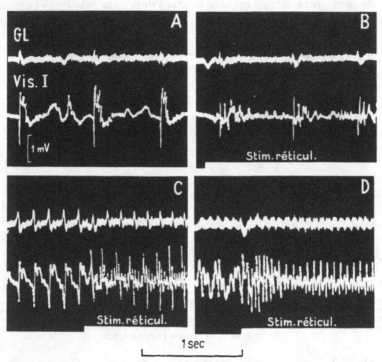

Fig. 6. *Action de l'éveil réticulaire sur la réponse de l'aire visuelle au stimulus lumineux rétinien.* Chat, encéphale
isolé; dérivations du corps genouillé et de l'aire visuelle, réponse à des éclairs stroboscopiques répétitifs de fréquence
croissante, avec superposition en *D*, *E* et *F* de stimulations réticulaires mésencéphaliques (200/sec; 0,3 msec; 1 V)
indiquées par le bloc-signal au bas des tracés; autres explications dans le texte

étroite entre l'activité régulière dominante de l'EEG et la post-décharge rythmique
de la réponse photique (à des éclairs stroboscopiques) chez le même sujet. Bien que
très voisines, les fréquences des deux rythmes corticaux ne sont cependant pas
identiques. COOPER et GREY WALTER (26), utilisant d'autres méthodes, sont
arrivés à des conclusions similaires.

La sommation temporelle réalisée par la répétition rythmique du stimulus
photique (brefs éclairs stroboscopiques) s'est révélée d'autre part d'un grand
intérêt physiologique, psychophysiologique et pathologique. Parmi les nombreux
problèmes qui ont été abordés grâce à la méthode, on peut mentionner l'étude des
irradiations extrastriaires de la réponse chez l'Homme et chez l'animal (19, 57),
l'existence d'une fréquence optimale pour ces irradiations cortico-corticales et
cortico-sous-corticales, l'analyse de leurs effets subjectifs et comportementaux (26,
31, 57), la signification pathologique de leurs effets électroencéphalographiques
et moteurs (photomyocloniques) et l'utilisation de ces effets pour la mise en évi-

dence et la catégorisation des épilepsies, (voir *50*) et pour le diagnostic de conditions psychopathiques et névrosiques (*36*).

Tout récemment, la stimulation lumineuse intermittente a permis de démontrer chez l'animal non anesthésié (chat, encéphale isolé) l'existence d'une facilitation réticulaire très nette des potentiels évoqués de l'aire visuelle et du corps genouillé au stimulus photique (*55*), facilitation que n'avait pu mettre en évidence l'enregistrement de la réponse à un éclair isolé ou à des flashs de très basse fréquence (inférieure à 5 éclairs/seconde). La dépression plus ou moins profonde du potentiel évoqué photique dans l'éveil réticulaire (fig. 6, A et B), dépression résultant vraisemblablement d'un processus d'«occlusion» (*15, 17*), fait place alors à une dynamogenèse, caractérisée à la fois par l'augmentation du voltage des réponses, la synchronisation plus marquées de leurs influx constitutifs et l'apparation d'une post-décharge rapide (fig. 6, C et D). L'absence de modification du potentiel évoqué de la bandellette optique a fait exclure (*55*), tout au moins en tant que facteur principal, un déterminisme rétinien du phénomène. On peut voir dans ces expériences l'aspect macrophysiologique des observations microphysiologiques de CREUTZFELDT et AKIMOTO (*27*) et de CREUTZFELDT et GRÜSSER (*28*).

La stimulation photique rétinienne a permis d'autre part, grâce à son caractère d'excitant naturel at à sa grande maniabilité, l'étude de divers facteurs de modification de la réponse de l'aire visuelle, que l'on peut qualifier de psychophysiologiques. Ces travaux, auxquels HERNANDEZ PEON et ses collaborateurs se sont particulièrement attachés, ont mis en évidence l'effet de la distraction sensorielle, qui réduit l'amplitude de la réponse (*38, 50* bis); celui de l'habituation résultant de la répétition monotone longtemps prolongée du stimulus photique qui a le même effet dépresseur (*39, 47, 48, 50* bis); celui de l'attention pour le stimulus, qui tend au contraire à augmenter l'amplitude de la réponse (*38, 41, 50* bis).

Les variations d'amplitude du potentiel évoqué — dans l'un ou l'autre sens — semblent être essentiellement le reflet de processus rétiniens, car elles s'observent déjà pour les potentiels de la bandelette optique (*50* bis), du corps genouillé (*47, 48*) et des radiations optiques (*41*). Le rôle de la formation réticulaire du tronc cérébral dans le déterminisme du processus d'inhibition active qui serait responsable de l'habituation n'est pas encore clair. HERNANDEZ PEON et ses collaborateurs l'avaient admis à la suite d'expériences de stimulation, de paralysie narcotique et de destruction de la formation réticulaire. On peut objecter à cette conclusion qu'il pourrait s'être agi, dans les expériences d'excitation, du phénomène de «masquage» qui caractérise la modification des réponses du corps genouillé et de l'écorce dans l'éveil réticulaire (*15*). Les lésions très larges de la formation réticulaire mésencéphalique faites par HERNANDEZ PEON (voir *39*) dans leur analyse de l'habituation acoustique pourraient avoir lésé la voie extraréticulaire (paralemniscale) dont DESMEDT et MECHELSE (voir *30*) ont montré qu'elle transmet des influx inhibiteurs corticifuges destinés notamment au noyau cochléaire. Enfin, les doses de pentobarbital utilisées pour abolir l'habituation sont très supérieures à celles qui suppriment l'éveil réticulaire. MANCIA, MEULDERS et SANTIBANEZ (*47, 48*) qui ont fait cette remarque, ont rejeté l'hypothèse du déterminisme réticulaire de l'habituation photique à la suite de leurs expériences; celles-ci leur ont montré, d'une part que l'habituation est encore présente — et est même beaucoup plus précoce que chez l'animal intact — chez le chat «cerveau isolé» (dont une grande partie de la formation réticulaire est déconnectée du telencéphale), d'autre part que la stimulation directe ou sensorielle (olfactive) de la formation réticulaire «ascendante» en avant de la transsection, a comme effet de supprimer l'habituation. Ce dernier argument nous parait le plus décisif.

Conclusion

L'étude des tracés du potentiel évoqué de l'écorce visuelle, enregistré en dérivation monopolaire de surface et interprété selon la théorie du volume conducteur permet d'obtenir des renseignements intéressants sur le déroulement des processus réactionnels, rétiniens, sous-corticaux et corticaux qui conditionnent la sensation visuelle élémentaire.

Pour l'analyse de ces processus, il est commode de commencer par l'examen de la phase ultime de la réponse en provoquant celle-ci par un stimulus électrique appliqué sur les radiations visuelles thalamo-corticales. La stimulation du nerf optique ou du corps genouillé introduit en effet la complication des transmissions interneuroniques à l'intérieur de ce noyau de relais: délai synaptique, période réfractaire neuronique, post-décharge rythmique.

Si l'on excepte l'éventualité d'une post-décharge, les configurations générales des réponses suscitées par un bref stimulus électrique pré- ou post-géniculé sont toutefois très semblables. Une de leurs caractéristiques communes réside dans l'interposition, entre le potentiel d'action des fibres thalamo-corticales et les potentiels post-synaptiques successivement positif et négatif traduisant l'activation des somas puis des dendrites superficiels des cellules pyramidales de l'écorce, de deux oscillations si brèves qu'ont les a qualifiées de *spikes*. La polarité, l' amplitude relative et l'intervalle de ces deux pointes sont d'une constance qui a justifié l'intérêt porté à leur signification physiologique. Leur attribution à la succession de réactions d'interneurones corticaux a suscité des objections théoriques et expérimentales et l'hypothèse a été émise qu'il s'agit d'évènements présynaptiques, encore qu'indubitablement intracorticaux.

La régularité morphologique si remarquable de la réponse élémentaire de l'aire visuelle a conduit à utiliser celle-ci dans des recherches de physiologie générale de l'écorce cérébrale, parmi lesquelles on peut citer celles concernant les processus initiaux de l'éveil réticulaire et les modifications fonctionnelles corticales caractérisant les états de veille et de sommeil, les narcoses, l'action de l'éclairement rétinien, celle des anticholinestérases et des drogues psychotropes.

L'analyse du potentiel évoqué de l'aire visuelle suscité par des stimuli photiques de paramètres variés a fourni, elle aussi, maintes informations importantes, mais qui concernent plus spécialement la physiologie sensorielle en raison de l'importance des processus intrarétiniens dans le déterminisme des caractéristiques de la réponse. Celle-ci, même dans le cas du stimulus photique le plus bref, se distingue du potentiel évoqué par un stimulus électrique appliqué sur les voies visuelles par sa plus grande latence, sa plus grande durée, la complexité de la configuration de sa phase négative terminale. Cette configuration typique s'observe déjà dans le potentiel dérivé de la bandelette optique, indication claire de son déterminisme rétinien.

La répétition rythmique de la stimulation lumineuse modifie considérablement la morphologie et l'amplitude de la réponse, son irradiation en dehors de l'aire visuelle, sa réactivité à la stimulation réticulaire d'éveil.

Un intérêt particulier s'attache à la réponse au stimulus photique en raison de la possibilité de la dériver de la surface cranienne chez l'homme grâce à un repérage actuellement précisé et à l'emploi d'intégrateurs électroniques. Les modifications expérimentales de la réponse visuelle corticale seront sans doute utilisées de plus en plus souvent pour la mise en évidence de la catégorisation des épilepsies et pour le diagnostic de conditions psychopathologiques.

Summary

The report is devoted to the analysis of the responses of the mammalian visual area, evoked by a brief photic or electrical stimulus, exciting the peripheral receptors or the optic pathway.

The wide variations of amplitude and wave form of the response to an invariant testing stimulus provide interesting informations on the first stages of the retinal and cortical processes that lead ultimately to perception. The validity of these informations is, for many purposes, increased by the fact that the gross electrode which records the activity of a large neural population is performing an averaging process.

The response evoked by an electrical stimulus applied on the optic pathway is characterized by a sequence of brief initial transients, preceding the positive-negative slow phases, obviously of postsynaptic origin. Spike 1 is the record of the radiation potential. But the nature of spikes 2 and 3 is still a matter of controversy. A significative feature of the spike sequence is the striking dependance of the spacing of its constituting potentials on the temperature of the cortex, a fact which, together with other data, suggests that spikes 2 and 3 contain important intracortical presynaptic components.

The complex configuration of the cortical response to a flash of light reflects essentially retinal organization.

The various factors that have proved responsible for correlated changes of retinal, geniculate and cortical reactivity are discussed. Special emphasis is placed on the facilitatory and suppressive processes which are operative during reticular arousal of the brain.

Bibliographie

1. ARDUINI, A., and T. HIRAO: Enhancement of evoked responses in the visual system during reversible retinal inactivation. Arch. ital. Biol. 98, 182—205 (1960).
2. BARLOW, J. S.: Rhythmic activity induced by photic stimulation in relation to intrinsic alpha activity of the brain in man. EEG Clin. Neurophysiol. 12, 317—326 (1960).
3. — M. A. B. BRAZIER and W. A. ROSENBLITH: The application of autocorrelation analysis to electroencephalography. 622—626. Proc. 1srt. Nat. Biophys. Conf. Columbus, Ohio, March 1957. New Haven: Yale University 1960.
4. BARTLEY, S. H.: Central mechanisms of vision, in: Handbook of Physiology, Section I, vol. I, 693—712 (1959).
5. BISHOP, G. H., and M. CLARE: Site of origin of electric potentials in striate cortex. J. Neurophysiol. 15, 201—220 (1952).

6. BISHOP, G. H., and M. CLARE: Sequence of events in optic cortex response to volleys of impulses in the radiation. J. Neurophysiol. **16**, 418—437 (1953).

7. BISHOP, P. O., D. JEREMY and J. C. MC LEOD: Phenomenon of repetitive firing in lateral geniculate in cat. J. Neurophysiol. **16**, 427—447 (1953).

8. BONNET, V.: La transmission synaptique d'influx au niveau des dendrites superficiels de l'écorce cérébrale. Arch. int. Physiol. **50**, 163—168 (1958).

9. BRAZIER, M. A. B.: The action of anesthetics on the nervous system, in: Brain Mechanisms and Consciousness, 162—199. Oxford: Blackwell 1954.

10. — A study of the late response to flash in the cortex of the cat. Acta physiol. pharmacol. neerl. **6**, 692—714 (1957).

11. BREMER, F.: Etude oscillographique des activités sensorielles du cortex cérébral. C. R. Soc. Biol. (Paris) **124**, 842—848 (1937).

12. — Considérations sur l'origine et la nature des « ondes » cérébrales. EEG Clin. Neurophysiol. **1**, 177—193 (1949).

13. — et N. STOUPEL: Interprétation de la réponse de l'aire visuelle corticale à une volée d'influx sensoriels. Arch. int. Physiol. **64**, 234—248 (1956).

14. — — Analyse oscillographique comparée des réponses des aires de projection de l'écorce cérébrale du chat. Arch. ital. Biol. **93**, 3—19 (1957).

15. — — Facilitation et inhibition des potentiels évoqués corticaux dans l'éveil cérébral. Arch. int. Physiol. **67**, 240—275 (1959).

16. — — Etude pharmacologique de la facilitation des réponses corticales dans l'éveil réticulaire. Arch. int. Pharmacol. **122**, 234—248 (1959).

17. — — et P. C. VAN REETH: Nouvelles recherches sur la facilitation et l'inhibition des potentiels évoqués corticaux dans l'éveil réticulaire. Arch. ital. Biol. **98**, 229—247 (1960).

18. BROOKHART, J. M., A. ARDUINI, M. MANCIA and G. MORUZZI: Thalamo-cortical relation as revealed by induced slow potentials changes. J. Neurophysiol. **21**, 499—525 (1958).

19. BUSER, P., et PH. ASHER: Mise en jeu du système pyramidal chez le chat. Arch. ital. Physiol. **98**, 123—164 (1960).

20. — et P. BORENSTEIN: Réponses somesthésiques, visuelles et auditives recueillies au niveau du cortex « associatif » suprasylvien chez le chat curarisé non anesthésié. EEG Clin. Neurophysiol. **11**, 285—304 (1959).

21. CASPERS, H.: Changes of cortical d. c. potentials in the sleep-wakefulness cycle. In: The nature of sleep, Ciba Foundation Symposium, juin 1960. London: Churchill 1961.

22. CHANG, H. T.: Functional organisation of central visual pathways. Res. Publ. Ass. Nerv. Ment. Dis. **30**, 430—463 (1952).

23. — and B. KAADA: An analysis or primary response of visual cortex to optic nerve stimulation in cats. J. Neurophysiol. **13**, 305—318 (1950).

24. CLAES, E.: Contribution à l'étude de la fonction visuelle. I., Analyse oscillographique de l'activité spontanée et sensorielle chez le chat non anesthésié. Arch. int. Physiol. **48**, 180—257 (1939).

25. COBB, W. A., and G. D. DAWSON: The latency and form in man of the occipital potentials evoked by bright flashes. J. Physiol. (Lond.) **152**, 108—121 (1960).

26. COOPER, R., and W. G. WALTER: Intracerebral responses to single flash stimulus. EEG Clin. Neurophysiol. **12**, 544—545 (1960).

27. CREUTZFELDT, O., u. A. AKIMOTO: Konvergenz und gegenseitige Beeinflussung von Impulsen aus der Retina und den unspezifischen Thalamuskernen in einzelnen Neuronen des optischen Cortex. Arch. Psychiat. Nervenkr. **196**, 520—538 (1958).

28. — u. O.-J. GRÜSSER: Beeinflussung der Flimmerreaktion einzelner corticaler Neurone durch elektrische Reize unspezifischer Thalamuskerne. Proc. of the First International Congress of Neurol. Sciences, Brussels, 1957, 349—355. London: Pergamon Press 1959.

29. DELL, P.: Discussion de la communication de F. BREMER à l'International Colloqium on EEG of higher nervous activity. Moscou 1958. EEG Clin. Neurophysiol. suppl. **13** (1960).

30. DESMEDT, J. E.: Contribution à l'étude des processus neurophysiologiques mis en jeu au cours de l'attention sensorielle. Mém. Acad. roy Méd. Belg. **4**, 133—157 (1959).

31. DONGIER, M., S. DONGIER, J. BARRABINO and H. GASTAUT: On the psychiatric significance of certain responses evoked by intermittent photic stimulation. EEG. Clin. Neurophysiol. **12**, 541 (1960).

32. DUMONT, S., et P. DELL: Facilitations spécifiques et non spécifiques des reponses visuelles corticales. J. Physiol. (Paris) **50**, 261—264 (1958).

33. ECCLES, J. C.: The physiology of nerve cells, pp. 270. Baltimore: Johns Hopkins Press 1957.

34. EVARTS, E. V.: Communication personelle.

35. — T. C. FLEMING and P. R. HUTTENLOCHER: Recovery cycle of visual cortex of the awake and sleeping cat. Amer. J. Physiol. **199**, 373—376 (1960).

36. GASTAUT, H., Y. GASTAUT, A. ROGER, J. CORRIOL et R. NAQUET: Etude électroencéphalographique du cycle d'excitabilité corticale. EEG Clin. Neurophysiol. **3**, 401—428 (1951).

37. GRANIT, R.: Neural activity on the retina. In: Handbook of Physiology, Section I, vol. I, 693—712 (1959).

38. HERNANDEZ PEON, R., C. GUZMAN FLORES, M. ALCARAZ and A. HERNANDEZ GUARDOLIA: Sensory transmission in visual pathway during attention. Acta neurol. lat.-amer. **3**, 1—8 (1957).

39. — — — — Habituation in the visual pathway. Acta neurol. lat.-amer. **4**, 121—127 (1958).

39a HIRSCH, R., F. BANGE, G. PULVER and J. STEFFENS: Evoked responses of the cat's visual cortex to optic tract stimulation at temperatures between 39° and 15° C. EEG Clin. Neurophysiol. **12**, 679—684 (1960).

40. HUGHES, J. R., E. V. EVARTS and W. H. MARSHALL: Post-tetanic potentiation in the visual system of cats. Amer. J. Physiol. **186**, 483—487 (1956).

41. JOUVET, M.: Etude neurophysiologique chez l'homme de quelques mécanismes sous corticaux de l'attention. Rev. Psychol. Franc. **2**, (1957).

42. LENNOX, M. A.: Geniculate and cortical responses to colored light flash in cat. J. Neurophysiol. **19**, 271—279 (1956).

43. — and A. MADSEN: Cortical and retinal responses to colored light flash in anesthetized cat. J. Neurophysiol. **18**, 424 (1955).

44. LI, C. L., C. CULLEN and H. H. JASPER: Laminar microelectrode studies of specific somatosensory cortical potentials. J. Neurophysiol. **19**, 113—130 (1956).

45. MADSEN, A., and M. A. LENNOX: Response to colored light flash from different areas of optic cortex and from retina in anesthetized cat. J. Neurophysiol. **18**, 574—582 (1955).

46. MALIS, L. C., and I. KRUGER: Multiple response and excitability of cats visual cortex. J. Neurophysiol. **19**, 172—183 (1956).

47. MANCIA, M., M. MEULDERS and H. G. SANTIBANEZ: Changes of photically evoked potentials in the visual pathway of the "cerveau isolé" cat. Arch. ital. Biol. **97**, 378—398 (1959).

48. — — — Changes of photically-evoked potentials in the visual pathway of the midpontine pretrigeminal cat. Arch. ital. Biol. **97**, 399—413 (1959).

49. MONNIER, M.: Le centre visuel cortical et l'organisation des perceptions visuelles in Problèmes actuels d'ophtalmologie 1, 277—301. Bâle-New York 1957.

50. NAQUET, R., L. FERGERSTEN and J. BERT: Seizure discharges localized to the posterior cerebral regions in man provoked by intermittent photic stimulations. EEG Clin. Neurophysiol. **12**, 305—316 (1960).

50a. PALESTINI, M., A. DAVIDOVITCH and R. HERNANDEZ-PEON: Functional significance of centrifugal influences upon the retina. Acta neurol. lat.-amer. **5**, 113—131 (1959).

51. POSTERNAK, J. M., I. C. FLEMING and E. V. EVARTS: Effect of interruption of the visual pathway on the response to geniculate stimulation. Science **129**, 39—40 (1959).

52. PURPURA, P. P., and H. GRUNDFEST: Physiological and pharmacological consequences of different synaptic organization on cerebral and cerebellar cortex. J. Neurophysiol. **20**, 494—522 (1957).

53. ROSENBLITH, W. A.: Some quantifiable aspects of the electrical activity of the nervous system (with emphasis upon responses to sensory stimuli). Rev. modern Physics **31**, 532—545 (1959).

54. SCHOOLMAN, A., and E. V. EVARTS: Responses to lateral geniculate radiation stimulation in cats with implanted electrodes. J. Neurophysiol. **22**, 112—119 (1959).

55. STERIADE, M., et M. DEMETRESCO: Phénomènes de dynamogenèse réticulaire aux divers niveaux de la voie optique pendant la stimulation lumineuse intermittente. J. Physiol. (Paris) **52**, 224—225 (1960).

56. Euler, C. v., J. D. Green and C. Ricci: Role of hippocampal dendrites in evoked responses and afterdischarges. Acta physiol. scand. **42**, 87—111 (1958).

57. Walter, V. J., and W. G. Walter: The central effects of rhythmic sensory stimulation. EEG Clin. Neurophysiol. **1**, 57—86 (1949).

58. Widén, L., and C. Ajmone Marsan: Unitary analysis of the response elicited in the visual cortex of cat. Arch. ital. Biol. **98**, 248—274 (1960).

Discussion

A. Arduini: It is suggested that possible mechanism of the facilitation of the evoked cortical activity obtained by reticular stimulation may also stem from the release from an inhibition.

R. Jung: Professor Bremers Deutung, daß die unspezifische Bahnung nach retinalen Licht-reizen durch Okklusion verdeckt wird, paßt zu den Befunden von Akimoto, Creutzfeldt u. Mitarb., die an einzelnen Neuronen auch bei adäquater Lichtreizung eine unspezifische Bahnung durch Thalamusreizung sahen. Synchrone afferente Impulse nach kurzen Lichtblitzen werden offenbar besser gefördert als länger dauernde Lichtreize. Die maximale Bahnung nach Opticusreiz betrifft abnorm synchronisierte Impulse einer reziprok organisierten Afferenz (on versus off, B versus D), die unter physiologischen Bedingungen niemals gleichzeitig erregt werden. Diese Bahnung unphysiologisch synchronisierter Impulssalven spricht für einen re-lativ undifferenzierten Mechanismus der reticulo-thalamischen Bahnung. Bei differenzierten Reizmustern ist die Bahnung weniger deutlich oder okkludiert.

Daß ponto-medulläre Strukturen am "tonus cortical" der visuellen Neurone beteiligt sind, geht aus Baumgartners Versuchen hervor: Nach retinaler Ischämie fehlen neuronale Ent-ladungen der Area 17 beim cerveau-isolé, aber nicht beim encéphale-siolé. Die anatomischen Grundlagen dieser Phänomene sind noch sehr unklar. Ist bekannt, ob die retikulären Afferen-zen auch nach Zerstörung des unspezifischen Thalamus wirksam bleiben, ferner ob und welche Verbindungen von der Reticularis zum Geniculatum gehen?

F. Bremer: Je ne crois pas que la potentiation des réponses des aires sensorielles corticales à un stimulus «central» puisse s'expliquer par une libération d'inhibition, ainsi que le suggère le docteur Arduini. Et cela pour les raisons suivantes: a) les quatre aires de projection que nous avons étudiées (la somesthésique, l'auditive, la visuelle, le gyrus suprasylvien activé par un stimulus pulvinarien) ont toutes présenté le phénomène, et non pas seulement l'aire visuelle; b) un stimulus réticulaire unique conditionnant la réponse au stimulus spécifique testant peut être très efficace; c) la potentiation s'observe encore sur la préparation *cerveau isolé* (stimulus «réticulaire» appliqué sur le n. centre médian).

Je remercie mon collègue Jung de l'intéressant commentaire dans lequel il rapproche les résultats des observations microphysiologiques, faites dans son laboratoire, de nos expériences sur le potentiel évoqué de l'aire visuelle. Ces observations indiquent très bien l'une des condi-tions dans lesquelles la potentiation de la réponse corticale peut-être remplacée par une dépres-sion, résultant sans doute d'un phénomène de compétition neuronique occlusive entre influx spécifiques et non spécifiques.

Je ne connais pas de données expérimentales permettant de répondre à sa question con-cernant la persistance ou non de la dynamogenèse réticulaire d'éveil après la destruction des noyaux non spécifiques du thalamus. De pareilles expériences seraient sans doute d'une exécution très difficile. Tout ce que je puis dire c'est que la stimulation de noyaux thalamiques non spécifiques (le n. centre médian en particulier) nous a donné le même effet de potentiation de la réponse de l'aire visuelle à un choc «nerf optique» ou «genouillé» que la stimulatiin du tegmentum mésencéphalique.

L'existence de connexions des formations réticulaires mésencéphalique et thalamique avec le corps genouillé latéral ressort des observations anatomiques des Scheibel et de nos obser-vations électro-physiologiques démontrant une facilitation de la transmission corticipète dans le noyau de relais thalamique sous l'influence de stimulations réticulaires.

Veränderung der Neuronaktivität des visuellen Cortex durch Reizung der Substantia reticularis mesencephali[1,2]

Von

Otto Creutzfeldt, Rainer Spehlmann und Dietrich Lehmann

Mit 5 Abbildungen

In früheren Untersuchungen (Akimoto, Baumgartner, Creutzfeldt, Jung, *1, 7, 8, 9, 11, 20*) konnte gezeigt werden, daß an den Neuronen des visuellen Cortex sowohl spezifische Impulse aus der Retina als auch unspezifische aus den intralaminären Thalamuskernen und der Substantia reticularis konvergieren. Die Antworten corticaler Neurone auf Lichtreize können durch vorausgehende Thalamusreizung gebahnt werden. Besonders ausgeprägt ist die Bahnung bei Verwendung von Flimmerlicht (*11, 20*): Durch gleichzeitige Reizung in den unspezifischen Thalamuskernen wird die Fusionsgrenze (CFF) der corticalen Neurone signifikant erhöht, wie der eine von uns (Cr.) mit Grüsser (*11*) zeigen konnte.

Nachdem Chang (*6*) gefunden hatte, daß das evoked potential im optischen Cortex nach Reizung des Corpus geniculatum laterale durch gleichzeitige spezifische Reizung mit Licht gebahnt werden kann, fanden Dumont und Dell (*12, 13*) und Bremer und Stoupel (*3, 4, 5*) eine Bahnung verschiedener Teile des evoked potential nach Opticusreizen bei physiologischen Weckreizen und elektrischer Reizung der Substantia reticularis mesencephali.

Angeregt durch diese elektrocorticographischen Befunde haben wir in Fortsetzung unserer Untersuchungen an einzelnen Neuronen jetzt die Beeinflussung der Neuronenentladungen des visuellen Cortex durch vorausgehende Reizung der Substantia reticularis mesencephali geprüft. Als Testreiz diente sowohl Licht als auch elektrische Reizung des Tractus opticus unmittelbar oberhalb des Chiasma opticum.

Methodik

Die Versuche wurden an neun nichtnarkotisierten Katzen durchgeführt, die nach hoher Halsmarkdurchtrennung (encéphale isolé nach Bremer) künstlich beatmet wurden. Insgesamt wurden 48 Neurone abgeleitet und ausgewertet.

Ableitung. Die Neuronaktivität wurde extracellulär mit Glasmikropipetten (Spitzendurchmesser 0,5—2 μ, Füllung mit 3molarer KCl-Lösung) abgeleitet, das epicorticale EEG (ECG) mit einem Silberdraht. Einzelheiten der Präparation siehe (*10*).

Reizung. *Licht.* Diffuses weißes Licht von etwa 400 Lux Stärke wurde auf das kontralaterale Auge gegeben. Es wurde im helladaptierten Zustand gereizt, die Lichtreize waren mehrere 100 msec lang. Bei Flimmerlichtreizung wurden die Hell- und Dunkelperioden etwa gleich lang gehalten.

Reizung des Tractus opticus. Der homolaterale Tractus opticus wurde einige Millimeter oberhalb des Chiasma opticum mit bipolaren Reizelektroden (Elektrodenabstand 0,5—1 mm, siehe *29*) gereizt. Die Elektroden wurden stereotaktisch eingeführt. Als Reizimpulse dienten Rechteckreize von 0,3—0,5 msec Dauer, die Reizstärke wurde so eingestellt, daß das jeweils abgeleitete Neuron gerade überschwellig gereizt wurde. Nur bei Neuronen, die nicht direkt auf

---

[1] Aus der Abteilung für klinische Neurophysiologie der Universität Freiburg i. Br.

[2] Die Arbeit wurde mit Unterstützung der Deutschen Forschungsgemeinschaft durchgeführt.

einen Tractusreiz reagierten (Gruppe 1 und 3, s. unten), wurde vor der reticulären Bahnung der Reiz so stark eingestellt, daß die Amplitude des corticalen Reaktionspotentials etwa 50 bis 75% seiner maximalen Ausprägung betrug.

Reizung der Substantia reticularis mesencephali. Auch hier wurde bipolar gereizt (Abstand der Elektrodenspitzen 0,5 mm). Die Elektroden wurden stereotaktisch supratentoriell eingesetzt und drangen zwischen den vorderen und hinteren Vierhügeln kontralateral zur Ableitungsseite in das Mittelhirn ein. Es wurde mit Rechteckreizen von 0.5 msec Dauer und einer Frequenz von 50—100/sec gereizt. Die Reizstärke wurde vor jedem Versuch so eingestellt, daß bei Aufsetzen der benutzten Reizelektrode auf die eigene Zunge der elektrische Tetanusreiz gerade unter der Schmerzschwelle an der Zungenspitze lag. Bei richtiger Lokalisation waren dann nur geringe Reaktionen, vor allem des motorischen Trigeminusanteils, an der Katze zu beobachten.

Nach jedem Experiment wurden die Reizpunkte durch die Reizelektroden elektrocoaguliert, die Elektroden in situ belassen und der Kopf durch intraarterielle Formalininfusion fixiert. Am folgenden Tag wurde das Gehirn herausgenommen und in Frontalschnitte zerlegt. Die Schnittebenen, in denen die Elektrodenspitze lag, wurden photographiert.

Ergebnisse

a) Reaktionen auf Reizung des Tractus opticus (40 Neurone). In Anlehnung an die Einteilung von Grützner u. Mitarb. (*18*) wurden die Reaktionen der corticalen Neurone nach Reizung des Tractus opticus in drei Gruppen eingeteilt:

Gruppe 1. Keine reizgekoppelte Reaktion nach dem Reiz im Tractus opticus. 5 Neurone = 12,5% gehörten dieser Gruppe an.

Gruppe 2. Frühe reizgekoppelte Reaktionen mit 1—2 Entladungen und einer inkonstanten postexcitatorischen Hemmung von 50—150 msec, der bei einigen Neuronen ein leichter rebound folgt. Die Latenzen sind bei den einzelnen Neuronen verschieden, die Mittelwerte liegen zwischen 1 und 6 msec. Nur ein Neuron hatte eine mittlere Latenz von 10 msec. Die Mittelwerte verteilen sich über den Bereich der ersten vier raschen Wellen des evoked potential (s. Abb. 4a). Die Einzelwerte streuen bei einigen Neuronen stärker, so daß auch manchmal während der 5. (negativen) Welle des evoked potential Entladungen auftreten (s. Abb. 4b und 2g). Im allgemeinen aber ist die Latenz nach Tractusreizung sehr konstant und streut nur stärker bei schwellennahen Reizen. 29 Neurone = 72,5% gehörten zur Gruppe 2.

Gruppe 3: Nach einer mehr oder weniger stark ausgeprägten primären Hemmung folgt eine *Spätaktivierung* mit einer Latenz von 40—100 msec. In dieser Gruppe haben wir die Typen 3 und 4 nach Grützner zusammengefaßt. 6 Neurone = 15% gehörten zu dieser Gruppe.

b) Reaktionen auf Lichtreize (27 Neurone). Nur bei 27 Neuronen konnte die Reaktion auf Licht genauer untersucht werden. Die Verteilung der verschiedenen Lichtreaktionstypen ist daher nur mit Vorbehalten den Verteilungen von Jung u. Mitarb. (*23, 24*) vergleichbar, soll aber hier der Vollständigkeit halber kurz aufgeführt werden:

A-Neurone (keine Reaktion auf monoculare Belichtung): 7 Neurone = 26%,

B-Neurone (on-Reaktion): 5 Neurone = 18,5%,

D-Neurone (off-Reaktion): 12 Neurone = 44,5%,

E-Neurone (on-off-Reaktion): 3 Neurone = 11%.

c) Reaktionen auf elektrische Reizung der Substantia reticularis (44 Neurone). Es ließen sich drei verschiedene Reaktionsmuster auf eine Reizung der mesencephalen Substantia reticularis mit 50—100/sec-Reizen unterscheiden:

Typ a: *Keine Reaktion* (16 Neurone = 26,5%),
Typ b: *Aktivierung* (neuronales arousal) (22 Neurone = 50%).

Die Latenz der Aktivierung nach Beginn des Tetanusreizes ist 60—90 msec und schwankt bei den einzelnen Neuronen um 10—50 msec. Sie ist bei höherfrequenten Reizen (100/sec) meist etwas kürzer als bei 50 oder 25/sec-Reizen. Am Anfang kann die Aktivierung bis zu einer Entladungsfrequenz von 100/sec gehen.

Die einzelnen Neurone können verschieden reagieren, behalten aber jeweils dasselbe Reaktionsmuster während der ganzen Untersuchung. Einige Neurone zeigen *während und nach der Reizung* eine den Reiz 0,5—1,0 sec überdauernde starke Aktivierung. Bei diesen Neuronen erscheint auch ein *Optimum der Reizdauer des tetanischen Reticularisreizes* bei etwa $^1/_5$ sec (150—250 msec Dauer bei 50/sec Reizfrequenz). Andere sind vorwiegend während der Reizung deutlich aktiviert (Abb. 1*A*), sowie nach 100—200 msec, und zeigen nach dem Reizende nur eine *leichte* Erhöhung der durchschnittlichen Entladungsfrequenz. Wenige zeigen eine leichte Aktivierung nur nach Aufhören der Reizung (Abb. 1 *B*). Eine weitere Gruppe von Neuronen ist nur im Beginn deutlich aktiviert und erscheint nach 100—200 msec sogar leicht gehemmt. Diese Verminderung der Entladungsfrequenz hält oft auch noch 0,5—1 sec nach Reizende an (Abb. 1, Abb. 3).

Typ c. *Hemmung* (6 Neurone = 13,5%). Bei diesen Neuronen bewirkt

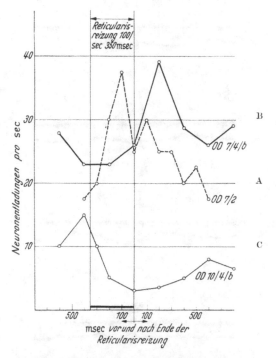

Abb. 1. Graphische Auswertung der Reaktionen dreier Neurone des optischen Cortex auf tetanische Reticularisreizung: A Aktivierung während und nach der Reizung (Typ b), B Aktivierung nach der Reizung (Typ b) und C Hemmung während und nach der Reizung (Typ c). Ordinate: Neuronentladungen pro Sekunde, Abszisse: Zeit in msec vor und nach Ende der Reticularisreizung. Der Balken zeigt die Dauer der 100/sec Reticularisreizung (350 msec)

der Reticularisreiz 60—100 msec nach Reizbeginn eine anhaltende Hemmung der Spontanaktivität, die den Reiz bei einigen Neuronen 0,5—1 sec (Abb. 1 *C*), bei anderen nicht überdauert.

Wiederholte *Tetanusserien* in Abständen von einigen Sekunden erhöhen die Spontanaktivität der meisten Neurone entsprechend einem leichten arousal, unabhängig davon, wie sie auf die einzelne Reizserie reagieren. Meistens waren die Tiere jedoch während des ganzen Versuches wegen der häufigen Reizungen dauernd wach. Die Wirkung von Reticularisreizung bei schlafenden Tieren wurde in dieser Versuchsserie nicht studiert. *Einzelreize* in der Substantia reticularis hatten meistens keinerlei Effekt auf die corticale Neuronaktivität. Es müssen mindestens 2—5 Reize mit einer Frequenz von 25—100/sec gegeben werden, um einen sicheren neuronalen Effekt zu erzielen. Das epicorticale *EEG* zeigt bei der encéphale isolé-

Katze meist schon ohne Reiz einen flachen Typ mit schnellen Wellen entsprechend dem arousal pattern. Nach Reticularisreiz ändert sich dieser EEG-Typ meistens nicht wesentlich. Nur wenn Alpha-Wellen vorkommen, werden diese blockiert.

Verwertbare *lokalisatorische Differenzen* bei Reizung der F. reticularis mesencephali wurden nicht gefunden. Die verschiedenen Reaktionstypen fanden sich

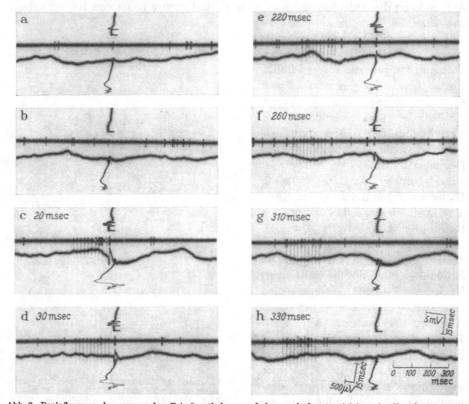

Abb. 2. Beeinflussung der neuronalen Primärentladung und des evoked potential im visuellen Cortex nach schwellennaher Reizung des Tractus opticus (Testreiz) durch in verschiedenem Abstand vorhergehende Reticularisreizung (Conditioning-Reiz). Area striata (OD 6/3 a). a und b Reizung des Tractus opticus allein. c—h Zunehmender Abstand zwischen Reticularis- und Opticusreizung. Waagerechte Zeilen: oben Neuronenaktivität, unten Corticogramm. Senkrechte Zeilen: die entsprechenden schnellen Ablenkungen. Beachte die Abnahme der Entladungswahrscheinlichkeit mit der Zunahme des Abstandes beider Reize (vgl. Abb. 3 a) und in g auch die längere Latenz der Primärentladung bei großem Abstand

sowohl bei Lokalisation der Reizelektrode in den medialen als auch den lateralen Teilen der Substantia reticularis mesencephali, sowohl bei Lokalisation an ihrer oberen Grenze als auch in einem Versuch, in dem die Elektrode außerhalb der Substantia reticularis im Nucl. interpeduncularis lag.

Die verschiedenen Reaktionstypen auf Licht-, Opticus- und Reticularisreiz sind nicht miteinander gekoppelt. Ein Neuron, das durch Reticularisreizung aktiviert wird, kann durch einen Opticusreiz primär gehemmt, ein anderes primär aktiviert werden usw. Da der Lichtreiz monocular gegeben wurde, waren auch einige nicht auf Licht reagierende Neurone (A-Neurone) durch einen Tractusreiz zu erregen.

d) Beeinflussung der Reaktionen nach Opticusreiz durch einen vorangehenden Reticularisreiz. Wie bereits von Dumont und Dell (*12, 13*) sowie Bremer und

STOUPEL (*3, 4*) beschrieben, wird das evoked potential durch eine vorausgehende Reticularisreizserie während und noch 300—500 msec nach der Reizung gebahnt. Sämtliche Komponenten des evoked potential sind in etwa gleichem Maße vergrößert. Alle corticalen Neurone der Gruppe 2, die also auf einen Opticusreiz mit einer primären Entladung nach kurzer Latenz reagierten, wurden durch eine vorausgehende Reticularisreizserie gebahnt, so daß es bei gerade unterschwelliger

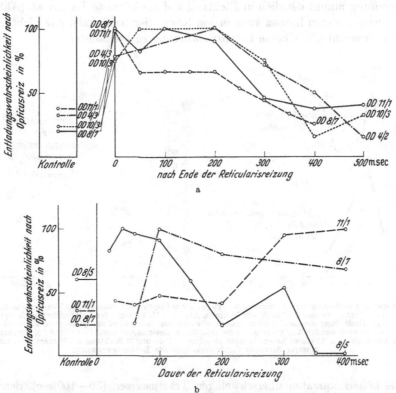

a

b

Abb. 3a und b. a Graphische Darstellung der Dauer der bahnenden Wirkung einer tetanischen Reticularisreizung (Conditioning-Reiz) auf die primäre Entladung mehrerer Neurone nach Opticusreiz (Testreiz). Ordinate: Wahrscheinlichkeit primärer Entladungen auf Opticusreiz. 100% = höchster vorkommender Wert an Primärentladungen auf Opticusreiz nach Reticularisreizung. Kontrolle: Wahrscheinlichkeit primärer Entladungen auf Opticusreiz allein. Abszisse: Abstand vom Ende der Reticularisreizung (100/sec) zum Opticusreiz. — b Graphische Darstellung der Entladungswahrscheinlichkeit mehrerer Neurone nach Opticusreiz in Abhängigkeit von der Dauer einer davor beendeten tetanischen Reticularisreizung. Ordinate: Wahrscheinlichkeit primärer Entladungen nach Opticusreiz. 100% und Kontrolle wie bei 3a. Abszisse: Dauer der Reticularisreizung (100/sec)

Opticusreizung nach vorausgehender Reticularisbahnung häufig oder regelmäßig zu einer Reaktion kommt. Wenn die Tractusreizung in der Kontrolle gerade überschwellig war, aber nicht in 100% eine Entladung erfolgte (bei gerade überschwelligen Tractusreizen liegt die Entladungswahrscheinlichkeit pro Reiz oft unter 50%), wurde die Entladungswahrscheinlichkeit durch vorangehende Reticularisreizung deutlich erhöht. Manche Neurone, die bei überschwelliger Opticusreizung mit nur einer Entladung antworten, entladen nach Reticularisbahnung mit 2—3 Entladungen pro Reiz (Abb. 2).

Die Bahnung beginnt 50—90 msec nach Beginn des Tetanusreizes und überdauert die Reticularisreizung 350—500 msec. 200 msec nach Reizende beginnt sie abzunehmen (Abb. 2 und 3). Bei sehr langen Tetanusserien über mehrere 100 msec nimmt die Bahnung im Verlauf der Reizung langsam ab, bei einigen Neuronen sogar bis auf den Ausgangswert (Abb. 3b).

Außer auf die Entladungswahrscheinlichkeit selbst wirkt sich die Reticularisbahnung bei einigen Neuronen auch auf die mittlere Reaktionslatenz aus. Die kürzeste Latenz dieser Neurone nach Tractusreiz wird nicht unterschritten, aber die Streuung nimmt deutlich in Richtung auf die kürzeste Latenz ab (Abb. 4b). Bei Neuronen, deren Latenz auch in den Kontrollen wenig oder gar nicht um den Mittelwert streute, war keine Latenzverkürzung zu beobachten.

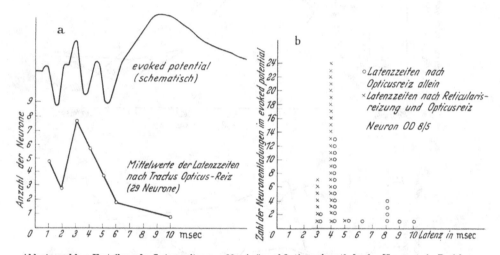

Abb. 4a und b. a Verteilung der Latenzzeiten von 29 primär auf Opticusreiz entladenden Neuronen in Beziehung zum evoked potential. Ordinate: Anzahl der Neurone, Abszisse: Mittelwerte der Latenzzeiten nach Opticusreiz. b Graphische Darstellung der Latenzzeiten eines primär erregten Neurons auf 23 Opticusreize allein (o) und auf 32 Opticusreize nach unmittelbar vorhergehender tetanischer Reticularisreizung (×) (OD 8/5). Ordinate: Zahl der Primärentladungen. Abszisse: Latenz in msec. Beachte die Bahnung in Richtung auf kürzere Latenzen mit geringerer Streuung durch vorausgehende Reticularisreizung.

Bei höherfrequenten überschwelligen Tractusreizen (30—100/sec), denen die corticalen Neurone häufig nicht mehr folgen können, bewirkt eine Reticularisreizung in der Regel keinerlei sichtbare Bahnung. Diese ist bei höherfrequenten Tractusreizen ebenfalls nur dann erkennbar, wenn die Tractusreize unterschwellig sind.

Eine Bahnung der Tractusreizreaktion ist bei einigen Neuronen auch durch einen *physiologischen Weckreiz* (akustische Reizung o. ä.) möglich. In Abb. 5a ist ein Neuron abgebildet, bei dem die Tractusreizung in der Kontrolle unterschwellig ist. In Abb. 5b wird ein arousal durch starke akustische Reizung (Klatschen und Pfeifen) hervorgerufen, wodurch die Spontanaktivität deutlich erhöht und die Tractusreizwirkung gebahnt wird. In der untersten Reihe (Abb. 5c) wird der Tractusreiz durch vorausgehende Reticularisreizung gebahnt. Man erkennt deutlich, daß die physiologische sensorisch-akustische Arousal-Wirkung auf das evoked potential stärker ist als die Reticularis-Reizwirkung.

Die *Nachentladung* nach der postexcitatorischen Hemmung bei Tractusreizung wird durch Reticularisreizung gewöhnlich mehr oder weniger stark *vermindert*. Wenn bei einigen Neuronen die Nachentladung bei der Kontrollreizung in rhythmischen Entladungsgruppen bestand, bewirkt die Reticularisreizung meistens, daß die Nachentladung stetig wird. In der Regel setzt sich die postexcitatorische Hemmung auch gegen eine Frequenzerhöhung infolge vorausgehender Reticularisreizung durch.

Entsprechend diesen Befunden bei den Neuronen der Gruppe 2 werden auch die Neurone der Gruppe 3, die eine primäre Hemmung und eine postinhibitorische Nachentladung nach Tractusreiz zeigen, beeinflußt. Die primäre Hemmung setzt sich auch gegen eine Aktivierung infolge vorausgehender Reticularisreizung durch,

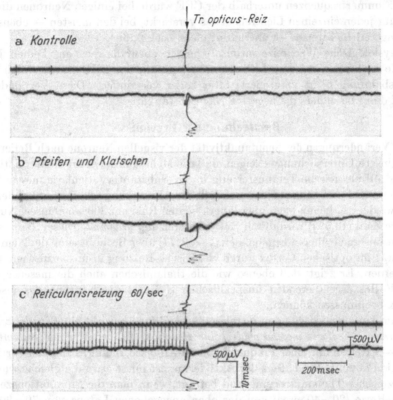

Abb. 5. Elektrische und sensorische Beeinflussung der Neuronenentladungen und des Reaktionspotentials nach Reizung des Tractus opticus durch akustische und Reticularisreizung (60/sec) (OD 10/3). a Für die Neuronentladung unterschwelliger Opticusreize. b Dasselbe während akustischer Reizung (Pfeifen und Klatschen). c Dasselbe nach Reticularisreizung. Waagerecht: oben Neuronaktivität kontinuierlich; unten Corticogramm. Senkrecht: oben und unten die entsprechenden schnellen Ablenkungen. Beachte die für akustische und Reticularisreizung gleiche Bahnung der Neuronenentladung und des Reaktionspotentials

wobei aber oft keine vollständige Entladungsruhe wie in der Kontrolle, sondern nur eine Verminderung der Frequenz eintritt. Die Nachentladung wurde bei etwa der Hälfte der Neurone der Gruppe 3 vermindert, bei den übrigen war sie in der Intensität gleich, manchmal wurde eine rhythmische Spätaktivierung in eine kontinuierliche umgewandelt.

Die Neurone der Gruppe 1 (keine Reaktion auf Tractusreizung) zeigen auch nach Reticularisreizung keine reizgebundene Reaktion auf den Tractusreiz.

e) **Beeinflussung von Lichtreaktionen durch Reticularisreizung.** Im Gegensatz zu den Reaktionen nach Tractusreiz werden die durch Lichtreizung ausgelösten

Reaktionen durch vorausgehende Reticularisreizung nur wenig oder nicht verändert. Bei D-Neuronen (off) setzt sich die Lichthemmung gegenüber einer Reticularisbahnung vollständig durch. Nur manchmal zeigen B- oder E-Neurone eine leichte Bahnung der on-Reaktion nach vorausgegangener Reticularisreizung.

Bei Flimmerlichtreizung ergeben sich ebenfalls keine konstanten Ergebnisse. Die CFF (Fusionsfrequenz) der corticalen Neurone wurde bei der Hälfte der Neurone überhaupt nicht verändert, bei der anderen Hälfte leicht erniedrigt. Diese Erniedrigung der CFF war vor allem bei D-Neuronen (off) zu beobachten. Bei mittleren Flimmerfrequenzen unterhalb der CFF wurde bei einigen Neuronen die Antwort auf jeden einzelnen Lichtreiz etwas verstärkt, bei den meisten — ebenso wie bei längeren Lichtreizen — überhaupt nicht beeinflußt.

Physiologische Weckreize (arousal) hatten ebenfalls meistens keinen Effekt auf die Lichtreaktion. Das Lichtreaktionspotential im EEG wurde durch Reticularisbahnung nicht vergrößert, öfter sogar vermindert. Diese Verminderung betraf dann besonders die negative Nachschwankung.

Besprechung der Ergebnisse

1. Veränderungen der Spontanaktivität der visuellen Neurone nach Reticularisreiz. Unsere Untersuchungen zeigen, daß die Mehrzahl der Neurone des optischen Cortex auf elektrische Tetanusreizung in der Substantia reticularis mesencephali aktiviert wird; bei einigen Neuronen fällt die Aktivierung schon während der Reizung wieder ab, bei anderen überdauert sie den Reiz um 300—500 msec. Nur eine geringe Zahl (13,5%) wird durch Reticularisreizung *gehemmt*. Dieser Befund entspricht unseren früheren Ergebnissen (*1, 7, 9, 11*) über Beeinflussung der Neuronenaktivität im optischen Cortex durch elektrische Reizung in unspezifischen Thalamuskernen. Er zeigt, daß ebenso wie die thalamischen auch die mesencephalen Anteile des ascendierenden · unspezifischen Systems die Neurone des visuellen Cortex beeinflussen können.

Zum Unterschied von den intralaminären Reizen bewirkt ein *Einzelreiz in der Substantia reticularis mesencephali keine Reaktion.* Es bedarf einer *Summierung* von 2—3 Reizen mit einer Frequenz von 50—100/sec, damit es zu einer corticalen Reaktion kommt. Die Latenz der Aktivierung ist meist etwa die gleiche wie nach unspezifischer Thalamusreizung und beträgt, wenn man die Summationszeit der ersten Reize (20—40 msec) von der oben angegebenen Latenz von 70—90 msec abzieht, etwa 30—50 msec. Es handelt sich also um einen langsam wirkenden Vorgang und nicht um eine direkte Übertragung über wenige Synapsen. Diese langsame Wirkung wird noch deutlicher bei Vergleich zwischen verschieden lang dauernden Tetanusreizen; ein Optimum des „neuronalen arousal" findet sich bei einer Reticularis-Reizungsdauer von etwa 150—250 msec. Bei kürzeren und längeren Tetanusreizen ist die Aktivierung oft geringer.

Über den Weg der reticulocorticalen Erregungsausbreitung läßt sich nichts Sicheres sagen. Arden und Söderberg (*2*) fanden beim Kaninchen, daß unspezifische Impulse bereits im Corpus geniculatum in die optische Afferenz einstrahlen. Grüsser u. Mitarb. (*9*) sahen jedoch bei der Katze eine Wirkung der Labyrinthpolarisation nur an corticalen und nicht an Geniculatumneuronen, obwohl der Reizeffekt wahrscheinlich über die Substantia reticularis mesencephali fortgeleitet wird.

Im Gegensatz zur Labyrinthpolarisation, die eine Nachwirkung von Sekundendauer auf die visuellen Cortexneurone hat, hält die Wirkung der Reticularisreizung dort nur bis zu etwa 400 msec an. Weder bei hohen noch bei niedrigen Reticularisreizfrequenzen folgen die corticalen Neurone mit reizgekoppelter Entladungsfrequenz. Die Entladungsfrequenz bei Reticularisreizung liegt meist unter der Reizfrequenz. Ferner zeigt die Mehrzahl der Neurone eine Zunahme der Entladungsfrequenz nur während eines Teils der gesamten Reizdauer; es handelt sich also um ein mehr phasisches Verhalten als um ein tonisches, das bei vestibulocorticalen Afferenzen zu erwarten wäre. Die verhältnismäßig kurze Wirkung der Reticularisreizung auf die corticalen Neurone unterscheidet sich ferner auch von der längeren auf das EEG (arousal), auf das evoked potential (Bahnung) und auf das Verhalten; in diesen Fällen überdauert die Wirkung meist mehrere Sekunden (*4, 13, 15, 28*).

2. Veränderungen der spezifischen neuronalen Reaktionen durch Reticularisreiz.
Die Reaktionen der corticalen Neurone auf Reizung des Tractus opticus entsprechen im wesentlichen den Befunden von GRÜTZNER, GRÜSSER und BAUMGARTNER (*17, 18*), allerdings mit dem Unterschied, daß nach Reizung des Tractus opticus etwa doppelt so viele Neurone mit einer Entladung reagieren wie nach Reizung des Nervus opticus, was nach den anatomischen Gegebenheiten zu erwarten ist. Unter Berücksichtigung dieses Umstandes stimmt die Verteilung der Reaktionstypen in beiden Versuchsreihen etwa überein, wie Tab. 1 zeigt.

Tabelle 1

Reaktionstyp	Reizung des Nervus opt. (GRÜTZNER u. Mitarb.)	Reizung des Tractus opt. (CREUTZFELDT u. Mitarb.)
1. Keine reizgekoppelte Reaktion	125 Neurone = 39%	5 Neurone = 12,5%
2. Frühe Primärentladung während des evoked potential . .	144 Neurone = 33%	29 Neurone = 72,5%
3. Primäre Hemmung und späte Entladung*	91 Neurone = 28%	6 Neurone = 15%
Summe	330 Neurone = 100%	40 Neurone = 100%

* Anmerkung: In Gruppe 3 sind die Reaktionstypen 3 und 4 von GRÜTZNER u. Mitarb. zusammengefaßt.

Die Neurone der Gruppe 3 (primäre Hemmung und Spätaktivierung), die etwa 15% der gesamten Neurone des optischen Cortex ausmachen, haben eine zu lange Latenz, als daß direkte Afferenzen aus dem Tractus opticus für sie angenommen werden könnten. Immerhin erhalten sie auf dem Umweg über andere Hirnregionen durch prä- oder postsynaptische Afferenzen noch späte reizgebundene Erregungen von der Retina.

Wenn man zu diesen Neuronen der Gruppe 3 die der Gruppe 1 (ohne reizgekoppelte Reaktion) hinzuzählt, so ergibt sich, daß insgesamt ein Drittel der Neurone des optischen Cortex keine direkten Afferenzen aus der Retina empfängt. Diese Zahl stimmt annähernd mit der früher (*17, 24*) festgestellten Anzahl corticaler A-Neurone (ohne Lichtreaktion) überein.

Es ist bemerkenswert, daß eine *deutliche reticuläre Bahnung nur an denjenigen Neuronen nachgewiesen werden kann, die auf Tractusreizung mit kurzer Latenz reagieren* (Gruppe 2). Das bestätigt die früher gemachte (*17, 18*) Annahme, daß die

Neurone der Gruppe 1 und 3 keine direkten Afferenzen von der Retina erhalten, welche durch Reticularisreizung gebahnt werden könnten.

Die bahnende Wirkung überdauert die Reticularisreizung für 300—400 msec; das ist kürzer als die Bahnung der evoked potentials (*4, 13*) und gilt auch für solche Neurone, deren Aktivität nur vorübergehend während der Reticularisreizung erhöht wird. Die neuronale Bahnung der Tractusreizreaktion durch die Reticularisreizung hält also oft länger an als die Verstärkung der Spontanaktivität, aber nicht so lange wie die Bahnung der mit Oberflächenelektroden abgeleiteten evoked potentials .

Es bleibt offen, ob die bahnende Wirkung der Reticularisreizung in einer längerdauernden Depolarisation der Neurone im Corpus geniculatum und Cortex besteht oder in der Freisetzung einer Überträgersubstanz, die eine Fortleitung spezifischer Impulse erleichtert und die dann während 300—400 msec, entsprechend der Dauer der Bahnung, abgebaut wird. Jedenfalls ist ein verhältnismäßig *langsamer Vorgang* anzunehmen, der nicht in unsere herkömmlichen Vorstellungen von der synaptischen Bahnung paßt, sondern mehr der posttetanischen Bahnung am Rückenmark ähnelt, die von Eccles (*14*) auf eine Freisetzung von synaptischen Überträgersubstanzen zurückgeführt wird.

Über den *Ort der Konvergenz* spezifischer und reticulärer Afferenzen läßt sich auf Grund unserer Versuche wenig sagen. Sicher ist nur, wie auch aus den Makroableitungen (*3, 12*) hervorgeht, daß neben einer corticalen Konvergenz auch eine Bahnung zumindest im Corpus geniculatum stattfindet. Arden und Söderberg (*2*) haben am Kaninchen eine Konvergenz spezifischer und unspezifischer Afferenzen bereits an Geniculatumneuronen nachgewiesen, doch scheint die unspezifische Geniculatumaktivierung bei der Katze geringer zu sein. Über entsprechende Untersuchungen an Geniculatumneuronen der Katze werden Kornhuber und Fonseca später berichten. Praktisch werden alle Neurone der Gruppe 2 gebahnt, darunter auch präsynaptische Neurone, also Fasern der Sehstrahlung, entsprechend den Untersuchungen von Widén und Ajmone Marsan (*32*). Rein corticale Bahnung ist ebenfalls wahrscheinlich, weil auch die Neurone der Gruppe 1 (ohne Beeinflussung durch spezifische Afferenzen) eine Erhöhung der Spontanfrequenz nach Reticularisreizung zeigen, die wahrscheinlich nicht über das Corpus geniculatum zustande kommt.

Der Unterschied zwischen starker Bahnung bei Opticusreizung und geringer Bahnung der Lichtreaktion durch Reticularisreizung ist bei Mikroableitungen ebenso auffällig wie bei Makroableitungen (*3, 12*).

Auch bei Reizung in unspezifischen Thalamuskernen (*1, 7*) fiel uns trotz häufiger Konvergenz spezifischer und unspezifischer Impulse an corticalen Neuronen (in etwa $^2/_3$ der Fälle) die verhältnismäßig geringe Beeinflussung der spezifischen corticalen Lichtreaktion auf. Sie ist nur bei wenigen Neuronen deutlich und äußert sich bei unspezifischer Thalamusreizung vor allem in einer Verlängerung der Dauerentladung während eines längeren Lichtreizes und einer Erhöhung der CFF bei Flimmerlichtreizen. Bei Reticularisreizung war in unseren Versuchen jedoch die CFF entweder gar nicht beeinflußt oder sogar herabgesetzt.

Eine Erklärung für diese Unterschiede können wir vorläufig noch nicht geben. *Jedenfalls scheinen stark synchronisierte afferente Impulssalven stärker gebahnt zu werden als funktionell organisierte Erregungsmuster.*

Summary

1. 48 neurons of the visual cortex of 9 cats (encéphale isolé) were recorded with microelectrodes and their responses to the following stimuli were examined: a) electrical stimulation of the optic tract, b) electrical stimulation of the mesencephalic reticular formation and c) light stimulation. The influence of conditioning reticular stimuli on the neuronal responses to optic tract stimulation was investigated in detail.

2. Single shock stimuli of the optic tract caused no reaction in 5 neurons of the visual cortex (group 1 after GRÜTZNER et al., *18*), an early primary discharge in 29 neurons (group 2) and, finally, a primary inhibition and/or a delayed activation (40—100 msec) in 6 neurons (group 3 = GRÜTZNER's group 3 and 4, *18*). The latent periods of the group 2 neuronal responses, although relatively constant in individual neurons, are for the total population evenly distributed over the first four phases of the evoked potential. Only a few neurons exhibited a greater variance of their latent periods, particularly in the threshold region.

3. Upon reticular stimulation about one half of the cortical neurons showed transitory activation with increase of their spontaneous frequency (type b). Only one third was not affected by reticular stimulation (type a) while the remaining 6 neurons were inhibited during the stimulation (type c). The neurons activated by reticular stimulation revealed various discharge patterns which remained quite constant for the same neurons: short transitory activation for 100—200 msec, or activation lasting through stimulation, or retaining activation for 300—500 msec after cessation of stimulation, or activation following cessation of stimulation. The latency before neuronal activation lasted 60—100 msec after the beginning of the stimulation volley.

4. Conditioning reticular stimulation facilitated the responses to optic tract stimulation in all group 2 neurons (early primary reactions after optic tract stimulation). The facilitation lasts 300—500 msec after cessation of stimulation and raised the discharge probability of subthreshold optic tract stimulation. The latent period is shortened only in those neurons which exhibit a greater variance at threshold stimulation. The reduction in latency is maximal with supramaximal stimulation.

5. Similarities and differences in the effects of intralaminar thalamic stimulation and possible mechanisms of nonspecific influence are discussed.

Literatur

1. AKIMOTO, H., u. O. CREUTZFELDT: Reaktionen von Neuronen des optischen Cortex nach elektrischer Reizung unspezifischer Thalamuskerne. Arch. Psychiat. Nervenkr. **196**, 494—519 (1958).
2. ARDEN, G. B., and U. SÖDERBERG: The relationship of lateral geniculate activity to the electrocorticogram in the presence or absence of the optic tract input. Experientia (Basel) **15**, 163 (1959).
3. BREMER, F., et N. STOUPEL: De la modification des résponses sensorielles corticales dans l'éveil réticulaire. Acta neurol. belg. **58**, 401—403 (1958).
4. — — Facilitation et inhibition des potentiels évoqués corticaux dans l'éveil cérébral. Arch. int. Physiol. **67**, 240—275 (1959).
5. — — et P. CH. VAN REETH: Nouvelles recherches sur la facilitation et l'inhibition des potentiels évoqués corticaux dans l'éveil réticulaire. Arch. ital. Biol. **98**, 229—247 (1960).

6. Chang, H.-T.: Cortical response to stimulation of lateral geniculate body and the potentiation thereof by continuous illumination of retina. J. Neurophysiol. 15, 5—26 (1952).
7. Creutzfeldt, O., u. H. Akimoto: Konvergenz und gegenseitige Beeinflussung von Impulsen aus der Retina und den unspezifischen Thalamuskernen an einzelnen Neuronen des optischen Cortex. Arch. Psychiat. Nervenkr. 196, 520—538 (1958).
8. — and G. Baumgartner: Reactions of neurons on the occipital cortex to electrical stimuli applied to the intralaminar thalamus. EEG Clin. Neurophysiol. 7, 664—665 (1955).
9. — — u. R. Jung: Convergence of specific and unspecific impulses on neurons of the visual cortex. EEG Clin. Neurophysiol. 8, 163—164 (1956).
10. — A. Kasamatsu u. A. Vaz-Ferreira: Aktivitätsänderungen einzelner corticaler Neurone im akuten Sauerstoffmangel und ihre Beziehungen zum EEG bei Katzen. Pflügers Arch. ges. Physiol. 263, 647—667 (1957).
11. — u. O.-J. Grüsser: Beeinflussung der Flimmerreaktion einzelner corticaler Neurone durch elektrische Reize unspezifischer Thalamuskerne. First International Congress of Neurological Sciences Brussels 1957. Vol. III, 349—355. London, New York, Paris 1959.
12. Dumont, S., et P. Dell: Facilitations spécifiques et non spécifiques des réponses visuelles corticales. J. Physiol. (Paris) 50, 261 — 264 (1958).
13. — — Facilitation réticulaire des méchanismes visuels corticaux. EEG Clin. Neurophysiol. 12, 769—796 (1960).
14. Eccles, J. C.: The physiology of nerve cells. Baltimore: Johns Hopkins Press 1957.
15. French, J. D.: Corticifugal connections with the reticular formation. In Jasper et al. (ed.). Reticular formation of the brain. Henry Ford Hospital Intern. Symposium 1957, 491—505, Boston-Toronto: Little, Brown & Co.
16. Grüsser, O.-J., U. Grüsser-Cornehls u. G. Saur: Reaktionen einzelner Neurone im optischen Cortex der Katze nach elektrischer Polarisation des Labyrinths. Pflügers Arch. ges. Physiol. 269, 593—612 (1959).
17. — u. A. Grützner: Reaktionen einzelner Neurone des optischen Cortex der Katze nach elektrischen Reizserien des Nervus opticus. Arch. Psychiat. Nervenkr. 197, 405—432 (1958).
18. Grützner, A., O. J. Grüsser u. G. Baumgartner: Reaktionen einzelner Neurone im optischen Cortex der Katze nach elektrischer Reizung des Nervus opticus. Arch. Psychiat. Nervenkr. 197, 377—404 (1958).
19. Hubel, D.H.: Cortical unit responses to visual stimuli in nonanesthetized cats. Amer. J. Ophthal. 46, 110—122 (1958).
20. Jung, R.: Coordination of specific and nonspecific afferent impulses at single neurons of the visual cortex. In: Jasper et al. (ed.). Reticular formation of the brain. Henry Ford Hospital Internat. Symposium 1957, p. 423—434. Boston-Toronto Little, Brown & Co.
21. — Microphysiologie corticaler Neurone: Ein Beitrag zur Koordination der Hirnrinde und des visuellen Systems. In: Tower and Schade (ed.), Structure and function of the cerebral cortex, proceed. IInd Intern. Meeting of Neurobiologists, Amsterdam 1959, pg. 204—233. Amsterdam: Elsevier & Co. 1960.
22. — Neuronal integration in the visual cortex and its significance for visual information. In: Rosenblith (ed.). Sensory communication. p. 627—674. Cambridge (Mass.): Technology press 1961.
23. — R. von Baumgarten u. G. Baumgartner: Microableitungen von einzelnen Nervenzellen im optischen Cortex. Die lichtaktivierten B-Neurone. Arch. Psychiat. Nervenkr. 189, 521—539 (1952).
24. — u. G.Baumgartner: Hemmungsmechanismen und bremsende Stabilisierung an einzelnen Neuronen des optischen Cortex. Pflügers Arch. ges. Physiol. 261, 434—456 (1955).
25. Li, C. L: The facilitatory effect of stimulation of an unspecific thalamic nucleus on cortical sensory neuronal responses. J. Physiol. (Lond.) 131, 115—124 (1956).
26. Monnier, M., M. Kalberer and P. Krupp: Functional antagonism between diffuse reticular and intralaminary recruiting projections in the medial thalamus. Exp. Neurol. 2, 271—289 (1960).
27. Moruzzi, G., and H. W. Magoun: Brain stem reticular formation and activation of the EEG. EEG Clin. Neurophysiol. 1, 455—473 (1949).

28. SEGUNDO, J. P., R. ARANA and J. D. FRENCH: Behavioral arousal by stimulation of the brain in the monkey. J. Neurosurg. 12, 601—613 (1955).
29. SPEHLMANN, R., O. CREUTZFELDT u. R. JUNG: Neuronale Hemmung im motorischen Cortex nach elektrischer Reizung des Caudatum. Arch. Psychiat. Nervenkr. 201, 332—354 (1960).
30. STOUPEL, N.: Etude de l'interaction dans l'écorce d'influx thalamo-corticaux spécifiques et non spécifiques. Acta neurol. belg. 58, 759—771 (1958).
31. VASTOLA, E. F.: An electrical sign of facilitation accompanying repetitive presynaptic activity. J. Neurophysiol. 22, 624—632 (1959).
32. WIDÉN, L., and C. AJMONE MARSAN: Unitary analysis of the response elicited in the visual cortex of cat. Arch. ital. Biol. 98, 248—274 (1960).

Diskussion

siehe S. 372

Effects of Arousal Stimuli on Evoked Neuronal Activities in Cat's Visual Cortex[1]

By

HARUO AKIMOTO, YOICHI SAITO and YUTAKA NAKAMURA

With 7 Figures

Although EEG arousal induced by stimulation of brain stem activating system is now a familiar phenomenon to us, and close relationship between consciousness and functional states of this structure has been established, much is left unknown about the details of changes in the level of cortical excitability induced by arousal stimulation.

We examined at first the effects of arousal stimulation on spontaneous discharge in the cortical area of relatively non-specific function, i. e. association cortex of cats (15, 16) and then investigated the effects on excitability of neurones in specific areas of cortex, i. e. sensory and motor areas (2, 13, 17).

This report is concerned mainly with our experimental results in the effects of arousal stimuli upon the excitability of neurones in cat's visual cortex. As the first step in our investigations influence of arousal stimulation on photically evoked cortical unit activity was examined. Then for the next step, changes in unit activities evoked by single shocks in optic radiation (RO) or lateral geniculate body (GL) were studied.

Methods

Cats immobilized with Succinyl-choline-chloride or d-Tubocurarine-chloride[2] were used throughout. After stimulating electrodes[3] were placed stereotaxically, a glass-pipette micro-electrode[4] was inserted into the middle part of lateral gyrus. Cortical unit discharges and

---

[1] From the Department of Neuro-Psychiatry, School of Medicine, Tokyo University.

[2] SCC or DTC was administrated intravenously or intramuscularly. No difference of the results was seen between two paralysing agents.

[3] Stimulating electrodes consisted of two steel needles cemented together. Tip of each needle had the diameter below 100 μ. Tips were separated 0.2—0.5 mm. Histological confirmation was obtained by electrolytic deposit of iron and the Prussian blue reaction.

[4] Glass capillary was filled with 3 M-KCl solution and with electrode resistance of 5—20 MΩ.

surface Electrocorticogram (ECoG) were simultaneously recorded with 2-beam CRO and long recording camera. General arousal state of the animal was observed by 8-channel inkwriting oscillograph. For arousal stimulation repetitive square pulses were applied to midbrain reticular formation, thalamic non-specific nuclei or sciatic nerve.

Results

A. Influence of arousal stimuli on cortical unit discharges photically evoked in the visual cortex. *I. Patterns of unitary responses.* In this series of observations patterns of unitary responses evoked by single intense flashes (12,000 Lux, 0.03 msec, 0.3—0.5/s) were classified into the following 5 groups on the basis of their relationship with evoked potential (Evp).

Group 1 (B-neurons after Jung and Baumgartner) (23/100 responsive units) started to fire in the surface-positive phase of primary response with short and constant latency, and were responsive to repetitive stimulations of relatively high frequency (20—30/s, or more).

Group 2 (E-neurons?) (36/100 units) started to fire in the surface negative phase of primary response with more variable latency and were irresponsive to repetitive stimulations over 3—6/s. They showed on-off-type or on-type response to continuous light stimulation.

Group 3 (B_2 or A-neurons?) (38/100 units) discharged with latency longer than group 2 in the period of after-waves of Evp. Latencies and discharging numbers were more variable than that of group 2, and were often unable to follow the flash rate above 1/s. They showed labile, long latency on-type response for continuous light stimulation.

Group 4 (A-neurons) were unresponsive to either single flash or repetitive stimulation.

Group 5 (D-neurons) (3/100 units) stopped firing during a few hundred msec. after flash and supressed during continuous illumination or high frequency flash stimulation.

II. Effects of arousal stimuli. The effects of arousal stimuli were examined on 50 units about 100 times.

1. Changes in spontaneous discharge: In most of the units, the mean discharging numbers increased, but in the case of group 1 and 2 neurons the augmenting effect was more "phasic" and transient than that observed in association area (*1*). A few showed arrest response.

2. Changes in after-discharge. The periodic repetitive-burst pattern of after-discharge changed into a tonic pattern and often became indistinguishable with increased spontaneous background discharge. Sometimes more marked tonic augmentation or supression of afterdischarge was seen.

3. Changes in evoked discharge. The changes were classified into 5 types.

a) Indifference: no marked changes in either latency or number of discharge.

b) Facilitation: shortened latency and/or increased discharge.

c) Suppression: elongated latency and/or decreased discharge.

d) Diphasic changes.

　　d-1) Facilitation-suppression type.

　　d-2) Suppression-facilitation type.

Type b response was seen most frequently. Fig. 1 shows an example of this type of change. Single flashes were given once for each 2 sec. In first colum (*1—4*), control records the unit showed 2, 3, 2 and 3 spikes in the period of surface positive primary responses. In second colum (*5, 6*), repetitive reticular stimulation was added. Numbers of primary discharges increased to 5, 5, 5, 4 in this colum. In this case evoked potential was also augmented remarkably. In general, however, surface Evp could be often depressed but peak latency of primary positive potential was usually shortened and surface negative phase of potential was divided into several wavelets. Facilitatory influence of the units by arousal stimulation was also recognized in the elevation of unitary critical fusion frequency.

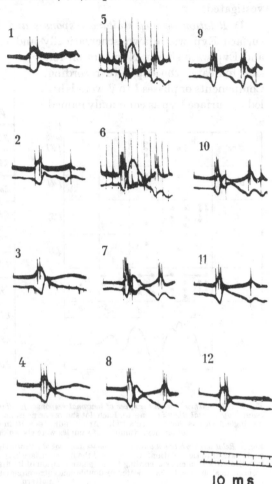

The same unit showed the same type of response to repeated arousal stimuli of varied intensity except for rare, untypical cases. No difference was found between the effects of reticular and of sciatic stimulation.

Relations between these 5 types of response to arousal stimuli (A) and types of flash response (F) are illustrated in Fig. 2. It indicates the summary of the results from 50 units. At the bottom of this figure surface evoked potential for single flash stimulation was shown schematically. Patterns of flash responses of the units were divided into 5 groups mostly according to its relation with Evp as above mentioned.

10 ms

Fig. 1. *Facilitatory effect on unitary response and Evp induced by flash stimuli.* Single flashes at a rate of 0.3/sec At 5, 6 reticular stimulation (150/sec) was applied. Upper channel: microelectrode record from the deep layer of visual cortex. Lower channel: surface Evp. In these and all subsequent records time constant of amplifying system is 100 msec unless otherwise mentioned. Time: 10 msec

Many of indifferent type units were that of the shortest latency group for photic stimulation. But because in these cases flash stimulation were of constant strength and not varied, there existed some doubt about whether these short latency group of neurons was truly indifferent as it appeared. And the levels in CNS where the effects of arousal stimuli acted on were not confirmed in this type of experiment.

B. **The effects of arousal stimuli upon unitary responses evoked by stimulation of thalamic relay nucleus or radiation afferents to the visual cortex.** In these experiments, first, the spatial distribution of intracortical Evp, and the relation between evoked unit discharge and intracortical Evp were studied, then the effects of arousal stimulation (stimulation of mesencephalic reticular formation and non-specific thalamic nuclei) upon these evoked discharges and Evp were investigated.

I) *Relation between unitary responses and Evp.* In Fig. 3 the time course of surface Evp was drawn schematically and relations between unitary response and Evp were shown. Numbers on left side indicates the depth of recording. Components or phases I to V were labelled on surface Evp as commonly named.

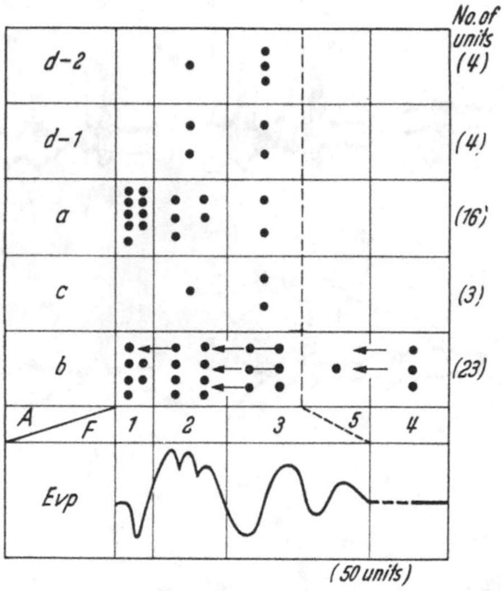

Fig. 2

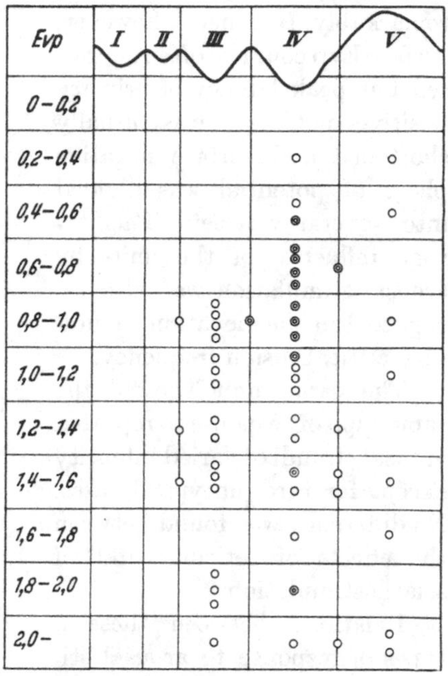

Fig. 3

Fig. 2. *Relationship between the types of neuronal responses for flash stimulation* (F, 1—5) *and the types of changes induced by arousal stimuli* (A, a—d). Each dot shows one neuronal sample. At the bottom of the figure surface Evp for single flash was shown schematically. Arrow indicates shift in flash response type of the unit due to shortening of latency. Numbers of samples were shown on the right side of the figure.

Fig. 3. *Relationship between unitary responses and evoked potential* induced by single electric shock applied on lateral geniculate or optic radiation. At the top of the figure surface Evp is shown schematically and each sample of units is indicated with a circle according to the phase relation of its first spike response to Evp and depth of recording from cortical surface. Units indicated by double concentric circle shows type IV response with repetitive discharging pattern

Results of laminar analysis of Evp confirmed that of Marshall's. Details of the discussion on the nature of these components were omitted in this paper. No difference was found in potential distributions among Evps from RO, GL, and TO (optic tract) stimulation. In the case of GL stimulation I and II had very short recovery times. Yet III, IV and V showed transient recovery or facilitation at shock intervals of 5 to 15 msec, followed by a long lasting depression of between 20—200 msec. The peak of this depression lay between 30 and 50 msec. The recovery cycles of the cortical unit response usually agreed with those of III and IV. Generally speaking, of these components, I and II stable and resistent to mechanical compression or asphyxia, but III, IV and V were labile and easily depressed. Component III could however, remain after the disappearance of IV and V.

Most of unitary response started in the third and fourth phase. No orthodromic soma-spike response was found during the first and second phase. Patterns of the unitary responses were divided into following 4 types.

1. Some units showed single spike response during the phase III with constant latency. In this type of response, shortening of latencies due to increasing the stimulus strength (to RO or GL) was within 0.5 msec. It was the same order with shortening of the peak latency of the third component of cortical neuron (Type III response = Typ 2 of GRÜTZNER et al. 7).

2. More labile, single or repetitive discharge during the fourth phase of evoked potential was found most commonly. Shortening of latencies at strong stimuli reaches a few milliseconds or more, acompanied with increase of discharging numbers (Type IV response = Typ 2b of GRÜTZNER et al. [7]).

3. Some of this type units fired in the third phase at strong stimulation (Type III—IV response).

4. The units which fired only in the fifth phase were found in relatively rare instances (Type V

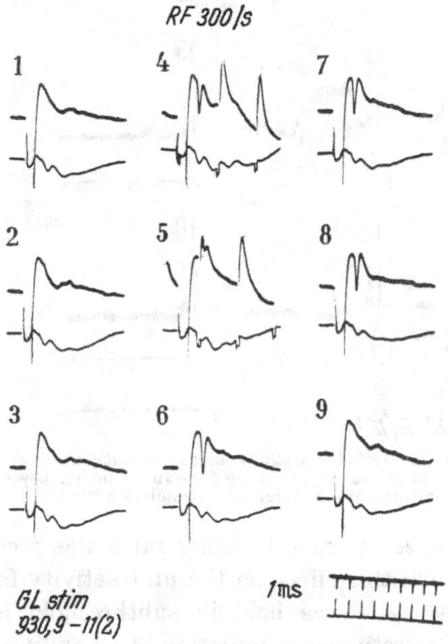

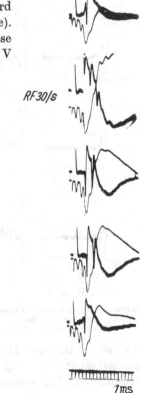

RF 300/s

1   4   7

2   5   8

3   6   9

GL stim
930,9 -11(2)

1ms

7ms

Fig. 4   Fig. 5

Fig. 4. *Type III response for geniculate shocks.* Upper channel: intracortical microelectrode record (time constant: 1 msec). Lower channel: surface Evp. Before arousal stimulation (1—3), strength of GL shocks was subthreshold. Note that threshold was lowered during (4,5) and several seconds after arousal stimulation (6—8). Time: 1 msec

Fig. 5. *Type IV response for geniculate shocks.* About the time of second sweep reticular stimulation (30/s) was given. Sweeps in sequence of 1 sec. Upper channel: intracortical microelectrode record (time constant 1 msec). Lower channel: surface Evp. Time: 1 msec.

response = Typ 3 of GRÜTZNER et al. [7]). Type III, IV, III— IV and V were considered as multisynaptic responses.

The IV and V type responses were found in the more superficial layers than that of the III type. This may be correlated to the fact, that the fourth and fifth components of evoked potential reverses its sign in more superficial layers than the third component. The units that send out long axons to white matter and respond antidromically to RO stimulation usually give an orthodromic response of type IV.

II. *Effects of arousal stimuli.* Stimulation of arousal system caused almost exclusively facilitatory effect on these evoked responses. Inhibitory effect was observed only in one exceptional case.

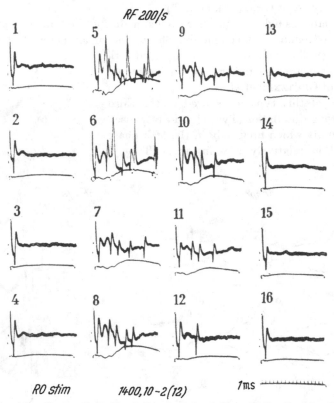

Fig. 6. *Facilitation of the unit responding antidromically and orthodromically to radiation stimulation.* Single Radiation (RO) stimulation. Upper channel: intracortical microelectrode record (time constant: 1 msec). Lower channel: surface Evp. Time: 1 msec. 1—4: control record, 5, 6: reticular stimulation 200/s

In the case of the type III response increase in firing ratio was recognized during arousal stimulation. Fig. 4 shows this effect on the unit activity for geniculate stimulation. The stimulus strength was held in subthreshold level in control records (*1—3*). During and after reticular stimulation (*4—5* and *6—8*) unit began to fire in its own phase relation to evoked potential. At threshold or suprathreshold shocks, the units did not show any signs of inhibition.

Fig. 5 shows an example of the type IV response. In this case repetitive reticular stimulation was given during the second record. Marked facilitatory effect was seen on both unitary response and evoked potential for geniculate stimulation.

Fig. 6 indicates the effect of reticular stimulation on both antidromically and orthodromically activated unit response for radiation stimulation. In the control records (*1—4*) strength of RO shocks was subthreshold for orthodromic response, and the unit showed only antidromic response. In 5 and 6 repetitive reticular stimulation (200/s) was given. Marked facilitation of orthodromic response was seen on this type units which were supposed to send out long axon to the white matter.

Unitary response and Evp for radiation or geniculate shocks preceeded by single conditioning shock of reticular formation were facilitated during shock

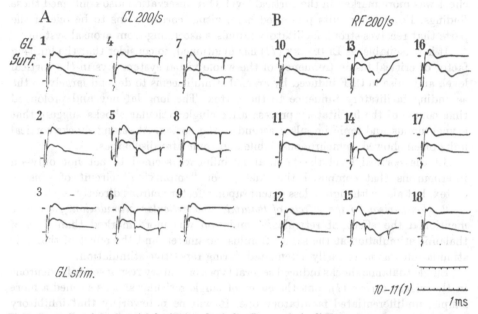

Fig. 7. *Comparison of the effect of thalamic (A) and reticular (B) arousal stimuli.* Upper channel: record from lateral geniculate. Lower channel: record from the surface of visual cortex. Repetitive stimulations (200/sec) of the same intensities were applied on thalamic CL and RF in second and fifth column. Time: 1 msec.

interval between 30 and 200 msec. Peak of the augmentation laid between shock interval of 40 and 80 msec. Inhibitory phase was not found. Augmentation of the fourth and fifth components of Evp were more marked than that of the third component.

By comparison of the augmenting effect of reticular and of thalamic stimulation, it was found that the effect was more prominent in the former than in the latter under the same conditions. Fig. 7 shows the Evp in lateral geniculate and Evp in visual cortex are enhanced more markedly by reticular stimulation than by thalamic stimulation of the same parameter. Augmentation of the cortical Evp was more prominent than that of lateral geniculate.

The time course of the facilitatory process induced by single reticular shocks agreed roughly with that of the slow potential change observed in ECoG following single strong reticular stimulation.

Comments

1. Comparison of the facilitatory effects induced by arousal stimuli in different levels of visual system. In the level of retinal ganglion cell (*6*), mainly facilitatory influence was observed after the stimulation of mesencephalic reticular formation.

Hernández-Peon et al. (8) observed that flash responses were augmented in the retina but supressed in the lateral geniculate. But after investigating the effect of arousal stimuli on cortical flash response we observed that the cortical evoked potential and unitary response for geniculate stimulation were augmented by arousal stimulation (14).

Recently Long (12) had shown that evoked potentials induced by optic nerve stimulation were enhanced both in lateral geniculate and visual cortex, and this effect was more marked in the cortical level. Our observation also confirmed these findings. From our results presented here, visual cortex seems to be one of the parts that receives strong facilitatory impulses ascending from arousal system.

It is reasonable, as Lindsley (11) has mentioned, to consider that the limiting factor of critical fusion frequency of the whole visual system lays in the cortical level, and raise in CFF induced by arousal stimuli seems to depend largely to the ascending facilitatory influence to the cortex. The long latency and prolonged time course of the facilitatory process after single reticular shocks suggest that asynchronous and tonic impulses ascend to the cortex. At strong shocks cortical units often showed asynchronous, labile and tonic afterdischarges.

In the cortical level the facilitatory influence seemed to act not only on interneurons that composed the "delay" or "amplifying" circuit of sensory cortex, but also, although to less extent, upon effector neurons directly.

2. *Comparison of the effects of thalamic and reticular stimulation.* As above mentioned the effect of reticular stimulation was more marked than that of thalamic stimulation at the same stimulus parameter, and the effect of thalamic stimulation was more easily attenuated during repetitive stimulation.

Single thalamic shocks induced several types of unitary response of the neurons in the visual cortex (1), but the effect of single reticular shocks seemed a more simple, undifferentiated facilitatory one. It will be noteworthy that inhibitory process was observed frequently in thalamic shocks and scarcely in reticular shocks.

3. *Comparison between visual cortex and other cortical areas.* In somato-sensory and auditory cortex (10) stimulation of thalamic relay nuclei or radiation afferents evoked similar complex of superposed wavelets as that described in the visual cortex. But *some difference seemed* to exist in our microelectrode observation (2). In short, in other sensory cortices than visual areas most of short latency response of the cortical neurons were of type IV and type III—IV, and single spike type III response could be scarcely obtained in these areas. Component III of Evp also showed most prominent and discrete feature in the visual cortex. The effects of repetitive stimulation of thalamic or reticular arousal system were of the similar direction, i. e. almost exclusively facilitatory as previously described in visual cortex.

In somato-sensory cortex, single conditioning shock of reticular formation gave not only the same interaction curves as in visual cortex, but sometimes different curves with inhibitory phase at shock intervals 50 to 120 msec. When stimulus frequency increased, however, this inhibitory phase reduced and finally disappeared. In auditory cortex, facilitatory effect by arousal stimuli was less prominent and the effect of single reticular stimulation were also less marked than other cortical areas.

Responses of pyramidal single fibre evoked synaptically by direct stimulation of pericruciate cortex were also facilitated by the stimulation of thalamic or reticular arousal system. Cortical unit response evoked from direct cortical stimulation in the areas other than motor cortex was also facilitated by repetitive or single reticular stimulation.

From these observations the cortical facilitation as was seen in visual cortex is not a specific and areal phenomenon but a manifestation of more general feature of cortical arousal.

4. Relationship between change in Evp and in unitary response. Evoked potential for flash stimulation was often depressed whereas unitary response was unchanged or facilitated. In somato-sensory cortex similar phenomena were frequently observed. In both cases, however, persistence or facilitation of very early surface positive component of Evp was often found.

The discrepancies between the effect on centrally, and peripherally induced evoked potentials may be caused from 1. superposition of arousal influence on upper and lower relays and/or peripheral receptors, 2. possible difference of arousal influence on well synchronized and dispersed impulses, 3. occlusion or supression in the activities of interneurons that formed by-path at lower levels including reticular formation. Some differences may correlate to the first factor. From our observations at various levels in CNS about the effect of arousal stimuli on the activities evoked by peripheral nerve stimulation, the third factor seemed to be concerned. There were little evidence to suggest the existence of the second factor, whereas the other kind of cortical activities i. e. thalamo-cortical recruiting activity could easily be depressed or blocked in both excitatory and inhibitory aspect and activities of units were dispersed and desynchronized tonically.

Summary

1. In the visual cortex of non-anesthetized and paralysed cats unitary responses evoked by single flash stimuli or single shocks in optic radiation or lateral geniculate body, and the effects of peripheral and central arousal stimuli upon these neuronal activities were examined.

2. Unitary responses for single flash stimuli were classified into 5 groups according to their relations with Evp. Relations between these types of flash responses and types of changes induced by arousal stimuli were described and discussed. Most common change observed under arousal stimuli was facilitation of the response.

3. Unitary responses for radiation or geniculate shocks were divided into several groups on account of relation with Evp. The nature of these types of responses and the effects of reticular or thalamic arousal stimuli were investigated. Most unitary responses were facilitated more clearly and uniformly in evoked responses after electrical stimulation than in flash responses.

4. Comparisons were made between the effects of thalamic and of reticular arousal stimuli, and between the changes of unitary response in the visual cortex with those in other cortical areas. The mechanisms of arousal effects on each level of visual pathway and the relationship between changes in unitary response and in Evp were discussed.

References

1. Akimoto, H., u. O. Creutzfeldt: Reaktionen von Neuronen des optischen Cortex nach elektrischer Reizung unspezifischer Thalamuskerne. Arch. Psychiat. Nervenkr. 196, 494 (1957).
2. — Y. Saito, Y. Nakamura, K. Maekawa and S. Kuroiwa: Effects of arousal stimuli on evoked unitary responses in cat's sensory and motor cortices. Proceedings of the IXth Annual Meeting of the Japan EEG Society (in press).
3. — — S. Takenaka, E. Koga, Y. Nakamura and K. Maekawa: Effect of arousal stimuli on cortical unit discharge photically evoked in visual cortex (in Japanese). Psychiat. Neurol. jap. 62, 1112 (1960).
4. Baumgartner, G.: Reaktionen einzelner Neurone im optischen Cortex der Katze nach Lichtblitzen. Pflügers Arch. ges. Physiol. 261, 457 (1955).
5. Creutzfeldt, O., u. O.-J. Grüsser: Beeinflussung der Flimmerreaktion einzelner corticaler Neurone durch elektrische Reize unspezifischer Thalamuskerne. The First International Congress of Neurological Sciences, Brussels 1957, Vol. III, 349. London, New York and Paris: Pergamon Press 1959.
6. Granit, R.: Centrifugal and antidromic effects on ganglion cells of retina. J. Neurophysiol. 18, 388 (1955).
7. Grützner, A., O.-J. Grüsser u. G. Baumgartner: Reaktionen einzelner Neurone im optischen Cortex der Katze nach elektrischer Reizung des Nervus opticus. Arch. Psychiat. Nervenkr. 197, 377 (1958).
8. Hernandez-Peon, R., H. Scherrer and M. Velasco: Central influences on afferent conduction in the somatic and visual pathways. Acta neurol. lat.-amer. 2, 8 (1956).
9. Jung, R., R. von Baumgarten u. G. Baumgartner: Mikroableitungen von einzelnen Nervenzellen im optischen Cortex der Katze. Archiv Psychiat. Nervenkr. 189, 521 (1952).
10. Landau, W. M., and M. H. Clare: A note on the characteristic response pattern in primary sensory projection cortex of the cat following a synchronous afferent volley. EEG Clin. Neurophysiol. 8, 457 (1956).
11. Lindsley, D. B.: The reticular system and perceptual discrimination, in: Reticular Formation of the Brain. London: Churchill 1957.
12. Long, R. G.: Modification of sensory mechanisms by subcortical structures. J. Neurophysiol. 22, 412 (1959).
13. Nakamura, Y.: Effects of arousal stimulation upon the evoked neuronal activity of visual cortex (in Japanese). Psychiat. Neurol. jap. 62, 1058 (1960).
14. Saito, Y.: Discussion in the Vth Symposium on Physiology of Central Nervous System at Kyoto. August 1958.
15. — Single cortical unit activity during EEG arousal (in Japanese). Psychiat. Neurol. jap. 61, 1665 (1959).
16. — K. Maekawa, S. Takenaka and A. Kasamatsu: Single cortical unit activity during EEG arousal. Proceedings of the VIth Annual Meeting of the Japan EEG Society, 95 (1957).
17. — Y. Nakamura, K. Maekawa, S. Takenaka, E. Koga, S. Jimbo and G. Hirano: Influence of arousal stimulation on photically evoked cortical unit activity. Proceedings of the VIIth Annual Meeting of the Japan EEG Society, 39 (1958).

Discussion to Creutzfeldt and Akimoto et al.

O. Creutzfeldt: Die Untersuchungen von Akimoto zeigen etwa gleiche Ergebnisse wie unsere eigenen. Nur ein Unterschied bei der Lichtreizung scheint bemerkenswert. Akimoto fand meistens auch eine Bahnung der Reaktion corticaler Neurone nach kurzen Lichtblitzen durch vorausgehende oder gleichzeitige Reticularisreizung, während wir meistens keine wesentliche Beeinflussung der Reaktion nach länger dauerndem Lichtreiz fanden. Dieser Unterschied könnte rein methodisch durch die in beiden Untersuchungen verschiedenen Lichtreize bedingt sein: Akimoto arbeitete mit kurzen Lichtblitzen von 1 msec, wir mit Dauerlichtreizen von mehreren 100 msec Dauer. Ähnliche Unterschiede sieht man zwischen der starken Bahnung von Opticusreizen und der geringen bei Dauerlichtreizung. Man muß annehmen, daß — wie wir bereits in unserem Vortrag diskutierten — *nur stark synchronisierte afferente Impulse* der Neurone des optischen Systems (A—E, on, off, on-off) *durch Reticularisreizung gebahnt werden,* während koordinierte Reaktionsmuster in ihrem Informationscharakter wenig verändert werden. Mich würde interessieren, ob Prof. AKIMOTO auch eine geringere Beeinflussung der Dauerlichtreaktionen durch Reticularisreizung beobachtet hat.

L. M. HURVICH: In the slide which compares facilitation and inhibition I can see the facilitation effects quite clearly. The inhibitory and control records are less clearly different. I also had difficulty in seeing some of the differentiating indices described by Mrs. GRÜSSER and Dr. VERZEANO in their talks. Are the conclusions based on actual counts of many such records or have I failed to understand the criteria that the electrophysiologists are using to analyze their records?

R. JUNG: Die Frage von Prof. HURVICH ist so zu beantworten, daß nicht nur die spike-Zahl und Frequenz, sondern auch das charakteristische Entladungsmuster (pattern of discharge) für manche Auswertung von Bedeutung ist. Dies kann bei etwa gleicher Grundfrequenz sehr verschieden sein; z. B. die gruppierten Entladungen im Schlaf, die Dr. VERZEANO gezeigt hat und die offenbar auch Ausdruck einer subcorticalen Beeinflussung von seiten des unspezifischen Systems sind. Für die quantitative Auswertung ist natürlich die Zahl und Frequenz der spikes die beste Methode, wie sie auch CREUTZFELDT und AKIMOTO verwendet haben.

F. BREMER: I have been pleased to see the confirmation by Dr. CREUTZFELDT researches, combining macro- and microphysiological recordings, of our conclusions based only on the study of the averging process represented by the evoked potential recorded from the pial suface. Such combined studies increase obviously the physiological significance of each category of records.

I should like to point out, once more, that the spatial cortical diffusion of the dynamogenic effect exerted, in our experiments, by reticular and sensory arousal designs it as a process involved in conscious awareness rather than in selective sensory attention.

W. A. BERESFORD: B is the cell in the visual cortex that gives a response Rn when the retina is light stimulated and response Rs when the retina is light stimulated with simultaneous electrical stimulation in the mesencephalon and diencephalon. Your responce difference Rn versus Rs you interpret as resulting from activation of fibres from non-specific nuclei by your electrical stimulus.

The results might be explained by the specific cortical efferents rather than by the non-specific afferents. The type of cell shown by A is common in the visual cortex (SHOLL gives a % for cats visual cortex). If your electrical stimulation activates the cortico-fugal fibres shown, as it passes through the thalamus, the collateral would propagate an abnormal pattern of firing to cell B. The response difference of cell B to light stimulation measures the difference between the normal firing in As collateral and that produced by antidromic stimulation. To exclude this possible explanation your stimulating electrode ought to be distant to the cortico-fugal fibres. Was it? I would like to know more specifically where in the di-and mesencephalon you stimulated.

O. CREUTZFELDT (zu BERESFORD): Die Reizelektroden waren bei den Thalamusversuchen in folgenden Kernen: N. centralis lat., paraventricularis centralis med., paramedialis, anteroventralis, parataenialis und medialis (s. AKIMOTO und CREUTZFELDT 1958). Die Substantia reticularis wurde im pontinen Abschnitt gereizt, einige Male war die Elektrode auch etwas unterhalb der Substantia reticularis am Nucl. interpeduncularis lokalisiert. Abgesehen von den Unterschieden zwischen intralaminärer Thalamusreizung und mesencephaler Reticularisreizung hatte die Lokalisation keinen wesentlichen Einfluß auf die corticalen Reizreaktionen. Die Möglichkeit gelegentlicher Reizung antidromer Fasern haben wir bereits 1958 diskutiert und kamen zu dem Ergebnis, daß eine antidrome Reizung aus lokalisatorischen Gründen sehr unwahrscheinlich ist. Auch waren im EEG keine antidromen Potentiale nachweisbar. Offen bleiben muß die Frage, ob die corticalen Effekte durch corticale Konvergenz oder über das Corpus geniculatum vermittelt werden.

R. Jung: Die Einwände von Beresford gelten nur für elektrische Reizexperimente. Antidrome Reizung kollateraler corticaler Efferenzen ist aber ausgeschlossen, wenn ein arousal ohne elektrische Reize ausgelöst wird oder die Reizelektrode weit von den spezifischen Bahnen entfernt liegt. Derselbe Bahnungseffekt nach akustischem arousal, wie ihn Creutzfeldt u. Mitarb. gezeigt haben (Abb. 5b, S. 357), beweist ohne jede elektrische Reizung, daß es sich nicht um ein antidromes Reizartefakt handeln kann.

Die Ergebnisse von Creutzfeldt u. Mitarb. und Akimoto u. Mitarb. beweisen, daß eine nicht-visuelle unspezifische Beeinflussung der Neurone der Sehrinde auch aus dem Hirnstamm unterhalb des Thalamus möglich ist. Akimoto und Creutzfeldt finden beide mehr aktivierende als hemmende Effekte nach Reticularisreizung. Daß neben einer Aktivierung aber auch *hemmende Wirkungen* enthalten sind, zeigt die von Creutzfeldt gefundene Hemmung der Spontanentladung beim Typ c und die Wechselwirkung mit Flimmerlicht: Im Gegensatz zum Thalamusreiz erzeugt Reticularisreizung auch eine Verminderung der Fusionsfrequenz, bis zu der corticale Neurone dem Flimmerreiz folgen können (neuronale CFF). Bei Thalamusreizen fanden Creutzfeldt u. Grüsser dagegen häufiger eine Erhöhung der neuronalen CFF.

Unklar ist noch der Weg der retikulären Afferenz und der Ort der spezifischen und unspezifischen Konvergenz. Wie wir gestern schon bei Söderberg diskutiert haben, scheint die Reticularis bei der Katze vorwiegend auf corticale Neurone, weniger auf Geniculatumneurone und noch weniger auf retinale Neurone einzuwirken. Dies geht auch aus Dumont-Dells und Bremers Analysen der Makropotentiale hervor.

H. Akimoto: Wir haben den Einfluß der „arousal"-Reizung auf verschiedene Rindenfelder mit gleichen Reizmethoden verglichen, d. h. mit elektrischer Reizung unspezifischer thalamo-reticulärer und spezifischer thalamischer Afferenzen. Nur bei den Untersuchungen im visuellen Cortex brauchten wir zustätzlich die Lichtblitzreizung. Aus den Versuchen mit elektrischen Reizen spezifischer Thalamuskerne und thalamo-reticulärer Reizung ergab sich, daß der visuelle Cortex einen stärkeren excitatorischen Einfluß aus der Reticularis erhält als andere Rindenfelder, z. B. senso-motorische, akustische und Assoziationsfelder.

Wie Creutzfeldt haben auch wir gefunden, daß Dauerlichteffekte nicht wesentlich durch Reticularisreize gebahnt werden. Die Erklärung möchte ich offen lassen.

F. Der Informationswert verschiedener Reaktionstypen der Neurone des visuellen Systems

Gruppendiskussion

Initial Remarks

By

H. BARLOW*

I think there are three aspects of this problem which people will have views about. The *first* is the question of what subjective experience is evoked by a discharge in "off" (or off-center) units. I agree with BAUMGARTNER and JUNG that it is probably the sensation of black, or darkness. A stimulus which causes a discharge in such units in the cat, evokes in us a sensation we would label black; the correspondence is quite close, and I cannot think of any facts which contravert it, but I do not feel too happy about it for this reason. The relation between "off" units and blackness involves processes which we do not understand the physiology of at all — the business of attaching the linguistic label "blackness" to the sensation, for instance. Where so much of the relation is beyond our understanding, I am reluctant about being too dogmatic.

The kind of difficulty one can run into can be exemplified by putting the *second question* of interest in what I consider to be a misleading way: What sensation corresponds to a decrease of resting discharge in an "on" unit? Not blackness, one is inclined to say, because we know that that is signalled by activity in "off" units. In a very short time one is lost in a linguistic fog of one's own manufacture — the same kind of fog as the colour vision experts are so good at creating by talking about Red and Green pathways. The fact of the matter is that we are not yet ready to attach labels that are normally used for *sensations* to physiological processes. I think the right way to put this second question is: Is the decrease of a resting discharge of any significance? Does it carry any information? Undoubtedly it does carry information, for it is correlated with certain specific changes in the pattern of stimulation of the visual field, but this does not necessarily mean that central structures utilise it. Possibly the information is always carried more efficiently by the reciprocal set of fibres.

The *third question* arises from the fact that the "off" system seems to be universal in visual pathways. Why, then, is it advantageous to an animal to have it?

* Physiological Dept. University of Cambridge, England

What are the engineering advantages of designing it in this way? If we had ideas about this we might make more pertinent observations on the visual system. Here are four possible answers:

1. Filtering. If one looks at visually aroused responses one sees that a positive action follows a decrease in intensity of a part of the visual field as often as it follows an increase. Think of the escape movements made when a shadow encroaches on the visual field of a frog, or the attack movements elicited by a small black moving object. When we bear in mind the complex information-filtering operations which must occur between the reception of light and the resulting muscular movement, it seems very naive to expect that increased impulse frequency will always signal increased incident energy.

2. Asymmetry of impulse frequency modulation. Information is transmitted along nerves by modulating the frequency of impulses, and such a transmission system is inherently asymmetrical. If there is no resting discharge, then obviously decreases in stimulus intensity could not be signalled at all without a separate "off" system. Where there is a resting discharge, this is rarely so high that there is as much room for a decrease in frequency as there is for an increase, and on top of this there is another kind of asymmetry. When the pulse frequency is increased the time resolution improves, whereas if it is decreased it gets worse. This is easily seen to be true if one considers how long one has to wait before one could tell if an impulse was missing, for obviously one has no indication of change until the next impulse is due. If increases and decreases of light are equally significant and the transmission system is asymmetric, inverting the signal would be a common-sense trick for combatting the difficulty.

3. Cancellation of previous pictures. The human eye executes several saccadic movements per second, and the brain needs to get a separate picture from each position. But we know that some of the effects of light are long-lasting; the time constant of regeneration of pigment, for instance, is several minutes. For any one part of the retina one would expect the impulse frequency to be gravely distorted by the intensity of light previously impressed upon that part, and particularly by the intensity of light in the previous fixation position. How can the brain separate out the contribution of the pattern of light in the present fixation position from the residual effects of the previous pattern? Possibly one function of the "off" discharge is to cancel the effect of the preceeding "on" discharge, and vice-versa.

4. Statistical testing hypothesis. Perhaps the retina is performing a statistical test on the incoming information, and signalling centrally when it obtains a significant P value. The information locally available is the number of quanta currently being absorbed. Successive values of this number will be scattered round a mean value, and there are three simple questions one could ask: i) Is the current number significantly different from the mean? ii) Is it significantly greater? iii) Is it signicantly less? It looks as though the frog's "on-off" units asked question i), the cat "on" centre unit question ii), and "off"-centre unit question iii). According to this notion impulses signify the degree of improbability of a null-hypothesis which is characterized by the spatial and temporal properties of the unit's receptive field. Obviously this is rather a wild idea, but I think the way of looking at c.n.s. function which it typifies may be helpful.

Der Informationswert der on-Zentrum- und off-Zentrum-Neurone des visuellen Systems beim Hell-Dunkel-Sehen und die informative Bedeutung von Aktivierung und Hemmung

Von

Günter Baumgartner

Mit 2 Abbildungen

Meine Auffassung über die informative Bedeutung habe ich schon in den beiden Referaten mitgeteilt (S. 45, 297). Hier soll sie noch einmal kurz zusammengefaßt werden, da weder hinsichtlich der informativen Leistung der einzelnen licht-beeinflußten Neurone noch in bezug auf die Bedeutung von Aktivierungs- und Hemmungsvorgängen die Ansichten der verschiedenen Untersucher überein-stimmen. Ich stütze mich dabei auf die oben geschilderten Helligkeits-Kontrast-untersuchungen an nicht narkotisierten encéphale-isolé-Katzen. Dabei ist noch einmal zu betonen, daß fast nur Lichtreize gleicher Intensität appliziert und mög-lichst konstante Adaptationsbedingungen angestrebt wurden. Ferner ist zu be-achten, daß bei der Interpretation der Kontrastversuche subjektiv sinnesphysio-logische Erfahrungen zur Erklärung mit herangezogen worden sind. Die Beschrän-kung auf weiße Lichtreize gleicher Intensität und das Heranziehen subjektiv-sinnesphysiologischer Daten bei der Deutung der Versuche vermindert zweifellos ihre allgemeine Gültigkeit. Dies vorausgesetzt, machen unsere Untersuchungen folgende Annahmen wahrscheinlich.

1. Die von Kuffler 1951 und 1953 in der Katzenretina beschriebene antagonisti-sche Organisation der rezeptiven Felder gilt in ähnlicher Weise auch für das Corpus geniculatum laterale und den primären optischen Cortex (Area 17) (Baumgartner S. 297—311, Hubel 1959 und 1960).

2. Die informative Bedeutung der verschiedenen Neurone wird durch ihr *Feldzentrum* bestimmt. Dies gilt auch für die Information der on-off-Neurone, je nach dem, ob sie ein off- oder on-Feldzentrum besitzen.

3. *On-Zentrum-Neurone* (B-Neurone des Cortex) melden dementsprechend bei Aktivierung stets eine Aufhellung, *off-Zentrum-Neurone* (D- und E-Neurone des Cortex) bei Aktivierung stets eine Verdunkelung im Bereich ihres rezeptiven Feld-zentrums.

4. Die Informationsübertragung von der Peripherie nach zentral erfolgt über-wiegend durch das jeweils *aktivierte System* (on- oder off-System). Ich halte es dar-über hinaus für wahrscheinlich, daß auch bei der zentralen Informationsbearbei-tung das aktivierte System bevorzugt wird, soweit Leitungsprozesse dabei eine Rolle spielen. Dagegen sind hemmende und erregende Synapsen für das Zustande-kommen einfacher formaler Operationen am einzelnen Neuron gleichwertig.

Die Punkte 1—3 ergeben sich aus meinen Ergebnissen (S. 45 und S. 297). Die Verwandtschaft der präexzitatorisch gehemmten on-off-Elemente (E-Neurone des Cortex) zu den reinen off-Zentrum-Neuronen zeigt ergänzend das präexzitatorisch gehemmte, corticale on-off-Neuron der Abb. 1. Das Neuron hat bei Belichtung mit vollerLichtintensität eine typische, präexzitatorisch gehemmte on-Reaktion und eine off-Reaktion mit kurzer Latenz. Bei Reduktion der Lichtintensität auf 10% der Ausgangslichtstärke reagiert das Neuron wie ein reines off-Element, was besagt, daß die geringere Empfindlichkeit der Umfeldzone bei verminderter Intensität nicht mehr für eine on-Aktivierung ausreicht. Nach 3 min, während denen wiederholt Lichtreize mit geringer Intensität appliziert wurden, reagiert das Neuron auch bei voller Lichtintensität als reines off-Neuron. Wiederholt man den Lichtreiz mit voller Intensität mehrfach, so zeigt das Neuron nach wenigen Belichtungen

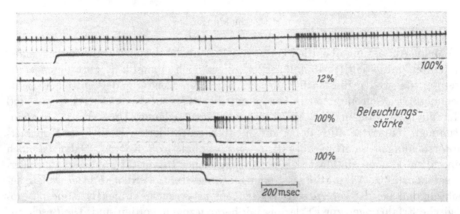

Abb. 1 a—d. a) Off-Zentrum-Neuron des Cortex mit on-off-Reaktion bei diffuser Belichtung voller Intensität (300 Lux). b) Reine off-Reaktion des gleichen Neurons bei Belichtung mit 12% der Ausgangslichtstärke. c) Reine off-Reaktion bei voller Lichtstärke nach vorausgehender intermittierender Belichtung mit 12% der Ausgangsintensität über 3 min. d) Wiederherstellung der on-off-Reaktion wie in a nach mehrfacher Wiederholung des Lichtreizes voller Intensität in Abständen von 1—2 sec

wieder ein reines on-off-Verhalten. Die Reaktionen dieses Elementes werden verständlich, wenn man berücksichtigt, daß die Umfeldgröße bei Dunkeladaptation kleiner wird, wie BARLOW et al. 1957 nachgewiesen haben. Bei Lichtreizen geringerer Intensität verändert sich das rezeptive Feld in Richtung zunehmender Dunkeladaptation, d. h. das Umfeld schrumpft, weshalb auch bei voller Lichtstärke eine off-Reaktion eintritt. Wird die volle Lichtstärke mehrfach wiederholt, so nimmt das Umfeld wieder zu und stellt die alte on-off-Reaktion wieder her (on-off-D-Neuron).

Die Abb. 2 zeigt umgekehrt ein on-off-Neuron mit on-Feld-Zentrum, welches bei geringer Lichtstärke als on-off-Element reagiert, jedoch mit einer on-Reaktion ohne präexzitatorische Hemmung und mit einer off-Aktivierung mit großer Latenz. Dieses Neuron reagiert bei intensiverer Belichtung nach mehrfachen Belichtungen mit geringer Intensität wie ein reines on-Neuron (on-off-B-Neuron).

Wegen des Überganges der präexzitatorisch gehemmten on-off-Neurone in off-Elemente und der mit kurzer Latenz on-aktivierten on-off-Neurone in on-Elemente sowie wegen des Kontrastverhaltens der präexzitatorisch gehemmten on-off-Neurone nehme ich an, daß diese beiden Neuronentypen zum Dunkel- bzw. Hellsystem gehören, d. h. off- bzw. on-Feldzentren besitzen.

Zu Punkt 4 ist zu ergänzen: Wenn eine aktive zentrale Hemmung existiert, so muß der Hemmungsvorgang über das aktivierte System erfolgen. Eine aktive zentrale Hemmung kann bei Wegfall der entsprechenden Afferenz nur über Kollateralen des jeweils aktivierten neuronalen Überträgers zustande kommen, die wahrscheinlich über Interneurone eine Hemmung der entsprechenden antagonistischen Neurone verursachen. Für die Informationsübertragung von der Peripherie nach zentral ist deshalb das aktivierte System allein ausschlaggebend. Aber auch für die zentrale Informationsauswertung halte ich die Aktivierung für wichtiger als die Hemmung. Bei der oft geringen Grundaktivität zentraler Neurone wäre bei informativ gleichrangiger Hemmung eine erhebliche Asymmetrie des Informationssystems zu erwarten, was nicht wahrscheinlich ist. Darauf hat schon BARLOW hingewiesen. Wir müssen zur Zeit annehmen, daß Informationen durch Modulationen der Impulsfrequenz der Neurone übertragen werden. Ist die Hemmung gleichrangig wie die Aktivierung, so ergäbe dies bei Zunahme der Hemmung eine progressive Informationsminderung, was unzweckmäßig wäre.

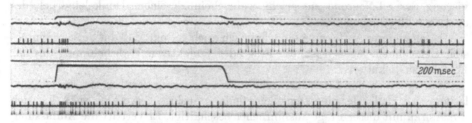

Abb. 2. On-Zentrum-Neuron des Cortex,welches bei geringer Lichtintensität (∼ 700 Lux) als on-off-Element mit später off-Aktivierung und einer on-Reaktion mit kurzer Latenz reagiert und bei starker Lichtintensität (∼7000 Lux) eine reine on-Reaktion zeigt

Wie bei der Vermischung von objektiv-physiologischen Fakten mit aus der subjektiv-psychologischen Erfahrung entliehenen Deutungen nicht anders zu erwarten, bleibt noch vieles unklar. So setzt beispielsweise die Annahme, daß die Aktivierung eines off-Zentrum-Neurons stets dunkler bedeutet, schon zwei verschiedene Aktivierungsmechanismen voraus. Die Aktivierung eines off-Neurons bei Verdunklung erfolgt über das Feldzentrum und muß anders gesteuert werden als die Aktivierung des gleichen Neurons im Kontrast bei Belichtung. Während sich die Aktivierung bei Kontrastbelichtung durch laterale Aktivierung erklären läßt, kommt dies für die Aktivierung bei Verdunkelung nicht in Frage. Ob bei der Aktivierung nach Verdunkelung rebound-Phänomene eine Rolle spielen, wie WOLBARSHT annimmt, oder ob Richtung und Steilheit der sog. R-C-Potentiale dafür verantwortlich sind, wie GRÜSSER diskutiert, wird so lange offenbleiben, wie wir über die intraretinale Verschaltung nicht besser orientiert sind.

BARLOW hat auch schon darauf hingewiesen, daß das off-System im visuellen Bereich überall vorkommt. Dies kann der Positivität der Dunkelempfindung zugrunde liegen, zu der ich kein Analogon aus anderen sensorischen Systemen kenne. Gestattet man sich hier eine teleologische Interpretation, so ist der visuelle Mechanismus der positiven Perzeption von Gesichtsfeldstellen mit fehlender energetischer Anregung von außen von großer Bedeutung. Denn nur dadurch werden uns beispielsweise dunkle Körper als Hindernisse bemerkbar und sind nicht nur einfach nicht vorhanden wie innerhalb eines Skotoms.

Über die subjektive Wahrnehmung des off-Effektes[1]

Von

W. Best

Mit 1 Abbildung

Auf dem Deutschen Physiologenkongreß in Bad Nauheim 1959 kam es im Anschluß an die Vorträge von Baumgartner und Grüsser zu einer Diskussion. Beim Zuhören hatte ich den Eindruck, daß die Freiburger Schule die Auffassung vertritt, daß der off-Effekt eine Dunkelempfindung auslöst. Ich habe dies in einer Arbeit von Grüsser und Grützner bestätigt gefunden. Sie schreiben, die Aktivierung der off-Neurone entspricht wahrscheinlich einem Dunkeleindruck des optisch Wahrgenommenen.

Da ich anderer Auffassung bin[2], habe ich mich gefreut, daß auf diesem Symposion Gelegenheit gegeben ist, die Frage der subjektiven Wahrnehmung des off-Effektes zu diskutieren.

Man findet in der Literatur verhältnismäßig wenig darüber, ob die off-Entladung eine Hell- oder eine Dunkelempfindung auslöst. Soweit ich weiß, hat sich nur Asher mit dieser Frage ausführlicher beschäftigt. Er vertritt die Auffassung, daß der off-Effekt als Helligkeit empfunden wird. Sein Hauptargument besteht darin, daß bei intermittierender Belichtung die Hellphase länger empfunden wird, als die Dunkelphase, obwohl objektiv beide Phasen gleich lang sind. Meines Erachtens ist dieses Argument nicht beweisend, da die längere Dauer der Hellphase auch auf Nachentladungen zurückgeführt werden könnte und nicht unbedingt auf den off-Effekt.

Auch die Versuche, die ich jetzt anführen will, sind kein Beweis, sondern nur ein Hinweis. Zusammen mit Bohnen habe ich vor einiger Zeit den Einfluß der Reizdauer auf das Elektroretinogramm des Menschen bei Helladaptation untersucht. Wir fanden, daß die positive Amplitude des Elektroretinogramms bei Verkürzung der Reizdauer größer wird (siehe Abb. 1).

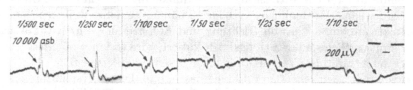

Abb. 1. Elektroretinogramm des Menschen im helladaptierten Zustand bei Variation der Reizdauer. Grundbeleuchtung: 700 asb, Reizfeld 110°. Zusatzlicht: 10000 asb, Reizfeld 110°. Die Kurven sind von links nach rechts zu lesen. Oberer Strahl: Reiz- und Zeitmarkierung (1/50 sec). Ausschlag nach oben: Licht an; Ausschlag nach unten: Licht aus. Die Pfeile kennzeichnen den Beginn des off-Effektes. Rechts oben Testwert von 200 μV [aus W. Best u. K. Bohnen: Albrecht v. Graefes Arch. Ophthal. 158, 568 (1957)]

Ich glaube, daß ein Zusammenhang besteht zwischen dieser Zunahme der positiven Amplitude des Elektroretinogramms bei Verkürzung der Reizdauer und

---

[1] Aus der Universitäts-Augenklinik Bonn.

[2] In der Diskussion zeigte sich, daß ein Mißverständnis als Folge der verschiedenen Nomenklatur vorlag. Baumgartner, Grüsser und Grützner sind, wenn ich richtig verstanden habe, der Ansicht, daß die Aktivierung der B-Neurone immer eine Lichtempfindung, und die der D-Neurone immer eine Dunkelempfindung auslöst, gleichgültig, ob es sich um eine on- oder eine off-Antwort handelt.

der Tatsache, daß kurze Lichtreize heller empfunden werden als längere. Das letztere wissen wir aus Arbeiten von Broca und Sulzer sowie Ebbecke. Die Zunahme der Amplitude des Elektroretinogramms bei Verkürzung der Reizdauer ist nun unseres Erachtens auf ein Hinaufwandern des off-Effektes auf den on-Effekt und außerdem auf ein echtes Größerwerden des off-Effektes zurückzuführen. Wir schließen dies einmal aus dem Aspekt. Zweitens findet sich die Zunahme der positiven Amplitude bei Verkürzung der Reizdauer nur im helladaptierten Zustand, nicht aber im Stadium der Dunkeladaptation, und wir wissen, daß der off-Effekt während der Dunkeladaptation kleiner wird bzw. verschwindet. Drittens schließlich ist aus Versuchen von Granit bekannt, daß die off-Entladung der Opticus-Ganglienzellen bei hoher Intensität und kurzer Reizdauer stärker sein kann als bei langer Reizdauer. Bei der on-Antwort findet sich dies nicht oder nur angedeutet.

Aus all diesen Gründen erscheint es mir sicher, daß die Zunahme der positiven Amplitude des helladaptierten Elektroretinogramms bei Verkürzung der Reizdauer auf einer Zunahme des off-Effektes beruht. Wenn wir aber wissen, daß bei Verkürzung der Reizdauer der off-Effekt und die subjektive Helligkeit zunehmen, während der on-Effekt gleich bleibt, so spricht dies meines Erachtens dafür, daß der off-Effekt eine Helligkeitsempfindung auslöst. Es wäre wünschenswert, die Zunahme der subjektiven Helligkeit und des off-Effektes bei Verkürzung der Reizdauer unter denselben Versuchsbedingungen zu vergleichen. Leider konnte ich diese Versuche bisher noch nicht ausführen.

Ich möchte noch kurz einiges zum off-Effekt bemerken. Wahrscheinlich versuchen ja viele von uns sich ein Bild vom Wesen des off-Effektes zu machen und ich glaube, ein Symposion ist der rechte Ort, darüber zu sprechen und die Gedanken der anderen kennenzulernen. Ich würde glauben, daß ein und dieselbe Nervenfaser nur eine Qualität der Information zu den höheren Zentren weitermelden kann, ich meine, weiß, rot, grün usw. und vielleicht auch schwarz[1]. Aber diese Information sollte dieselbe bei der on- und bei der off-Entladung sein. Die Amplitude der einzelnen spikes ist dieselbe, der Frequenz schreiben wir die Information des Helligkeitswertes zu und das Muster der Entladungsfrequenz kann durch intermittierendes Licht vielfältig geändert werden, ohne daß sich im allgemeinen die Qualität der Information ändert. Darum ist es mir unverständlich, wie es dem folgenden Neuron möglich sein sollte, zwischen on- und off-Antwort zu unterscheiden.

Ferner glaube ich, daß man den off-Effekt unter zwei ganz verschiedenen Aspekten betrachten kann. Der eine wesentliche Punkt scheint mir zu sein, daß die Hemmung der Entladungen während der Belichtung einen Informationsweg blockiert, der vermutlich sonst eine falsche Information liefern würde. Wenn es nach Schluß der Belichtung zur off-Entladung und damit zu einer kurzdauernden falschen Information kommt, so hat dies möglicherweise mit dem Sukzessivkontrast und Nachbildern zu tun und ist nicht sehr wesentlich. Während aus diesem Blickwinkel die Hemmung der Entladungen während der Belichtung das Wichtige darstellt, ist unter einem anderen Blickwinkel der off-Effekt selbst von

---

[1] Durch die Diskussion wurde ich überzeugt, daß theoretisch die Möglichkeit besteht, daß durch eine einzelne Nervenfaser zwei verschiedene Qualitäten der Information geleitet werden können. Eine Steigerung der Spontanaktivität könnte z. B. die Ursache einer Helligkeitsempfindung, eine Erniedrigung der Spontanaktivität die Ursache einer Dunkelempfindung sein.

Bedeutung. Zum Beispiel könnte der off-Effekt dazu beitragen, daß kurze Licht-reize besser wahrgenommen werden und daß durch kleine Augenbewegungen der Simultankontrast erhöht wird. Ich bin sehr daran interessiert, Ihre Gedanken über den off-Effekt zu hören.

Summary

In light adapted states shortening of the stimulus duration gives bigger off-effects in the electroretinogram. Perhaps, there is a correlation to the fact that short flashes of light seem to be brighter than longer ones.

The question is discussed which sensation is caused by the off-effect. The author believes that one and the same neuron gives the same sensation at "on" and at "off".

Literatur

Asher, H.: Contrast in eye and brain. Brit. J. Psychol. (Gen. Sect.) 40, 187—194 (1950).
Best, W., u. K. Bohnen: Über den „off-Effekt" im Elektroretinogramm des Menschen. Albrecht v. Graefes Arch. Ophthal. 158, 568—577 (1957).
Broca, A., et D. Sulzer: La sensation lumineuse en fonction du temps. J. Physiol. Path. gén. 4, 632—640 (1902); zit. n. Granit, R.: Sensory mechanism of the retina. London: Oxford Univ. Press 1947.
Ebbecke, U.: Über das Augenblicksehen. Mit einer Bemerkung über rückwirkende Hemmung. Pflügers Arch. ges. Physiol. 185, 181—195 (1920).
Granit, R.: The antagonism between the on- and off-systems in the cat's retina. Ann. psychol. (Paris) 50, 129—134 (1951).
Grüsser, O.-J., u. A. Grützner: Neurophysiologische Grundlagen der periodischen Nachbild-phasen nach kurzen Lichtblitzen. Albrecht v. Graefes Arch. Ophthal. 160, 65—93 (1958).

Diskussion

D. Hurvich-Jameson: Dr. Barlow stated that to derive correlations between electro-physiological responses and perceptual responses what is really needed is a direct estimate of the apparent brightness of a light of known stimulus intensity. Direct estimates of brightness magnitudes are indeed available, by the psychological scaling technique of direct magnitude estimation in which numerical values are assigned to various stimuli in accordance with their apparent brightnesses. Some quantitative functions obtained in this manner were re-ported by us earlier in this meeting to demonstrate the dependence of the perceptual Inten-sity vs. Response function on various parameters, and to raise the question of comparable dependencies in electrophysiological functions. The psychophysical functions obtained for different surround intensities show that brightness magnitude is related to stimulus intensity by a simple power function when the surround intensity is low, but that there is a break in the function with a marked increase in slope below the surround intensity when the surround level is high.

H. Barlow: I would like to modify slightly my remarks about the difficulty of relating nerve discharges to subjective sensations. I have no quarrel with the type of psycho-physical experiment in which one finds out what physically different stimuli give rise to indistinguish-able sensations. But as soon as the sensations experienced are admitted by the subject to distinguishable *in any way*, then in order to find out how or in what way they differ you have to get involved in a tricky process which I, as a physiologist, have little confidence in. But it does seem to me possible that one might be able to quantify perceived differences in the sort of way that George Miller has quantified the accuracy of making metrical judgements. One could use the sensations to obtain an estimate of information transfer, and one might then find how the efficiency of transfer varied under different conditions. These results could be compared with the information transfer given by a physiological preparation in similar conditions, or with the transfer predicted according to some postulated physiological mechanism. The experiments on colour contrast reported by Dr. and Mrs. Hurvich may fall into this class, though I am sure they would agree that the numbers attached to a stimulus by a subject cannot be directly compared with the numbers of nerve impulses in a physiological preparation, or anything as simple as that. But the efficiency of information transfer may be the common currency which is so badly needed.

Another point I feel strongly about is that if psycho-physical data are to be considered in connection with results of physiological experiments one must make sure that the conditions are comparable. For instance the number of jnd's of intensity is not what one wants when discussing the question whether the decrease of a resting discharge can convey a sufficient number of gradations of "blackness". It would be more relevant to consider the number of reliably distinguishable levels of blackness, and this must be far fewer than the number of jnd's (vide MILLER).

F. BREMER: The vestibular system represents a case where the normal existence of a spontaneous activity of the receptors implies necessarily an asymmetry in the spans of the central informations resulting from the increase or decrease of the tonic excitatory background. This was clearly shown in LOWENSTEIN's and LEDOUX's experiments on the fish and frog semicircular canals. There was apparently no limit for the increase of the ampullar discharge (recorded by ballistic integration in LEDOUX's experiments), produced by ampullopetal pressure in the horizontal canal, while the decrease of the same tonic discharge — equally important behaviourly — induced by ampullofugal pressure has its obvious limit at the zero level.

When, in the experiments by Dr. DE VALOIS, in the monkey, the *on* response of a geniculate neuron to a specific wave length has been by experimental manipulations, f. i. by bleaching, transformed in an *off* response, what becomes of the spectral information conveyed to the *area striata*?

R. L. DE VALOIS: Professor BREMER raises a very interesting point here. The transformed off-response may convey the same color as former on-responses. I can only speculate that the on discharge conveys the same information in both cases, but that in the light-adapted state additional information about complementary color is being carried now by inhibition.

With regard to the discussions of Drs. BARLOW and BAUMGARTNER, I would like to point out that we often find that the threshold for inhibition in an off-cell is often one or two log units below the threshold for an off-response. This would appear to suggest that the inhibition itself is carrying important information.

H. BARLOW (to DE VALOIS): The fact that the threshold for suppression of resting discharge may be lower, by one or two log units, than the threshold for the off discharge in your monkey geniculate units does seem to suggest that such suppression is important in carrying information. However one should really compare the threshold for decrease of resting discharge with the threshold for increase of impulse frequency in reciprocal units, if such exist. It must be very hard to be sure that there are none.

I am also a bit dubious about drawing this kind of conclusion from nembutalised animals. Barbiturates in anaesthetic concentrations play havoc with the cat's retina.

Are there enough gradations between a resting discharge of, say, 20/sec and zero to account for all the gradations of subjective blackness one can experience? This continuous gradation over a big range makes me doubt whether it could be carried by a decrease in discharge frequency.

R. L. DE VALOIS: In evaluating whether there are enough gradations between the resting discharge level and complete inhibition for the inhibition to be carrying brightness information, one should remember that brightness (or color) discrimination becomes extremely poor as the area and duration of a spot of light is decreased. The many gradations you mention are found only when there is the possibility of an integration over thousands of neurones for several seconds, with repeated samplings as one looks back and forth betwen the two areas being compared. A further point is that the number of brightnesses which one can discriminate from a given adaptation level is quite limited (see W. H. MARSHALL and S. A. TALBOT, *Biological Symposia*, Vol. 7, pg. 130, Jacques Cattell Press). I think it is clear that a single neurone over a short period of time at a given adaptation level *is* carrying but little information.

R. Jung: 1. *Zur dualistischen Terminologie der neuronalen Hell- und Dunkelsysteme:* Der verschiedene Informationswert der visuellen Neurone und Baumgartners Trennung in zwei antagonistische Systeme mit reziproker Funktionsbeziehung scheint einleuchtend und kann viele Phänomene des Hell-Dunkel-Sehens befriedigend erklären: Sukzessivkontrast durch reziproke Hemmung antagonistischer Neurone im selben Feld mit rhythmisch-sukzessiver Abwechslung des Überwiegens des einen oder anderen Systems und Simultankontrast durch laterale Hemmung synergistischer Neurone in den Nachbarfeldern. Die Bezeichnung der Neurone nach ihren Feldzentren ist physiologisch exakt und für Punktlichtreize zweifellos zweckmäßiger als die alte Bezeichnung on-Elemente, off-Elemente und on-off-Elemente, da dieselben Neurone je nach ihrer Situation im Kontrastfeld mit verschiedenen on-, off- oder on-off-Entladungen antworten können. Gerade dieses verschiedene Verhalten und seine Übereinstimmung mit dem subjektiven Kontrastsehen beweist die *informatorische Konstanz dieser Systeme für das Hell- und Dunkelsehen.* Da unsere Bezeichnung der corticalen Neuronentypen mit B- und D sowohl im Deutschen wie im Englischen gut mit disem Informationswert übereinstimmt (B-Belichtungsaktivierung, Brightness information; D-Dunkelaktivierung, Darkness information), scheint es mir zweckmäßig, das dualistische System der hell dunkel meldenden Neurone allgemein mit diesen beiden Buchstaben B und D zu bezeichnen: *B-System für Hellinformation und D System für Dunkelinformation.* Die Bezeichnung B-Neuron und D-Neuron, die wir zunächst nur für den Cortex vorgeschlagen haben, würde dann auch für die unteren Stationen von Retina und Geniculatum passen. Diese Termini sind kürzer und sinnesphysiologisch verständlicher als „on Feldzentrum-Neuron" oder „off-Feldzentrum-Neurone", und sie sind zweckmäßiger dann, wenn man keine einzelnen rezeptiven Felder untersucht und ihre Zentrumsaktivierung erst indirekt aus diffusen oder Kontrastlichtreizen ableiten muß. Die mit on-off-Entladungen antwortenden E-Typen wären dann je nach Überwiegen der on- oder off-Komponente nach ihrem Feldzentrum und Informationswert dem B- oder D-System zuzuteilen, etwa als on-off D (sehr häufig) oder on-off B (sehr selten) oder als D_E und B_E.

2. *Zur Informationsleitung und Hemmung:* Ich glaube, daß Baumgartner die Bedeutung der Hemmungsmechanismen unterschätzt, wenn er eine Bevorzugung des aktivierten Systems für die zentrale Informationsverarbeitung annimmt. Zweifellos muß die *Leitung* der Information über ein aktiviertes System erfolgen. Doch kann auch Hemmung einer Dauerentladung Information bedeuten. Diese Hemmung kann in einem reziproken System auch auf der nächsten Stufe eine Aktivierung des Antagonisten auslösen.

Vielleicht kann man fast alle Befunde neuronaler Wechselwirkung im visuellen System durch *zwei Hemmungsmechanismen* befriedigend erklären: 1. *Reziproke Hemmung* antagonistischer Neurone in demselben Erregungsgebiet, 2. *Laterale Hemmung* synergistischer Neurone im Nachbargebiet. Laterale Aktivierung des off-Zentrums kann dann Enthemmung sein. Veränderungen der lateralen Hemmung können auch die neuronale Dunkeladaptation erklären, wenn diese nach den Befunden von Barlow u. Mitarb. eine Verminderung bis zum Verschwinden des hemmenden Umfeldes erzeugt und damit größere Feldzentren und weitere Irradiation für den Stäbchenapparat ermöglicht.

Glaubt Dr. Baumgartner, daß außer diesen beiden Hemmungsmechanismen noch andere Wechselwirkungen der Hell-Dunkel-Neuronensysteme notwendig sind, und welche wären es?

G. Baumgartner: Für die Korrelation des on-Systems zur Hellempfindung und des off-Systems zur Dunkelempfindung scheint relative Übereinstimmung zu bestehen. Doch wird die informative Bedeutung von Aktivierungs- und Hemmungsvorgängen noch verschieden interpretiert. Wie Dr. Barlow schon betonte, könnte ein gehemmtes Neuron Informationswert besitzen, da seine Hemmung mit Belichtungsänderung innerhalb seines rezeptiven Feldes korrespondiert. Diese Hemmung ist jedoch für die Übertragung uninteressant und bleibt in der Peripherie lokalisiert. Unter der Voraussetzung aktiver zentraler Hemmungen wird die ihr korrespondierende Information über das aktivierte System nach zentral weiter gegeben. Auch Prof. Jung stimmt bis dahin überein, daß die Informations*übertragung* lediglich über aktivierte Neurone erfolgen kann. Wird dies aber akzeptiert, so ist es nicht konsequent, in die zentrale Informations*auswertung* die Hemmung wieder als gleichrangig einzuführen, sofern Leitungsprozesse dabei mitgemeint sind.

Ob eine Hemmung in einem reziproken System eine Aktivierung des Antagonisten auslöst, ist eine Schaltungsfrage. Wenn die Hemmung vom aktivierten System aus erfolgt, wird der

Antagonist zunächst nicht aktiviert. Ich halte deshalb die Hemmung des Antagonisten vom informativen Gesichtspunkt lediglich für ein Begleitphänomen, das für die Signifikanz der Information erforderlich ist. Darin liegt meines Erachtens auch ihr möglicher Informationswert und vielleicht der Grund der gegenseitigen Verständnisschwierigkeit. Wenn eine Gesichtsfeldstelle hell erscheint, darf sie nicht gleichzeitig dunkel gemeldet werden. Dies kann durch begleitende Hemmung des Antagonisten erreicht werden.

Man könnte also von einer *negativen Informationsfunktion der Antagonisten-Hemmung* sprechen und sie als einen Löschvorgang betrachten, der die Tafel „schwärzt" und für eine neue Beschriftung vorbereitet. Die positive Empfindung „heller" oder „dunkler" erfolgt jedoch vermutlich stets über die Aktivierung entsprechender Neurone des on- oder off-Systems. Gleichwertig sind inhibitorische und excitatorische Prozesse nur innerhalb der beiden Systeme.

Neben den Hemmungsmechanismen im visuellen System, die Prof. JUNG erwähnt, ist die laterale Aktivierung des off-Systems zur Erklärung der Kontrastwirkung erforderlich. Die on-Aktivierung der off-Neurone erfolgt durch sie und ist ohne laterale Aktivierung nicht verständlich. *Im on-System ist die laterale Hemmung, im off-System die laterale Aktivierung der Mechanismus, der jeder Simultankontrastbildung zugrunde liegt.*

R. JUNG: Laterale Aktivierung des off-Systems ist *Enthemmung* eines auch im Dunkeln vor völliger Adaptation dauernd wirksamen Hemmungsprozesses des rezeptiven Umfeldes.

G. BAUMGARTNER: Die laterale Aktivierung als Enthemmung aufzufassen, ist meines Erachtens nicht möglich, da Enthemmung Hemmung voraussetzt. Die Hemmung der off-Zentrum-Neurone erfordert aber Licht. Im Dunkeln besteht keine Hemmung dieser Neurone. Trotzdem erfolgt im Kontrast bei Belichtung durch laterale Aktivierung eine on-Reaktion der off-Zentrum-Neurone. Wie ich schon betonte, ist deshalb anzunehmen, daß der Aktivierungsmechanismus eines off-Zentrum-Neurons im Kontrast von den Aktivierungsvorgängen bei Verdunkelung im diffusen Licht verschieden ist. Nur bei der Aktivierung bei Verdunkelung kann formal eine Enthemmung angenommen werden, für die Kontrastaktivierung ist eine laterale Aktivierung des off-Systems ausschlaggebend.

R. JUNG: Fassen wir die Ergebnisse der Diskussion zusammen, so besteht Einigkeit über die *relative Informationskonstanz der visuellen Neurone*, sowohl für das Hell-Dunkel-Sehen wie nach DE VALOIS auch für das Farbsehen. Ferner sind wir einig, daß die *on-, off- oder on-off-Antworten je nach Reizart wechseln und allein nicht die Neurone charakterisieren können.* Zurückhaltung und Bedenken wurden geäußert gegen die Überschätzung des Informationswertes einzelner Neurone und gegen eine zu enge und dogmatische Korrelation zwischen psychophysischen und neuronalen Daten.

BARLOW hat mit Recht gewarnt, subjektive psychophysische Daten ohne vergleichbare Bedingungen auf die Neuronenphysiologie zu übertragen. Dennoch hätte ich keine Bedenken durch solche terminologische Korrelationen die Anschaulichkeit unserer physiologischen Ergebnisse zu verbessern. Man braucht dabei nicht der Äquivokation zu verfallen. Wir dürfen Neuronentypen, deren Informationswert mit neurophysiologischen Methoden wahrscheinlich gemacht wurde, auch kurz in ihrer Bedeutung bezeichnen: Beim Hell-Dunkel-Sehen kann man kurz vom *B- oder Hellsystem* oder vom *D- oder Dunkelsystem* sprechen (vgl. S. 412). Auch bei Farbenuntersuchungen erleichtert es die Verständigung, wenn man nicht Wellenlängen und on-off-Korrelationen umständlich erklären muß, sondern einen kurzen Terminus hat. Auch hier genügt die *Bezeichnung der positiven Informationsbedeutung*, z. B. würde man bei DE VALOIS' on-or-off-cells die red-on, green-off-Zellen als *Rot-Neurone* kurz bezeichnen können und die blue-on und yellow-off-Zellen als *Blau-Neurone* oder, entsprechend BAUMGARTNERs on-off-D-Neuronen, als *on-off-Blau-Neurone. Die Informationsbedeutung bleibt für die on- und off-Antwort eines Neurons die gleiche*, sowohl bei BAUMGARTNERs on-Zentrum-Neuronen wie bei DE VALOIS' red-on-cells. „Hell" oder „Rot" bezeichnet in beiden Fällen am kürzesten ihre Informationsbedeutung.

G. Synopsis von subjektiver und objektiver Sinnesphysiologie des Sehens

A Clarification of Some of the Procedures and Concepts Involved in Dealing with the Optic Pathway[1,2]

By

S. Howard Bartley

Methods of producing brightness enhancement. The purpose of the present paper is to clarify some of the principal procedures and concepts in dealing with the optic pathway and then to proceed to examining the facts that have to do with accounting for brightness enhancement. This clarification first has do with stating what is involved in the use of certain kinds of *photic stimulation*, the results obtained from them, and the labeling of the results. Secondly and thirdly the clarification pertains to the inferences made from diverse forms of information, namely photochemical, neuroretinal, and cortical phenomena. There have been continuing confusions and misconceptions in all these matters and it is therefore imperative that we pause to eradicate them before expecting to understand each other.

As was said, the specific purpose at hand is the understanding of brightness enhancement. Brightness enhancement is the fact that intermittent stimulation may produce a greater sensory end-result, namely greater brightness, than continuous stimulation of the same intensity. Its occurrence is not in question, except by a few who have made only incidental attempts to produce it. Various workers report what, on the surface, seem to be conflicting results and make diverse and conflicting statements in interpreting what they find. One factor underlying this discord seems to be the assumption that all means of supplying photic stimulation are essentially equivalent. There are two dissimilar methods commonly in use. One is the use of revolving disks with alternating unlike sectors. The other is the use of two stationary, adjacent translucent targets made intermittent by interrupting the radiation that is transmitted through them. The first is a complex moving target of wide visual angle; the second is a stationary target of restricted visual angle. The first produces a great variety of sensory end-results in association with which is some brightness enhancement. The second produces a much more limited variety of results, of which brightness enhancement is salient.

In dealing with brightness enhancement, the rate of intermittency needed to produce it is one of the main quantitative determinations dealt with. It turns out

[1] From the Department of Psychology, Michigan State University, East Lansing, Mich., USA.

[2] The work was done under Resarch Grant NSF-G 5821 from the National Science Foundation

that in this respect the two modes of producing brightness enhancement are quite unlike. That is, the minimal rates at which brightness enhancement just begins to occur, the ranges of enhancement rates and number of other features are quite incomparable in the two cases. This should be no surprise, since the two sets of stimulus conditions are so different. Yet despite this, the findings in the two cases are used interchangeably, and sometimes the findings under one method are used in an attempt to refute those obtained by the other. The sector-disk method was the one used long ago by BRÜCKE (1864) and the brightness increases obtained by the method have been called, in recent years, the Brücke effect. The second method, the one in which intermittent photic radiation is passed through an opal glass target to make it visible, or an electronic circuit alternately turns on and off a photic source, is the method BARTLEY and colleagues and others as well have used. The brightness increase produced in this way has been called the Bartley effect (HALSTEAD, 1941). Furthermore, the two effects, since they both involve brightness increases over that produced by steady stimulation, have been considered totally identical and have been called the Brücke-Bartley effect (GRÜSSER and CREUTZFELDT, 1957; REIDEMEISTER and GRÜSSER, 1959). In keeping with this identification, the terms Brücke effect and Bartley effect were used separately and interchangeably in the same articles. And even before the term Bartley effect appeared in the literature, BARTLEY (1939) erroneously identified his brightness enhancement with the Brücke effect. It should be recognized that in the beginning, BARTLEY simply used the term brightness enhancement for the results he obtained by the means he used. The term had not been in technical usage prior to that time as far as we know. Other workers began to call brightness enhancement the Bartley effect. Still others began to remind us that BRÜCKE had produced brightness increases a long time ago. Both they and BARTLEY have erred in identifying the two effects. Since a distinction between various ways of producing increased brightness is necessary because of the difference in relations between stimulus conditions and end-result, and since the two terms Brücke effect and Bartley effect have been introduced, they should be retained exclusively to label the effects obtained by the two methods, respectively. When this usage is not adhered to, the terms add to confusion rather than to precision and clarity.

Only the results obtained by the stationary target method should be considered usable for most purposes, especially the relating of sensory effects and the neural activities of the various parts of the optic pathway from retina to cortex. Hence it must be understood why we would ignore findings from the use of revolving disks as sources of luminous flux.

Principles and methods of studying and interpreting neurophysiological data. The second matter to be dealt with here pertains to how to compare data obtained from the retina with those obtained from points further along the optic pathway, the optic cortex, for example.

It is an old rule, that when one wishes to understand a sensory mechanism such as visual apparatus (optic pathway), the first step is to study the peripheral rather than the central portion of the mechanism so as not to assign to the central nervous system some discriminatory or selective function that is actually performed at the periphery (in the sense organ). Although this, in general, is a good rule and is used by many people, it does possess some limitations. For example, if two portions of the pathway are studied and analytical data obtained from both, there are proper and inproper inferences that can be made regarding which portion of the pathway accounts for given aspects of the ultimate sensory end-result such as brightness. In some cases, the pattern of the sense organ functions may seem to be quite well reflected in the sensory end-result and hence it would be tempting to say that the sense organ activity *accounts* for the sensory end-result. The implication would be that nothing in addition is necessary to account for it. Some workers sometimes go so far as to ignore the contribution of the central end of the pathway. At least, where they find something seemingly contradictory between the two sets of data, they use the peripheral data to invalidate the central data. This very procedure has been used in dealing with findings of the optic pathway where it is said that the pattern of retinal discharge frequency relating to stimulus intermittency accounts for brightness enhancement.

The recent occasions in which neuroretinal data have been used to "invalidate" the central data or interpretations regarding central phenomena are but a new example of the curious procedure that was common several decades ago among the workers who were primarily interested in receptor photochemistry (Hecht and colleagues). These workers did not want to consider the facts then on hand regarding neuroretinal and cortical activity. They regarded the portion of the pathway beyond the receptors themselves as simply a conductor system. Now we are several decades further along and the tendency to center on the data from the neuroretina as the definitive information and put the central data in a secondary place is simply a new example of the same pattern of interpretation made earlier by the photochemists and which has since been seen to be inappropriate.

There is a third principle that is not always properly taken into account. It has to do with the interpretation of the findings from two diverse kinds of neurophysiological recording. The one is microelectrode sampling of the activity of various kinds of individual elements and the making of deductions about how the cell masses function as units. The second is the direct recording from cell masses and describing the overall pattern of function manifested by the masses as totals. It should be obvious that both kinds of recording are needed but it also should be obvious that the microelectrode sampling method is not as direct and accurate a way of determining the overall activity pattern of cell groups as the mass recording method is. The latter method, of course, has many serious limitations, but this is not particularly the case when recording from a structure such as the optic nerve which is a longitudinal bundle of extended parallel channels, as it is when the mass is a volume of complex circuits running in various directions.

Brightness enhancement findings. In continuing our clarification, i. e., in dealing with principles two and three, we shall first consider the findings in regard to the stimulus frequencies at which brightness enhancement (the Bartley effect) is obtained. Originally Bartley (1938, 1939) obtained enhancement (using two targets somewhat separated from each other) which reached a maximum at about 8—10 per second as he reduced photic pulse frequencies from the region of CFF (critical flicker frequency). This was so plain that he was able to obtain consistent results from a 12-year old boy. Shortly following this Halstead (1941) obtained fully similar results on normals and patients with cerebral lesions. It should be noted both in BARTLEY's and in HALSTEAD's study, the two targets were well separated, HALSTEAD's being 25 degrees apart. The intensity was 22 ft. lamberts or about 7 c/ft². HALSTEAD's frequency range was 4.2 to 42 per second. The PCF (pulse-to-cycle fraction) was 0.5 and binocular viewing was used.

BARTLEY (1951) at a later date made another study in which photic pulse frequency was varied and the intensity of the targets was quite low (standard at .007 c/ft²). The 11 × 7 inch targets also covered a wide visual angle (14° 48'). For one observer, he did not obtain any brightness enhancement, for others only at frequencies much below 10 per second. Maximum enhancement for those who manifested any at all was at 3.6 cycles per second which was the lowest rate used. It is thus not known what would have been found at still lower rates. BARTLEY in this article discussed the various sorts of results that might be expected when such factors as visual angle of target, photic intensity, etc., are varied. He thus did not, by any means, claim that all conditions would produce enhancement nor that maximum enhancement would be produced only at 10 per second as it has frequently been implied in more recent literature.

Stroud, in a master's thesis (Stanford University), found maximum brightness at 2 per second falling to an asymtote at 10 per second. He studied frequencies from 2 to 20 per second with an intensity of 0.41 c/ft² using Wratten filter no. 29. The maximum did not, however, amount to enhancement. In this respect, the results were like those manifest by one of BARTLEY's subjects in the study just referred to.

In another thesis (COLGAN, 1951, University of Florida), frequency of photic stimulation was varied in the study of brightness enhancement (called in this case, the Bartley effect). SYLVANIA's glow modulator tubes (type R 1130 B) were used as photic sources. In COLGAN's case, red filter were used (612—668 mμ). The resulting intensity was about 2.2 c/ft². The results, in general, showed that brightness enhancement was obtained over a wide range of frequencies but began to materialize at about 20 per second and increased until a rate of 2 per second was reached. This was a study in which large numbers of naive subjects rather than a few trained subjects were chosen as observers. It is our experience (NELSON, BARTLEY and DeHARDT, 1960) that although such subjects do well enough to provide gross general information, they do not serve to provide the kinds of results needed in many precise investigations.

LINDSLEY, in the discussion of BARTLEY's paper in a recent symposium on vision (BARTLEY, 1958), indicated that he, LINDSLEY, had varied frequency and found enhancement peaked at 2 per second for some subjects. It occurred down to 5 per second in a study of his that was conducted "by BARTLEY's own method or very similar to his method." He also indicated that enhancement could occur from 5 per second up to 20 per second with the "predominant range being about five to eleven, and more enhancement occurring in the range from five to eight than in the range from eight to twelve." It should be kept in mind that it is not clear whether in the various reports, brightness enhancement means simply an effect greater than the Talbot effect, or greater than the effect of steady stimulation.

REIDEMEISTER and GRÜSSER (1959) also varied the stimulus frequency to determine its relation to brightness enhancement (which they unfortunately call the Brücke effect). They found the maximum enhancement at 5 per second. They also varied the PCF using not only the usual value of 0.5 but also 0.33 and 0.143. They found greater effects with 0.5 than with the others. This is opposite to the effects of Bartley (1939), Bartley, Paczewitz and Valsi (1957), and Valsi, Bartley and Bourassa (1959).

It is obvious that not only have a variety of results been reported but the means of obtaining these have been diverse. This would also include a variety of the kinds of observers and the instructions given them. This variety has particular significance in the light of the supposed necessity of a frequency rate of 8—12 for supporting Bartley's alternation of response theory. It also is relevant in considering the retinal theory of Grüsser and colleagues for explaining brightness enhancement. While no necessary special range of frequencies was stated by the retinal theory proponents, a maximum within the range from 0 to CFF was assumed and that the retinal behaviour was said to be the basis for it.

It is apparent that we do not have at our command detailed enough information concerning all of the studies to make as good an analysis as desired. It would seem better on this account to begin by stating expectations based upon certain well known facts and principles including the retinal information and the cortical information epitomized in the alternation of response theory. It is to be hoped that this will furnish a usable beginning understanding of what is happening in the optic pathway.

Some guiding principles in arranging targets for studying brightness enhancement. The first thing to be aware of is the existence of stray illumination in the eye (Bartley, 1935, Boynton, 1953) which activates not only the area of the retina covered by the image of the target but considerable areas outside. At times this forms an activating blanket over the whole retina (Bartley and Fry, 1934; Fry and Bartley, 1935). Actually it is this blanket rather than the image of a small target that may produce the electroretinogram (ERG) in some cases (Boynton and Riggs, 1951; Boynton, 1953; Fry and Bartley, 1935).

The conclusions to be drawn from the active existence of stray illumination is that when intense photic impingements are used, the scatter will be intense enough to be effective. Thus areas of the retina not intended will be activated. In using intermittent stimulation in the comparison target and steady illumination in the standard target, the retinal area supposedly at rest during the "dark" periods of the intermittency cycle will be stimulated by the stray illumination of the steady target. If then the test situation is one requiring this rest, the experiment will be biased by the stray illumination. There are ways in which this bias can be minimized if not fully eradicated. *The separating of the two targets by a considerable visual angle will help,* because the stray illumination tapers away from the retinal image and thus is at a minimum beyond a certain number of degrees of visual angle. The placement of the image of the standard target on one eye and the comparison image on the other is a way of attempting to obviate the difficulty, but in turn introduces others such as the inequality in function of the two sides of the visual apparatus (Bartley, 1952).

The various studies cited in the previous section did not all use the same amount of separation between targets, hence they would differ in the degree to which they allowed the retina to rest between pulses. According to the neurophysiological findings of BISHOP and BARTLEY in all of their relevant studies, this rest is one of the crucial factors in the degree of effectiveness in obtaining cortical response. And, of course, in producing brightness enhancement we are concerned with distinguishing the effective from the less effective conditions, because it is assumed that what produces intense cortical activity produces high brightness.

Another factor is target area. The greater the area, the greater the stray illumination for a given target intensity. Hence increasing target area should work in the same direction as putting the two targets closer together.

We have already mentioned the factor of the sensory end-result itself. The same sensory end-results are not obtained at all frequencies below CFF. When photic pulse frequency is high, flicker is low and insignificant or even absent. When frequency is reduced, the observer ultimately comes to the point of seeing not a lighted field which is fluctuating somewhat and whose average brightness can be dealt with, but seeing alternations of light and dark. VALSI, BARTLEY and BOURASSA (1959) encountered this sensory shift and the results were considered to be two very different phenomena. They believe that in plotting brightness enhancement, one is not justified in putting them on the same graph, at least not without calling attention to this distinction. When alternations go much below 10 per second, one comes to this disjunction where light and dark are now seen. BARTLEY in his original work and in his later studies halted before he came clearly to the point of producing distinct alternations of light and dark. Hence he did not carry his work down to low frequencies except in a few cases.

We do not claim it is improper to do so and thus improper to deal with the brightness of a series of flashes. It is only that these measurements must be kept separate from those in which virtually steady (average) fields are being viewed.

The neurophysiological findings in dealing with the activity of optic pathway. Before we can make sense out of diverse findings such as already mentioned we must describe the findings that have led to the statement of the alternation of response theory. This theory is an intermingling of these findings with inferences which serve to tie them together in the most plausible way we can conceive at present.

BARTLEY and BISHOP (1933a, 1933b), BISHOP (1933) and BARTLEY (1933) reported work on stimulating the stub of the optic nerve and recording responses from the optic cortex of the rabbit. From these and subsequent studies they developed an understanding of the relation of stimulus intensity, duration, spacing of pairs of stimuli, and the repetition rate of trains of stimuli to the effects recorded at or within the optic cortex.

It will be noted first, that although at times, photic stimulation was used, much of the work was done with the eye removed and thus *without retinal patterning of discharge* being involved. From this array of information the alternation of response concept was evolved.

The following facts that are relevant to our discussion were observed.

1. Midst the so-called spontaneous activity recorded on the cortex, a definite wave conformation called the *cortical response* could be recorded.

2. Equal repeated electrical stimuli to the optic nerve did not elicit equal cortical responses.

3. Successive responses seem to wax and wane in a manner suggesting some sort of rhythmicity in the inherent cortical activity.

4. By a tuning process, consisting of varying the temporal separation of trains of electrical stimuli and shifting these trains forward and backward in time until uniformly sized responses were elicited, the suspected intrinsic periodicity of the cortex was fully confirmed. By this method, either all small, all large, or all medium sized responses were elicitable.

5. This rhythm was found to approximate 5 per second in the rabbit.

6. The cortical response consisted of several components, among which was a very sizeable diphasic component, and a late monophasic longerlasting component which might be either single or repeated.

7. The temporal features of the late component when repeated appeared to be the same as the alpha waves in the same animal.

8. A further analysis between the stimulus, the wave composition of the cortical response and the intrinsic periodicity (including the alpha rhythm) was accomplished by Dusser de Barenne's strychnine technique. The conclusion from this analysis was that the spontaneous and the elicited activity were expressions of the same set of elements.

9. Bartley (1936) continued the analysis of the temporal relations of the electrical stimulation of the optic nerv eand the cortical response. For this purpose he used paired shocks, and varied their temporal separation. He found that the second of two stimuli could not evoke a response equal to that of the first unless the two stimuli were separated by one-fifth second. If the separation were made progressively less, the size of the second response declined, if the separation were made progressively more, the response declined to a minimum and then rose to a maximum at two-fifths of a second. He thus determined that the size of the cortical response is dependent upon the separation and again confirmed the five per second rhythm of individual channels of the optic pathway for accepting stimulations. In the same study, he also used photic stimulation to the eye and found that the same five per second rhythmicity prevailed.

This finding is one of the pivotal points in the understanding of the activity of the optic pathway. It shows that the rhythmicity dealt with later on in the alternation of response theory is not something growing out of the patterning of activity of the retina, but a fundamental feature of the pathway further along stream.

Such consequences of stimulation were not only produced again and again in the early studies of Bishop and Bartley in the rabbit, but were repeated in the work of Bishop and O'Leary on the cat (1938a, 1938b).

Jasper (1937), using repetitive photic stimulation in which the pulse rates varied up to 55 to 60 per second found evidence in the occipital cortex for the very same kind of activity that we have just been describing. Although he obtained cortical waves following the repetitive frequencies up to 55 or 60 per second, he did not interpret this as a driving of the cortex. This was based on the fact that he found that the amplitude of the cortical waves at 20 per second was about one-half what it was at 10 per second. Waves at 40 per second were about one-fourth as high as those obtained at 10 per second. Furthermore, as the photic train was slowly increased in frequency, at some stages the waves underwent what he termed "desynchronization". For instance, at frequencies of from 14 to 15 per second, this happened, the result including a shift in response wave amplitude so that at from 18 to 20 per second, the amplitude would rather rapidly drop to one-half the previous value. These results and interpretation not only fit in with the material we have been presenting, but very obviously contribute to the interpretation about to be given in the following section.

The integration of the neurological findings into a unitary concept. This concept not only describes the behaviour of the optic pathway as a neurological mechanism but provides for a set of expectations regarding sensory outcomes, particularly the property called brightness. This integration is called the *alternation of response theory*.

The alternation of response theory consists first in a set of statements regarding the way the optic pathway responds in relation to the quantitative (intensive, durational and distributional) features of the photic impingement. It consists, second, in what is expected in the sensory end-result as related to the recorded features of the cortical response.

The theory includes the following assertions, some of which are factual and some purely inferential:

1. There is a fixed number of parallel channels in the optic pathway. In the section of the pathway composed of the optic nerve, this idea is most clearly recognizable. Each nerve fiber there is one of these channels.

2. After a short initial facilitational period, each channel possesses a finite time during which it cannot be reactivated. This may be called a refractory period, but here refractoriness is many times longer than the refractoriness of a single nerve axon (here an optic nerve fiber). In the rabbit this period is about $^1/_5$ second. In the cat it is shorter and in the human it is about $^1/_{10}$ second.

3. Stimuli applied to the optic nerve may activate all, many, or few of the fibers and thus activate a maximal number of channels, or some fraction of that number, depending upon the strength of the impingement.

4. Brief maximal impingements activate all or nearly all the channels of the pathway *simultaneously*. The channels having been activated together, tend to recover together but recovery time may differ somewhat from channel to channel. The greatest opportunity to keep the maximal number of channels in phase with each other occurs with a stimulus repetition of the same rate as the cortical rhythmicity of the particular species or animal used.

5. To use brief maximal stimuli is to get results pretty much like those manifested by a single channel and thus the nature of a single channel may be studied in this manner.

6. To use other temporal patterns of impingement is to activate various channels in various temporal relations to each other. If one disregards the inherent rate of rhythmicity of the cortex, a motley group of sizes of response may occur to trains of impingements of equal strength. If impingement is made continuous rather than repetitive or intermittent, there will be as many channels going into action as are going into the recovery phase at any and all instants. This amounts to saying that uniform, prolonged impingements will elicit uniform overall response of the pathway.

7. This uniformity in overall response is brought about by the principle of alternation of response. For example, if a second impingement is presented before all of the channels originally activated by the first one have recovered, it will be able to activate only those channels that have recovered. The third impingement will find still other channels in the recovered or resting state and will be able to activate them. Hence depending upon impingement strength and repetitive rate in relation to the inherent periodicity of the central part of the optic pathway, one impingement will activate a certain fraction of the total number of channels, a second still other channels and a third still another group of channels. Actually the third impingement may be delivered at such a time as to activate most of the channels activated by the first impingement. This alternation of response reaches its limit when impingments become uniform and indefinitely prolonged. The first brief portion of the prolonged impingement sets a number of channels into action. If the impingement is maximal, the number activated will be maximal. If not, some lesser number will be activated. If the maximal number is activated simultaneously, no more activation can occur until some recovery has taken place. Sooner or later a uniform rotation in the activation and coming to rest of the various channels will be accomplished. This is one of the commonest examples of alternation of response.

8. Thus, no continuous impingement can be as effective per unit time as a very brief one.

9. Under many circumstances, there is a parallelism between the size of the cortical response and the sensory end-result. That is, the factors tending to produce cortical responses

of high amplitude should likewise result in high brightness. This is the fact that correlates neurophysiology and sensation.

10. Various rates of repetition of photic impingement should possess various degrees of effectiveness in producing brightness.

11. Brief photic pulses should be more effective in producing brightness enhancement than longer ones for the latter come to function as "continuous stimulation" (already mentioned) rather than as simultaneous activators of large groups of channels. Hence up to a point low PCF's (in repetitive photic stimulation) should be more effective than higher ones.

12. We should take into account the possibility that not all conditions in the optic pathway related to the emergence of the experience of brightness may be measurable as something occurring at a single point in the tissue system. To the extent that the energy ("message") arriving at the first synapse of the visual cortex is closely related to experiential outcome, the single point registration may be useful and fairly representative in the way implied by the present assertion. But to the extent that brightness is a function of the *pattern* of activity of a more widespread tissue area or volume, item (9) requires qualifications.

The present theory has nothing to do with the principles that govern the strength and other characteristics of the afferent input sent from eye to brain. It also ignores the influences from other parts of brain upon the cortical projection area for vision. These two factors are among the salient ones determining the overall output. Certainly cases could occur in which the retinal factors become critical, even though the alternation of response principles are in operation at the same time.

Conclusions regarding the various brightness enhancement studies. The alternation of response theory, including its corollaries provides a basis for attempting to make some rime and reason out of the varied results we reported in a previous section pertaining to the pulse frequencies and other conditions which produce brightness enhancement.

A full consideration of the facts and principles involved should make it apparent that under the most favorable conditions, the optimal repetition rate for the application of stimulation is in the neighborhood of 10 per second in man, the rate implied by the intrinsic rhythmicity of the optic cortex. It should be obvious that some sub-multiple of this rate such as 5 per second ought also to be a favorable rate for enhancement. Hence when it is reported in the literature that the maximum rate found was 5 per second, no surprise ought to result. Furthermore, if a rate as low as 2 per second is reported, here again it ought not to be surprising, for 2 is also a sub-multiple of 10, and furthermore, the slower the rate, the nearer one comes to using what could be called isolated single stimuli, which, in general, produce vigorous responses.

The alternation of response theory is a core framework by which to relate the many complex and diverse phenomena that are constantly being reported. One cannot ignore the central portion of the pathway by preclusive statements regarding what the periphery (retina) does. We must either retain the present alternation of response theory, or obtain something else to take its place. It would seem that with the many facts for which it forms a kind of integration, it is useful as a means of understanding what is going on in the visual apparatus. It seems fortunate that experimental conditions could have been found to lay bare enough of the hidden activities of the optic pathway to enable the formation of any worthwhile theory of function whatsoever.

If an experimenter is unaware of the nature of the optic pathway activity epitomized in the alternation of response theory, or disregards it and uses a random combination of conditions in an experiment, almost any outcome that has been clearly obtained by BARTLEY and colleagues, can be matched with some other sort of one seeming to contradict it. One of the most likely factors in masking or bringing out seeming contractions is the use of weak stimulation, or the use of photic ranges in which the experimenter is either innocent of or ignores the role of entoptic stray radiation (stray "light"). It should be noted that using less than maximal strengths of stimulation provides for only *some*, *not all* the channels in the pathway to be used and to be stimulated simultaneously (i. e., synchronized). In this event, the nature of single channels is thus not disclosed (unmasked) and many of the positive aspects of statements in the alternation of response theory are *not tested*, but are taken to be *contradicted* by the findings. Indeed, it is only when proper conditions are set up to test the theory, that *any* statements regarding its validity or falsity should be made. The statements in the theory are clear enough to be tested, if they are examined carefully and sympathetically. A number of the statements in the literature which seem to conflict with the theory show that experiments were not properly designed to test it. To take each of these cases individually and find out what was or was not done in accord with the proper testing procedures, would be a wild-goose chase rather than a fruitful scientific procedure. Let those who claim to be interested in this area seek to find out what is necessary for the testing procedure.

The complementary roles of microelectrode and mass recording studies. Using the third principle to which attention was called in the beginning of the paper, certain conclusions in regard to necessary differences in the interpretation of microelectrode findings from mass recording should be called to attention.

There are times when, not having any more direct evidence, samplings by microelectrodes serve as a basis for inferring what tissue masses or systems will do. But this is by statistical inference rather than by direct observation. There are other times when direct recordings are available. The latter has been the case in all of the neurophysiological findings used by BARTLEY to construct his interpretations. In this way, for example, he and BISHOP have found that it requires a much feebler impingement ("stimulus") to evoke overall on responses in optic nerve discharges than to evoke a material off response (BARTLEY and BISHOP, 1942). This does not seem to be the type of impression gained by microelectrode sampling of types of response in individual units. Explanatory dependence upon the statistical or micro-sampling procedure and the overall direct recording procedure sometimes may lead to opposite conclusions. This distinction would sometimes be crucial as is true in the following case.

The example has to do with understanding the relation of PCF to the production of CFF, i. e., the relation of PCF to just producing steady sensation. It has long been generally believed that only one PFC will just provide this for a given intensity and a given CFF. The argument is that for an intermittency cycle of a given length, a certain fraction of it has to be occupied by the photic pulse. If one lengthens the pulse, one has provided more than enough energy to just eliminate flicker. Hence only one PCF will be just right. This idea has been proved to be erroneous despite its general acceptance. BARTLEY provided direct evidence (1936, 1937, 1939) which has since been corroborated to show without doubt that several PCF's can be equivalent in this respect (BARTLEY and NELSON,

1960a, 1960b). The explanation lies in using the off response as a signal for flicker under some conditions. Were we to believe that the very same stimulus conditions evoke off responses that evoke on responses in all cases, the explanation that proved effective could not have been suggested in the first place. The fact that short, and weak stimuli do not evoke a material off discharge in the optic nerve whereas longer stimuli do, as evidenced by overall recording of the optic nerve discharge (BARTLEY and BISHOP, 1942) was used in the explanation. It appears that the kinds of evidence provided by microelectrode recording of single elements leaves the matter in doubt as to whether both the off and on discharge occur in material amounts under the distinguishing conditions in question. Here is a single example of the third principle stated earlier.

On the other hand, we should expect the use of information from microelectrode recording to embark us on a new phase in the understanding of the finer details of neurophysiological function. This will be true if we do not overlook the conditions under which occasional direct overall information about tissue masses is needed. For example, GRÜSSER and CREUTZFELDT (1957), GRÜSSER and RABELO (1957), and JUNG (1958) report that a maximal discharge in most of the responsive neurones of the optic cortex occurs when the frequency of intermittent photic stimulation a series of brief flashes is about 10 per second in the cat. This fact along with the many other fine details of cortical function disclosed by the micro-electrode technique begins to account for the rhythmic nature of the optic path-way's selective acceptance of various temporal patterns of stimulation that we have been discussing in this paper. This cortical rhythmicity, of course, is aided under some conditions by the very fact that certain retinal elements have been shown to be selectively susceptible to various frequencies of intermittent stimula-tion (GRÜSSER and CREUTZFELDT, 1957). Cortical behaviour alone seems to be the foundational core of brightness enhancement, and the very greatest enhancement is brought about when the maximal discharge frequency of cortex and retina become synchronous.

No matter what the discharge rate in the retina happens to be, the input has to be favorably received by the cortex before sensory effects will be maximal and be ex-pressions of brightness enhancement. This is the logic for our saying all we have said regarding the notion of cortical acceptance.

Summary

The paper attempts to clear up some misunderstandings regarding the basis for brightness enhancement, sometimes called the "Brücke-Bartley Effect." The failure to adhere to three general principles is the basis for this confusion. The first of these principles pertains to distinguishing the Bartley effect from the Brücke effect. The second pertains to how to interpret peripheral and central data. The third principle pertains to the proper interpretation of microelectrode sam-pling and overall mass recording.

The paper shows that a number of investigations of various authors which seem to conflict do not actually do so. The paper concludes by suggesting that the alternation of response theory is a core foundation for the next step, namely the use of the fine detail information obtained by the microelectrode technique.

References

BARTLEY, S. H.: Action potentials of the optic cortex under the influence of strychnine. Amer. J. Physiol. 103, 203—212 (1933).
— The comparative distribution of light in the stimulus and on the retina. J. comp. Psychol. 19, 149—154 (1935).
— Temporal and spatial summation of extrinsic impulses with the intrinsic activity of the cortex. J. cell. comp. Physiol. 8, 41—62 (1936).
— The neural determination of critical flicker frequency. J. exp. Psychol. 21, 678—686 (1937).
— A central mechanism in brightness discrimination. Proc. Soc. exp. Biol. (N. Y.) 38, 535—536 (1938).
— Some factors in brightness discrimination. Psychol. Rev. 46, 337—358 (1939).
— Intermittent photic stimulation at marginal intensity levels. J. Psychol. (Princetown) 32, 217—223 (1951).
— Brightness comparisons when one eye is stimulated intermittently and the other eye steadily. J. Psychol. (Princetown) 34, 165—167 (1952).
— Some facts and concepts regarding the neurophysiology of the optic pathway. A. M. A. Arch. Ophthal. II, 60, 775—791 (1958).
— and G. H. BISHOP: The cortical response to stimulation of the optic nerve in the rabbit. Amer. J. Physiol. 103, 159—172 (1933a)
— — Factors determining the form of the electrical response from the optic cortex of the rabbit. Amer. J. Physiol. 103, 173—184 (1933b).
— — Some features of the optic nerve discharge in the rabbit and cat. J. cell. comp. Physiol. 19, 79—93 (1942).
— and G. A. FRY: An indirect method for measuring stray light within the human eye. J. Opt. Soc. Amer. 24, 342—347 (1934).
— and T. M. NELSON: Some relations between pulse-to-cycle fraction and critical flicker frequency. Percept. Mot. Skills 10, 3—8 (1960a)
— — Equivalence of various pulse-to-cycle fractions in producing critical flicker frequency. J. Opt. Soc. Amer. 50, 241—244 (1960b)
— G. PACZEWITZ and E. VALSI: Brightness enhancement and the stimulus cycle. J. Psychol. (Princetown) 43, 187—192 (1957).
BISHOP, G. H.: Cyclic changes in the excibility of the optic pathway of the rabbit. Amer. J. Physiol. 103, 213—224 (1933).
— and J. L. O'LEARY: Potential records from the optic cortex of the cat. Proc. Soc. exp. Biol. (N. Y.) 38, 532—535 (1938a).
— — Potential records from the optic cortex of the cat. J. Neurophysiol. 1, 391—404 (1938b).
BOYNTON, R. M.: Stray light and the human electroretinogram. J. Opt. Soc. Amer. 43, 442—449
— and L. A. RIGGS: Effect of area and intensity upon the human retinal response. J. exp. Psychol. 42, 217—226 (1951).
BRÜCKE, E.: Über den Nutzeffekt intermittender Netzhautreizungen. Akad. Wiss. Wien 49, 2, 128—153 (1864).
FRY, G. A., and S. H. BARTLEY: The relation of stray light in the eye to the retinal action potential. Amer. J. Physiol. 111, 335—340 (1935).
GRÜSSER, O.-J., u. O. CREUTZFELD: Eine neurophysiologische Grundlage des Brücke-Bartley-Effektes: Maxima der Impulsefrequenz retinaler und corticaler Neurone bei Flimmerlicht mittlerer Frequenzen. Pflügers Arch. ges. Physiol. 263, 668—681 (1957).
— u. C. RABELO: Die Wirkung von Flimmerreizen mit Lichtblitzen an einzelnen corticalen Neuronen. I. Internat. Congr. Neurol. Sci. Vol. III: IV. International EEG Congress, Brussels, 1957, 371—375. London: Pergamon Press 1959.
HALSTEAD, W. C.: A note on the Bartley effect in the estimation of equivalent brightness. J. exp. Psychol. 28, 524—528 (1941).
JASPER, H. H.: Reports and communications. XI. Internat. Congr. Psychol. 1937, 226.
JUNG, R.: Excitation, inhibition and coordination of cortical neurones. Exp. Cell. Res. Suppl. 5, 262—271 (1958).
LINDSLEY, D. B.: In discussion of Bartleys paper. A. M. A. Arch. Ophthal. II, 60, 775—791 (1958).

Nelson, T. M., S. H. Bartley and D. deHardt: A comparison of three sorts of observers in
    a sensory experiment. J. Psychol. (Princetown) 49, 3—11 (1960).
Reidemeister, C., u. O.-J. Grüsser: Flimmerlichtuntersuchungen an der Katzenretina I.
    Z. Biol. 111, 241—253 (1959).
— — Flimmerlichtuntersuchungen an der Katzenretina II. Z. Biol. 111, 254—270 (1959).
Valsi, E., S. H. Bartley and C. Bourassa: Further manipulation of brightness enhancement.
    J. Psychol. (Princetown) 48, 47—55 (1959).

Discussion

W. Metzger: I am happy to see that one of my first scientific attempts[1] continues by these researches on flicker stimulation in a way that I never expected. My old observations in 1926 about the phenomena of apparently increased number of series of stripes running across the field of vision of a fixated eye, suggested something like a natural period of neural processes. But I did not attach to that so much importance, because my physiological knowledge was then so poor that I did not dare to express any opinion. I think there should be a common condition for the Brücke effect and the Bartley effect. Close similarities between these two conditions are apparent. I would like to stress the point that there occurs *not only brightness enhancement under these conditions but also an increase of darkness in the intervals.* In my experiments this enhancement of darkness was much more impressive than the enhancement of brightness.

G. Svaetichin: Differences in the optimum of the Brücke- or Bartley-effect in light and dark adaptation may be explained by the different flicker fusion and slope of the receptor processes in rods and cones. The horizontal cell potentials will be cut off by higher flicker frequencies. This means that the amplitude of the recorded response is reduced to such lower values at higher flicker frequencies. In the rods the time course and the decay is much longer and this may be the reason, why Bartley gets lower frequencies in dark adapted eyes.

O.-J. Grüsser: Die von Bartley vorgeschlagene Trennung der Bezeichnung Brücke-Effekt und Bartley-Effekt ist, wenn man beide Reizarten (projiziertes Flimmerlicht und Betrachtung einer rotierenden Sektorenscheibe) streng auseinander hält, berechtigt. Diese Trennung wird jedoch in der Regel auch für die kritische Flimmerfusionsfrequenz (CFF) nicht gemacht, da doch sehr ähnliche physiologische Mechanismen unter beiden Reizbedingungen in Funktion treten. Wie bei der CFF bestehen unter beiden Reizbedingungen auch für das "brightness-enhancement" nur quantitative Unterschiede, da phänomenal unter den von Brücke beschriebenen Bedingungen Bewegungseindrücke praktisch keine Rolle spielen.

Ebbecke[2] hat schon 1920 den Brücke-Effekt als retinales Phänomen erklärt und beschrieben, daß die subjektive Helligkeitssteigerung und die Flimmerfrequenz, bei der das Helligkeitsmaximum eintritt, von verschiedenen Reizbedingungen (Beleuchtungsstärke, Adaptationsgrad, Helldunkelverhältnis) abhängt. Er hat auch beobachtet, daß im scotopischen Helligkeitsbereich kein Brücke-Effekt eintritt. Der Effekt wird von Ebbecke als Folge der Ausschaltung der retinalen Momentanadaptation durch das Flimmerlicht erklärt. Diese Deutung Ebbeckes korrespondiert mit den Ergebnissen an einzelnen retinalen und corticalen Neuronen.

Wird der N. opticus elektrisch gereizt, so findet man ebenfalls eine Abhängigkeit der Entladungsfrequenz der Neurone im visuellen Cortex und Geniculatum lat. von der Reizfrequenz. Das Entladungsfrequenzmaximum wird jedoch unter diesen Reizbedingungen zwischen 70 und etwa 300 Reizen pro sec erreicht[3].

H. Schober: Auch ich wollte darauf aufmerksam machen, daß wir in der deutschen Literatur den von Bartley beschriebenen Effekt als Ebbecke-Effekt bezeichnen, z. B. auch in

---

[1] W. Metzger: Über die Vorstufen der Verschmelzung von Figurenreihen, die vor dem ruhenden Auge vorüberziehen. Psychol. Forsch. 8, 114—221 (1926).

[2] Ebbecke, U.: Über das Sehen im Flimmerlicht. Pflügers Arch. ges. Physiol. 185, 196—221 (1920).

[3] Grüsser, O.-J., u. A. Grützner: Reaktionen einzelner Neurone des optischen Cortex der Katze nach elektrischen Reizserien des Nervus opticus. Arch. Psychiat. Nervenkr. 197, 405—432 (1958).

meinen Büchern. Der wesentliche Unterschied zwischen dem Brücke-Phänomen und dem Bartley-Ebbecke-Phänomen ist doch offensichtlich der, daß das erste sich auf einen Wechsel in zeitlicher Reihenfolge an verschiedenen Netzhautstellen (Wandern des Sektors über das Gesichtsfeld) das zweite aber immer auf die gleiche Netzhautstelle bezieht. Deshalb bestehen für beide Effekte unterschiedliche physikalische und physiologische Grundlagen.

E. BAUMGARDT: Prof. BARTLEY as well as Dr. GRÜSSER use constant intensity stimulation and varying light-dark ratios. In these conditions, a small light-dark ratio corresponds to a lower mean of photic stimulation and thus necessarily provokes decrease of the CFF and of the discharge frequency as well as increase of the latency. Neither of the authors used *constant* photic stimulation, that is to say light intensity inversely proportional to the light-dark ratio. If one does this experiment (cf. HENRI PIÉRON, 1928) one observes an increase of the CFF when decreasing the light-dark ratio and, naturally, no Brücke-effect (one would observe no Bartley-effect as well).

An analysis of both of the effects without considering the result of varying photic stimulation must entertain confusion. In fact, it is easy to understand that these effects may be observed at any frequency depending only on the experimental conditions as, for instance, field-brightness, field-diameter, retinal location etc., that they must necessarily be detectable on the retinal level and, as a consequence, on higher levels. Speculations on rhythms located in higher centers should be ruled out.

H.-L. TEUBER: BARTLEY's hypothesis is certainly testable and that makes it so useful. If it is right or wrong can be decided by experiments. And this is more than one can say for some other correlations with the physiological basis of vision.

R. JUNG: Retinale und corticale Lokalisation von Sehfunktionen sind kein Entweder-oder, sondern ein Sowohl-als-auch. Neurophysiologisch sind "brightness enhancement" oder besser elektrophysiologische Grundlagen dafür in der Retina nachweisbar, sowohl an langsamen Potentialen (SVAETICHIN, GRÜSSER) wie auch an Neuronen (GRÜSSER u. CREUTZFELDT). BARTLEYs eigene Versuche über niedere Frequenz und Verminderung der brightness enhancement bei schwacher Beleuchtungsstärke sprechen für einen retinalen Faktor photopischer Prozesse.

Alles dies schließt corticale Komponenten nicht aus, vor allem nicht bei Flimmerreizung mit kurzen Lichtblitzen, bei der das Hell-Dunkelverhältnis extrem über 1:1000 verschoben ist. Hier ist ein Optimum der Neuronenentladungen bei 10/sec und neuronale Hemmung bei höheren Frequenzen am Cortex viel deutlicher als in der Retina, entsprechend der 1955 beschriebenen Überlastungshemmung[1], obwohl die Lichtmenge der Flimmerfrequenz proportional ansteigt. Die *Lichtblitzreizung* ist eine von den Brückeschen und den Bartleyschen Versuchen verschiedene *dritte Methode*. Dennoch glaube ich nicht, daß man neurophysiologisch Brücke-, Bartley- und Jung-Baumgartner-Effekt allzu scharf trennen soll, da sie ähnliche Optima der Neuronenfrequenz zeigen. Ich denke, daß alle diese Phänomene auf ähnliche neurophysiologische Ursachen zurückgehen: *ein langsames Glied in der Kette der visuellen Erregungsprozesse*, sei es an den Receptoren oder zentral, *begünstigt die mittleren Frequenzen um 10/sec.*

S. H. BARTLEY: *Closing remarks.* It seems quite apparent from the remarks made by some of the discussants that I have failed to say what I had actually intended. I had intended to point out certain facts and principles which would clear up what seems to be a diversity of opinion. This diversity of outlook or opinion rests partly on the fact that all of us are not using the same phenomena from which to draw conclusions.

It would seem first that I am interpreted as saying or implying that the neuroretina is to be ignored. I do not mean that at all and will indicate, before I am through, how I interpret its role. Secondly, I may say that many remarks made by the discussants indicate a determination to focus on what happens in the retina to the exclusion of anything that may occur in the cortex.

Let me say now, if I have not said it before, that I believe certain kinds of experiments although significant and good in themselves are not the sort to bear upon and settle the

---

[1] JUNG, R., u. G. BAUMGARTNER: Hemmungsmechanismen und bremsende Stabilisierung an einzelnen Neuronen des optischen Cortex. Pflügers Arch. ges. Physiol. **261**, 434—456 (1955).

problem at issue, namely the *nature of central nervous function* as regards response to intermittent stimulation. No retinal information, regardless of what it is, can by itself tell us the
answer to this problem. So discussion of findings and interpretations of retinal function taken
by themselves is beside the point.

What BISHOP and I found in 1931 when we first began to stimulate the optic nerve by a
series of equal-intensity electric shocks was a random-sized series of cortical responses. These
gave us the notion of a possible cortical periodicity of a kind accounting for this randomness.
We tested our hypothesis by a tuning process and confirmed it. Much work was done following
this first confirmation to arrive at further details of relationship between stimulus and cortical
response all of which added further confirmation.

Now, to come to one of the major points. We used photic stimulation of the retina and
found that this same rhythmicity of the cortex showed up in general essentials under repeated
stimulation. This means that with either very brief electrical shocks to the stump of the optic
nerve or to very brief photic pulses to the retina, the rhythmicity is essentially the same. This
rules out the rhythmicity being due to some peculiarity of the way the retina organizes the
input over the optic nerve. All I am trying to describe is the nature and implications of this
rhythmicity. Once this is understood we can go to dealing with the various kinds of retinal
input as have so ably been described by GRÜSSER and others. We certainly could expect the
inherent functional properties of the neuroretina to determine what the intensity of the optic
nerve discharge will be and also what the temporal distribution of the impulses will be. Of
course, what this distribution is like makes a difference in cortical response. If a brief grouping
of many impulses (a burst) is exchanged for a more extended one, such a distribution will feed
into the cortical machinery in a different way and in accord with the principles described in the
alternation of response theory will bring about a very different result.

What seems to happen according to the information we have is that the slower frequencies
(in some cases a range of intermediate frequencies) of intermittent stimulation cause *both*
the retina *and* the cortex to produce a series of bursts and form the neural basis for brightness
enhancement. One more point, the recording from single neurons by the microelectrode techniques tells us what individual neurons are doing, not how their activity is grouped and
what the transmission across synapses and along chains of neurons is like, so that when we
find that single neurons fire at high frequencies we are not thereby able to deny the existence
of slow rhythms. By saying this, I hope I have now made my position clear.

Absolute Schwelle und Differentialschwellen*

Von

E. BAUMGARDT

Mit 1 Abbildung

Einleitung. Die Verfeinerung der elektrophysiologischen Methoden ist nun so
weit vorgeschritten, daß man den Eindruck gewinnen könnte, die Psychophysik
sei eine notwendig im Verschwinden begriffene Form der sinnesphysiologischen
Forschung. Gewiß, wenn z. B. am Primaten alle zur Zeit vorliegenden Probleme
elektrophysiologisch lösbar wären, dann könnte dieser Eindruck gerechtfertigt
erscheinen. Wir sind aber von diesem Stand der Dinge noch weit entfernt und
nur in relativ so einfach organisierten Augen wie diejenigen von LIMULUS, beginnt
die Elektrophysiologie uns klare Aussagen darüber zu liefern, welche Folgen z. B.
die Absorption eines Lichtquantes in einem Rhabdomer zeitigt, und wieviel solcher
Absorptionen nötig sind, nur einen Impuls zu erzeugen.

---

* Laboratoire de Physiologie Générale, Université de Paris; Groupe de Recherches de
Physiologie des Sensations.

Sind es aber nicht gerade diese ganz peripheren Vorgänge, deren Kenntnis unentbehrlich ist, um das höchst komplizierte Zusammenwirken der zwischen Empfängern und Cortex eingeschalteten Neurone zu begreifen? Auf diesem Gebiet kann die Psychophysik mit Hilfe von Schwellenmessungen wertvolle Dienste leisten, unter der Voraussetzung, daß sie der diskreten Natur der Lichtenergie (Quanten) und Empfänger bzw. der Empfängergruppen Rechnung trägt. Die derart gewonnenen Erkenntnisse und begründeten Hypothesen können häufig im Tierversuch elektrophysiologisch kontrolliert werden. Wenn mein Beitrag zu diesem Kolloquium dazu dienen sollte, zu diesem oder jenem Kontrollversuch auf elektrophysiologischem Gebiet anzuregen, dann hätte er sein Ziel erreicht.

Die Schwelle ist ein Maß des Adaptationszustandes. Die Adaptation ihrerseits ist durch die Konzentration an lichtempfindlichen Pigmenten und durch das „Funktionspattern" retinaler und extraretinaler Neurone bestimmt. Das Funktionspattern ist zeitlichen und räumlichen Begrenzungen unterworfen. So kann z. B. an der absoluten Schwelle die Schwellenenergie im Laufe von bis zu 100 msec zugeführt werden und sich auf ein Gebiet von bis zu 1° Sehwinkeldurchmesser erstrecken. Dahingegen ist bei Lichtadaptation (Tagessehen) ein Ansteigen der Differentialschwelle zu beobachten, sobald die Schwellenenergie im Verlauf von mehr als etwa 30 msec zugeführt wird (11 A) und sobald der Winkeldurchmesser des zusätzlich gereizten Gebietes wenige Winkelminuten übersteigt.

Wir benutzen den Begriff *Schwellenenergie* anstelle von Schwellenleistung (Intensität). An der absoluten Energieschwelle z. B. nützt die Retina die sie erreichenden Lichtquanten am besten aus. Hingegen ist die absolute Intensitätsschwelle dann erreicht, wenn der Energiefluß per Flächen- und Zeiteinheit den geringsten Wert annimmt. In ersterem Fall erreicht das gesamte Sehsystem seinen höchsten Wirkungsgrad, wohingegen in letzterem Fall der Wirkungsgrad äußerst schlecht ist. Wenn also in der Praxis die Benutzung langer Reizdauern und großer Testdurchmesser von Nutzen sein kann, so kann einzig die Energieschwelle die theoretischen Unterlagen liefern, deren wir zur Kenntnis der retinalen Mechanismen bedürfen, denn sie allein charakterisiert jene im mathematischen Sinn diskreten Vorgänge, welche in der Retina zur Auslösung von Potentialen und in den höheren Zentren zur Sinneswahrnehmung führen.

Die absolute Schwelle: *Tatsachen.* HECHT, SHLAER und PIRENNE (11) zeigten, daß die Absorption eines Lichtquantes durch ein Stäbchen letzteres aktiviert und daß eine geringe Zahl solcher Aktivierungen zur Schwellenempfindung führen kann. Die hohe theoretische Bedeutung dieses Versuches gerechtfertigte in meinen Augen seine Wiederholung unter folgenden Bedingungen: 1 Std Dunkeladaptation, kurzdauernde quasi monochromatische Reize kleiner Winkeldurchmessers, 20° extrafoveal. Das Ergebnis, durch 4 erprobte und mittels einer großen Anzahl von Blindreizungen (Fallen) dauernd kontrollierte Beobachter erhärtet, unterscheidet sich im wesentlichen nur durch eine größere Homogenität von dem HECHTs et al.: Die Absorption von 7 Quanten kann eine Schwellenwahrnehmung auslösen (5).

Wie kurz muß ein solcher Schwellenreiz sein, und welchen Winkeldurchmesser darf er erreichen, damit seine Ausnützung optimal wird, d. h. damit die an der Hornhaut gemessene Lichtquantzahl zum Minimum wird?

Betreffs der Summation in der Zeit herrscht augenblicklich noch keine völlige Übereinstimmung darüber, ob sie vom Reizdurchmesser unabhängig ist oder nicht. Graham und Margaria (*10*) fanden eine komplizierte Abhängigkeit, derart, daß mit großen Reizen die zeitliche Summationsgrenze sehr klein ist, mit kleinen Reizen dagegen 100 msec erreicht. Die theoretische Bedeutung dieses Resultats ist beträchtlich, denn man könnte versucht sein, anzunehmen, daß verschiedene Neurone mit verschiedenen Zeitkonstanten am Werk sind, je nachdem man kleinere oder größere Retinabereiche reizt. Nun ist aber bekannt, daß Licht- und Radartechniker allgemein erfolgreich mit 100 msec totaler Summationszeit rechnen, ohne auf den Reizdurchmesser zu achten. Barlow (*2*) fand diese selbe Summationszeit für Reize von 0,011 (Grad)^2 und 27,6 (Grad)^2.

Noch einmal glaubte ich ein grundlegendes Experiment wiederholen zu sollen. Mit Fräulein Beverly Hillmann führten wir (*6*) an 4 Beobachtern eine eingehende Untersuchung in quasimonochromatischem blaugrünen und roten Licht aus, und zwar von 3′ bis zu 8° Testdurchmesser, bei extrafovealer Reizung (15° und 20°). In der Tat ist die zeitliche Summation von der Testgröße völlig unabhängig. In der Veröffentlichung, die in J. opt. Soc. Amer. erscheinen wird, werden die Versuchsbedingungen der amerikanischen Autoren analysiert, um zu zeigen, wie sie durch Anwendung weißen Lichtes und nicht neutraler Filter ihre sehr komplizierten Ergebnisse erhalten konnten.

Ich fasse zusammen: Für periphärische Schwellenreize von höchstens 100 msec Dauer ist die Reizmenge allein bestimmend, unabhängig von der Reizgröße, d. h. Blochs Gesetz (gewöhnlich in Anlehnung an die Photochemie Bunsen-Roscoes Gesetzt genannt) trifft zu.

Das entsprechende Gesetz der räumlichen Summation ist Riccos Gesetz. Im peripherischen Sehen, zwischen 12° und 20° extrafoveal, wo seine Prüfung sorgfältig vorgenommen wurde (*3*), gilt es bis zu etwa 1° Winkeldurchmesser.

Die Histologie der Primatenretina zeigt, daß ein solcher Reiz etwa 10000 Stäbchen und einige hundert Zapfen erreicht. Andererseits fand Polyak (*13*) in dieser Retinazone viele Riesenganglionzellen, deren Verästelungen etwa 70′ Durchmesser aufweisen. Man darf also annehmen, daß 7 Quanten im Bereich einer solchen Riesenganglionzelle absorbiert werden müssen, um die Sehschwelle zu erreichen.

Gehen wir nun zu längeren Reizdauern und zu größeren Testdurchmessern über. An der absoluten Schwelle sind die beobachteten Summationsgesetze inverse Quadratwurzelgesetze. Pipers Gesetz besagt, daß die Intensitätsschwelle der Wurzel aus der gereizten Retinafläche — Piérons Gesetz, daß sie der Wurzel aus der Reizdauer umgekehrt proportional ist. Jedoch gelten diese Gesetze niemals gleichzeitig: Damit Piérons Gesetz zutrifft, muß der langdauernde Reiz geringe Ausdehnung (< 1°) haben, und Pipers Gesetz trifft nur dann streng zu, wenn die Reizdauer kurz genug, d. h. ≦ 100 msec ist. Für sehr lange Dauer (etwa 5 sec) und für sehr große Testdurchmesser (etwa 40°) wird die Schwelle konstant. Es existiert z. Z. keine befriedigende Erklärung für diese Tatsachen. Bouman et van der Velden zeigten, daß für gleichzeitig langdauernde und ausgedehnte Reize das quadratische Gesetz in ein kubisches und schließlich sogar in ein Gesetz der vierten Potenz übergeht. Diese Begrenzung gleichzeitig räumlicher und zeitlicher Summation läßt daran denken, daß mehrere lokale, also dekrementielle

Potentiale um so schwerer zu einem Impuls führen, je weiter voneinander in Raum und Zeit entfernt sie entstehen. Dies ist ein wichtiger Punkt.

Riccos und Blochs Gesetze werden verständlich, wenn man die Existenz quasi unabhängiger Empfängereinheiten postuliert, deren räumliche Ausdehnung und deren Zeitkonstante die oberen Grenzen der Gültigkeit dieser Gesetze bestimmen. Diese Einheiten sind in der Peripherie mit dem System der Riesenganglionzelle zu identifizieren, ausgenommen in rotem Licht, wo sehr viel kleinere Ganglionzellen die Einheit bestimmen; die Summationsgrenze erreicht hier etwa 6′.

Wie erklärt sich nun der Übergang von Blochs und Riccos zu Piérons und Pipers Gesetzen?

Theorien

Zur Erklärung der inversen Quadratwurzelgesetze der räumlichen und zeitlichen Summation liegen z. Z. zwei Hypothesen vor. Die eine ist auf der Koincidenz zweier Quantenabsorptionen begründet, die andere besagt, daß ein Signal nur dann wahrgenommen werden kann, wenn die durch es erzeugten Nervenimpulse die im Opticus bestehende Spontantätigkeit eindeutig überschreiten.

VAN DER VELDEN (16) nimmt an, daß die Absorption zweier Quanten in einer quasi unabhängigen Einheit zur Schwellenempfindung führt, wenn diese Absorptionen innerhalb der Totalsummationszeit stattfinden. Mittels statistischer Überlegungen, die er auf Quantenabsorptionen – die ja Zufallsereignisse sind – anwendet, sagt er die Gültigkeit der inversen Quadratwurzelgesetze voraus. Nun besteht aber nicht mehr der geringste Zweifel daran, daß stets mehr als zwei Quantenabsorptionen zu einer Schwellenempfindung benötigt werden. Die klassische 2 Quanten-Hypothese muß also aufgegeben werden.

Nach BAUMGARDT (4) genügt eine leichte Abänderung der 2 Quanten-Hypotese, um alle beobachteten Gesetze sowie die Tatsache, daß mehr als 2 Quanten-Absorptionen zu einer Schwellenempfindung nötig sind, zu erklären. Wenn man ansetzt, daß nicht nur eine, sondern mehrere Doppelabsorptionen notwendig sind, dann ergeben sich mit sehr großer Annäherung die beobachteten Summationsgesetze. Es genügt dabei, als erste Doppelabsorption die erste und die zweite, als zweite Doppelabsorption die zweite und die dritte, als dritte Doppelabsorption die dritte und die vierte Quantenabsorption usw. zu betrachten. Diese Hypothese steht mit keiner bekannten Tatsache in Widerspruch.

BARLOWs allgemeine Schwellentheorie. BARLOWs (1) Störpegelhypothese beruht auf dem Postulat, daß die absolute Schwelle in Wirklichkeit eine Differenzialschwelle sei. BARLOW hatte gezeigt, daß im Opticus der Katze auch bei Dunkeladaptation spontane Impulse auftreten. Andererseits beobachtet man in Dunkeladaptation das bekannte Eigengrau. BARLOW postuliert, daß dies Eigengrau durch die spontane Opticustätigkeit erzeugt wird und definiert ein „Eigenlicht", welches eben derjenigen Opticustätigkeit entspricht, welche von einem Reizlicht von X Quanten/sec (Grad)^2 ausgelöst werden würde. Sei I die Intensität (in Quanten) des Adaptationsfeldes, ΔI die Differentialschwelle, A die gereizte Retinafläche und T die Reizdauer, dann errechnet er $I = K \cdot A^{-1/2} \cdot T^{-1/2} (I + X)^{1/2}$, wobei K eine Konstante ist. Der Faktor $(I + X)^{1/2}$ ist der durchschnittlichen Variabilität von $I + X$ proportional; dies ergibt sich zwingend aus der Tatsache, daß Quantenabsorptionen ein Zufallsereignis darstellen.

Um seine Hypothese zu prüfen, hat BARLOW Differentialschwellen von skotopischen Adaptationszuständen bis zu ausgesprochen photopischen Intensitäten
gemessen. Dabei zeigte sich (2), daß seine Formel den Tatsachen nicht entspricht,
denn $I = K' (I + X)^{1/2}$ nur, wenn A und T gleichzeitig klein und $I = K'' A^{-1/2}$
oder $K'' T^{-1/2}$ nur, wenn A bzw. T groß.

Das bedeutet, daß andere Mechanismen notwendig mitspielen müssen, und
einer unter ihnen ist sicher die von ihm bei der Katze beobachtete "lateral inhibition". Auch die zeitliche Summation läßt ja bei wachsender Intensität nach und
zwar sowohl für Stäbchen- als auch für Zapfentätigkeit.

Könnten noch andere Mechanismen die Differentialschwelle mitbestimmen?
Wenn die Störpegelhypothese zutrifft, ist das möglich, wenn nicht, sogar notwendig.

Die Gültigkeit der Störpegelhypothese kann geprüft werden. Wenn man beweisen könnte, daß ΔI abnehmen kann, selbst wenn I zunimmt, dann wäre sie
ad absurdum geführt. Eine solche Möglichkeit liegt vor, wenn I unterschwellig ist
und der Testreiz sowohl in Anwesenheit als auch in Abwesenheit des Hintergrundes der Intensität I gegeben wird. Wenn man annimmt, daß die Schwelle
erreicht wird, sobald eine genügend große Menge von Lichtquanten innerhalb
einer gegebenen Retinafläche und einer gegebenen Zeitdauer absorbiert worden ist,
dann könnten die während der Reizdauer im Reizfelde von dem unterschwelligen
Hintergrundfelde I erzeugten Quantenabsorptionen sich mit denjenigen des
Testfeldes ΔI vereinen, um die Schwelle zu erreichen. Dann würde also ΔI in
Gegenwart von I kleiner als in seiner Abwesenheit sein.

Ich habe mit zwei Beobachtern diese Messung bei 15° extrafoveal durchgeführt, und zwar mit Hintergrundfeldern von 2° und 4° Durchmesser. Diese
Felder blieben 4 sec lang sichtbar. Vor ihrem Verschwinden wurde ihnen ein Testreiz von 1° Durchmesser während 1 sec überlagert. Es ergab sich eine ganz erhebliche Senkung der Schwelle in Anwesenheit des unterschwelligen Hintergrundes.
Bei einer Versuchsperson wurden 74 positive Antworten auf 190 Darbietungen in
Abwesenheit des 2°-Hintergrundfeldes und 413 positive Antworten auf 670 Darbietungen bei seiner Anwesenheit beobachtet, d. h. eine Erhöhung von 38,7%
auf 61,6%. Bei dem zweiten Beobachter waren diese Zahlen 44 auf 150 und 177
auf 350 bzw. 29,4% und 50,6%. Mit einem Feld von 4° Durchmesser war der
Effekt, wie zu erwarten ist, geringer, denn die Intensität des ersteren betrug nur
60% derjenigen des 2°. Feldes, um unterschwellig zu bleiben. Somit konnte der
Beitrag an Quanten in diesem Fall auch nur 60% desjenigen sein, der dem 2°-Feld
entspricht, was den beobachteten Effekt verringern mußte. Immerhin wurden
selbst in diesem ungünstigeren Fall in Anwesenheit des Hintergrundfeldes noch
20% mehr positive Antworten gegeben als in seiner Abwesenheit.

Dieses Experiment sollte kontrolliert werden, da sein Ergebnis eindeutig
gegen die Störpegelhypothese entscheidet, somit von erheblicher theoretischer
Bedeutung ist. Jedoch bestehen noch andere, gewichtige Gründe, die gegen diese
Hypothese sprechen.

BARLOW wollte eine allgemeine gültige Schwellentheorie schaffen, und
da er sie auf den Begriff des Störpegels, d. h. der Zufallsschwankungen in der Zahl
der Quantenabsorptionen begründete, so mußte die Dunkellichtintensität X notwendig eingeführt werden, damit die absolute Schwelle nur als Grenzfall der

Differentialschwelle aufträte. Er betrachtet X als diejenige Aktivität, welche das Eigengrau erzeugt. Dagegen ist einzuwenden, daß letzteres kein schnell fluktuierendes Phänomen ist. Es besteht im Gegenteil aus stetig wechselnden Mustern, die zuweilen langsam pulsieren können. Wahrscheinlich ist das Eigengrau extraretinalen Ursprungs.

Rhythmische Schwellenänderungen mit einer Zeitkonstante von mehreren Minuten gehen parallel mit Eigengrauintensitätsänderungen (8), dieses spricht gegen die Hypothese schnell wechselnder Zufallsereignisse. Daß es sich um spontane Sehpurpurzersetzung handeln könne, ist wohl auszuschließen, denn dieselben Phänomene werden beim Gehörsinn beobachtet.

Entwurf einer allgemeinen Schwellentheorie. Könnte man die modifizierte 2 Quanten-Hypothese verallgemeinern, so daß sie im gesamten Adaptationsbereich Gültigkeit erhielte? Ich möchte hier nur kurz skizzieren, wie ein solcher Versuch zu unternehmen wäre und eine eingehende Behandlung bis zu einem Zeitpunkt verschieben, wo genügend Beobachtungsmaterial vorliegen wird.

Wir postulieren, daß die Zahl der Impulse, die innerhalb der totalen Summationszeit (100 msec an der Schwelle, etwa 30 msec beim Tagessehen) von einer Einzelfaser des Opticus den höheren Zentren zugeführt wird, das Niveau der Sinnesempfindung bestimmt, welche die Reizung der dieser Faser zugeordneten Retinafläche auslöst. Nun erreicht die Impulsfrequenz im Opticus der Katze etwa 500/sec. So darf man annehmen, daß eine photopische funktionelle Retinaeinheit, die in der Peripherie etwa 6′, in der Fovea wahrscheinlich etwa 1′ Durchmesser aufweist, nur ungefähr 15 verschiedene Intensitäten der Sinneswahrnehmung vermitteln kann. Diese Annahme könnte im Prinzip mittels Flickerphotometrie kontrolliert werden. Das Niveau der Sinneswahrnehmung erhöht sich, wenn man bei konstanter Reizintensität die Reizfläche vergrößert, aber diese Summation ist nur partiell, und ihr biologischer Untergrund ist nicht bekannt. Immerhin weiß man, daß die Zahl der Empfindungsstufen bei mäßig großen Testfeldern von der Größenordnung 1000 ist, wenn man sich mit Reizintensitäten von etwa 10^9 facher Schwelle begnügt.

BLACKWELLs (7) ausführliche Messungen der Differentialschwelle in Abhängigkeit von Adaptationsniveau und Testdurchmesser erlauben eine annähernde Kontrolle meines Postulats. Sie gestatten aber außerdem eine wenn auch nur sehr rohe Kontrolle des Konzeptes einer allgemeinen auf die modifizierte 2 Quanten-Hypothese begründeten Schwellentheorie.

Abb. 1 zeigt, in logarithmischem Maßstab aufgetragen, die relative Differentialschwelle $\Delta I/I$ in Abhängigkeit von der Adaptationsleuchtdichte in Millilambert. Was uns interessiert, sind retinale Leuchtdichten. Da ohne künstliche Pupille gearbeitet wurde, müssen wir nachträglich diese Korrektur durchführen, indem wir die durchschnittliche Pupillenöffnung in Abhängigkeit von der Leuchtdichte berücksichtigen. Wir drücken uns also besser in *Troland* aus, indem wir Millilamberts in Meterkerzen umrechnen und mit der jeweiligen Pupillenfläche (mm²) multiplizieren.

Die Beobachtungsdauer ist 5 sec, also praktisch unbegrenzt. Der kleinste Test hat 3,6′ Durchmesser, der größte 121′. Mit Hilfe der Tafeln III und IV der genannten Veröffentlichung kann man folgende Daten errechnen:

406   E. BAUMGARDT:

Testdurchmesser 3,6′			Testdurchmesser 121′			
Troland	0,086	12	430	0,00023	0,086	12	430
$\Delta I/I$	16,5	0,39	0,075	1,66	0,056	0,0107	0,0079
Differentialstufen	1	6	43	1	19	234	762

Sei I_s die Schwellenenergie in Troland. Bei 12 Troland ist $(I/I_s)_{3,6'} =$ 12:0,086 = 140, dagegen $(\Delta I_s/I_s)_{3,6'} : (\Delta I/I)_{3,6'} = 16,5:0,39 = 42$. Für den größten Test ergibt sich $(I/I_s)_{121'} = 52000$ und $(\Delta I_s/I_s)$: $(\Delta I/I)_{121'} = 155$.

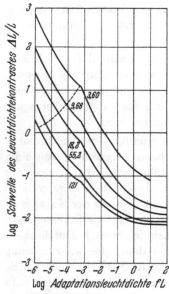

Abb. 1. Differentialschwelle in Abhängigkeit vom Adaptationszustand und vom Testdurchmesser. Gestrichelt: absolute Schwellen. Beidäugiges Sehen ohne Fixierpunkt und künstliche Pupille. Darbietungszeit 5 sec (nach BLACKWELL)

Für den kleinsten Test ist also die beobachtete Differentialschwelle 140/42 = 3,34mal, für den größten Test 52000/155 = 336mal höher als die erwartete. In beiden Fällen erklärt sich ein Faktor 1,6 durch die bei höheren Adaptationsniveau kürzere Totalsummationszeit $(II A)$. Ferner kann bei 12 Troland die räumliche Summation geringer als an der Schwelle sein. Dort ist sie total bis zu etwa 50′ Testdurchmesser, wohingegen sie es bei starker Lichtadaptation nur bis zu ungefähr 1′ ist (genaue Werte sind schwer zu bestimmen, da die diversen optischen Eigenschaften des Auges eine experimentell sehr schwierige Situation bewirken). Der räumliche Faktor kommt bei dem 3,6′ Test noch nicht ins Spiel, da bei so mäßigen Leuchtdichten die Totalsummation sich selbst bei fovealem und parafovealem Sehen noch merklich oberhalb des Tiefpunktes befindet. Bei dem 121′ Test dagegen bleibt ein Faktor übrig, der einer Totalsummation bis etwa 8′ entspricht (zwischen 121′ und 50′ Testdurchmesser ist selbst an der Schwelle die Summation nicht mehr ganz vollständig).

Bei 430 Troland bleibt für den 3,6′ Test ein weiterer Faktor von etwa 7 übrig, der durch eine Beschränkung der Totalsummation auf ein Gebiet von etwa 1,4′ Durchmesser erklärt werden kann. Für den 121′ Test bleibt ein Faktor 26,6 übrig. Dividiert man 8′ durch $\sqrt{25,6}$, so erhält man 1,55′, was wenig von 1,4′ verschieden ist.

Wenn bei 430 Troland Totalsummation für Reize bis zu 35 msec Dauer $(II A)$ und bis zu etwa 1,5′ Durchmesser (bei fovealer Betrachtung) angesetzt werden, dann sind die Blackwellschen Messungen in vollem Einklang mit unserer Annahme. Von der Dunkeladaptation ab bis zu diesem photopischen Niveau entspricht jede Differentialschwelle der Absorption von ebensoviel Lichtquanten − weniger als 10 − wie an der absoluten Schwelle selbst, innerhalb der durch zeitliche und räumliche Totalsummation definierten funktionellen retinalen Einheit.

Bei höherem Adaptationsniveau treten ständig wachsende Abweichungen auf. Dies stimmt überein mit der weithin gültigen Regel vom konstanten Quotienten $\Delta I/I$ (Gesetz von BOUGUER-WEBER). Auf die Retina und die höheren Sehzentren angewandt, ergibt seine Interpretation, daß immer höhere lokale Erregungen (durch Quantenabsorptionen verursachte dekrementielle Potentiale) nötig werden, um einen zusätzlichen Impuls in den Opticus zu senden, aber auch, daß nicht mehr jeder zusätzliche Impuls die Überwindung einer zusätzlichen Stufe der Intensität der Sinneswahrnehmung bewirkt. Nur letztere Hypothese macht es verständlich, daß das Bouguer-Webersche Gesetz erst viel später bei kleinen als bei großen Testen Gültigkeit gewinnt. In letzterem Fall ist also eine zusätzliche extraretinale Hemmung vorhanden, die durch schwierige räumliche Summation im *Geniculatum* oder in der Hirnrinde oder auch in beiden Zentren erklärt werden könnte.

Es erscheint nach vorstehendem berechtigt, Differentialschwellen und absolute Schwellen einheitlich als Ausdruck der geringstmöglichen Erhöhung der peripheren Neuronentätigkeit zu betrachten, sofern man unterhalb der Leuchtdichten bleibt, für welche $\Delta I/I$ konstant wird. Jegliche Störpegelhypothese ist überflüssig.

Mathematische Analyse der Differentialschwelle. C. JONES (*12*) hat eine mathematische Analyse der Blackwellschen Ergebnisse durchgeführt, wobei er den wichtigen Begriff der "Quantum efficiency", bereits von ROSE benutzt, strenger definierte. Ähnlich wie BARLOW und, vor ihnen beiden, ROSE (*14*) sucht er die Detektoreigenschaften des gesamten visuellen Systems zu beschreiben, das er mit einem idealen Detektor vergleicht. Dabei begnügt er sich aber mit ausgesprochen überschwelligen Adaptationsniveaus und vermeidet damit die Schwierigkeit, der BARLOW mit der Hypothese der Spontantätigkeit (Eigengrau usw.) zu begegnen trachtet.

Man kann seine Resultate wie folgt zusammenfassen. Die Funktion $\dfrac{\Delta I_i}{I}$ erreicht ein Minimum für ein und nur ein Wertepaar der Parameter A und T. Diesem Wertepaar entspricht die höchste Quanteneffizienz. Außerdem existiert für jeden beliebigen Wert I_i der Leuchtdichte I ein Wertepaar A_i und T_i derart, daß $\dfrac{\Delta I_i}{\sqrt{I_i}} = $ min. Diesem Wertepaar entspricht also ein relatives Maximum der Quanteneffizienz.

Dieses Ergebnis ist einwandfrei. Es sagt aber nichts über die Physiologie des Sehens, es sei denn, daß es sowohl mit der 2 Quanten-Hypothese als auch mit der Störpegelhypothese vereinbar ist. Letzteres nimmt nicht wunder, denn JONES schließt gerade die niedrigen skotopischen Niveaus aus, bei denen Barlows Eigengeräuschhypothese numerisch eine Rolle spielt.

Das Limulusauge als Modell. YEANDLE (*16*) hat gezeigt. daß die Absorption eines Lichtquantes in einem Rhabdomer eines Ommatidiums aus dem Facettenauge von *Limulus* ein dekrementielles Potential erzeugt und daß einige dieser Potentiale genügen, um in der excentric cell dieses Ommatidiums einen Impuls auszulösen.

Wenn wir im Primatenauge eine Ganglionzelle mit dem ihr vorgeschalteten Empfänger- und Neuronenapparat als Äquivalent eines Ommatidiums betrachten, dann entspricht Yeandles Beobachtung unserer Grundhypothese. Die Absorption eines Lichtquantes löst ein dekrementielles Potential aus; zwei solche Potentiale können einen Impuls bewirken, wenn sie nahe genug in Raum und Zeit auftreten. Hoffentlich kann YEANDLEs Versuch an Limulus und vielleicht auch einmal an anderen Organismen wiederholt werden. Seine ganz besondere Bedeutung macht das äußerst wünschenswert.

Eine kurze Bemerkung noch zum Begriff der zeitlichen Differentialschwelle. Die Unterbrechung eines Lichtreizes wird nur dann wahrgenommen, wenn sie lange genug dauert. Mehrere Forscher stellten fest, daß diese Maximaldauer äußerst kurz sein kann und unter geeigneten Bedingungen nur 0,6 ms beträgt (15). Eine elektrophysiologische Untersuchung dieses Phänomens erscheint lohnend. Messungen an der einzelnen Ganglionzelle oder einer Einzelfaser des Opticus von z. B. Katze oder Taube könnten wichtige Aufschlüsse liefern, besonders was die speziellen sinnesphysiologischen Funktionen von off — aber auch von on-Antworten betrifft.

Summary

It is emphasized that the energy threshold of vision is reached when the dark-adapted eye is exposed to a stimulus whose duration and angular size are within certain limits. It is shown that at the absolute threshold of energy about 7 light quanta are absorbed in the rods, if the angular size of the test stimulus is below 1° and its duration does not exceed 0,1 second. The latter condition is shown to be independant of the angular size of the stimulus. Spatial summation (Riccos and Pipers laws) and temporal summation (Blochs and Piérons laws) are discussed.

The inverse square root laws of summation (PIPER, PIÉRON) may be derived from two essentially different hypothesis. One of them is a noise hypothesis (BARLOW), the other one a modified 2 quanta hypothesis (BAUMGARDT). It is proved experimentally that the former one has to be ruled out.

A tentative general theory of contrast threshold is developed. It is postulated that the number of light quanta to be absorbed in order to raise the sensation level just by one step, is constant over the scotopic and part of the photopic adaptation ranges, if these quanta are absorbed within the spatial and temporal limits of validity of total summation (Riccos and Blochs law). This is in satisfactory agreement with Blackwells experimental results.

With beginning logarithmic response of visual pathway (constancy of the Weber-Fechner fraction), the efficiency of light quanta absorption decreases, as well as it does as a consequence of the bleaching of the photosensitive pigments at higher adaptation levels.

YEANDLE's findings on the *Limulus* eye prove that the absorption of one quantum in the rhabdomere of a given ommatidium evokes one graded response and that some of these latter are needed in order to fire the eccentric cell. It is probable that the vertebrate eye is functioning in a similar way; YEANDLE's experiment should be repeated — if possible — on the vertebrate retina, in order to clarify this fondamental question.

Literatur

1. BARLOW, H. B.: Retinal noise and absolute threshold. J. Opt. Soc. Amer. **46**, 634—639 (1956).
   — Increment thresholds at low intensities considered as signal noise discrimination. J. Physiol. (Lond.) **136**, 469—488 (1957).
2. — Temporal and spatial summation in human vision at different background intensities. J. Physiol. (Lond.) **141**, 337—350 (1958).
3. BAUMGARDT, E.: Les théories photochimiques classiques et quantiques de la vision et l'inhibition nerveuse en vision liminaire. Rev. opt. 28, 453—479, 661—690 (1949).
4. Sehmechanismus und Quantenstruktur des Lichtes. Naturwissenschaften **39**, 388—393 (1952).

5. — Mesure pyrométrique de seuil visuel absolu. Optica Acta 7, 305—316 (1960).
6. — and B. M. HILLMANN: Duration and size as determinants of peripheral retinal response. J. Opt. Soc. Amer. 51, 340—344 (1961).
7. BLACKWELL, H. R.: Contrast thresholds of the human eye. J. Opt. Soc. Amer. 36, 624—643 (1946).
8. BORNSCHEIN, H.: Die absolute Lichtschwelle des menschlichen Auges. Albrecht v. Graefes Arch. Ophthal. 151, 466 (1951).
9. BOUMAN, M. A., and H. A. VAN DER VELDEN: The two-quanta explanation of the dependence of the threshold values and visual acuity on the visual angle and the time of observation. J. Opt. Soc. Amer. 37, 908—919 (1947).
10. GRAHAM, C. H., and R. MARGARIA: Area and the intensity-time relation in the peripheral retina. Amer. J. Physiol. 113, 302—305 (1935).
11. HECHT, S., S. SHLAER and M. H. PIRENNE: Energy, quanta and vision. J. gen. Physiol. 25, 819—840 (1942).
11A. HERRICK, R. M.: Foveal luminance discrimination as a function of the duration of the decrement or increment in luminance. J. comp. physiol. Psychol. 49, 437—443 (1956).
12. JONES, R. C.: Quantum efficiency of human vision. J. Opt. Soc. Amer. 49, 645—653 (1959).
13. POLYAK, S. L.: The retina. Chicago: The University of Chicago press 1941.
14. ROSE, A.: The sensitivity performance of the human eye on an absolute scale. J. Opt. Soc. Amer. 38, 196—208 (1948).
15. SIMONSON, E.: Flicker between different brightness levels as determinant of the flicker fusion. J. Opt. Soc. Amer. 50, 328—331 (1960).
16. YEANDLE: Discussion to the paper of John C. Armington and George H. Crampton: Comparison of spectral sensitivity at the eye and the optic tectum of the chicken. Amer. J. Ophthal. 46, 72—87 (1958).

Diskussion

H. BARLOW: If I have understood correctly, Dr. BAUMGARDT has obtained a figure for the limit of complete temporal summation which agrees approximately with what I found, but he does not find any change with the area of the stimulus. GRAHAM and MARGARIA got different figures with large and small stimuli, but they were considerably shorter than either BAUMGARDT's or mine.

Have you any explanation of these discrepancies? The only things I can suggest are that we are investigating different retinal regions, and that the properties of the retina may vary in different zones. And I believe your figures did show a difference between large and small stimuli in the amount of summation beyond the limit of complete summation; could this have mislead GRAHAM and MARGARIA and me?

My second question is about the drop below the absolute threshold which you find when a weak background light is present. STILES and CRAWFORD also found this, and I believe they thought it might be caused by the background light enabling the eye to focus more accurately on the target. I don't myself feel that this is a very likely explanation in your case, but I wondered if you have tried a control using homatropine? In addition to this there are two other factors which ought to be considered before your finding is taken as conflicting with the idea that intrinsic noise limits the absolute threshold.

1. I assumed that the signal/noise ratio was constant at threshold [i. e. K is constant in the equation $\Delta I = K (I + X)^{1/2} A^{1/2} T^{1/2}$]. This amounts to saying that threshold are responses of constant reliability, or that the false positive rate is constant. It would not be surprising if a weak background *did* change the reliability, especially if the subject was unaware of its presence: have you measured the false positive rate, and is it the same with and without background? Unfortunately false positives occur so rarely that it is exceedingly tedious to get a reliable numerical estimate of their frequency.

2. The weak background may afford a cue to the subject indicating where the stimulus is to be expected. In may own formulation of the signal/noise hypothesis I assumed that the subject knew both the size and locality of the stimulus, so this factor would not affect the prediction. But one could test its importance experimentally, and if it is the factor responsible for lowering threshold, than the hypothesis could be modified.

Finally I would like to point out that Dr. BAUMGARDT's interpretation in terms of double hits being required for a response, and several such responses being required for threshold,

410   R. Jung:

is not necessarily in conflict with my own views. The formula quoted above represents the performance of an ideal light detector with a source of intrinsic noise like the dark current of a photo-cell. This intrinsic noise is an added assumption which accounts satisfactorily for part of the discrepancy between the human eye's performance and that of an ideal device *without* intrinsic noise. But it does not account for all of the discrepancies, and I think that Dr. BAUMGARDT's suggestion that a double hit is required to initiate a response at an early level in the visual pathway may account for others.

E. BAUMGARDT: My figure for the limit of complete temporal summation is the same you found and, at threshold, does not vary with stimulus area. This agrees with your own finding (see [2], p. 340). GRAHAM and MARGARIA using white light and so-called neutral filters whose spectral transmission factors they did not know, got aberrant figures (see [6]).

The drop below the absolute threshold in the presence of an *infraliminal* background light can hardly depend on eye focus, even for foveal stimulus projection, whereas I used 15° peripheral projection, without homatropine.

Following your own suggestions of May 58, I measured the reliability in the presence of a slightly supraliminal background field as compared with the reliability in the absence of a background field.

Using 402 "blancs" mixed with 1000 stimuli, I observed a highly significant threshold drop in the presence of a background field of somewhat more than the double of the test field area. There was only one false positive in the absence of the background field, none in its presence.

I tested also your suggestion that a weak background may afford a cue to the subject, thus facilitating the detection of the stimulus. 1250 observations in the presence of an annular red mark located around the tested area showed clearly that threshold does not vary for weak red light, and increases in the presence of more intense red marks. Thus, there seems to be no *a priory* reason to consider that my experiment is not a crucial one. But I hope that it will be repeated, for its result, if confirmed, is conclusive.

Korrelationen von Neuronentätigkeit und Sehen[1, 2]

Von

RICHARD JUNG

Mit 5 Abbildungen

Die Sinnesphysiologie des visuellen Systems entwickelte sich auf zwei getrennten Wegen und zu verschiedenen Zeiten. Die *subjektive Richtung* hat seit der Psychophysik FECHNERs und seit HELMHOLTZ' und HERINGs Entdeckungen vorwiegend im 19. Jahrhundert die Sehphänomene beschrieben, experimentell untersucht und, soweit sie meßbar waren, gemessen. Die noch heute gültigen Grundlagen der Physiologie des Sehens beruhen auf diesen psychophysiologischen Untersuchungen. Die *objektive Richtung* kam später und hat sich in den letzten 25 Jahren durch mikrophysiologische Registrierungen in der Retina wie im zentralen visuellen System als fruchtbar erwiesen.

---

[1] Abteilung für Klinische Neurophysiologie der Universität Freiburg.
[2] Herrn Prof. W. R. HESS, Zürich, dem Förderer der experimentellen Psychophysiologie, zum 80. Geburtstag gewidmet.

Der von HERING und seiner Schule vertretene und von TSCHERMAK (*120*) klar formulierte „exakte Subjektivismus" in der Sinnesphysiologie ist zwar für eine genaue Terminologie notwendig. Dennoch darf man nicht die zahlreichen objektiven Korrelate dieser subjektiven Phänomene übersehen.

Schon bei unseren ersten Mikroableitungen von lichtaktivierten B-Neuronen im Cortex der Katze (*82*) 1951/52 fielen uns die regelmäßigen Nachentladungen dieser Neurone nach Verdunkelung auf, die wir im Laborjargon „Nachbilder" nannten (*8*). Damals haben wir die Beziehung zum Sukzessivkontrast nur kurz diskutiert (*82*) und eine echte Korrelation von subjektiver und objektiver Sinnesphysiologie erschien noch verfrüht. Inzwischen haben systematische Untersuchungen von BAUMGARTNER (*10–13*), CREUTZFELDT (*22*), GRÜSSER (*37–43*) und anderen Mitarbeitern so gute Übereinstimmungen zwischen Neuronenentladungen bei der Katze und subjektiven Sehphänomenen beim Menschen ergeben, daß sich eine systematische Korrelation lohnt.

Unter Hinweis auf frühere Darstellungen (*78–80*) zeige ich in einer Tabelle einige Korrelationen subjektiver und objektiver Sinnesphysiologie und bespreche Bedeutung und Grenzen dieses Vergleichs. Ich beschränke mich zunächst auf das *Hell-Dunkel-Sehen*, da unsere eigenen Untersuchungen bei der Katze nichts über den Farbensinn aussagen können und bisher nur wenige Untersuchungen bei farbsehenden Fischen (*112–115*) und Affen (*91, 121–123*) vorliegen.

Reaktionstypen der Neurone des visuellen Cortex. Nach diffusen Lichtreizen der Retina zeigen die corticalen Neurone *5 verschiedene Reaktionstypen* (*74–81*), lichtrefraktäre (*A*) oder lichtbeeinflußte (*B, C, D, E*) entsprechend Abb. 3 (links unten). Sie haben bestimmte Beziehungen mit den von KUFFLER (*90*) und seiner Schule (*5, 70*) beschriebenen Organisationen der rezeptiven Felder und geben Hinweise auf eine spezifische Informationskonstanz.

Der *A-Typus* zeigt keine Reaktion auf diffusen Lichtreiz eines Auges. Ein Teil von diesen Neuronen kann aber durch Reizung des anderen Auges aktiviert oder gehemmt werden und die Reaktionstypen B bis E zeigen. Als „*A-Neuron*" bezeichnen wir nur solche Neurone, die keine Reaktion auf *binoculare* Lichtreizung zeigen. Die A-Neurone können sowohl durch Labyrinthreize, wie durch unspezifische Thalamusreize aktiviert oder in ihrer Entladungsfrequenz verändert werden. Einige A-Neurone reagieren auf bewegte Lichtreize (HUBEL 68, 69).

Der *B-Typus* entspricht den *on-Zentrum-Neuronen* der Retina und wird durch Licht aktiviert, durch Dunkel gehemmt. Bei Kontrastlichtreizung reagieren diese Neurone mit on- oder off-Entladungen, je nachdem die Projektion ihres rezeptiven Feldzentrums auf ein helles oder dunkles Objekt fällt (Abb. 3 rechts).

Der *C-Typus* wird sowohl durch Licht wie durch Dunkel gehemmt.

Der *D-Typus* entspricht den *off-Zentrum-Neuronen* der Retina und wird durch Licht gehemmt, durch Dunkel aktiviert. Bei Kontrastlicht werden diese Neurone bei on oder off aktiviert, wenn der Reiz einer Verdunkelung ihres Feldzentrums entspricht (Abb. 3 rechts).

Der *E-Typus* entspricht den on-off-Neuronen der Retina und wird sowohl durch Licht wie durch Dunkel aktiviert. Die Mehrzahl der E-Typen hat *off-Zentren*. Bei diesen *on-off-D* oder E_D-Neuronen hat die stärkere off-Reaktion der Dunkelaktivierung eine kürzere Latenz, die schwächere on-Reaktion der Lichtaktivierung erfolgt verspätet nach einer präexzitatorischen Lichthemmung. Eine seltene Minderzahl von E-Typen hat *on-Zentren* meistens mit großem hemmenden Umfeld *(on-off B* oder E_B) und zeigt kürzere Latenz der stärkeren Lichtaktivierung, aber meistens längere präexzitatorische Dunkelhemmung.

Die durch Licht und Dunkel beeinflußten Neurone B bis E erhalten meistens monoculare spezifische Afferenzen und werden vom anderen Auge entweder nicht beeinflußt oder leicht gehemmt (*45*). Der Reaktionstyp der Neurone wird am eindeutigsten durch simultane Reizung *beider Augen* bestimmt. Bei binoculärer Reizung sprechen wir von A-Neuronen, B-Neuronen

usw. Bei getrennter Reizung des linken und rechten Auges finden sich kompliziertere Verhältnisse mit Kombinationen der Reizantworten, die durch die Reaktionen vom ipsilateralen oder
kontralateralen Auge genauer definiert werden (80) (A-B-Neurone, A-C-Neurone, B-A-Neu-
rone usw.).

**Das reziprok-antagonistische B- und D-System und sein Informationswert für
das Hell-Dunkelsehen.** Die verschiedenen corticalen Reaktionstypen A—E nach
monocularer und binocularer Belichtung erscheinen zunächst kompliziert und
schwer verständlich. Ihre Funktion ist einfacher zu verstehen, wenn wir uns auf
das Hell-Dunkelsehen beschränken und die A-Neurone [deren Zahl in der Sehrinde
kleiner ist als früher (76, 83) angenommen und deren Funktion heterogen erscheint]
und die seltenen C-Neurone (deren Informationswert noch nicht bekannt ist)
unberücksichtigt lassen. Dann bleiben zwei *reziprok-antagonistische Neuronensysteme:* B-System (belichtungsaktivierte Neurone als *Hell-System,* brightness
system) und D-System (dunkelaktivierte Neurone als *Dunkelsystem,* darkness
system) mit den Reaktionstypen D und E.

Wie früher dargestellt (81, 83), besteht im Cortex eine reziprok-antagonistische
Funktionsbeziehung zwischen den lichtaktivierten B-Neuronen und den primär
lichtgehemmten D- und E-Neuronen mit Erregung des einen und simultaner
Hemmung des anderen Systems und etwa eine gleiche Zahl beider Gruppen, so daß
in der Sehrinde neuronale Erregung und Hemmung in relativem Gleichgewicht
bleiben. Wenn wir, wie BAUMGARTNERs Kontrastuntersuchungen (11—13) gezeigt
haben, einen konstanten *Informationswert „heller" für die B-Neurone und „dunkler"
für die D-Neurone und Mehrzahl der E-Neurone* annehmen, so wird die Funktion
dieser reziprok arbeitenden beiden Neuronengruppen im ganzen Sehsystem allgemein verständlich.

Alle hellaktivierten Neurone bezeichnen wir dann allgemein als *B-System*
(on-center-Neurone der Retina und des Geniculatum und B-Neurone des Cortex),
da sie unter allen uns bekannten Bedingungen durch Hellreize ihres rezeptiven
Feldzentrums erregt und durch Dunkelreize gehemmt werden. *Alle dunkelaktivierten Neurone* nennen wir allgemein *D-System* (off-center-Neurone von
Retina und Geniculatum, D-Neurone und Mehrzahl der E-Neurone des Cortex),
da sie durch alle Dunkelreize ihres Feldzentrums erregt werden. Bei Annahme
einer solchen Informationskonstanz der beiden reziproken B- und D-Systeme
verstehen wir die neuronale Grundlage des Hell-Dunkel-Sehens unter den verschiedensten Bedingungen diffuser und kontrastgestalteter Lichtreize: Abb. 3
zeigt die Korrelationen dieses reziproken B- und D-Systems mit der subjektiven
Hell- und Dunkel-Empfindung bei fehlendem Lichtreiz, bei Belichtung und folgen-
dem Sukzessivkontrast und beim Simultankontrast.

Dieses Postulat eines konstanten Informationswertes des B- und D-Systems
ergibt sich übereinstimmend aus den Punktlichtuntersuchungen von KUFFLER
(90) und seiner Schule (5, 70) mit ihrer Zweiteilung von on-center- und off-center-
Neuronen wie aus den Kontrastlichtuntersuchungen von BAUMGARTNER (11—13)
u. Mitarb. (15). Bei gleichzeitiger Registrierung von B- und D-Neuronen im
visuellen Cortex der Katze ist die reziprok-antagonistische Entladungsfolge
dieser Neurone bei Licht- und Dunkel-Reizen eindrucksvoll darzustellen (Abb. 1a,
b). Bei fehlenden Lichtreizen zeigen beide Neurone eine unregelmäßige Ruheentladung ähnlicher Frequenz. Eine alternierend-reziproke Ruhetätigkeit kann

aber im Schlafzustand mit abwechselnden Gruppenentladungen erkennbar werden (Abb. 1c).

Die reziproke Funktion der B- und D-Neurone und die Prävalenz des B-Systems zeigt sich noch deutlicher nach kurzen Lichtblitzen (Abb. 2) wie BAUMGARTNER (9)

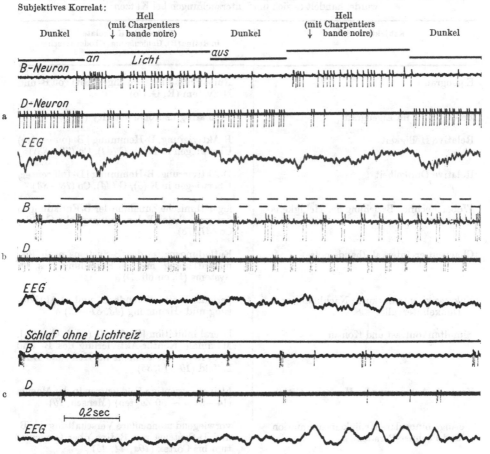

Abb. 1. *Antagonistisch-reziproke Tätigkeit von zwei Neuronen des B- und D-Systems im visuellen Cortex bei Lichtreizung (50 Lux) und im Schlaf.* Weniger als 2 mm benachbarte corticale Neurone werden durch 2 Mikroelektroden gleichzeitig registriert. (Experiment von LEHMANN und SPEHLMANN, Katze encéphale-isolé A 7/2).
a und b *Licht-Dunkel-Reizung zunehmender Frequenz.* Bei Licht-an wird das B-Neuron und bei Licht-aus das D-Neuron aktiviert. Das lichtgehemmte D-Neuron zeigt wie die E-Typen (on-off D) bei längerem Lichtreiz verspätete on-Entladungen mit reziproker Entladungspause des B-Neurons. Bei schnellerer Flickerfrequenz wird die Latenzzeit des B-Neurons verlängert, so daß es später scheinbar nach Licht-aus entlädt, doch behält es seinen reziproken Entladungstypus gegenüber dem D-Neuron bei.
c Die periodischen Gruppenentladungen im Schlaf sind zunächst annähernd reziprok verteilt und werden während der Spindelgruppe im EEG in Einzelentladungen aufgelöst

1955 nachgewiesen hat. Obwohl bei diesen weniger als $^{1}/_{1\,000}$ sec dauernden Blitzreizen die *on- und off-Reizung fast gleichzeitig eintritt,* entsteht immer *zunächst eine Aktivierung des B-Systems mit gleichzeitiger Hemmung des D-Systems* und dann erst eine späte Entladung der D-Neurone.

Auch nach Blitzreizen zeigt sich eine gute *Korrelation mit dem subjektiven Sehen* beim Menschen: Die erste B-Entladung entspricht dem primären Bild, die späte D-Entladung dem dunklen Intervall vor dem Purkinjeschen Nachbild, das

Tabelle 1. *Korrelationen von subjektiven Phänomenen des Hell-Dunkel-Sehens und neuronalen Vorgängen.* Auf der Neuronenseite ist das Substrat, in dem das Phänomen neurophysiologisch nachgewiesen ist, durch einen Buchstaben in Klammer bezeichnet: R für *Retina*, G für *Geniculatum* und Co für *Cortex*. Die entsprechenden Publikationen sind in Zahlen des Literaturverzeichnisses angegeben. Wenn keine Literaturnummern angegeben sind, handelt es sich um unveröffentlichte Arbeiten unseres Laboratoriums. Wenn keine Speciesbezeichnung verwendet wurde, handelt es sich um Untersuchungen bei Katzen

Subjektives Sehen	Neuronale Korrelate in Retina (R), Geniculatum (G) oder visuellem Cortex (Co)
Eigengrau	Ruhe-Entladung (Gleichgewicht) von B- und D-System (R, G, Co)
Bewegungen im Eigengrau	circulating neuronal activity (G) (*24*)
Relative Helligkeit	B-Aktivierung, D-Hemmung [B- (on-center) Überwiegen in R (*5*), G (*44*), Co (*78—83*)]
Relative Dunkelheit	D-Aktivierung, B-Hemmung [D- (off center) Überwiegen in R (*5*), G (*44*), Co (*78—83*)]
Weber-Fechner-Beziehung der Helligkeitszunahme	logarithmische Zunahme der B-Entladungen bei vermehrter Beleuchtungsstärke G (*121*) Co (*31, 78*)
Charpentier-Intervall (bande noire)	Entladungspause des B-Systems nach Primärentladung mit on-Entladung des D-Systems (E, on-off, D)
Sukzessivkontrast (kurze Nachbilder und Dunkelintervalle)	periodisch alternierende B- und D-Aktivierung und -Hemmung (*43, 81—83*)
Simultankontrast und Kontur	lateral inhibition [R (*90*), G (*69a*), Co (*70*)]. Maximale Kontur-Aktivierung des B- und D-Systems mit Umkehr im Hell- und Dunkelfeld (*10—13, 35*)
Zentrale Aussparung im Hermann-Gitter	kleinere rezeptive Feldzentren in der Macula (14—24 $\mu \sim$ 50 Zapfen) (Mensch, *10*)
Geringe binoculare Helligkeitssummation und Fechner-Paradox	vorwiegend monoculare Verschaltung des B- und D-Systems von Retina über Geniculatum bis Cortex (*40a, 44, 45*)
Binocularer Wettstreit	gegenseitige Hemmung monocularer Impulse [G (*44*), Co (*45*)]
Flimmerfusion	maximale neuronale CFF corticaler Neurone (*39, 78, 79*)
Brücke- und Bartley-Effekt	maximale B-Entladung bei mittlerer Flimmerfrequenz [R (*39*), Co (*39*)]
Ähnliche monoculare und binoculare CFF	vorwiegend monoculare neuronale CFF corticaler Neurone mit geringer binocularer Beeinflussung (*40a, 45*) oder Hemmung
Lokaladaptation (bis zum Eigengrau)	Angleichung der B- oder D-Entladungen bei längeren Licht- oder Dunkelreizen bis zur Ruheentladung [R (*5*), G, Co (*81, 84*)]
Subjektive Lichterscheinungen bei Weck- und Schreckreizen (Weckblitz, Schreckblitz)	unspezifische Aktivierung corticaler Neurone, vorwiegend des B-Systems (*81*)

Tabelle 1. (Fortsetzung)

Subjektives Sehen	Neuronale Korrelate in Retina (R), Geniculatum (G) oder visuellem Cortex (Co)
Aufmerksamkeitssteuerung des Sehens	Konvergenz retinaler und thalamo-reticulärer Impulse an corticalen Neuronen (2, 21, 23)
Höhere CFF bei Wachheit und Aufmerksamkeit als bei Ermüdung	Erhöhung der neuronalen CFF durch thalamo-reticulare Reize (22, 77, 81, 84)
Hell- und Dunkelempfindung bei anodischer und kathodischer galvanischer Retinareizung	umgekehrte Beeinflussung der on-off-Entladung des retinalen B- und D-Systems bei Umpolung der Retina-Polarisation (34, 36)

der Nachentladung des B-Systems korreliert ist (43) (Abb. 2a u. ähnlich 3). Die on-off-reagierenden E-Neurone zeigen eine kürzere primäre Hemmung und frühere Entladung nach 40—60 msec. Da die Mehrzahl der E-Neurone ein off-Zentrum und den Informationswert „dunkler" haben und daher zum D-System gehören (on-off-D), ist es wahrscheinlich, daß sie nach Blitzreizen *nur das erste dunkle Intervall vor dem Heringschen Nachbild bedingen* und nicht, wie GRÜSSER und GRÜTZNER

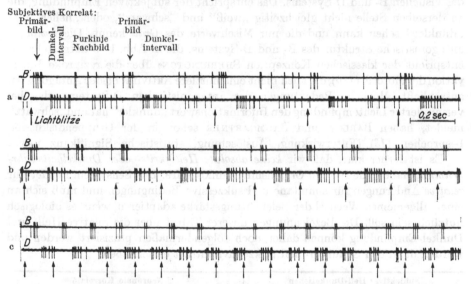

Abb. 2. *Reziprok-antagonistische Entladung von corticalen B- und D-Neuronen nach Lichtblitzen verschiedener Frequenz* (0,5 msec + 12000 Lux). Montage nach einem Experiment von BAUMGARTNER mit successiver Registrierung benachbarter Neurone durch geringe Verschiebung der gleichen Mikroelektrode in der Area 17 (Katze encéphale-isolé, M B K 41/40, 42)
Obwohl der on- und off-Reiz des weniger als 1 msec dauernden Lichtblitzes fast gleichzeitig wirkt, arbeiten die Neurone streng reziprok: Primäre B-Entladung mit gleichzeitiger reziproker D-Hemmung, dann 80 msec nach dem Reiz reziproke postinhibitorische D-Entladung mit B-Hemmung.
Bei langsamem Blitzintervall entstehen rhythmisch alternierende Nachentladungen beider Neurone, entsprechend dem subjektiven Dunkelintervall (erste D-Entladung) und dem Purkinjeschen Nachbild (sekundäre B-Entladung) (vgl. Abb. 3)

(43) diskutiert haben, das Heringsche Nachbild selbst. Allerdings ist das Heringsche Nachbild (58) noch nicht genügend geklärt, um seine neuronale Grundlage sicherzustellen. Ob es durch die seltenen E-Neurone mit on-Zentren des B-Systems (on-off-B) oder durch B_2-Neurone langer Latenz bedingt ist, muß offenbleiben.

Bei *längeren Lichtreizen* erzeugt die on-Entladung der E-Neurone mit off-Zentren, die mit der ersten Hemmungsphase der B-Neurone koinzidiert, wahrscheinlich CHARPENTIERs (*19*) «bande noire» (Abb. 1a u. 3 vgl. S. 417).

Das Helligkeitssehen und die Schwarzempfindung. HERINGs sinnesphysiologische Konzeption des Hell-Dunkel-Sehens mit eigenen Qualitäten von zwei positiven Empfindungen „*weiß*" und „*schwarz*" als Gegenfarben (*56, 59, 60*) ist erst durch neuronale Befunde objektiv begründet worden: HARTLINEs Entdeckung der off-Neurone (*48*) 1938 und KUFFLERs Nachweis der Feldorganisation der off-Zentren (*90*) 1953 haben ein eigenes Neuronensystem für die Dunkelinformation festgestellt, das wir *D-System* nennen. Daß „Schwarz" und „Dunkel" nicht einfach Fehlen einer Hellempfindung ist und eine eigene biologische Bedeutung für die Schattenreaktionen hat, wird auch für das tierische Verhalten anerkannt. Es ist also nicht nur ein subjektives Postulat für den Menschen. Die hier vertretene *Korrelation der Dunkelempfindung und Schwarzqualität mit einer Aktivierung des D-Systems der off-Zentrum-Neurone* wurde in unserer Gruppendiskussion über den Informationswert (vgl. S. 375) gestern ohne viel Widerspruch angenommen. Daß neben der D-Aktivierung auch eine *Hemmung des B-Systems der on-Zentrum-Neurone* mit Dunkelinformation gekoppelt ist, liegt an der reziproken Struktur des visuellen B- und D-Systems. Das entspricht der subjektiven Empfindung, die an derselben Stelle nicht gleichzeitig „weiß" und „schwarz", oder „heller" und „dunkler" sehen kann und die nur Mischwerte des *Grau* kennt. Die reziprok-antagonistische Struktur des B- und D-Systems, die in Abb. 1–3 dargestellt ist, entspricht der klassischen Konzeption SHERRINGTONs über die reziproke Innervation der Motorik (*110*), die auch nicht eine mittlere Aktivität beider Antagonisten ausschließt. Mögliche Bedeutungen des antagonistischen D-Systems, das bei verminderter Lichtempfindung den Informationswert „dunkler" hat und „schwarz" meldet, haben BARLOW und BAUMGARTNER schon in der Gruppendiskussion besprochen (*13*) (Filterwirkung, Auslöschung, statistische Signifikanz usw.).

Es ist ferner klar, daß wir *keine absolute Helligkeits- oder Dunkelheitswahrnehmung* haben, die für den Organismus sinnlos wäre. Das Sehsystem meldet nur *relative* Änderungen für simultane und sukzessive Bedingungen und muß sich an einen allgemeinen Wechsel der Beleuchtungsstärke adaptieren, wenn es biologisch nützlich sein soll. Die Bezeichnungen unserer Tab. 1 über die relative Hell- und Dunkel-Empfindung können daher noch folgendermaßen präzisiert werden und würden dann den Simultan- und Sukzessivkontrast einschließen:

Subjektives Hell-Dunkelsehen	Neuronale Korrelate
„*heller*": als die Umgebung (simultan), als die vorangehende Empfindung (sukzessiv)	Lokale B-Aktivierung mit reziproker Hemmung des D-Systems und lateraler Umfeldhemmung des B-Systems in Retina, Geniculatum und Cortex
„*dunkler*": als die Umgebung (simultan), als die vorangehende Empfindung (sukzessiv)	Lokale D-Aktivierung mit reziproker Hemmung des B-Systems und lateraler Umfeldhemmung des D-Systems in Retina, Geniculatum und Cortex

Das B- und D-System informiert also nur über *relative Helligkeit* und *relative Dunkelheit*, relativ für räumliche Kontraste zum Umfeld und für zeitliche

Änderung im selben Feld (entsprechend dem Simultan- und Sukzessivkontrast). Die subjektive Empfindung „grau" entsteht offenbar als Zwischenwert und entspricht einer Mischung gleichzeitiger B- und D-Aktivität mittlerer Intensität, die zu einem relativen Erregungsgleichgewicht der beiden Systeme B und D führt: Bei fehlendem Lichtreiz Ruheentladung und diffuse Spontanaktivität im Eigengrau wie in Abb. 3 links, bei längerer Belichtung durch Lokaladaptation verminderte B-Entladung, bei geformten Grauflächen eine mittlere Aktivität des B- und D-Systems im Kontrast zu helleren oder dunkleren Flächen mit B- oder D-Überwiegen.

Der periodische Ablauf der Lichtaktivierung bei den on-Elementen und B-Neuronen nach „Licht-an" mit anfänglich starker Primärentladung und folgender kurzer Hemmungsphase vor der anschließenden geringeren Dauerentladung entspricht etwa der subjektiven Helligkeit (Abb. 3): Unsere Hellempfindung hat anfangs ähnliche periodische Veränderungen, die wir allerdings beim täglichen Sehen kaum beachten: Ebbeckes *Augenblickssehen (26)*, Charpentiers *bande noire (19)*, und Herings *Lokaladaptation (59)* sind subjektive Korrelate dieser Neuronentladungen. Entsprechend dem Frequenzverlauf der B-Neurone bei zunehmender Lichtstärke mit höherfrequenten Spikes der Primärentladung und folgender Pause zeigt auch die subjektive Helligkeit eine ähnliche zeitliche Entwicklung: *Vermehrte Anfangshelligkeit, danach früheres und ausgeprägteres Charpentier-Intervall bei zunehmender Beleuchtungsstärke* [s. Fröhlich *(32)*, Fig. 43].

Das der maximalen Primärentladung folgende Abklingen der Dauerentladung der B-Neurone mit allmählich vermehrter D-Neuronaktivität entspricht der zunehmenden *Lokaladaptation*. Diese lokale Adaptation wird nur durch Augenbewegungen verhindert und führt bei konstant erhaltenem Bild zu einer allmählichen Helligkeitsverminderung in wenigen Sekunden *(24, 106)*, die zeitlich der Verminderung der B-Neuronentladung bei Dauerlicht korreliert ist.

Die von Charpentier *(19)* beschriebene *bande noire*, die Fröhlich *(32)* 1929 *Charpentiersches Intervall* nannte, ist nur bei heller Beleuchtung deutlich und erscheint bei geringeren Lichtstärken schwächer und später.

Das zeitliche Verhalten wurde sehr verschieden beschrieben. Während Charpentier *(19)* an der optischen Drehscheibe im Sonnenlicht eine sehr kurze Latenz von $1/_{60}$ sec nach der ersten Hellempfindung angibt mit einem Intervall von $1/_{30}$ sec bis zum nächsten schwächeren Dunkelband, fand Fröhlich *(32)* bei am Lichtschlitz bewegten Farbreizen und abnehmender Lichtintensität längere Latenzzeiten von 0,1—0,2 sec. C. Hess *(63)* gibt mit verschobenen Flächenreizen keine genauen Zeiten an, fand aber bei abnehmender Belichtung eine mehr als dreifache Verlängerung der Latenz.

Das neuronale Korrelat des Charpentier-Intervalls ist offenbar die erste Entladungspause der B-Neurone, die der Primärentladung nach Licht-an folgt, und die gleichzeitig mit der B-Pause eintretende *Aktivierung* der *E-Neurone* (on-off-D-Neurone des D-Systems, vgl. Abb. 1 u. 3).

Bei starkem Lichtreiz erscheint diese B-Hemmung und on-off-D-Entladung etwa 15 bis 40 msec nach Beginn der ersten B-Entladung. Da die Latenzzeiten der B-Neurone meist zwischen 18 und 60 msec wechseln, bleibt das B-System auch während dieser Zeit dominant und verhindert ein Überwiegen des D-Systems. Die hochfrequente Primärentladung und die folgende Entladungspause ist ausgeprägter bei den corticalen B-Neuronen als bei on-Neuronen der Retina und des Geniculatum. Ob diese Entladungspause durch die von Grüsser *(37, 38)* beschriebene H-Welle retinaler Receptorpotentiale ausgelöst wird, kann hier offenbleiben. Die wesentlich stärkere corticale Ausprägung der Primärentladung und Hemmungspause des

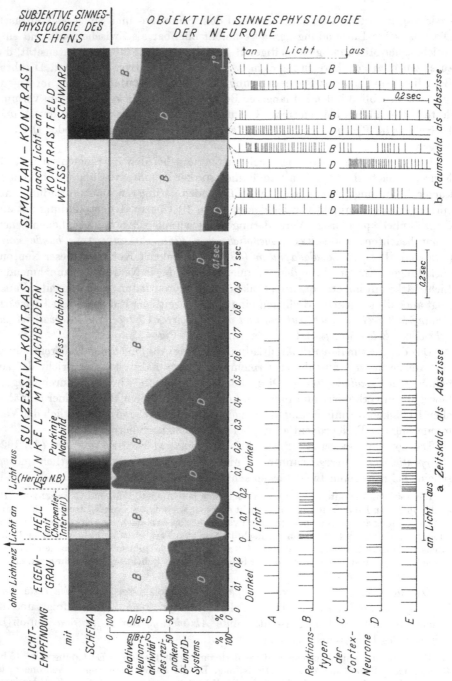

Abb. 3. *Schema der subjektiven und objektiven Phänomene des Hell-Dunkel-Sehens.* Oben die *Lichtempfindung beim Menschen*, unten die entsprechende *Neuronentätigkeit bei der Katze*. Das neuronale Korrelat wird auf *zwei reziproke Neuronensysteme B und D* mit konstantem Informationswert vereinfacht: Das *B-System gibt Hellinformation* durch die B-Neurone und die seltenen E-Neurone mit on-Zentren (on-off B). *Das D-System gibt Dunkelinformation* durch die D-Neurone und häufigen E-Neurone mit off-Zentren (on-off D). Lichtreiz 500 Lux am helladaptierten Auge.

Links sind in *zeitlicher* Reihenfolge der Abszisse dargestellt: Eigengrau, Licht- und Dunkeleffekte mit Sukzessiv-kontrast der Nachbilder. Darunter die verschiedenen Reaktionstypen der corticalen Neurone. Das *Überwiegen des*

B-Systems spricht trotz zeitlicher Korrelation mit retinalen Vorgängen für eine Mitwirkung *zentraler* Erregungs- und Hemmungsvorgänge im reziproken B- und D- System mit postinhibitorischem rebound im D-System. Ähnlich wie das subjektive Charpentier-Intervall erscheint auch die Entladungspause der B-Neurone am frühesten und deutlichsten bei starkem Lichtreiz, aber später und geringer bei schwacher Belichtung.

Zur Weber-Fechner-Relation. *Die logarithmische Beziehung von Reizstärke und Neuronenreaktion* gilt vor allem bei mittleren Beleuchtungsstärken für die B-Aktivierung und D-Hemmung. Die exakte Untersuchung wird durch Adaptationsvorgänge erschwert, so daß man die besten Ergebnisse bei Variationen der Lichtintensität um eine mittlere Beleuchtung erhält. Unveröffentlichte Untersuchungen von BAUMGARTNER und FRANGOS (*31*) ergaben folgendes: Bei einer größeren Variation der Beleuchtungsstärken von schwellennahen Lichtreizen bis zur 5. Potenz findet sich eine durchschnittlich logarithmische Beziehung im mittleren Bereich, wenn man die Neuronentladungen in der ersten halben Sekunde nach „Licht an" auszählt. Unter- und oberhalb des Bereiches der 2.—4. Potenz der Reizstärke, nahe dem Schwellenbereich und bei sehr hohen Lichtstärken, zeigt sich eine Abflachung der logarithmischen Kurve mit S-förmiger Gestalt. Ähnliche Kurven wurden von DE VALOIS an on-Neuronen des Geniculatums (*121*) und früher von KÖNIG für das Helligkeitssehen (*86*) und von HECHT (*53*) für die photochemischen Prozesse erhalten. Doch ist noch nicht erwiesen, daß dies nur eine Folge photochemischer Prozesse ist. Auch neuronale Wechselwirkungen, insbesondere die laterale Hemmung, müssen für die Intensitätsbeziehung eine Rolle spielen, wie aus BAUMGARTNERs Kontrastuntersuchungen hervorgeht (*12, 13*).

Das Eigengrau. Das bei fehlenden Lichtreizen und geschlossenen Augen sichtbare subjektive „Eigengrau" oder „Eigenlicht" entspricht neuronal offenbar einer *Ruheaktivität der B- und D-Systeme,* die sich dann in relativem Gleichgewicht befinden (Abb. 3 links). Die seit PURKINJE (*103*), 1819, oft beschriebenen entoptischen Erscheinungen schwacher Helligkeitsänderungen und Bewegungserscheinungen im Eigengrau (*3, 27*) sind offenbar Ausdruck kleiner Abweichungen der Neuronaktivität vom mittleren Gleichgewicht des B- und D-Systems. Dieses Gleichgewicht kann sowohl durch spezifische Lichtreize wie durch akustische und andere Schreckreize (Weckblitz und Schreckblitz) (*28*) verändert werden, offenbar infolge Konvergenz dieser verschiedenen Afferenzen im visuellen Cortex (vgl. S. 423, Abb. 4). *Regelmäßig gestaltete Veränderungen des Eigengraus* ohne geformte Lichtreize sieht man bei diffuser Flimmerbelichtung der geschlossenen Lider. Meist sind es konzentrisch um das foveale Zentrum bewegte Ringe, die mit der von VERZEANO und NEGISHI (*124*) registrierten vermehrten Tätigkeit ihrer Neuronenkreise nach Flimmerlicht und mit der Wechselwirkung verschiedener Sehfeldstellen korreliert werden können (vgl. d. Symposion, S. 288 u. 295).

B-Systems über das D-System (Verhältnis B/(B + D) > 0,5) entspricht der *Hellempfindung,* das *Überwiegen des D-Systems* (Verhältnis D/(B + D) > 0,5) der *Dunkelempfindung:*
Bei starker *Belichtung* eines größeren Sehfeldes folgt der Primäraktivierung des B-Systems eine kurze Hemmungsphase der B-Neurone mit reziproker Aktivierung des D-Systems (on-Entladung der E-Neurone), die der «bande noire» CHARPENTIERs entspricht. Nach „Licht-aus" mit Aktivierung des D-Systems folgt der *Sukzessivkontrast:* Die periodischen *Nachbilder* entsprechen einer wiederkehrenden *B-Entladung,* die *Dunkelintervalle* einer vermehrten *D-Entladung.* Das 1. Heringsche Nachbild ist weniger deutlich als bei sehr kurzen Blitzreizen. Das sekundäre Purkinjesche Nachbild und das tertiäre Hess'sche Nachbild erscheint etwa gleichzeitig mit der *periodischen B-Aktivierung.*
Rechts bildet die *räumliche* Anordnung des *Simultankontrastfeldes* die Abszisse in Sehwinkelgraden. Der *zeitliche Ablauf* der Erregung ist darunter senkrecht in den reziprok-antagonistischen Neuronensystemen B- und D für die verschiedene Lage des Rezeptivfeldes im Kontrastfeld bei „Licht-an" und „Licht-aus" dargestellt. Der neuronale Grenzkontrast korreliert nach BAUMGARTNER jeweils mit der Summe der Neuronentladungen in der ersten halben Sekunde nach Licht-an. Die verschiedene Intensität der B-Entladung entspricht etwa der Hellempfindung im Kontrastfeld.

Der Sukzessivkontrast. Neuronale Korrelate des Sukzessivkontrastes können für die ersten periodischen Nachbilder sowohl in der Retina wie im Cortex objektiv registriert werden (*43*) (Abb. 3). In ihrem Neuronenmechanismus unsicher bleibt nur die späte, über 10 sec anhaltende dunkle oder komplementäre Phase VI von Hess, die nach dem tertiären Hess-Nachbild auftritt, und die noch länger dauernden Nachbilder nach langer Belichtung. Diese späten Nachbilder (Blendungsbilder Purkinjes *103*) sind vielleicht photochemisch bedingt (*43, 83*). Für die kurz dauernden Nachbilder sind periodisch alternierende Entladungen der reziproken B- und D-Neurone nachgewiesen. Dies entspricht den älteren Theorien Fröhlichs (*32*) und Ebbeckes (*26, 27, 29*) über Nachbilder in reziprok geschalteten Neuronensystemen. Zwar haben sich Herings Postulate entgegengesetzt gerichteter Stoffwechselvorgänge als Grundlage der Kontrastphänomene bisher nicht beweisen lassen, doch ist Herings Vorstellung eines vorwiegend retinalen Mechanismus der Nachbilderscheinungen jetzt neuro-physiologisch gut begründet (*43*). Ein doppelter peripherer und zentraler Anteil der Nachbildphänomene ist im experimentell-sinnesphysiologischen Versuch beim Menschen mit Retina-Ischämie (*20*) wie durch Neuronenableitungen bei der Katze (*43*) nachgewiesen. Abb. 3 gibt eine schematische Darstellung der *Korrelationen zwischen Nachbildern und periodischer Entladung des B- und D-Systems*. Da unsere Neuronenbefunde von der farbenblinden Katze stammen, sind nur die Nachbilder des Hell-Dunkel-Sukzessivkontrastes berücksichtigt. Ich bespreche hier nur die *Helligkeit der Nachbilder nach kurzen Lichtreizen* (< 0,2 sec) und ihre neuronalen Grundlagen. Die konstanten Farbverhältnisse bestimmter Nachbilder (Komplementärfarbe des Purkinjeschen Nachbildes und Urbild-Farben des Heringschen und Hess'schen Nachbildes) geben *Hinweise auf ähnliche gesetzmäßige neuronale Vorgänge des Farbensehens*, über die wir bisher noch nichts wissen.

Für die *Terminologie der Nachbilder*, die in der Literatur sehr verschieden benannt werden und die je nach Dauer, Intensität und Bewegung des Lichtreizes auch verschieden sind, folgen wir der letzten ausführlichen Studie von Fröhlich (*32*) 1929. Fröhlich unterscheidet nach kurzen Lichtreizen die Nachbilder von Hering, Purkinje (sekundäres Bild) und Hess (tertiäres Bild). Purkinjes und Hess' Nachbilder sind fast immer deutlich. Herings Nachbild (*58*) dagegen ist nur nach sehr kurzen Lichtreizen und rascher Reizbewegung erkennbar und wird deshalb in unserer Darstellung vernachlässigt. Für unsere Neuronenuntersuchungen bei der Katze verwenden wir nur die periodischen Helligkeitserscheinungen, die durch dunkle Intervalle getrennt sind ohne Rücksicht auf die Farbe der Nachbilder (z. B. die relativ konstante Komplementärfarbe des Purkinjeschen Nachbildes). Das zeitliche Auftreten dieser Nachbilder wurde mit bewegten, meist farbigen Lichtreizen beim Menschen untersucht. Die Frage, welche Komplikationen der bewegte Lichtreiz bringt und wieweit noch eine Wechselwirkung von Simultan- und Sukzessivkontrast vorliegen kann, ist hier nicht zu erörtern. Hering (*59, 60*) und Fröhlich (*32*) haben dies mehrfach diskutiert, und die Momentanadaptation wird von Hering als Mechanismus der simultanen Wechselwirkung der Sehfeldstellen aufgefaßt.

Der Simultankontrast. Die subjektive Sinnesphysiologie des 19. Jahrhunderts stritt lange über den Simultankontrast und die Alternative zwischen Helmholtz' (*54*) psychologisch-zentraler Deutung als Urteilstäuschung und Machs (*93*) oder Herings (*56*) physiologisch-peripherer Erklärung als retinale Wechselwirkung. Dieser Streit ist heute neurophysiologisch zugunsten von Hering entschieden. Retinale Vorgänge sind zweifellos die primären Kontrastmechanismen durch die von Hartline (*50*) am Limulus entdeckte *laterale Hemmung* und Kufflers (*90*)

antagonistische *Feldorganisation der Retinaneurone.* Doch ist HELMHOLTZ' (*54*)
Deutung nicht nur psychologisch aufzufassen, sondern impliziert auch einen
zentralen physiologischen Vorgang. Solche zentralen Kontrastmechanismen sind
ebenfalls neuronal als Umorganisation der corticalen rezeptiven Felder mit Verkleinerung oder Formänderung der Feldzentren (*12, 70*) und psychophysiologisch als
binocularer Kontrast (*59*) nachgewiesen. Da BAUMGARTNER seine Kontrastuntersuchungen auf diesem Symposion selbst ausführlich mitgeteilt hat (*11—13*),
kann ich auf eine nochmalige Darstellung verzichten. Ich möchte nur auf die allgemeine Bedeutung der Kontrastmechanismen als Bildverschärfung in verschiedenen Ebenen des visuellen Systems hinweisen.

Die Kontrastuntersuchungen an einzelnen retinalen und corticalen Neuronen
der Katze von KUFFLER (*90*) und seiner Schule (*4, 70*), BAUMGARTNER u. a.
(*11—13*) haben die von HERING postulierten Mechanismen der Bildverschärfung durch laterale Hemmung und dadurch bedingte mediale Bahnung der
Licht- und Dunkelerregung objektiv nachweisen können. Das von TSCHERMAK (*119*)
1903 nach HERINGs Vorstellungen und subjektiven Untersuchungen entworfene
Schema der Kontrastvorgänge entspricht daher ziemlich genau dem neuronalen
Mechanismus der lateralen Hemmung synergistischer und der reziproken Hemmung
antagonistischer Neurone, wenn man eine Informationskonstanz des B- und D-
Systems annimmt (*13, 81*).

Simultankontrast ist nicht nur in retinalen (*5, 11, 15, 90*), geniculären (*69a*) und corticalen
(*12, 35, 70*) Neuronen nachgewiesen, sondern auch in den receptornahen langsamen Potentialen
erkennbar, wie MOTOKAWA auf diesem Symposion berichtet hat (*102*). Zwar bleibt die Natur
der sog. Receptorpotentiale noch ungeklärt und nach SVAETICHINs neuesten Untersuchungen
(*116*) können auch Gliaelemente daran beteiligt sein, doch ist eine Lokalisation dieser Potentiale *vor* den retinalen Ganglienzellen unbestritten (*37, 38, 114—117*). Eine präganglionäre Verschaltung reziproker Vorgänge des Hell- und Dunkelsystems mit gegenseitiger Hemmung ist
durch hyperpolarisierte Membranpotentiale mit intracellulären Ableitungen retinaler Neurone
nachgewiesen (*117*). Wie die zentrale Schaltung der Umfeldhemmung und der reziproken
Hemmung des antagonistischen B- und D-Systems und die Membranveränderung ihrerNeurone
verläuft, bleibt noch offen. Intracelluläre Ableitungen von corticalen Neuronen der Area 17
durch LI u. Mitarb. (*92*) haben die ersten Hinweise auf hyperpolarisierende synaptische Membranpotentiale der Hemmung ergeben.

Neuronal ungeklärt ist die von MOTOKAWA nach subjektiven Untersuchungen beschriebene
retinale Induktion (*98*), durch die er auch komplexe Phänomene wie die figuralen Nacheffekte
von KÖHLER und WALLACH erklärt (*100*). KÖHLERs eigener Deutungsversuch durch elektrische
Feldeffekte (*85*) ist neurophysiologisch nicht bewiesen und wenig wahrscheinlich.

Sinnesphysiologisch interessant ist vor allem BAUMGARTNERs Befund, daß die
neuronalen Feldzentren bei corticalen Neuronen einen kleineren Querdurchmesser
haben als bei retinalen und Geniculatum-Neuronen (*12*). Ob dies allein durch die
von HUBEL und WIESEL (*70*) festgestellten Formveränderungen der corticalen
rezeptiven Felder bedingt ist, kann offenbleiben. Sicher ist danach jedenfalls ein
auch zentral von der Retina wirksamer Kontrastmechanismus. Ob eine weitere
Verstärkung der lateralen Hemmung synergistischer Neurone im zentralen visuellen System diese Feldverkleinerung allein erklären kann, ist noch nicht sicher.
Doch ist damit nachgewiesen, daß ein weiterer Verschärfungsvorgang des
Sehens im corticalen System stattfindet, wie er von HERING (*60*) und TSCHERMAK
(*119*) postuliert wurde. Vereinfacht und paradox formuliert könnte man sagen,
daß die *Cortexneurone schärfer sehen als die Retina- und Geniculatumneurone.*

Die subjektive Sinnesphysiologie hat durch diese Befunde eine erneute Anregung erhalten, auch mit psychophysiologischen Methoden analog den experimentellen Ergebnissen den neuronalen Simultankontrast zu untersuchen: BAUM-
GARTNERs indirekte Bestimmung des rezeptiven Feldzentrums der fovealen Neurone beim Menschen durch die Hermannsche Gittertäuschung (*10, 12*) ist eine
solche neue Anwendung der klassischen Methoden der beobachtenden Sinnesphysiologie auf die Analyse analog erschlossener Neuronen-Mechanismen beim
Menschen. Sie zeigt wie objektive und subjektive Sinnesphysiologie sich gegenseitig
anregen und ergänzen.

Das binoculare Sehen. Die bisher möglichen Korrelationen binocularen Sehens
mit neuronalen Befunden beschränken sich auf das *Helligkeitssehen*. Die entsprechenden Befunde für den binocularen Wettstreit, die Helligkeitssummation mit dem
Fechnerschen Paradox und für das binoculare Flimmersehen habe ich an anderer
Stelle (*78, 79, 81*) besprochen. Sie sind in Tab. 1 zusammengefaßt und wurden
von GRÜSSER-CORNEHLS und GRÜSSER (*45*) auf diesem Symposion dargestellt.

Die *neuronalen Vorgänge beim binocularen Sehen* sind im visuellen Cortex bisher
nur mit diffusen Lichtreizen untersucht [GRÜSSER-CORNEHLS und GRÜSSER (*40a,
45*)]. Der biologische Zweck des Binocularsehens, die stereoskopische Entfernungs-
schätzung beim Tiefensehen wird bei solchen diffusen Reizen verfehlt und muß
noch genauer mit Punkt- und Kontrastreizen untersucht werden, über die nur
wenige Beobachtungen HUBELs und WIESELs (*70*) vorliegen. Die beiden monocularen Bilder, wie wir beim Doppelsehen durch Koordinationsstörungen der Augen
erkennen, zeigen übereinstimmend mit den Neuronenableitungen GRÜSSERs (*45*)
eine *monoculare Durchschaltung von der Retina bis zum Cortex (Area 17)*. Daher
muß die Information der Entfernung beim stereoskopischen Sehen durch Auswertung der disparaten monoculären Bilder frühestens im visuellen Cortex oder
später in höheren Koordinationszentren entstehen. *Die Tiefenwahrnehmung bildet
dann eine neue Information*, die aus den beiden *monocularen disparaten Bildern
errechnet wird*, ähnlich wie dies in der Rechenmaschinentechnik geschieht. Das
stereoskopische Sehen ist daher ein gutes Modell für kybernetische Untersuchungen
am ZNS, doch fehlen noch neuronale Befunde über disparate Gestaltbilder.

Die Rolle zeitlicher Faktoren beim räumlichen und Bewegungssehen zeigt auch das
Fertsch-Pulfrich-Phänomen. Sein neuronales Korrelat ist offenbar die *einseitige retinale Latenz-
verzögerung der Neuronentladung bei schwächeren Lichtreizen*.

Neuronale Korrelationen visueller Aufmerksamkeitsvorgänge. In früheren
Arbeiten (*2, 76, 77*) sind die Korrelationen der Aufmerksamkeitsregulierung mit
der Konvergenz spezifischer und unspezifischer Afferenzen an den Neuronen des
visuellen Cortex mehrfach diskutiert worden. Die vorwiegend bahnende Wirkung
der reticulo-thalamischen Afferenzen auf den visuellen Cortex ist auf diesem Symposion von BREMER (*16*) für die Makropotentiale und von CREUTZFELDT (*23*),
AKIMOTO (*2a*) und ihren Mitarbeitern für die Neuronenentladungen dargestellt
worden. Eine genaue sinnesphysiologische Korrelation wird erst möglich sein,
wenn die optokinetischen und vestibulären Regulationen, die ebenfalls über das
reticuläre System laufen, neuronal exakter untersucht sind. *Die Aufmerksamkeitsvorgänge und visuellen Zuwendungsbewegungen sind eng mit dem optokinetisch-
vestibulären System verbunden* und bilden, wie schon HERING (*57*) betont hat, eine
Grundlage der Raumkonstanz der Sehdinge. Die Regelung von Optokinetik und

Aufmerksamkeit durch dasselbe morphologische Substrat der F. reticularis ist daher funktionell sinnvoll und entspricht einem Parallelismus von psychischen und Verhaltensregulationen. Bei Tieren können wir Verhalten und Neuronenvorgänge untersuchen, beim Menschen sind Verhalten und innerseelische Vorgänge durch Beobachtung und Introspektion erkennbar.

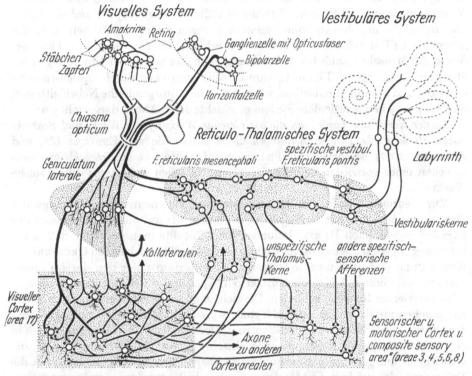

Abb. 4. *Schema der Erregungskonvergenz des vestibulären, visuellen und reticulo-thalamischen Systems im visuellen Cortex* (modifiziert nach JUNG, 1960). Die möglichen anatomischen Verbindungen sind nach den Ergebnissen von Mikroableitungen corticaler Neurone bei der Katze konstruiert. Neben den genannten 3 Systemen sind im sensomotorischen Cortex auch andere spezifisch-sensorische Afferenzen eingezeichnet, deren Einfluß auf die Sehrinde noch nicht genauer untersucht ist.

Das visuelle System sendet die durch Licht- oder Dunkelreize des Auges ausgelösten spezifisch-visuellen Impulse über das Geniculatum zur Hirnrinde, wo sie vorwiegend monocular verschaltet werden. Nur wenige Zellen erhalten binoculare Impulse.

Neben diesen spezifischen retino-genikulären Afferenzen werden die Neurone der Sehrinde durch vestibuläre und reticulothalamische Afferenzen beeinflußt. Das *unspezifische ascendierende reticulo-thalamische System,* in dem bereits eine Konvergenz verschiedener Sinnesmodalitäten stattfindet, erregt oder hemmt mit längerer Latenz die gleichen Neurone, die vom optischen System beeinflußt werden. Das *vestibuläre System* erregt von den Bogengangs- und Macularreceptoren über die Vestibulariskerne ebenfalls die Formatio reticularis der Pons und regelt in diesem spezifisch-vestibulären Teil der Reticularis die differenzierte Optomotorik und den Nystagmus. Teils über nicht berücksichtigte Bahnen spezifischer Thalamuskerne, teils über unspezifische thalamo-reticuläre Strukturen gelangen ascendierende Impulse in die corticalen vestibulären Endstellen des sensorischen und motorischen Cortex sowie in den visuellen Cortex der Area 17. Dort und zum Teil vorher im reticulo-thalamischen System konvergieren die vestibulären Impulse mit unspezifischen und spezifischen retinalen Afferenzen.

Die Kreuzungsverhältnisse sind nur für den N.opticus berücksichtigt. Die Zahl der Synapsen und Neuronenschaltungen ist schematisch-hypothetisch und soll nur ein Bildmodell für die Koordination verschiedener afferenter Erregungen im optischen Cortex geben

HUBELs Neuronenbefunde an der freien Katze (*68, 69*) und HERNÁNDEZ-PEÓNs Untersuchungen über den Einfluß von Aufmerksamkeit und Gewöhnung auf die evoked potentials (*61*) zeigen Wege für die neuronale Untersuchung des Verhaltens. Als Negativ zu diesen Befunden fand W. R. HESS (*64a*) nach Coagulationen im mesodiencephalen Hirnstamm Veränderungen des visuellen Aufmerksamkeitsverhaltens mit Nichtbeachtung von Hindernissen ohne Gesichtsfeld-störung. Die neurophysiologischen Mechanismen dieser Regulationen hat HESS (*64*) schon früher als Parallelschaltung von Blickbewegung und Aufmerksamkeit gedeutet. Ein vorläufiges Schema der Neuronenverbindungen dieser Regulationen zeigt Abb. 4 als Synopsis unserer Untersuchungen an der Katze.

Psychologisch interessant ist die *Veränderung der Flimmergrenze einzelner Neurone* (neuronale CFF) *durch thalamische (22), reticuläre (23, 77) und vestibuläre (40) Reize*, die unabhängig von Augenbewegungen eintreten. Meistens wird die neuronale CFF durch diese Reize deutlich erhöht, wie die sensorische Flimmer-fusion der Menschen auch bei Aufmerksamkeit höher ist als bei Ermüdung. Eine ähnliche Erhöhung der Flimmergrenze ist allerdings auch durch Opticusreize zu erhalten, und es muß offenbleiben, wieweit dies über unspezifische Nebenleitungen des N. opticus in das reticuläre System geschieht, die in Abb. 4 dargestellt sind.

In der Ermüdung kann man die aktivierende Wirkung von Weck- und Schreck-reizen als schwache Lichterscheinungen direkt sehen: die von EBBECKE (*28*) und AHLENSTIEL (*1*) beschriebenen Phänomene des *Weck- und Schreckblitzes* ent-sprechen einer vorwiegenden Aktivierung des fovealen B-Systems durch solche Weckreize.

Zur Neurophysiologie des Bewegungssehens. Die neuronalen Vorgänge des *Bewegungssehens* und der *Raumlokalisation* haben wir auf diesem Symposion nur kurz behandelt. Nach HUBELs Befunden (*68, 69*) sollte man erwarten, daß es ein für Bewegungsreize spezialisiertes Neuronensystem gibt. Doch haben GRÜSSER (*42*), KORNHUBER (*87*) u. Mitarb. in unserem Laboratorium unter den durch diffuses Licht unbeeinflußten A-Neuronen bisher keine spezifisch durch optische Bewegungs-reize aktivierten Neurone gefunden. Die richtungsspezifisch reagierenden Neurone entsprachen meist dem D- oder E-Typus, waren also vorwiegend durch *Dunkel-reize* zu erregende Neurone mit off-Zentrum. Doch schließt dies nicht aus, daß es in der wohl heterogenen A-Gruppe auch einzelne Zellen (Interneurone?) gibt, die vorwiegend auf gerichtete Bewegungsreize ansprechen. Wahrscheinlich sind die E-Neurone, die auf jede Lichtänderung, sei es hell oder dunkel, mit on-off-Ent-ladungen antworten und in der peripheren Retina stärker vertreten sind, enger mit dem Bewegungssehen verbunden. Weitere Untersuchungen über das Bewegungs-sehen und seine Beziehung zu Augenbewegungen und optisch-vestibulären Reaktionen sind erforderlich.

Eine theoretische Darstellung an Hand von Modellversuchen haben v. HOLST und MITTELSTAEDT in ihrem Reafferenzprinzip gegeben (*66*). v. HOLST hat dieses Prinzip dann auch für die Untersuchung der Konvergenz und Akkommodation und ihren Einfluß auf die Größenwahrnehmung der Sehdinge angewandt (*67*). Er fand, daß sowohl Akkommodation wie Konvergenz mit etwa gleichen Teilen zur Größen-schätzung beim Nahesehen beitragen. Die Rolle der Propriozeptivität der Augen-muskeln und ihrer zentralen Verwertung, ihr Bahnverlauf und ihre Koordination mit den Sehvorgängen ist neurophysiologisch noch unerforscht. Ungeklärt bleibt ferner das neurophysiologische Korrelat der „Efferenzkopie" v. HOLSTs. Vielleicht können Untersuchungen über die optisch-vestibuläre Koordination (*40, 41*) und ihre Beziehungen zu Augenbewegungen und Nystagmus (*25*) weiterführen.

Eine Beobachtung über den optokinetischen Nystagmus, die ich 1953 mit-geteilt habe (*75*), zeigt mit Abb. 5 die enge *Beziehung der Augenbewegungen zur optischen Aufmerksamkeit und Bewegungswahrnehmung:* Der optokinetische Nystagmus vermindert sich parallel mit der willkürlich steuerbaren visuellen Aufmerksamkeit. Bei verminderter Aufmerksamkeit (*5a* unaufmerksam), wenn die Augenbewegungen hinter dem bewegten Reiz zurückbleiben, entsteht gleichzeitig ein Eindruck vermehrter Drehgeschwindigkeit der bewegten Umwelt. Wir schließen daraus auf eine doppelte Regulation der subjektiven Geschwindigkeit bewegter Sehdinge sowohl durch Augenfolgebewegungen (relative Bildgeschwindigkeit auf der Retina = 0 bei perfektem optokinetischen Nystagmus) wie durch Bildverschiebungen auf der Retina (relative Bildgeschwindigkeit > 0 bei gegen die Reizbewegung zurückbleibendem Nystagmus).

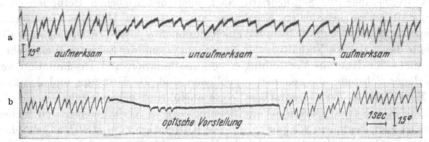

Abb. 5a u. b. *Hemmung des optokinetischen Nystagmus und Veränderung der subjektiven Bewegungsgeschwindigkeit durch Willküränderung der optischen Aufmerksamkeit nach* JUNG (*75*) (1953).
a *Visuelle Unaufmerksamkeit.* Im Beginn bei „interessiertem" Blick auf die Streifen sehr ausgeprägter optokinetischer Nystagmus, da die einzelnen Streifengrenzen foveal fixiert und verfolgt werden. Zwischen den Markierungen in der Mitte der Kurve „*desinteressierter*" *Blick* mit deutlicher *Verminderung der Amplitude und Frequenz des Nystagmus.* Bei erneutem interessiertem Hinsehen erreicht der Nystagmus wieder seine alte Intensität. *Während der verminderten optischen Aufmerksamkeit erschien die Streifengeschwindigkeit subjektiv etwa um das Doppelte schneller,* objektiv war sie unvermindert 90°/sec. Die Winkelgeschwindigkeit der langsamen Nystagmusphasen beträgt bei Unaufmerksamkeit weniger als die Hälfte des aufmerksamen Nystagmus (R. J. Nr. 378/48).
b *Visuelle Vorstellung* eines stehenden Objektes hinter dem Drehschirm. Die Hemmung ist fast ebenso stark wie bei willkürlicher Fixation eines unbewegten Sehdinges und ist mit wechselnden Änderungen der Drehempfindung der Umgebung und eigenen Person verbunden. Nur kurz dringen einige kleine Nystagmusschläge durch. (A. M. Nr. 415/48)

Diese Ergebnisse optokinetischer Reizung beim Menschen zeigen, wie die alten Versuche HERINGs (*55, 57*), MACHs (*94*) und HOFMANNs (*65*), daß die Bewegungswahrnehmung sowohl durch Augenbewegungen wie durch Bildbewegungen auf der Netzhaut gesteuert wird und daß vestibuläre Einflüsse nur sekundäre Regulationen bei Kopf- und Körperbewegungen sind (*25*). Über die neuronalen Grundlagen der optokinetischen Effekte können wir noch nicht viel aussagen. Man kann nur vermuten, daß die unterschiedliche Ausdehnung der rezeptiven Felder beim Bewegungssehen eine Rolle spielt. HUBELs interessante Befunde von bewegungsspezifischen Neuronen an der frei beweglichen Katze (*68, 69*) sind durch mangelnde Kontrolle der Augenbewegungen schwer zu interpretieren. GRÜSSERs neuere Ergebnisse über richtungsspezifische neuronale Regulationen bei Reizung mit optokinetischen Streifenmustern (*42*) zeigen, daß wir in unseren Erkenntnissen noch sehr im Anfang stehen. Weitere Untersuchungen über die Konvergenz verschiedener Sinnesmodalitäten an einzelnen Cortexneuronen, mit denen sich KORN-HUBER u. FONSECA (*87*) jetzt beschäftigen, sind daher notwendig.

Das eigentümliche Phänomen, daß nicht zu schnell bewegte Reize auch in ihrer Form deutlicher werden können, spricht für eine Koordination des Bewegungssehens mit dem Simultan- und Sukzessivkontrast, die beide eine gewisse Zeit brauchen. Die rasche Lokaladaptation des Auges, die neuronal als Verlangsamung der Impulsfrequenz bei längerer Belichtung erkennbar ist (vgl. Abb. 1 u. S. 414,

Tab. 1), erklärt, wie Augenbewegungen das Scharfsehen erhalten und durch wechselnde Kontraste immer wieder neu anregen (*24, 106*).

Modelle für die Neuronenmechanismen des Bewegungs- und Kontrastsehens zeigt die vergleichende Physiologie. Die speziellen Mechanismen des Facettenauges der Insekten (*4*) wurden von Hassenstein (*52*) und Reichardt (*105*) an einem Käfer mit einfachen Bewegungsreizen genau analysiert. Richtungsspezifische Bewegungseffekte, die bei verschiedener Lichtstärke konstant sind, haben Maturana, Lettvin u. Mitarb. (*96*) in bestimmten Tectumneuronen mit marklosen Axonen beim Frosch gefunden. Ihr starkes und spezifisches Ansprechen auf Kontrastsituationen könnte auch für unser Sehsystem bedeutungsvoll sein. Die Korrelationen von Kontrast- und Bewegungssehen müssen beim Säuger noch genauer studiert werden.

Neuronbefunde und Sehtheorien. Nach allen beschriebenen Befunden ist es klar, daß unsere neuronalen Ergebnisse am besten zu Herings *Gegenfarbentheorie* (*56, 59, 60*) für die Schwarz-Weiß-Komponente passen. Allerdings gilt dies nur für das reziproke Verhältnis der Neuronensysteme des Schwarz-Weiß-Sehens und nicht für Herings Vorstellungen von Assimilation und Dissimilation verschiedener Sehstoffe, die spekulativ geblieben sind. Da Hurvich und Jameson die Korrelationen der Gegenfarbentheorie ausführlich behandelt haben (*71, 72*) und die Katze trotz Purkinje-Verschiebung (*73*) im Verhaltensversuch farbenblind ist (*46*), begnügen wir uns mit dieser Korrelation zum Hell-Dunkel-Sehen.

Da wir über das Farbensehen bei der Katze nichts aussagen können, brauchen wir hier auch die Young-Helmholtz-Theorie nicht zu diskutieren. Ihre Geltung kann zunächst auf photochemische Prozesse in den Receptoren (*118, 125*) beschränkt werden, für die sie nach Rushtons Pigmentbestimmungen beim Menschen (*107, 108*) wahrscheinlich gemacht wurde. Eine gemeinsame Deutung aller Phänomene würde v. Kries' *Zonentheorie* (*89*) ermöglichen, wenn man für die Peripherie mit Photopigmenten und Receptoren eine 3-Farben-Theorie annimmt, aber bereits nach der ersten Synapse in Retina und Gehirn für alle neuronalen Vorgänge mit ihren reziproken Beziehungen die Gegenfarbentheorie als gültig ansieht.

Grenzen der neuronalen Korrelationen. Es ist natürlich hoffnungslos, durch einzelne Neuronentladungen die zahlreichen Gestaltphänomene des Sehens zu erklären, die etwa in Metzgers Buch (*97*) in vielen treffenden Bildern zusammengestellt sind. Dennoch werden manche zunächst unverständlichen Phänomene wie gewisse optische Täuschungen durch neurophysiologische Vorgänge relativ einfach erklärt (*10, 12, 67, 95*). Korrelationen zwischen Neurophysiologie und Sehen sind aber nur für *elementare visuelle Funktionen* möglich. Wir können nicht neurophysiologisch erklären, wie eine Katze eine Maus oder einen Kater sieht oder wie der Mensch ein Gesicht erkennt. Selbst wenn uns alle neuronalen Daten solcher Sehleistungen bekannt würden, wären diese zu kompliziert, um sie verstehen zu können. Komplexe visuelle Phänomene können wir im Tierversuch besser durch Verhaltensbeobachtung untersuchen oder beim Menschen psychologisch als höchstintegrierte Vorgänge in der Wahrnehmung selbst erfassen und durch sprachliche Kommunikation oder anschauliche Schemata mitteilen. Mit wenigen Worten, einer Skizze oder mit Schriftzeichen können wir rasch ein Bild verständlich machen, aber nicht mit der Beschreibung von vielen Neuronentladungen, die daran beteiligt sind. Beim Menschen fehlen noch mikrophysiologische Befunde, und nur wenige zentralvisuelle Vorgänge sind durch corticale (*33*) und EEG-Ableitungen (*97a*) untersucht.

Schluß

Dieser Vortrag hat zwei Ziele. Erstens wollte ich mit positiven Ergebnissen zeigen, daß die Neurophysiologie des Hell-Dunkel-Sehens mit ihren neuronalen Korrelaten in zwei antagonistischen Neuronensystemen für Hell- und Dunkelinformation relativ einfach verständlich ist. Zweitens möchte ich mit einer vorläufigen Synopsis der subjektiven und objektiven Sinnesphysiologie auf die Lücken unserer neurophysiologischen Kenntnisse hinweisen. Es ist zu hoffen, daß auch für das Bewegungssehen bei Berücksichtigung optomotorischer und vestibulärer Vorgänge mit ihren kybernetischen Regelkreisen entsprechende neuronale Korrelate gefunden werden können wie für das Hell-Dunkel-Sehen. Doch sind hier noch viele unbekannte Faktoren zu untersuchen, vor allem die Propriozeptivität der Augenmuskeln. Für das Farbensehen ergeben sich schon vielversprechende Ansätze nach SVAETICHINs *(111—116)* reziproken receptornahen Potentialen, nach Neuronentladungen *(91, 126)* und DE VALOIS' *(121—123)* reziproken on- oder off-Entladungen bei Gegenfarben, die dem Verhalten der on- und off-Erregung beim Schwarz-Weiß-Kontrast ähnlich sind. Für das komplexe Sehen und Erkennen von Gestalten sind die neuronalen Grundlagen noch zu kompliziert, um sie verstehen zu können. Ob die Modellvorstellungen, die W. R. HESS zuerst für die Wechselwirkung von Sehen, Augenmuskelapparat und Motorik *(64, 64b)* entwickelt hat, oder Parallelen mit dem Farbfernsehen (MÜLLER-LIMMROTH *102*) oder kybernetische Erklärungen, wie v. HOLSTs Modelle *(66, 67)* und MACKAYs Vermaschungsprozesse *(95)*, später auf neuronaler Basis weiterführen werden, muß offenbleiben.

Die genannten neuronalen Korrelationen genügen vielleicht zur Widerlegung des psychologischen Einwands, daß die Neurophysiologen mit ihren Ableitungen von Einzelelementen eine atomistische Forschung treiben, die nichts mit dem eigentlichen Sehen zu tun hat. Zwar ist es richtig, daß die Registrierung einzelner Neurone nur eine sehr begrenzte Auswahl der Millionen funktionierender Nervenzellen eines geordneten Systems geben kann. Diese Auswahl bringt aber mehr als zufällige Resultate, wenn die registrierten Neuronenpopulationen repräsentativ gesammelt und ihre Funktionen in gut geplanten Experimenten analysiert werden. Die Mikrophysiologie hat mehr brauchbare Korrelate des Sehens geliefert als die Elektrophysiologie mit Makroelektroden. Nur durch Mikroelektrodenuntersuchungen an einzelnen Neuronen war es möglich, gewisse Grundmechanismen neuronaler Koordination in dem regulierten komplexen System des Cortex aufzudecken. Um seine Experimente richtig zu planen, braucht der Neurophysiologe die Vorarbeit und theoretische Basis der subjektiven Sinnesphysiologie. Die psychophysiologische Untersuchung des Sehens ist der neurophysiologischen Analyse um mehr als 100 Jahre vorausgegangen. Diese alten subjektiv-sinnesphysiologischen Erfahrungen können auch heute bei neurophysiologischen Experimenten Richtung und Weg zeigen.

Alle subjektiv-sinnesphysiologischen Erscheinungen des Sehens sind als ganzes Phänomen unmittelbar anschaulich, wenn auch zeitlich weniger exakt bestimmbar. Die objektiven Registrierungen neuronaler Vorgänge sind zwar zeitlich völlig exakt zu messen, aber unanschauliche Teilausschnitte komplexer Vorgänge und müssen durch Analysen und Auszählungen erst indirekt erschlossen werden. Diese Verschiedenheit anschaulicher subjektiver Sinnesphänomene und indirekt erschlossener objektiver Registrierungen machen die gegenseitige Ergänzung beider Untersuchungsmethoden der Sinnesfunktionen notwendig und fruchtbar.

Unsere Ergebnisse zeigen, daß die Korrelation von subjektiver und objektiver Sinnesphysiologie ein aussichtsreicher Forschungsweg ist. Daraus ergibt sich die Notwendigkeit, *psychophysische und neurophysiologische Experimente miteinander zu koordinieren.*

Die Kombination beider Methoden weist uns auf diese doppelte Via regia für die Untersuchungen menschlicher Sinnesleistungen und ihre Begründung durch den Tierversuch. Der Neurophysiologe kann und darf nicht auf die anschaulichen Ergebnisse des subjektiven Sehens verzichten, wenn er gut geplante Experimente machen und sich nicht in Einzelheiten verlieren will. Ebensowenig darf der Psychologe physiologische und kausal erklärbare Vorgänge außer acht lassen, die seine begrifflichen Kriterien kontrollieren und korrigieren. Einseitige Untersuchungen des subjektiven oder objektiven Aspekts der Sinnesfunktionen ohne Rücksicht auf die Ergebnisse des anderen Forschungsgebietes führen entweder zu uninteressanten und unverständlichen Einzelergebnissen neurophysiologischer Registrierungen oder zu phantasievollen, somatisch nicht begründbaren psychologischen Hypothesen. Diese Seitenwege enden daher früher oder später in einer wissenschaftlichen Wildnis, entweder in zusammenhanglosen, trockenen Tatsachen oder in üppig wuchernder Spekulation. Nur die gemeinsam gebahnten Wege der psychophysischen und neurophysiologischen Forschung führen aus dieser Wildnis heraus zu koordinierter Erforschung der Sinnesleistungen bei Mensch und Tier.

Summary

1. Correlations of neuronal discharges in the visual system of animals with vision in man are discussed. Correspondent phenomena for brightness and darkness sensation in the visual neuronal system of the cat are summarized in a table. These results favour the assumption of two antagonistic neuronal systems (B and D) which signal "brighter" (B) or "darker" (D) respectively.

2. The B-system (retinal and geniculate on-center neurons and cortical B-neurons) and the D-system (retinal and geniculate off-center neurons and cortical D- and E-neurons) are interrelated reciprocally from retina to visual cortex. B-prevalence corresponds with relative brightness sensation in human vision and D-prevalence with relative darkness sensation (fig. 1 and 2). These correlations are valuable under various conditions: for absence of light stimuli (Eigengrau), for uniform field illumination as well as for patterned stimuli with simultaneous and successive contrast (fig. 3).

3. The on-off-responding neurons including cortical E-neurons mostly have shorter latency and stronger off-responses than on-responses. They belong to the D-system (on-off D), signalling relative darkness or moving patterns. Only a few on-off-neurons belong to the B-System (on-off B).

4. Most neurons of the visual cortex receive a convergence of retinal, labyrinthine and thalamo-reticular afferents (fig. 4). However, the neuronal activation or inhibition following nonspecific or labyrinthine stimuli does not change the B or D-type of neuronal responses to light stimulation which seems to be a specific fixed pattern of retino-cortical neuronal activity. The correlation of this neuronal

convergence with the alteration of visual perception by ocular movements, vestibular stimuli and attention is discussed.

5. Many features of visual neuronal activity can be explained satisfactorily by four mechanisms, which are demonstrated by experiments: 1. Reciprocal inhibition of antagonistic neurons (B versus D). 2. Lateral inhibition of synergistic neurons (organization of receptive fields within the B-system or D-system). 3. Constant information value of the light-activated neuronal B-system and the light-inhibited neuronal D-system. 4. Sensomotor integration of these basic neuronal informations with cybernetic regulation of the vestibulo-oculomotor-apparatus related to the ascending reticular system. This fourth mechanism probably regulates movement perception, visual space constancy and attention.

6. The relations of neuronal findings with some theories of vision are discussed. The necessity of parallel experiments with psychophysical and neurophysiological methods and the limits of psychophysiological correlations are stressed.

Literatur

1. AHLENSTIEL, H.: Der Weckblitz als hypnagoge Vision. Nervenarzt 20, 124—127 (1949).
2. AKIMOTO, H., u. O. CREUTZFELDT: Reaktionen von Neuronen des optischen Cortex nach elektrischer Reizung unspezifischer Thalamuskerne. Arch. Psychiat. Nervenkr. 196, 494—519 (1957—58).
2a. AKIMOTO, H., Y. SAITO and Y. NAKAMURA: Effects of arousal stimuli on evoked neuronal activities in cat's visual cortex. Dieses Symposion 363—374 (1961).
3. AUBERT, H.: Physiologie der Netzhaut. Breslau: E. Morgenstern 1865.
4. AUTRUM, H.: Das Sehen der Insekten. Stud. Gen. 10, 211—214 (1957).
5. BARLOW, H. B., R. FITZHUGH and S. W. KUFFLER: Change of organization in the receptive fields of the cat's retina during dark adaptation. J. Physiol. 137, 338—354 (1957).
6. BARTLEY, H.: Subjective brightness in relation to flash rate and the light-dark ratio. J. exp. Psychol. 23, 313—319 (1938).
7. BARTLEY, S. H.: Central mechanisms of vision. In Handbook of Physiology. Neurophysiology I, Pp. 713—740. Washington, D. C.: American Physiological Society 1959.
8. BAUMGARTEN, R. v., and R. JUNG: Microelectrode studies on the visual cortex. Rev. neurol. 87, 151—155 (1952).
9. BAUMGARTNER, G.: Reaktionen einzelner Neurone im optischen Cortex der Katze nach Lichtblitzen. Pflügers Arch. ges. Physiol. 261, 457—469 (1955).
10. — Indirekte Größenbestimmung der rezeptiven Felder der Retina beim Menschen mittels der Hermannschen Gittertäuschung. Pflügers Arch. ges. Physiol. 272, 21 (1960).
11. — Kontrastlichteffekte an retinalen Ganglienzellen: Ableitungen vom Tractus opticus der Katze. Dieses Symposion, 45—55 (1961).
12. — Die Reaktionen der Neurone des zentralen visuellen Systems der Katze im simultanen Helligkeitskontrast. Dieses Symposion, 297—313 (1961).
13. — Der Informationswert der on-Zentrum- und off-Zentrum-Neurone des visuellen Systems beim Hell-Dunkel-Sehen und die informative Bedeutung von Aktivierung und Hemmung. Dieses Symposion (Gruppendiskussion), 377—379 (1961).
14. — O. CREUTZFELDT and R. JUNG: Microphysiology of cortical neurones in acute anoxia and in retinal ischemia. In: Cerebral Anoxia and the Electroencephalogram (ed. J. S. MEYER and H. GASTAUT), Chapter 1, p. 5—34. Springfield, Ill.: C. Thomas 1961.
15. — u. P. HAKAS: Reaktionen einzelner Opticusneurone und corticaler Nervenzellen der Katze im Hell-Dunkel-Grenzfeld (Simultankontrast). Pflügers Arch. ges. Physiol. 270, 29 (1959).
16. BREMER, F.: Le potentiel évoqué de l'air visuelle corticale. Dieses Symposion, 335—350 (1961).
17. BRINDLEY, G. S.: Physiology of the retina and visual pathway. London: E. Arnold Ltd. 1960.

18. BRÜCKE, E.: Über den Nutzeffekt intermittierender Netzhautreizungen. Sitzber. Akad. Wiss. Wien (Math.-Nat. Kl.) **49 (II)**, 128—153 (1864).
19. CHARPENTIER, A.: Réaction oscillatoire de la rétine sous l'influence des excitations lumineuses. Arch. Physiol. (Paris) **24** (V, 4), 541—553 (1892).
20. CIBIS, P., u. H. NOTHDURFT: Experimentelle Trennung eines zentralen und eines peripheren Anteils von unbunten Nachbildern. Lokalisation der Leitungsunterbrechung, die bei experimenteller Netzhautanämie zu temporärer Amaurose führt. Pflügers Arch. ges. Physiol. **250**, 501—520 (1948).
21. CREUTZFELDT, O., u. H. AKIMOTO: Konvergenz und gegenseitige Beeinflussung von Impulsen aus der Retina und den unspezifischen Thalamuskernen an einzelnen Neuronen des optischen Cortex. Arch. Psychiat. Nervenkr. **196**, 520—548 (1957—58).
22. — u. O.-J. GRÜSSER: Beeinflussung der Flimmerreaktion einzelner corticaler Neurone durch elektrische Reize unspezifischer Thalamuskerne. In: Proc. 1st int. Congr. neurol. Sci., Brussels, Vol. III. EEG. Clinical Neurophysiology and Epilepsy. Pp. 349—355. London: Pergamon 1959.
23. — R. SPEHLMANN u. D. LEHMANN: Veränderungen der Neuronaktivität des visuellen Cortex durch Reizung der Substantia reticularis mesencephali. Dieses Symposion,351—363.
24. DITCHBURN, R. W., and B. L. GINSBORG: Involuntary eye movements during fixation. J. Physiol. **119**, 1—17 (1953).
25. DUENSING, F., u. K.-P. SCHAEFER: Die Aktivität einzelner Neurone der Formatio reticularis des nicht gefesselten Kaninchens bei Kopfwendungen und vestibulären Reizen. Arch. Psychiat. Nervenkr. **200**, 97—122 (1960).
26. EBBECKE, U.: Über das Augenblickssehen mit einer Bemerkung über rückwirkende Hemmung. Pflügers Arch. ges. Physiol. **185**, 181—195 (1920).
27. — Receptorapparat und entoptische Erscheinungen. In: Handbuch der Physiologie (Hrsg. BETHE, BERGMANN usw.) **12**, 1, 233—265. Berlin: Springer 1929.
28. — Über ein entoptisches Phänomen bei Schreck. Klin. Mbl. Augenheilk. **109**, 190—193 (1943).
29. — Experimentelle Beobachtungen über Kontrast und Adaptation. Z. exp. angew. Psychol. **7**, 366—391 (1960).
30. FECHNER, G. T.: Elemente der Psychophysik, Teil 1 und 2. Leipzig: Breitkopf und Härtel 1860.
31. FRANGOS, P.: Reaktionen corticaler Neurone bei verschiedener Lichtintensität und ihre Beziehung zum Weber-Fechner-Gesetz. Inaug.-Diss. Med. Fakultät Freiburg, 1961.
32. FRÖHLICH, F. W.: Die Empfindungszeit. Jena: Gustav Fischer 1929.
33. GASTAUT, H.: Enregistrement sous-cortical de l'activité électrique spontanée et provoquée du lobe occipital humain. EEG clin. Neurophysiol. **1**, 205—221 (1949).
34. GERNANDT, B., and R. GRANIT: Single fibre analysis of inhibition and the polarity of the retinal elements. J. Neurophysiol. **10**, 295—302 (1947).
35. GRAFSTEIN, B., B. D. BURNS and W. HERON: Activity of cortical neurons in response to patternd visual stimuli. In Structure and function of the cerebral cortex. Proc. of 2. Internat. Meeting of Neurobiologists: Amsterdam, Sept. 1959, p. 234—238. Amsterdam: Elsevier Publishing Comp. 1960.
36. GRANIT, R.: Receptors and sensory perception. New Haven: Yale University Press 1955.
37. GRÜSSER, O.-J.: Receptorpotentiale einzelner retinaler Zapfen der Katze. Naturwissenschaften **44**, 47 (1957).
38. — Receptorabhängige Potentiale der Katzenretina und ihre Reaktionen auf Flimmerlicht. Pflügers Arch. ges. Physiol. **271**, 511—525 (1960).
39. — u. O. CREUTZFELDT: Eine neurophysiologische Grundlage des Brücke-Bartley-Effektes: Maxima der Impulsfrequenz retinaler und corticaler Neurone bei Flimmerlicht mittlerer Frequenzen. Pflügers Arch. ges. Physiol. **263**, 668—681 (1957).
40. — u. U. GRÜSSER-CORNEHLS: Mikroelektrodenuntersuchungen zur Konvergenz vestibulärer und retinaler Afferenzen an einzelnen Neuronen des optischen Cortex der Katze. Pflügers Arch. ges. Physiol. **270**, 227—238 (1960).
40a.— — Entladungsmuster der Neurone des visuellen Cortex bei monocularer und binocularer Belichtung. Pflügers Arch. ges. Physiol. **272**, 51 (1960).

41. GRÜSSER, O.-J., U. GRÜSSER-CORNEHLS u. G. SAUR: Reaktionen einzelner Neurone im optischen Cortex der Katze nach elektrischer Polarisation des Labyrinths. Pflügers Arch. ges. Physiol. **269**, 593—612 (1959).

42. — — Reaktionsmuster einzelner Neurone im Geniculatum laterale und visuellen Cortex der Katze bei Reizung mit optokinetischen Streifenmustern. Dieses Symposion, 313—326.

43. — u. A. GRÜTZNER: Neurophysiologische Grundlagen der periodischen Nachbildphasen nach kurzen Lichtreizen. Albrecht v. Graefes Arch. Ophthal. **160**, 65—93 (1958).

44. — u. G. SAUR: Monoculare und binoculare Lichtreizung einzelner Neurone im Geniculatum laterale der Katze. Pflügers Arch. ges. Physiol. **271**, 595—612 (1960).

45. GRÜSSER-CORNEHLS, U., u. O.-J. GRÜSSER: Reaktionsmuster der Neurone im zentralen visuellen System von Fischen, Kaninchen und Katzen auf monoculare und binoculare Lichtreize. Dieses Symposion, 275—287.

46. GUNTER, R.: The discrimination between lights of different wave lengths in the cat. J. comp. physiol. Psychol. **47**, 169—172 (1954).

47. HARMS, H., u. E. AULHORN: Studien über den Grenzkontrast. Albrecht v. Graefes Arch. Ophthal. **157**, 3—23 (1955).

48. HARTLINE, H. K.: The response of single optic nerve fibers of the vertebrate eye to illumination of the retina. Amer. J. Physiol. **121**, 400—415 (1938).

49. — The receptive fields of optic nerve fibers. Amer. J. Physiol. **130**, 690—699 (1940).

50. — Inhibition of activity of visual receptors by illuminating nearby retinal areas in the Limulus eye. Fed. Proc. **8**, 69 (1949).

51. — and F. RATLIFF: Inhibitory interaction of receptor units in the eye of Limulus. J. gen. Physiol. **40**, 357—376 (1957).

52. HASSENSTEIN, B.: Optokinetische Wirksamkeit bewegter periodischer Muster. Z. Naturforsch. **14b**, 659—674 (1959).

53. HECHT, S.: The visual discrimination of intensity and the Weber-Fechner-law. J. gen. Physiol., **7**, 235—267 (1925).

54. HELMHOLTZ, H. VON: Handbuch der physiologischen Optik. 2. Aufl. Hamburg und Leipzig: G. Voss 1896.

55. HERING, E.: Beiträge zur Physiologie. I. Zur Lehre vom Ortssinn der Netzhaut. Leipzig: W. Engelmann 1861.

56. — Zur Lehre vom Lichtsinne. Wien: C. Gerold u. Söhne 1878.

57. — Der Raumsinn und die Bewegungen der Augen. In Hermanns Handbuch der Physiol. **3**, 343 (1879).

58. — Eine Methode zur Beobachtung und Zeitbestimmung des ersten positiven Nachbildes kleiner bewegter Objekte. Pflügers Arch. ges. Physiol. **126**, 604—609 (1909).

59. HERING, E., †: Grundzüge der Lehre vom Lichtsinn. Berlin: Springer 1920.

60. — Wissenschaftliche Abhandlungen. Leipzig: G. Thieme 1931.

61. HERNÁNDEZ-PEÓN, R., C. GUZMÁN-FLORES, M. ALCARAZ and A. FERNÁNDEZ-GUARDIOLA: Sensory transmission in visual pathway during "attention" in unanesthetized cats. Acta neurol. lat.-amer. **3**, 1—7 (1957).

62. HESS, C.: Untersuchungen über das Abklingen der Erregung im Sehorgan nach kurzdauernder Reizung. Pflügers Arch. ges. Physiol. **95**, 1—16 (1903).

63. — Untersuchungen über den Erregungsvorgang im Sehorgan bei kurzer und bei länger dauernder Reizung. Pflügers Arch. ges. Physiol. **101**, 226—262 (1901).

64. HESS, W. R.: Die Motorik als Organisationsproblem. Biol. Zbl. **61**, 545—572 (1941).

64a. — Induzierte Störungen der optischen Wahrnehmung. Nervenarzt **16**, 57—66 (1943).

64b. — Vom Lichtreiz zur bildhaften Wahrnehmung. Helv. Physiol· Acta. **10**, 395—402 (1952).

65. HOFMANN, F. B.: Die Lehre vom Raumsinn des Doppelauges. Ergebn. Physiol. **15**, 238—339 (1915).

66. HOLST, E. VON, u. H. MITTELSTAEDT: Das Reafferenzprinzip. Naturwissenschaften **37**, 256—272 (1950).

67. — Aktive Leistungen der menschlichen Gesichtswahrnehmung. Stud. Gen. **10**, 231 (1957).

68. HUBEL, D. H.: Cortical unit responses to visual stimuli in nonanesthetized cats. Amer. J. Ophthal. **46**, 110—122 (1958).

69. — Single unit activity in striate cortex of unrestrained cats. J. Physiol. **147**, 226—238 (1959).

69a. HUBEL, D. H.: Single unit activity in lateral geniculate body and optic tract of unrestrained cats. J. Physiol. **150**, 91—104 (1960).

70. — and T. N. WIESEL: Receptive fields of single neurones in the cat's striate cortex. J. Physiol. **148**, 574—591 (1959).

71. HURVICH, L. M., and D. JAMESON: An opponent process theory of color vision. Psychol. Rev. **64**, 384 (1957).

72. HURVICH-JAMESON, D., and L. M. HURVICH: Opponent colors theory and physiological mechanisms. Dieses Symposion, 152—163 (1961).

73. INGVAR, D. H.: Spectral sensitivity, as measured in cerebral visual centres. Acta physiol. scand. **46**, Suppl. 159 (1959).

74. JUNG, R.: Neuronal discharge. EEG clin. Neurophysiol., Suppl. 4, 57—71 (1953).

75. — Nystagmographie: Zur Physiologie und Pathologie des optisch-vestibulären Systems beim Menschen. In Handb. inner. Med., Bd. V. S. 1325—1379. Berlin-Göttingen-Heidelberg: Springer 1953.

76. — Excitation, inhibition and coordination of cortical neurons. Exp. Cell Res., Suppl. **5**, 262—271 (1958).

77. — Coordination of specific and nonspecific afferent impulses at single neurons of the visual cortex. In H. H. JASPER et al. (Editors), Reticular Formation of the Brain. Pp. 423—434. Boston: Little, Brown 1958.

78. — Mikrophysiologie des optischen Cortex: Koordination der Neuronenentladungen nach optischen, vestibulären und unspezifischen Afferenzen und ihre Bedeutung für die Sinnesphysiologie. 15. Gen. Assembly Jap. med. Congr., Tokyo **5**, 693—698 (1959).

79. — Microphysiology of cortical neurons and its significance for psychophysiology. In Festschrift Prof. C. ESTABLE. An. Fac. Med. Montevideo **44**, 323—332 (1959).

80. — Microphysiologie corticaler Neurone: Ein Beitrag zur Koordination der Hirnrinde und des visuellen Systems. In (D. B. TOWER and J. P. SCHADÉ, eds.) Structure and function of the cerebral cortex. Proc. 2. Intern. Meet. Neurobiol., Amsterdam 1959, p. 204—233. Amsterdam: Elsevier Publishing Company 1960.

81. — Neuronal integration in the visual cortex and its significance for visual information. In (ROSENBLITH, W., ed.) Sensory communication, p. 627—674. New York, London: M. I. T. Press and J. Wiley 1961.

82. — R. VON BAUMGARTEN u. G. BAUMGARTNER: Mikroableitungen von einzelnen Nervenzellen im optischen Cortex: Die lichtaktivierten B-Neurone. Arch. Psychiat. Nervenkr. **189**, 521—539 (1952).

83. — u. G. BAUMGARTNER: Hemmungsmechanismen und bremsende Stabilisierung an einzelnen Neuronen des optischen Cortex: Ein Beitrag zur Koordination corticaler Erregungsvorgänge. Pflügers Arch. ges. Physiol. **261**, 434—456 (1955).

84. — O. CREUTZFELDT u. O.-J. GRÜSSER: Die Mikrophysiologie corticaler Neurone und ihre Bedeutung für die Sinnes- und Hirnfunktionen. Dtsch. med. Wschr. **82**, 1050—1059 (1957).

85. KÖHLER, W., and H. WALLACH: Figural after-effects: An investigation of visual processes. Proc. Amer. Phil. Soc. **88**, 269—357 (1944).

86. KÖNIG, A., u. E. BRODHUN: Experimentelle Untersuchungen über die psychophysische Fundamentalformel in bezug auf den Gesichtssinn. I. S.-B. Akad. Wiss. Berlin 1888/II, 917—934.

87. KORNHUBER, H. H., u. S. DA FONSECA: Unveröffentlichte Untersuchungen.

88. KORNMÜLLER, A. E.: Eine experimentelle Anästhesie der äußeren Augenmuskeln am Menschen und ihre Auswirkungen. J. Psychol. Neurol. **41**, 354—366 (1931).

89. KRIES, J. V.: Die Gesichtsempfindungen. In Nagels Handbuch der Physiologie des Menschen. Pp. 109 ff. Braunschweig: Vieweg 1905.

90. KUFFLER, S. W.: Discharge patterns and functional organization of mammalian retina. J. Neurophysiol. **16**, 37—68 (1953).

91. LENNOX-BUCHTHAL, M.: Some findings on central nervous system organization with respect to colour. Dieses Symposion, 191—199 (1961).

92. LI, CH.-L., A. ORTIZ-GALVIN, S. N. CHOU and S. Y. HOWARD: Cortical intracellular potentials in response to stimulation of lateral geniculate body. J. Neurophysiol. **23**, 592 to 601 (1960).

93. MACH, E.: Über die Wirkung der räumlichen Verteilung des Lichtreizes auf die Netzhaut. I. S.-B. Akad. Wiss. Wien, math.-nat. Classe, **52/2**, 303—322 (1865).

94. MACH, E.: Die Analyse der Empfindungen und das Verhältnis des Physischen zum Psychischen. Jena: Gustav Fischer-Verlag 1903.

95. MACKAY, D. M.: Towards an information-flow model of human behavior. Brit. J. Psychol. **47**, 30—43 (1956).

96. MATURANA, H. R., J. Y. LETTVIN, W. S. McCULLOCH and W. H. PITTS: Anatomy and physiology of vision in the frog (Rana pipiens). J. gen. Physiol. **43**, 129—176 (1960).

97. METZGER, W.: Gesetze des Sehens. Frankfurt/Main: W. Kramer & Co. 1936.

97a. MONNIER, M.: Mesure de la durée d'un processus d'integration corticale: Temps d'intégration opto-motrice chez l'homme. Helv. Physiol. Acta **7**, C 52—53 (1949).

98. MOTOKAWA, K.: Physiological induction in human retina as basis of color and brightness contrast. J. Neurophysiol. **12**, 475—488 (1949).

99. — D. NAKAGAWA and T. KOHATA: Figural after-effects and retinal induction. J. gen. Psychol. **57**, 121—135 (1957).

100. — T. OIKAWA and K. TASAKI: Receptor potential of vertebrate retina. J. Neurophysiol. **20**, 186—199 (1957).

101. — E. YAMASHITA and T. OGAWA: The physiological basis of simultaneous contrast in the retina. Dieses Symposion, 32—45 (1961).

102. MÜLLER-LIMMROTH, W.: Elektrophysiologie des Gesichtssinns. Berlin-Göttingen-Heidelberg: Springer 1959.

103. PURKINJE, J.: Beiträge zur Kenntnis des Sehens in subjektiver Hinsicht. Prag: J. G. Calve 1819.

105. REICHARDT, W., u. D. VARJU: Übertragungseigenschaften am Auswertesystem für das Bewegungssehen. Z. Naturforsch. **14 b**, 674—689 (1959).

106. RIGGS, L. A., F. RATLIFF, J. C. CORNSWEET and T. N. CORNSWEET: The disappearance of steadily fixed visual test objects. J. opt. Soc. Amer. **43**, 495—501 (1953).

107. RUSHTON, W. A. H.: The physical analysis of cone pigment in the living human eye. Nature (Lond.) **179**, 571—573 (1957).

108. — Kinetics of cone pigments measured objectively on the living human fovea. Ann. N. Y. Acad. Sci. **74**, 291—304 (1958).

109. SCHUBERT, G.: Ein entoptisches Hypoxie-Phänomen. Z. Biol. **110**, 232—235 (1958).

110. SHERRINGTON, C.: The integrative action of the nervous system. London: Constable 1906.

111. SVAETICHIN, G.: The cone action potentials. Acta physiol. scand. **29**, Suppl. 106, 565 to 610 (1953).

112. — Spectral response curves from single cones. Acta physiol. scand. **39**, Suppl. 134, 17—46 (1956).

113. — Receptor mechanisms for flicker and fusion. Acta physiol. scand. **39**, Suppl. 134, 47—54 (1956).

114. — and E. F. MACNICHOL: Retinal mechanisms for chromatic and achromatic vision. Ann. N. Y. Acad. Sci. **74**, 385—404 (1958).

115. — Origin of the R-Potential in the mammalian retina. Dieses Symposion, 61—64 (1961).

116. — M. LAUFER G. MITARAI, R. FATEHCHAND, E. VALLECALLE and J. VILLEGAS: Glial control of neuronal networks and receptors. Dieses Symposion, 445—456 (1961).

117. TOMITA, T., M. MURAKAMI, Y. HASHIMOTO and Y. SASAKI: Electrical activity of single neurons in the frog's retina. Dieses Symposion, 24—31 (1961).

118. TRENDELENBURG, W.: Quantitative Untersuchungen über die Bleichung des Sehpurpurs in monochromatischem Licht. Z. Psychol. Physiol. Sinnesorgane **37**, 1—55 (1904).

119. TSCHERMAK, A.: Über Kontrast und Irradiation. Ergebn. Physiolog. **2**, 2, 726—798 (1903).

120. — Der exakte Subjektivismus in der neueren Sinnesphysiologie. Pflügers Arch. ges. Physiol. **188**, 1—20 (1921).

121. DE VALOIS, R. L.: Color vision mechanisms in the monkey. J. gen. Physiol. **43**, 115—128 (1960).

122. — C. J. SMITH and S. T. KITAI: Electrical responses of primate visual system. II. Recordings from single on-cells of macaque lateral geniculate nucleus. J. comp. physiol. Psychol. **52**, 635—641 (1959).

123. de Valois, R. L., and A. E. Jones: Single cell analysis of the organization of primate color vision system. Dieses Symposion, 178—191 (1961).

124. Verzeano, M., and K. Negishi: Neuronal activity in cortical and thalamic networks. A study with multiple microelectrodes. J. Gen. Physiol., **43**, 177—195 (1960).

125. Wald, G.: The photoreceptor process in vision. In Handbook of Physiology Neurophysiology I, (Hrg. J. Field, H. W. Magoun, V. E. Hall), p. 671—692. Washington, D. C.: American Physiological Society 1960.

126. Wolbarsht, M. L., H. G. Wagner and E. F. Mac Nichol jr.: Receptive fields of retinal ganglion cells: Extent and spectral sensitivity Dies. Symposion, 170—177 (1961).

Diskussion

L. M. Hurvich: Dr. Jung has presented an impressive set of specific correlations. I am of course, in agreement with his basic viewpoint, although there are some details that I might question. More important, I think, is the fact that despite the rapid strides being made by the electrophysiologists, some elementary problems still need looking into. Particularly for those organisms which have color vision, the nature of the so-called "white" stimulus still needs clarification. As far as I know, what the electrophysiologist usually calls "white" is any convenient tungsten light source, probably about 2800° K. We know from our psychophysical work on this problem — our papers on the question appeared in the Journal of the Optical Society of America of 1951 — that broad band distributions of different color temperatures differentially affect the chromatic response mechanisms of humans with demonstrable consequences for the specification of "white" or truly achromatic stimuli. Has there been any systematic exploration of this problem with respect to the color systems of animals?

F. Bremer: I have some hesitation, to use the word „Aufmerksamkeit" or "attention" and would prefer "awareness", „Wachheit" or "vigilance" to describe the behavioral and psychological state which you mean in your experiments.

W. A. Beresford: Three papers at this symposium, those of Bremer, Akimoto and Creutzfeldt, have claimed to provide electrophysiological evidence of a non-specific projection system to the visual cortex of the cat. The experimental method has used the responses of the visual cortex or of visual cortical neurones to light stimulation of the retina or sometimes by Bremer to electrical stimulation of the LGB, both with and without electrical stimulation of "non-specific" regions in the di- and mes- encephalon.

The cortical neurones that give rise to cortical efferent fibres often give off axonal collaterals in the cortex. The patterns of firing in these collaterals are probably very different when the cell is firing normally orthodromically and when its efferent axon is activated antidromically. This could produce a difference in influence upon the firing of the cortical cell from which Creutzfeldt takes his record. The response differences claimed to be due to non-specific afferents could be due to *specific cortical efferents* fired antidromically.

To exclude this possibility the stimulating electrode should be in a region not traversed by visual cortical efferents.

H. Schober: In der modernen deutschen und russischen Literatur spricht man jetzt immer vom Fertsch-Phänomen, da diese Erscheinungen nicht von Pulfrich, sondern von Fertsch entdeckt und beschrieben wurden. Auch die Deutung stammt von Fertsch. Pulfrich konnte das Phänomen schon deshalb nicht finden, weil er in früher Jugend sein eines Auge verloren hatte.

W. Sickel: Es läßt sich in speziellen Fällen zeigen (Abbildungsgüte — Netzhautraster) und ist allgemein anzunehmen, daß Teilfunktionen des Sehprozesses nach den Prinzipien optimaler Systeme verknüpft sind und Leistungsbegrenzungen an mehreren Stellen einer Kausalkette zugleich auftreten.

W. Metzger: 1. Lassen sich aus den bisherigen objektiven Beobachtungen über binoculare Prozesse schon Hinweise auf gewisse Eigentümlichkeiten des binocularen Wettstreits entnehmen (z. B. die Dominanz der Konturen). Andererseits gibt es schon Möglichkeiten, objektiv zu erklären, wieso beim Wettstreit größerer homogener Farbflächen die beiden Farben zuerst *in zwei verschiedenen Ebenen* und in zwei verschiedenen Erscheinungsweisen (Oberflächenfarbe und Raumfarbe bzw. verdeckende, teils durchsichtige Nebelschicht) gesehen werden.

2. Ist schon nachgeprüft, wie weit die Befunde von Ditchburn u. Mitarb. über gesehene Objekte, deren Bild sich auf der Netzhaut nicht verschiebt, sich mit den hier vorgetragenen Beobachtungen über on- und off-Effekte usw. vereinbaren lassen?

R. Jung (zu Hurvich): Die Qualität des „weißen" Lichtes ist bei unseren Versuchen nicht von Bedeutung, weil die Katze keine farbspezifischen Reaktionen zeigt. Nach Katzenexperimenten ist das Farbensehen neuronal noch nicht korrelierbar. Auch andere Sehphänomene lassen sich noch nicht psychophysisch und neuronal korrelieren und man wird sicher manche quantitativen und qualitativen Abweichungen finden. Aber wenn wir die neuronalen Korrelatioen einfacher psychophysiologischer Phänomene untersuchen, so finden sich doch sehr eindrucksvolle Parallelen.

Ich stimme Prof. Bremer gerne zu, daß bei neurophysiologischen Versuchen besser von „Wachheit" oder "awareness" gesprochen wird als von „Aufmerksamkeit". Doch ist der Aufmerksamkeitsbegriff bei der Untersuchung spezieller Sinnesfunktionen nicht ganz zu entbehren, weil "attention" besser die *aktive* Ausrichtung eines bestimmten Sinnes bezeichnet als awareness. Im visuellen Gebiet zeigt dies der optokinetische Nystagmus, dessen Stärke von der *gerichteten* visuellen Aufmerksamkeit abhängig ist (Abb. 5), nicht nur von der allgemeinen Wachheit.

Beresfords Einwände gegen die Reizversuche im thalamo-reticulären System sind zwar für elektrische Reizung beachtenswert, können aber nicht für natürliche Aktivierung durch andere Sinnesreize gelten. Diese sensorischen Weckeffekte zeigen die gleichen Phänomene wie die elektrische Reizung und haben sicher nichts mit antidromer Erregung zu tun.

Ich danke Professor Schober für seinen Hinweis auf Fertsch. Aber da der Effekt unter Pulfrichs Namen bekannter ist, möchte ich zur besseren Verständigung Fertsch-Pulfrich-Phänomen sagen.

(Zu Metzger): 1. Der binoculare Wettstreit hat offenbar bestimmte Gestaltdominanzen in den Konturen. Dies wird neurophysiologisch verständlicher durch Baumgartners Befunde maximaler Erregung und reziproker Hemmung im Kontrastfeld der Kontur. Durch doppeläugige Kontrastuntersuchungen könnten auch die neuronalen Grundlagen des binocularen Wettstreits und binocularen Glanzes genauer erforscht werden. Außer wenigen Beobachtungen von Hubel und Wiesel über doppeläugige Punktlichtreize wurden binoculare Untersuchungen an corticalen Neuronen aber nur mit diffusen Lichtreizen durchgeführt, über die Grüsser berichtete (vgl. S. 275). Eine neurophysiologische Grundlage des binocularen Wettstreites ergab sich aus dem vorwiegenden Hemmungseffekt bei binocularer Reizung. Ob man, wie Grüsser diskutiert hat, auch die stärkere Hemmung des Flimmerlichtes als Hinweis auf die Konturdominanz verwenden kann, möchte ich offenlassen. Diffuses Flimmerlicht ist natürlich nicht mit lokalen Flimmerregungen an Konturen bei Augenunruhe gleichzusetzen, aber vielleicht ergibt dies einen Hinweis für spätere Untersuchungen.

Der verschiedene Raumwert der Farben ist neurophysiologisch noch nicht zu erklären, da wir über das zentrale Farbensehen bei unseren Katzenversuchen nichts aussagen können. Vielleicht werden de Valois' und Frau Lennox' Affenversuche weiterführen.

2. Die Lokaladaptation von Ditchburn u. Mitarb. entspricht ziemlich genau dem allmählichen Rückgang der Neuronenentladung des B- und D-Systems bei länger dauerndem Licht- oder Dunkelreiz. Die nach „Licht-an" maximale Aktivierung der B-Neurone vermindert sich bei gleichbleibendem Licht in wenigen Sekunden auf die Ruheaktivität, die auch im Dunkel vorhanden ist und die ich für das Äquivalent des Eigengraus halte.

Aporien der Psychophysik*

Von

Wolfgang Metzger

Man kann in diesem Jahr nicht gut über Psychophysik sprechen, ohne Gustav Theodor Fechners (*1*) zu gedenken, der das bahnbrechende Werk dieses Namens vor genau 100 Jahren veröffentlicht hat. Was davon am besten im Gedächtnis

---

* Psychologisches Institut der Universität Münster i. W.

geblieben ist, ist sein Bemühen, die möglichen Abstufungen einer gegebenen
elementaren Sinnesqualität als Funktion bestimmter Änderungen der zugrunde
liegenden Sinnesreizung darzustellen und die Meßmethoden zu entwickeln, ver-
mittels derer man die zahlenmäßigen Daten gewinnen kann, die zur Erhellung der
gesuchten Funktionen erforderlich sind. Gefragt wird also nach dem Verhältnis
zwischen Reizgrößen und gewissen Größen anschaulicher Art. Man kann diese
Frage auch auf das Verhältnis zwischen Reiz*mustern* (patterns) und anschaulichen
Strukturen ausdehnen, wie das z. B. J. J. Gibson bei seiner Theorie des Sehraumes tut. Für diese Art der Psychophysik ist es kennzeichnend, daß man sich
über die mehr oder weniger lange Kausalkette zwischen der gereizten Sinnesfläche
und dem anschaulich Erlebten keine Gedanken macht. Es wird vielfach übersehen,
daß dies schon für Fechner nicht der ganze Sinn der Psychophysik gewesen ist.
Die andere Hälfte seines Anliegens ist am kürzesten ausgedrückt in einer (wesentlich älteren) Bemerkung Johannes Müllers, daß sich in der anschaulichen
Beschaffenheit unserer Wahrnehmungen das Wesentliche der zugrunde liegenden
somatischen Prozesse verrate. Fechner unterscheidet diese beiden Anliegen als
„äußere" und „innere" Psychophysik. Er sagt wörtlich: „Es ist aber die äußere
Psychophysik nur die Unterlage und Vorbereitung für die tiefer führende innere
Psychophysik ... Nicht der Reiz erweckt unmittelbare Empfindung, sondern
zwischen ihn und die Empfindung schiebt sich noch eine innere körperliche Tätigkeit, wir nannten sie kurz die *psychophysische*, ein, die vom Reiz erweckt wird, und
die nun erst unmittelbar Empfindung mitführt oder nachzieht ... Und die gesetz-
liche Beziehung zwischen dem äußeren und dem inneren Endglied dieser Kette,
Reiz und Empfindung, übersetzt sich notwendig in eine solche zwischen dem
Reize und diesem Mittelgliede einerseits und zwischen diesem Mittelgliede und
der Empfindung andererseits." Fechner läßt keinen Zweifel, daß er sich die
Beziehung zwischen dem Reiz und dem psychophysischen Prozeß kausal, die zwischen diesem und der Empfindung parallelistisch denkt. Ebenso bemerkenswert
erscheint mir die Tatsache, daß er die Annahme sogenannter „rein seelischer"
Erscheinungen in aller Schärfe ablehnt. Es gibt nach Fechner *keine* Bewußt-
seinserscheinungen ohne speziell zugehörige körperliche Prozesse. Er unterscheidet
also *nicht*, wie später Wundt und Helmholtz, zwischen Bewußtseinserscheinun-
gen, die man physiologisch erklären kann, und solchen, die nur psychologisch
erklärt werden können. Auch das, was wir heute als Arbeitshypothese des
„konkreten Parallelismus" bzw. der „Isomorphie" Wolfgang Köhler zuzu-
schreiben pflegen, finden wir bei ihm schon klar ausgesprochen. Er selbst spricht
hier von einem „Funktionsprinzip" und führt dazu aus: „Zwar können wir in
keiner Weise aus der Natur der geistigen Bewegungen auf die Natur der unterliegenden körperlichen Bewegungen schließen, d. h. schließen, welches Substrat
und welche Form diesen Bewegungen zukommen, wohl aber schließen, daß dem
psychischen Zusammenhang ein psychophysischer Zusammenhang, der psychischen Auf- und Auseinanderfolge eine psychophysische, der psychischen Ähnlichkeit und Verschiedenheit eine psychophysische, der psychischen Stärke und
Schwäche eine psychophysische entspreche ..." und zur Erläuterung fährt er
fort: „Erinnerungen tragen noch die Form der Anschauungen; auch die den
Erinnerungen unterliegenden Prozesse werden noch die Form der Prozesse tragen,
die den Anschauungen unterliegen." Und er schließt: „Nun würde es sehr müßig

sein, diese Art Übersetzung des Psychischen in das Psychophysische breit aus-
zuführen, solange sie uns eben nicht weiter als zur bloßen Übersetzung führt.
Aber sie bezeichnet den *Weg des Entgegenkommens* gegen das, was wir von der
äußeren Psychophysik her und nach anatomischen, physiologischen und pathologischen Tatsachen erschließen können, und nur, wo sich ein solches Entgegenkommen zeigt, werden wir näher darauf einzugehen haben und etwas dadurch gefördert sehen dürfen . . .‟

Sie werden mir zugeben, daß diese Gedankengänge FECHNERs erheblich
klarer sind, auch erheblich moderner, als die seiner unmittelbaren Nachfolger,
EWALD HERING ausgenommen. Wieder ist bemerkenswert, daß schon FECHNER
sein Isomorphieprinzip, d. h. seine Vermutung, man könne aus dem Anschaulichen
auf das Physiologische schließen, *nicht* auf das *Substrat* und die Mikrostruktur
der psychophysischen Prozesse, sondern nur auf ihre raum-zeitliche Makrostruktur
für anwendbar hält. G. E. MÜLLER hat dann in seinem Beitrag „Zur Psychophysik
der Gesichtsempfindungen‟ von 1896 das Fechnersche Prinzip zu präzisieren
versucht, in dem er 5 psychophysische Axiome aufstellte, von denen ich hier in
etwas zusammengefaßter und verallgemeinerter Form die drei wichtigsten nenne:

1. Jedem *Zustand* des Bewußtseins entspricht ein materieller *Vorgang*, der
sogenannte psychophysische Prozeß, an dessen Stattfinden das Vorhandensein
des Bewußtseinszustandes geknüpft ist; es kann weder der körperliche Vorgang
ohne den psychischen noch der psychische ohne den körperlichen stattfinden.

2. Einer Gleichheit, einer größeren oder geringeren Ähnlichkeit, einer Verschiedenheit psychischer Zustände entspricht eine Gleichheit, eine größere oder geringere Ähnlichkeit, eine Verschiedenheit der psychophysischen Prozesse und
umgekehrt.

3. Ist ein psychischer Zustand in n-facher Richtung variabel, so muß auch der
zugehörige psychophysische Prozeß in n-facher Richtung variabel sein.

Das Modell, auf das sich G. E. MÜLLER bei diesen Formulierungen bezieht,
ist offenbar HERINGs Annahme von drei je in sich antagonistischen Paaren von
Farbprozessen, und sein Verdienst ist, diese Annahme aus dem Zusammenhang
mit Stoffwechselprozessen gelöst zu haben. Hiermit hängt es zusammen, daß der
Anwendungsbereich des Vorgehens bei G. E. MÜLLER erheblich enger ist, als er
bei FECHNER vorgesehen war. Er beschränkt sich auf abstrakte Mannigfaltig-
keiten von Qualitäten – Beispiel: das Farbsystem –; die räumliche Verteilung
von Zuständen und Vorgängen bleibt ausgeschlossen. Da man angesichts des
Baues des Großhirns niemals erwarten kann, daß räumliche Eigenschaften des
anschaulich Erlebten in identischen räumlichen Eigenschaften von Hirnvorgängen
abgebildet sind, hält er es vorläufig für sinnlos, hierüber Vermutungen anzustellen.

Seine Bedenken wurden erst von W. KÖHLER beseitigt: 1920 in seinen „Physischen Gestalten‟ und nochmals in seinem Aufsatz „Ein altes Scheinproblem‟
in den „Naturwissenschaften‟ 1929. Die Bedenken G. E. MÜLLERs bestehen
danach nur so lange, als man erwartet, daß die psychophysischen Korrelate die
räumlichen Verhältnisse der Wahrnehmungsinhalte in einem von außen durch den
Kopf gelegten Cartesischen Koordinatensystem wiedergeben. Der Vortrag des
Herrn WHITTERIDGE hat uns aufs Eindrucksvollste veranschaulicht, wie unmöglich diese Erwartung ist. (Man denke z. B. daran, daß die Projektion der ganzen
äußersten Netzhautperipherie *nicht viel mehr als ein Punkt ist*, mindestens ein

kleineres Gebiet als die Projektion der Fovea, und daß die Feststellung seiner
Ringstruktur ziemliche Mühe macht.) Dieser Eindruck wird noch vertieft, wenn
man versucht, sich klar zu machen, wie die beiden corticalen Gesichtsfeldhälften
zu einer bruchlosen Einheit zusammengefaßt werden sollen, wovon Herr WHITTE-
RIDGE nicht mehr gesprochen hat. KÖHLER hat nun in durchaus einleuchtender
Weise erläutert, daß in diesem Gebiet z. B. gleiche Längen und gleiche Krümmun-
gen nicht geometrisch, sondern nur „dynamisch" definiert werden dürfen, was
ich aber hier nicht näher erläutern kann. Damit war die Psychophysik grundsätzlich ungefähr auf den Stand gebracht, der FECHNER von Anfang an vorschwebte,
und den Herr HURVICH vorgestern, wenn ich ihn recht verstanden habe, in die
Worte faßte: „Wir sehen unmittelbar, was sich in unserem psychophysischen
Niveau abspielt: so wie es aussieht, so ist es." Ich halte diesen Ausspruch nicht
für ein geistreiches bon mot, sondern für eine ernste und durchaus diskutable
These. Denn auf dem normalen Weg der physikalischen und der physiologischen
Beobachtung sind uns ausnahmslos nur *höchst kompliziert vermittelte Abbildungen
und Symptome* des beobachteten Sachverhalts, z. B. der Vorgänge im Cortex,
zugänglich. Dagegen sind unsere Wahrnehmungen mit allen ihren Eigenschaften
die einzigen Tatbestände der Welt, die ohne vermittelnde Abbildungsvorgänge
selbst, d. h. *im Original, offen* vor uns liegen, d. h. das einzige, was unserer *unmittelbaren* Kenntnis zugänglich und verfügbar ist. Sie stellen daher auch denjenigen Bereich des Seins dar, dem wir alles entnehmen müssen und entnommen
haben, was wir für das Verständnis der Welt im Ganzen an Gesichtspunkten
besitzen. BERTRAND RUSSEL hat das einmal so ausgedrückt: „Die scheinbare
Öffentlichkeit unserer Welt ist zum Teil eine Täuschung und zum Teil erschlossen.
Das gesamte Rohmaterial unseres Wissens besteht aus seelischen Vorgängen im
Leben einzelner Menschen." Und wenn unsere anschaulichen Erlebnisse solcherart
das Rohmaterial *unseres gesamten Wissens* sind, so sind sie es im besonderen Maß
für unser psychologisches Wissen. Ich möchte keineswegs so weit gehen wie der
Freiburger Entwicklungsmechaniker SPEMANN in einem Vortrag, den er 1937 in
Halle gehalten hat, und in dem er die Meinung äußerte, die Biologie und Physio-
logie hätten für ihre Theoriebildung bis auf weiteres von der Psychologie mehr
Anregung zu erwarten als umgekehrt. Ich bin, genau wie mein Lehrer KÖHLER,
nie der Meinung gewesen, man könne eine geschlossene Theorie der seelischen
Erscheinungen entwickeln, ohne die Physiologie zu Rate zu ziehen. Ganz abgesehen davon, daß noch nie eine Seele ohne ein Nervensystem beobachtet worden
ist, und daß jeder Eingriff in ein solches Nervensystem höchst charakteristische
Veränderungen an den seelischen Erscheinungen und Funktionen zur Folge hat,
stoßen wir in einem fort auf Eigentümlichkeiten auch der normalen Bewußtseins-
erscheinungen, die aus sich selbst nie verstanden werden können, sondern uner-
bittlich nach einer *physiologischen Erklärung* verlangen, ja, man möchte sagen,
geradezu danach schreien.

Trotzdem hat es einen guten Grund, bei der psychophysischen Theoriebildung
auf einem methodischen Primat der *psychologischen* Beobachtung zu bestehen,
d. h. auf der methodischen Forderung, daß über die unmittelbaren materiellen
Korrelate des Psychischen keinerlei Annahme erlaubt sein soll, die nicht in jeder
Beziehung den Gesetzmäßigkeiten des anschaulichen Erlebens und des Seelischen
überhaupt entspricht. Wir befinden uns nämlich am Ende einer fast hundert-

jährigen Periode, in der man aus sehr geringen anatomischen und physiologischen Kenntnissen sehr bestimmte psychologische Folgerungen zu ziehen pflegte: Man versuchte aus den bekannten objektiven Daten zu *konstruieren*, von welcher Art die *psychischen* Korrelate nervöser Vorgänge, das heißt die Erlebnisse und Wahrnehmungserscheinungen, eigentlich sein müßten bzw. nur sein *könnten*. Denken Sie an das, was EBBINGHAUS zur Theorie des Sehraumes äußerte. Nach seiner Meinung dürfte dieser *keine* Tiefe besitzen, weil die Netzhautzellen ebenfalls nur eine zweidimensionale Mannigfaltigkeit darstellen.

Oder mit seinen Worten: Nur die Breite und Höhe des Sehraumes wird „empfunden", seine Tiefe wird nur „vorgestellt". Auch die gesamte Wahrnehmungslehre des großen HELMHOLTZ unterliegt dieser Kritik. Wenn die Eigenart der psychischen Erscheinungen nicht mit dem übereinstimmte, was er auf Grund der bescheidenen anatomisch-physiologischen Kenntnisse seiner Zeit erwartete, so folgte daraus für ihn zwingend, es könne für sie keine streng zugeordneten materiellen Begleitvorgänge geben, es müsse vielmehr durch das Eingreifen eines außerphysischen, rein geistigen Agens aus dem nicht beobachtbaren, aber nach seiner Meinung gleichwohl unbemerkt vorhandenen, *unmittelbaren* psychischen Korrelat der gewissermaßen letzten vorpsychischen Station der gesamten körperlich-seelischen Kausalkette in entsprechender Weise umgewandelt worden sein.

Dabei handelt es sich offenbar, um in einem hier schon in den letzten Tagen gebrauchten Bild zu bleiben, um eine Tunnelbohrung, die nicht genügend auf das Klopfen der von der anderen Seite vordringenden Kolonne geachtet hat und daher ihr Ziel verfehlte.

Sehen wir nun zu, was für Erwartungen in den letzten Jahren von der psychischen Seite an die Neurophysiologie gerichtet wurden.

1. Da ist zunächst die *Heringsche Farbenlehre*, die viele Jahrzehnte lang als psychophysisches Postulat in der Luft schwebte und, wie man wohl sagen kann, gerade in der angelsächsischen Psychologie nie ganz ernst genommen wurde. Mir scheint der Hauptertrag *dieses* Symposiums u. a. in der Fülle und Vielseitigkeit physiologischer Beobachtungen zu bestehen, die objektive Gesetzmäßigkeiten zeigen von der Art, wie HERING sie von den Phänomenen her postulierte, und durch die z. B. die Urteilstheorie des Kontrastes sich endgültig als überflüssig erweist.

2. Das zweite große psychophysische Postulat, dessen Bestätigung sich in etlichem, was hier vorgetragen wurde, andeutet, ist das (wohl zuerst von MAX WERTHEIMER 1912 ausgesprochene) Postulat der *Querfunktionen*, d. h. der unmittelbaren gegenseitigen Beeinflussung gleichzeitiger corticaler Prozesse. Ich sehe diese Bestätigung in dem, was Herr TEUBER als *"lateral interaction"* bezeichnet und an der Ausfüllung zentraler Skotome und ihrer Überbrückung durch stroboskopische Bewegungen erläutert hat.

3. Wie weit damit schon eine relative *Freizügigkeit*, d. h. die Variabilität des Weges der afferenten Prozesse anerkannt ist, vermag ich nicht zu beurteilen. Jedenfalls ist diese Freizügigkeit ein *drittes psychophysisches Postulat*, dessen Formulierung, soviel ich sehe, auf WOLFGANG KÖHLER (1913) zurückgeht: Es muß danach eine und dieselbe Reizmannigfaltigkeit, je nach Umständen, auch figural, nicht nur qualitativ, sehr verschiedene zentrale Prozesse veranlassen können, wie auch umgekehrt ein und dasselbe zentrale Prozeßgebilde aus sehr

verschiedenen peripheren Reizmannigfaltigkeiten hervorgehen kann, wie die zahlreichen Konstanzphänomene in der Wahrnehmung es fordern.

4. Ein viertes, hiermit zusammenhängendes Postulat, das LASHLEY 1930 ausgesprochen hat, ist die *Bildung von funktionalen*, d. h. *Prozeß-Einheiten*, deren Grenzen sich von Fall zu Fall neu bilden, also nicht auf Gewebsstrukturen begründet, sondern vielmehr gegen die anatomischen Strukturen verschieblich sind. Im Zusammenhang damit werden Eigenschaften psychophysischer Prozesse gefordert, die zu spontanen (wechselnden!) Grenzflächenbildungen führen, Prozesse, die zweifellos bei rein elektrophysiologischer Untersuchung verborgen bleiben müssen.

5. Ein besonders kühnes und bei unserer gegenwärtigen Kenntnis des Nervensystems unerfüllbar erscheinendes Postulat ist das *eines gemeinsamen Sinnesraumes*, eines Sensorium commune, in das die Daten sämtlicher Sinne einmünden und in welchem sie in die verschiedensten räumlichen Beziehungen zueinander treten können.

6. Als letzte sei nur noch die Forderung erwähnt, auch für die Sachverhalte des Beurteilens, des Strebens, des Wertens, der Forderung usw. psychophysische Korrelate zu finden, und W. KÖHLERs Vermutung (1938) angeführt, daß diesen Sachverhalten bestimmte vektorielle Zustände im körperlichen Geschehen zuzuordnen seien.

In verschiedenen dieser Hinsichten ist schon mehr oder weniger von dem wechselseitigen „Entgegenkommen" der physiologischen und psychologischen Befunde zu bemerken, auf das wir seit FECHNER hoffen. In anderen sind zwar psychologische Versuche schon durchgeführt, u. a. zur Psychophysik der Größenkonstanz und der anschaulichen Distanz überhaupt (JACOBS, MADLUNG, SCHNEHAGE, OGASAWARA, KLEINBUB), haben aber bisher keine Resonanz gefunden. Auch zur Frage der Bedeutung von Konturen für die „laterale Interaktion" gibt es schon zerstreute Beobachtungen. Und Versuche zur Psychophysik des sensorium commune wären unschwer zu entwickeln.

In einigen anderen Hinsichten sieht es im Augenblick so aus, als ob Psychologie und Neurophysiologie niemals zusammenkommen könnten, ja als ob sie sich mehr und mehr voneinander entfernten.

Von Anfang an mußte man sich mit der Tatsache abfinden, daß nicht Zustand gleich Zustand und Prozeß gleich Prozeß ist, sondern daß auf der physischen Seite *ausschließlich Prozesse* in Frage kommen, daß also auch psychischen *Ruhezuständen* ausnahmslos psychophysische *Vorgänge* zugeordnet sind, den wahrnehmungsmäßig starren oder festen Gebilden also durchweg stationäre Zustände bzw. Fließgleichgewichte entsprechen. Andere Widersprüche sind erst im Verlauf der anatomisch-physiologischen Forschung in aller Schärfe hervorgetreten. Dazu gehört

a) der Widerspruch zwischen der (von den wechselnden anschaulichen Grenzverläufen abgesehen) *grundsätzlich kontinuierlichen* räumlichen Verteilung der Sinnesgegebenheiten — und der (auch abgesehen von der letztlich atomistischen Struktur der Materie) höchst komplizierten Mikrostruktur und *Diskontinuität* des nervösen Feldes, in dem sich die zugehörigen Prozesse abspielen (die Verflechtung von Nerven- und Gliazellen, die Unterbrechung durch Gefäße usw.).

b) Der Widerspruch zwischen der zeitlichen Kontinuität des seelischen Geschehens und der zeitlichen Diskontinuität des physiologischen, sofern dieses – wie Hunderte von Diagrammen während dieser Woche gezeigt haben – durchweg aus mehr oder weniger dichten Serien von offenbar isolierten Einzelereignissen (spikes, shots) besteht. Es war bis heute auch nicht möglich, irgendeine spezielle Bewußtseinserscheinung zu finden, die den *niedrig frequenten* (Bergerschen oder Kornmüllerschen) Schwingungen streng parallel verlief: Eine erste Andeutung davon stellen *vielleicht* die Befunde BARTLEYs über Flimmerphänomene dar, in denen er eine Resonanz auf eine "intrinsic fluctuation of cortical process" mit einer Schwingungsdauer von $^1/_{10}$ sec oder einfachen Vielfachen davon vermutet.

c) Die härteste Nuß für den Psychophysiker ist aber wohl das Alles- oder Nichtsgesetz der Nerventätigkeit, das man geradezu eine physiologische Quantentheorie nennen könnte, und demzufolge der stufenlosen Graduierung von psychischen Intensitäten (z. B. auch muskulären Anstrengungen) wieder die Dichte von Entladungssalven im räumlichen Querschnitt und in der Zeitfolge gegenübersteht.

Ob und wie diese drei Formen des Widerspruches zwischen anschaulicher Kontinuität und neurophysiologischer Diskontinuität aufgelöst werden können, wissen wir noch nicht.

Ich beobachte mit einiger Sorge, daß man unter diesen Umständen dazu neigt, sich auf die Terminologie der *Informationstheorie* zurückzuziehen, wie es hier besonders konkret GRÜSSER in seiner Demonstration von richtungsspezifischen Erregungsmustern getan hat, die ich meinen Ausführungen als Beispiel zugrunde legen will. Es ist richtig, daß diese Muster „ausreichenden Informationswert" besitzen; d. h., daß sie für einen Adressaten, der den Code kennt und zu entschlüsseln vermag, alle notwendigen Unterlagen enthalten. Sie sind Ereignisse, die *als Anzeichen* („Kriterien") für bestimmte Bewegungsrichtungen *dienen können* für denjenigen, der ihre Bedeutung versteht. Bei allen diesen informationstheoretischen Betrachtungen ist, wie man sieht, stets ein Empfänger oder Adressat impliziert, der selber *jenseits der psychophysischen Vorgänge steht*, wie ein Techniker neben dem Elektronenhirn, und die von ihm gelieferten Meldungen abliest und interpretiert. Dabei kehrt man aber, genau besehen, zu dem reinen, d. h. nicht mehr physiologisch repräsentierten, urteilenden Geist von HELMHOLTZ zurück; d. h. man führt durch die Hintertür wieder psychologische Vorgänge ein, die *kein* physiologisches Korrelat besitzen. Das psychophysische Problem ist so nicht lösbar: Was wir zu erklären haben, ist *nicht*, wie ein neben der Natur stehender Geist mehr oder weniger eindeutige „Meldungen" oder Nachrichten über irgendwelche dahinter verborgenen Sachverhalte oder Ereignisse (z. B. als Meldungen über Bewegungen, die sich auf der Sinnesfläche abspielen) *interpretiert*, sondern – z. B. im Falle GRÜSSERs – daß in einer anschaulichen Welt *Bewegungen* (Drehungen, Verlagerungen, Wachsen, Schrumpfen, Sichkrümmen, Sichstrecken) *selbst stattfinden*, die zwar unter günstigen Bedingungen eine wirkliche Bewegung in der physikalischen Umgebung des Organismus richtig *abbilden*, aber als solche keiner weiteren Interpretation bedürfen. Durch die gegenwärtig versuchten informationstheoretischen Gedankengänge wird also das hier vorliegende Problem nicht gelöst, sondern nur umgangen oder zurückgeschoben.

Ob die geschilderten Paradoxe sich auflösen lassen, oder ob es echte und endgültige Aporien sind, wissen wir noch nicht. Vielleicht bekommen wir in unseren elektrophysiologischen Beobachtungen *gar nicht die psychophysischen Prozesse selbst zu Gesicht*, sondern nur ihre Ursachen (oder einen Teil davon), oder gewisse Begleiterscheinungen davon. Vielleicht endeckt man eines Tages erst die „eigentlichen" psychophysischen Prozesse, die möglicherweise dem Alles-oder-Nichts-Gesetz gar nicht unterworfen sind und von den anatomischen Strukturen des Cortex nicht unterbrochen werden.

Aber selbst wenn es gelänge, diese Schwierigkeiten aufzulösen, dürften wir nicht erwarten, daß die beiden Ansichten der psychophysischen Vorgänge, die subjektive und die objektive, sich einmal in jeder Hinsicht zur Deckung bringen lassen. Wir müssen auf jeden Fall damit rechnen, daß auf dem verwickelten Weg der vermittelnden physikalischen und physiologischen Vorgänge, auf denen alle „objektive" Beobachtung beruht, wesentliche Eigenschaften der beobachteten Objekte unwiederbringlich verlorengehen, daß wir aber auf der anderen Seite dabei auf Eigenschaften der Objekte stoßen, die ihrer Natur nach psychisch nicht repräsentiert werden können.

So hat die im Kleinsten atomistische Struktur der physikalisch untersuchten Materie im Bewußtsein kein Korrelat. Andererseits wird sich aber auch der Traum des Mystikers FECHNER nie verwirklichen lassen: etwas der Buntheit der Sinnesqualitäten, der Gefühle und der Ausdruckserscheinungen Entsprechendes — aber auch schon so einfache Sachverhalte wie die *Nichtbeliebigkeit* anschaulicher Bezugssysteme — mit physikalischen Verfahren aufzuspüren oder zu bestätigen.

Summary

In a first part it is pointed out that the principle of isomorphism, which is usually considered as a last step of development of psychophysics, has been clearly formulated already by the founder of psychophysics, G. TH. FECHNER, and by E. HERING; W. KÖHLER, to whom the principle of isomorphism is often attributed, has instead the merit of eliminating some difficulties which were so far an impediment to the concrete application of the principle.

In a second part six postulates or expectations of the psychologist concerning the nature of the psychophysical correlates of perception are formulated. Three of them (the HERING color-theory, WERTHEIMER's assumption of lateral interaction („Querfunktionen"), and W. KÖHLER's assumption of „Freizügigkeit" or of variability of the pathways of afferent process) are substantiated by several physiological contributions to this symposion, while the three remaining postulates (LASHLEY's assumption of the formation of "functional units" independent of anatomical structures, v. WEIZSÄCKER's assumption of a "sensorium commune", and a postulate of W. KÖHLER concerning the psychophysics of higher mental processes) are still open.

In a 3rd part some divergencies between physiological and introspective findings are discussed, which in recent time seem to have rather increased than diminished (e. g. the spatial discontinuity of neural microstructure, the temporal discontinuity of nervous discharges, the all-or-none-law, the process character of correlates even of static percepts).

It follows a criticism of some actual attempts at solving these problems by means of information theory.

Literatur

1. FECHNER, G. TH.: Elemente der Psychophysik. Leipzig: Breitkopf u. Härtel 1860.
1a. GIBSON, J. J.: The perception of the visual world. Boston und New York 1950.
2. JACOBS, M. H.: Über den Einfluß des phänomenalen Abstandes auf die Unterschiedsschwelle für Helligkeiten. Psychol. Forsch. 18, 98—142 (1933).
3. KLEINBUB, M.: Über die Unterschiedsschwelle für Helligkeiten bei verschiedenen Abständen der Vergleichsobjekte und Fixationswechsel. Diss. Berlin 1933.
4. KÖHLER, W.: Über unbemerkte Empfindungen und Urteils-Täuschungen. Z. Physiol. 66, 51—80 (1913).
5. — Die physischen Gestalten in Ruhe und im stationären Zustand. Braunschweig: Fr. Vieweg & Sohn 1920.
6. — Ein altes Scheinproblem, Naturwissenschaften 17, 395—401 (1929).
7. — Zur Psychophysik des Vergleichs und des Raumes. Psychol. Forsch. 18, 343—360 (1933).
8. — The place of value in a world of facts. New York: Liveright Publ. Corporat. 1938.
9. LASHLEY, K. S.: Basic neural mechanisms in behavior. Psychol. Rev. 37 (1930).
10. MADLUNG, K.: Über anschauliche und funktionale Nachbarschaft von Tasteindrücken. Psychol. Forsch. 19, 193—236 (1934).
11. METZGER, W.: Zum gegenwärtigen Stand der Psychophysik. Stud. Gen. 3, 261—270 (1950).
12. MÜLLER, G. E.: Zur Psychophysik der Gesichtsempfindungen. Z. Psychol. 10, 1—82, 321—413 (1896).
13. OGASAWARA, I.: Über den Einfluß des phänomenalen Abstandes auf das Auftreten von β (stroboskopischer) Bewegung. Jap. J. Psychol. 11, 109—122 (1936).
14. SCHNEHAGE, H. I.: Versuche über taktile Scheinbewegung bei Variation phänomenaler Bedingungen. Arch. Psychol. 104, 175—228 (1939).
15. WERTHEIMER, M.: Experimentelle Studien über das Sehen von Bewegungen. Z. Psychol. 61, 161—265 (1912).

Diskussion

L. M. HURVICH: 1. Isn't it true, that MACH the eminent physicist also played a prominent role in the development of the psychophysiological axioms ?

2. The all-or-none principle no longer presents the difficulties it once did. Graded potentials — as much of the work presented here gives evidence of — are important components of the electrophysiological responses.

E. BAUMGARDT: Prof. METZGER hat die Begriffe Information, Codage und Urteil zueinander in Beziehung gebracht. Welcher Natur auch die Information, die in codierter Sprache den höheren Zentren zugeführt wird, sei, so kann ein Urteil, d. h. eine bewußte Reaktion, ausschließlich dank einer vorher gewonnenen *Erfahrung* erfolgen. Letztere aber verbindet eben diese codierte Information mit einer gegebenen Situation. So erschwert das Tragen einer Umkehrbrille die Bewegung im Raum, bis die neu codierte Information ohne zusätzliche Latenz verstanden wird. Ohne auf die praktische Anwendbarkeit der Informationstheorie auf den Sehmechanismus eingehen zu wollen, möchte ich doch feststellen, daß betreffs der Urteilsbildung keinerlei Bedenken vorzuliegen scheinen.

W. SICKEL: Die Informationstheorie erschöpft sich keineswegs in der Codierung von Nachrichten. Zu den aufgeworfenen Problemen liefert sie Rahmengesetze und läßt Mögliches von Unmöglichem trennen. Insbesondere werden eine Reihe von Phänomenen einer quantitativen Behandlung zugängig (Alles- oder Nichts-Gesetz). Der scheinbare Widerspruch objektiv zu verzeichnender Aktivität ohne subjektive Wahrnehmung beinhaltet den Begriff der Funktionsbereitschaft.

H. SCHOBER: Ich stimme sehr mit Prof. METZGER überein, daß man die Begriffe und Gesetze der Informationstheorie nicht ohne weiteres auf die Physiologie und Psychologie des Sehens anwenden kann. Diese Gesetze sind ursprünglich nur für die Hochfrequenzphysik geschaffen worden und haben die Unabhängigkeit und lineare Addierbarkeit der Meldungen als Voraussetzung. Gerade das ist aber beim Sehorgan nicht der Fall. Trotz mancher Erfolge, die die Informationstheorie im Bereich der Optik hatte, glaube ich, daß ihre gute Zeit hier bereits vorüber ist.

H.-L. Teuber: One can readily agree with Prof. Metzger's warnings against abuses of information theory in physiology and psychology, but there are some uses. The most important one is very simple (though often overlooked): Information theory permits us to specify our stimuli in a new way — not only in terms of the stimuli that are present at any one moment, but also in terms of those stimuli that might have been there but were not. Considerations of this sort (e. g. Broadbent[1]) can be quite helpful. The same, of course, is true of description of responses: We can and ought to describe them in terms, not only of the present response, but in terms of the ensemble of responses possible for the system.

W. Metzger: Zu Herrn Hurvichs Bemerkung möchte ich sagen, daß ich mich außer seinem Buch über die Analyse der Empfindungen zwar keiner ausdrücklichen Ausführungen von Ernst Mach über psychophysische Axiome entsinnen kann, wohl aber einiger kühner und unbekümmerter Versuche ihrer Anwendung, z. B. in der Theorie des monocularen Raumsehens sowie seiner ersten originellen Arbeiten über den Simultan-Kontrast, die für Herings Axiome richtunggebend waren.

Da die folgenden Bemerkungen sich sämtlich auf die Frage der Anwendbarkeit der *Informationstheorie* beziehen, will ich versuchen, sie im ganzen zu erörtern, muß mich dabei aber auf einige ganz allgemeine Bemerkungen beschränken: Die Wahrnehmung *ist* ein typischer Fall von Nachrichtenübermittlung, und ich bin mit Herrn Teuber der Meinung, daß es nur sinnvoll und höchst anregend ist, wenn man versucht, festzustellen, ob und wie weit die in der technischen Nachrichtenübermittlung entwickelten und dort bewährten Modi auch beim biologischen Organismus Anwendung finden. Daß dabei, z. B. beim Durchgang durch die Nerven, kontinuierlich variable Vorgänge in diskontinuierliche übersetzt und am anderen Ende wieder zurückübersetzt werden (was wohl Herr Sickel vor allem im Auge hatte), entspricht grundlegenden Verfahren der technischen Übermittlung. Daß trotzdem wesentliche Vorgänge in einer in der modernen Nachrichtentechnik bisher noch *nicht* bekannten Weise ablaufen, haben u. a. Millers Untersuchungen über die mystische Zahl 7 gezeigt; (an Abweichungen der dort beschriebenen Art hat wohl Herr Schober in erster Linie gedacht).

Aber von allen diesen Erwägungen bleibt das eigentlichste Problem der Psychophysik der Wahrnehmung unberührt, das Problem, das Herr Baumgardt in seiner Bemerkung andeutet: nämlich *welcher Natur die Vorgänge sind*, die in den höheren Zentren — also am Ende des Informationskanals — sich abspielen, und dieses Problem ist, wie mir scheint, einer informationstheoretischen Erklärung unzugänglich, da es unabhängig davon besteht, ob diese Vorgänge Information über die physikalische Außenwelt enthalten oder nicht. Sofern sie aber bestimmte und lebenswichtige Information enthalten, haben gerade die kürzlich bekannt gewordenen Versuche von Eleanor J. Gibson und R. D. Walk über die Grundlagen der Tiefenwahrnehmung[2] gezeigt, daß dazu erstaunlicherweise *keine* vorher gewonnene Erfahrung erforderlich ist, daß man also mit empirischen Ansätzen hier nicht weiterkommt.

---

[1] Broadbent, D. E.: Perception and Communication. New York: Pergamon Press 1958.

[2] The "Visual Cliff". Scientific American, April 1960, p. 64—71.

Nachtrag zu AII:
Receptoren, Gliazellen und Retinaneurone

Glial Control of Neuronal Networks and Receptors*

By

Gunnar Svaetichin, Miguel Laufer, Genyo Mitarai, Richard Fatehchand,
Edmundo Vallecalle and Jorge Villegas

With 6 Figures

Our experimental findings which showed the glial origin of the retinal S-potentials and their behavior were for the first time presented and discussed at this symposium. The conference, concerning the same subject, given by Svaetichin (October 26, 1960) at Washington, stimulated his old friend and colleague Robert Galambos to write a paper concerning "a glia-neural theory of brain function" [Proc. Nat. Acad. Sci. 47, 129 —136 (1961)]. This exciting article is a much better introduction to our work than anything we could have written ourselves, since it emphasizes the problem faced by the conventional "millisecond" neurophysiology and the neuron theory when trying to explain complex functions of our nervous system, as for instance sleep, alertness, learning, memory, inborn instinctive behavior, etc., and also gives a historical review of earlier thought, suggesting an important role for the glia in brain function. Anatomical and biochemical studies (Nansen, Holmgren, Kornmüller, Hydén, Sjöstrand, de Robertis, G. Villegas and others) suggest the existence of interactions between the neuron and the glia; however, our studies directly demonstrate that the glial cells exert a metabolic excitability control on the neurons. Actually, all investigations on the S-potentials which have been carried out since 1953 are studies on the functional mechanisms of the glial cells, although this had not been realized before we definitely localized the recording site of the micro-electrode to individual Müller fibers and (glial) horizontal cells of the Teleost retina. Thus, there already exists considerable information concerning the physiological aspects of the glia-neuron interaction.

In the following, we describe our histological determination of the recording sites of the S-potentials, and review present knowledge of the glial-neuronal structures of the retina. Finally, we consider this information in the light of our recent physiological findings on the glial-neuronal interactions.

1. Histological determination of the recording site of the micro-electrode

The lack of accurate localizations of micro-electrodes introduced into the depths of central nervous structures has for long complicated the interpretation of the recordings obtained. Numerous attempts have been made to localize the recording sites of the retinal potentials, but as far as we know, no one has been able to demonstrate exactly from which individual cell the actual intra-cellular recording has been obtained. For localization purposes,

* Department of Physiology, Instituto Venezolano de Investigaciones Científicas, Caracas, Venezuela.

MacNichol, Macpherson and Svaetichin (7) and MacNichol and Svaetichin (8) used capillary micro-electrodes filled with crystal violet. At the recording site, the stain was passed electrophoretically out of the electrode, the retina then being fixed and sectioned by the freezing technique. The above mentioned authors had been able to show that the L-response originated at the level of the large horizontal cells, whereas the C-response was produced by structures 20—30 μ deeper, corresponding to the level of the bipolars. However, definite localization to an individual cell was not achieved. Mitarai (9, 10) obtained similar results using lithium carmine as the marking dye and working with paraffin embedded material.

On the basis of the experience obtained by Mitarai and our own laboratory, new efforts were made to localize histologically the site of the micro-electrode tip. The main obstacle in all of our experiments had been the fast disappearance of the spot of stain due to diffusion. Furthermore, ordinary histological procedures involving washing in water, alcohol, xylene, etc., usually dissolved the deposited stain, except when the dye showed a specific affinity for certain cell structures. A large number of different stains were tested, and lithium carmine proved to have the most favorable properties for the marking purpose since 1. it dissolved well in a neutral or alkaline medium, while it was insoluble in acid media, and 2. it diffused at a slower rate than any other stain.

In our present experiments, the capillary-type micro-electrode was filled with an almost saturated neutral or weakly alkaline solution of lithium carmine, without the addition of any other electrolyte. Under these conditions the dye had a positive charge and moved electrophoretically towards the cathode. The stain solution was first centrifuged, and then introduced into the wide upper shaft of the electrode, the thin branch and the tip being previously filled with distilled water. Electrodes showing a 10—20 megohm resistance were selected, and a successfully prepared electrode could be used for all the markings done in one retina. In the localization experiments, the isolated retina was deprived of its pigment layer and examined in transmitted light under the dissecting microscope. When a current of 10^{-8} to 10^{-9} amp. ways passed through the electrode for about half a minute, the formation of a just visible spot around the tip of the micro-electrode could be observed. For the marking experiments, the isolated retina was spread out on a filter paper in which a pattern of small holes had been cut, and all markings were done within one of these holes. The use of filter paper kept the retina flat and easy to handle. In a restricted area of the retina, 10—20 markings corresponding to a certain type of response were made, whereupon the retina was fixed in Bouin's solution. After fixation for one hour in this solution, the small parts containing the markings were separated from the rest of the retina, and the filter paper removed, the pieces then being embedded in a 20% gelatine solution to which 5% glycerol had been added. Serial sections, 20—30 μ thick, were cut with a freezing microtome and spread out on the surface of slightly acid ice-cold water. The sections were then mounted in glycerol.

The difficulty in using heavy metal salts for marking purposes has been pointed out by several investigators, since these salts coagulate the cytoplasm and adhere to the tip of the electrode, pulling out the cell when the electrode is removed. An excess of current also coagulates the cytoplasm, the outcome being the same as when heavy metal salts are used.

The micrographs shown in A and B of Fig. 1 illustrate the results obtained from these experiments, in which we succeeded in determining the intra-cellular recording site of the electrode in an individual cell. The cell, into which the micro-electrode was inserted, was stained in a reddish color and showed up clearly in our color micrographs. In black and white reproductions, the stained cell appeared with a higher optical density than those surrounding it. Fig. 1, A illustrates the results corresponding to markings of the L-type of response, i. e., a horizontal cell (arrow). The C-response, i. e., the Müller fiber, can be seen in Fig. 1, B. Our recordings from the Müller fiber were obtained at the level of the internal bipolars, where this cell has its largest expansion. In the fish retina the Müller fiber apparently is large enough to permit an intra-cellular recording to be obtained at the level of the internal bipolars. The horizontal cell always remained intact and evenly stained during the marking experiments, whereas the Müller fiber "explodcd" during the electrophoretic procedure. The typical picture observed when a C-response marking was made was a deeply stained nucleus with granulated cytoplasm spread around it, as well as a proximal broken end of a Müller fiber which had a slight reddish stain (Fig. 1, B, arrow below). Paraffin embedded material showed this same feature in markings done for the C-response, although we never succeeded in preserving the stain in the horizontal cell due to all the different treatments necessary for the inclusion in paraffin. The Müller cell seems to have a specific affinity to lithium carmine, while the horizontal cell does not.

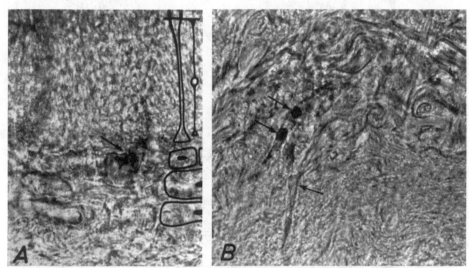

Fig. 1. *A* Localization of L-response in retina of fish (Centropomidae) retina. The horizontal cell (He) indicated by arrow was stained by the marking dye. Right: boundaries of the three layers of horizontal cells are indicated, and also a rod and a cone. *B* Localization of C-response (Centropomidae). Typical picture: deeply stained Müller cell nucleus (upper arrow), surrounded by scattered granulated cytoplasm originating from cell "explosion," and broken end of Müller fiber (arrow below).

Therefore, we only used freezing sectioning, a method which was found to perfectly preserve the tissue without shrinking, and which also gave a very clear picture of the glial structures. On examination of our serial sections with a magnification of 400 times, we were able to find more than 50% of the deposited marking spots.

2. Glial-neuronal structures in the retina

Ultrastructural studies on the retina of a shallow water fish (Centropomus) have been carried out by Dr. GLORIA VILLEGAS at this Institute (*18, 19*), whose research and whose numerous discussions with us have been of paramount importance for our work. The following general description is mainly based on her studies, and for additional information we refer to her original papers.

a) **The Müller fibers.** The Müller fiber is beyond any doubt a glial cell and was classified as such by CAJAL. The Müller fiber (Fig. 2, M) is radially oriented, extending between the internal and external limiting membranes of the retina, which two membranes in fact are formed by these cells. At the level of the internal bipolars the Müller fibers show expansions which are interspersed in the inner-most layer of the internal horizontal cells (Fig. 2, Hi). The Müller fibers are in membrane to membrane contact in their expanded parts, forming in this way a tangential net which is partly interwoven with the one composed by the internal horizontal cells.

   b) **The horizontal cells.** The large horizontal cells of the fish retina are a kind of glial cell (*19*); in any case, they are definitely not neurons, since their cytoplasmic structure is of the glial type and further, they have no axons or any synaptic

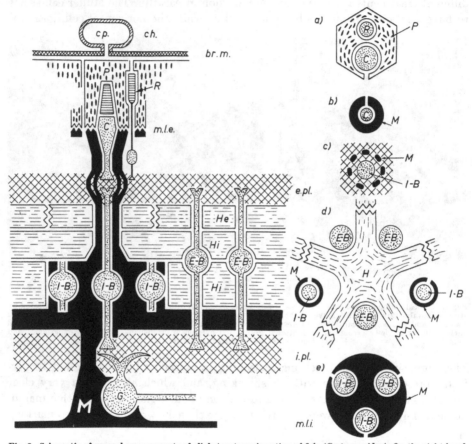

Fig. 2. Schematic of general arrangements of glial structures in retina of fish *(Centropomidae)*. On the right hand side, the relations of glial cells to receptors (*a, b*) and to bipolar cells (*c, d, e*) are shown at different levels. *C* cones. *E—B* external bipolars. *G* ganglion cell. *H* horizontal cell. *He* external horizontal cell. *Hi* internal horizontal cell. *I-B* internal bipolar cell. *M* Müller fiber. *P* pigment cell. *R* rods. *br. m.* Bruch's membrane. *ch.* choroid. *cp* capillary vessel. *e. pl.* external plexiform layer. *i. pl.* internal plexiform layer. *m. l. e.* external limiting membrane. *m. l. i.* internal limiting membrane

connections. These horizontal cells of the fish should not be confused with those which POLYAK (*12*) calls "horizontal cells" of the primate retina, these latter cells being tangentially oriented neurons.

   The horizontal cells of the fish retina are divided into three layers; adopting CAJAL's terminology (*13*), the horizontal cells of the first layer are termed external horizontal cells (Fig. 2, He), while those of the second and third layers are called internal horizontal cells (Fig. 2, Hi). The external horizontals clearly differ in their cytoplasmic structure from the internal ones. The short processes of the first row of small horizontal cells are in membrane to membrane contact with each other forming a continuous net, the interspaces containing the dendritic processes of the bipolars, most of which are enveloped by the Müller fibers. The large star-shaped internal horizontal cells have long processes, the large meshes of the continuous net they form being filled up by the bipolars, most of the bipolars being surrounded by a thin mantle of Müller fiber cytoplasm and only a few of them being directly in contact with the horizontal cells (see Fig. 2).

In her studies on the primate and human retina, G. VILLEGAS (19) discovered in the extra-foveal regions cellular structures equivalent to the horizontal cells of the fish retina, those cells being situated between the external plexiform layer (Fig. 2, e. pl.) and the bipolars, where they form a continuous net similar to those made up by the horizontal cells of fish. However, these elements are of such small dimensions that they were missed by the light microscopists, and are lacking in the fovea, where only the Müller fiber glia exists. It is probable that this glial network of the primate and human retina is also involved in a glial mechanism of adaptation (11), having a function similar to the one described below for the horizontal cells of the fish retina.

c) The glial networks and barriers. From the description given above it is seen that the retina, which is a central nervous tissue, is infiltrated by a number of tangential glial nets, those of the horizontal cells and of the Müller fibers having been described above. The Müller fibers also simultaneously constitute the radial glia of the retina. At the level of the internal limiting membrane the expansions of the Müller fibers together form a continuous glial barrier in which the ganglion cell bodies are totally embedded. In the retina of another fish (Mugillidae) studied in this laboratory, light microscopy shows the existence of two more tangential glial nets situated at the external and internal margins of the inner plexiform layer (Fig. 2, i. pl.). According to G. VILLEGAS (personal communication) the network seen at the external margin is built up of extensions from amacrine cells of glial character, the cytoplasmic structure of these cells being similar to that of the Müller fibers, which differs to some extent from the fibrillar cytoplasm of the horizontal cells. The pigment cells form another "glial" barrier, the outer segments of the photo-receptors being embedded in this layer. Hence, the retina is built up not only of receptors and neurons but to a great, and as will be shown below, functionally important extent of glial cells, which form intricate nets and barrier layers (six tangential nets and two barriers), the glial cells being in intimate membrane to membrane contact with one another and with the receptors and the neurons.

Ultra-structural studies by G. VILLEGAS (18, 19 and personal communication) show that these tangentially oriented glial networks are continuous, extending throughout the whole retina, the membrane to membrane contacts between the glial processes being very close indeed. From electron-micrographs which show these inter-glial contacts, one has the impression that there is something peculiar with the cell membranes of these regions, since they seem to be partly discontinuous. This question needs further attention; however, there is an indication of a syncytium-like continuity of the glial networks. Our studies on the functional activity described below definitely show that the metabolic reaction of the horizontal cell, and also of the Müller fiber, spreads to neighboring cells bringing into action wide areas of the retinal networks. This tangential spreading of the glial reaction constitutes (see MITARAI et al. this symposium) an important mechanism for controlling the level of adaptation (excitability) of the retina.

The transfer of matter from the vasal circulatory system to the neurons and receptors is beyond any doubt bound to be carried out by the glial cells. Even without taking into account the support for such a view obtained from ultra-structural studies of nervous tissues (1, 2, 15, 19), this is self-evident when one considers the fact that in the Teleost vasal circulation is completely lacking inside the retina (14, 20). It is therefore necessary for the pigment cells (glia) to transfer substances from the chorioid plexus, the Müller fibers carrying out a corresponding mission on the vitreous side, where the circulation is either supplied by the capillary nets of the falciform body (e. g. *Centropomidae*) or by the hyaloretinal vessels (e. g. *Mugillidae*), neither vasal system entering the retina. Thus the two glial barrier layers, limiting the retina towards the vasal circulatory systems on both sides, function as blood-brain barriers, this being in agreement with views earlier expressed by several authors (1, 2, 15, 19). These are anatomical facts which further stress the importance of an inter-glial and glial-neuronal transfer and inter-action.

The glial networks as seen in the retina, which in itself is a central nervous tissue, have their anatomical and certainly also their functional counterparts in the cortex. (The structural similarity is strikingly seen when comparing the retinal Müller fibers, ref. 13, Fig. 187, p. 300 with the cortical glial cells, ref. 13, Fig. 51, II, p. 70.) We are therefore convinced that our observations concerning the retinal glial networks can be generalized, offering a new approach to the understanding of the functional mechanisms of the nervous system.

3. Glial networks controlling excitability levels and integrative functions of neuronal circuits

Here we discuss the results of our recent studies on glial-neuronal behavior, and the new approach these offer to several of the unsolved problems of classical neurophysiology. When the glial cell and the neuron were normally interacting the intracellularly recorded membrane potentials were always found to behave in opposite ways. These opposite reactions of the glial and neuronal membranes have been tested under physiological conditions and stimulation, and during exposure to temperature changes, CO_2, NH_3, etc. (4). The intracellular recordings were obtained for the following types of glia: Müller fiber, horizontal cell and other retinal glial cells, and from the following neuronal structures: perikaryon, dendrite and myelinated axon. It should be noticed that a nerve cell membrane which lacked glia in its normal functional state (the glial function having been abolished by exposure to NH_3, cocain, etc., or by absence of 5% CO_2), showed the conventional behavior well known from all work up to now, as for instance the studies on axons isolated by dissection. Under these conditions the amplitudes of the membrane resting and action potentials of the neuron varied very little with the temperature. According to the Nernst formula only a membrane potential change of 3% would be expected to be produced by a 10°C change of temperature, although with the glia in its normal functional state striking changes due to temperature variations were produced in the membrane potentials recorded from the neuron and the glial cell. Under these normal experimental conditions a temperature change of $10°C$ caused a more than 50% change of the GMP (glial membrane potential), the resting and acting membrane potentials of myelinated axons changing by about 25%, while corresponding amplitude alterations of up to 60% were observed in the perikaryon of the spinal ganglion cell. The changes of the neuronal membrane potentials were always opposite to the ones observed in the retinal glial cells.

These experiments demonstrate that the glial membrane potential (GMP) is directly dependent on metabolic processes, which processes we have shown to be promptly and vigorously modified in opposite directions by CO_2 and NH_3 (H, OH, CO_3, NH_4 and other ions having no comparable effect). The membrane potentials of neuronal structures lacking glia in their normal functional state, and of the muscle cell which has no glial envelope, reacted under the corresponding experimental conditions in a way which indicated the absence of a similar direct metabolic dependence.

The neuronal circuits including their synapses, and the receptors, were found to be excitation carriers exclusively. A graded excitability control of the neurons is performed by the hyperpolarizing, metabolic reaction of the glial networks (alpha-adaptation in the retina), this corresponding to a graded setting of the membrane potential levels of the nerve cells. The hyperpolarizing "plastic" (HERNÁNDEZ PEÓN) excitability control process spreads in the glial networks with a velocity of 0.35 m/sec, while the inhibitory depolarizing process (Müller fiber) spreads with a velocity of 0.15 m/sec (Isolated Teleost retina, at $25°C$). The Müller fiber controls the excitability of the chain: ganglion cell-bipolar-receptor, with which cells the Müller fiber is closely related (Fig. 2). After abolishing the glial function with NH_3 the receptor action potential showed an amplitude higher than before the exposure (see MITARAI et al. this symposium). It might be suggested that there exists a glial sensitivity control of the photoreceptors, at least of the cones. Possibly such a glial control also is important for the regulation of the sensitivity of the auditory receptors.

In the intact sciatic nerve kept in $O_2 + 5\%\ CO_2$, LORENTE DE NÓ (5) demonstrated a striking correlation between the excitability and the slow electrotonus (L-fraction). Our work, in which full-sized intracellular resting and action potentials were recorded from sciatic axons, shows that the slow L-fraction of the electrotonus corresponds to the glial (Schwann cell) control of the excitability of the neuron. This glial control did not operate in the absence of $5\%\ CO_2$, neither did it function more than 10 minutes after opening the peri-neuronal sheaths. Consequently, all work which has been done on isolated myelinated axons shows the functional characteristics of the axon alone in the absence of the metabolic excitability control exerted by the Schwann cell.

Only EPSP's were found in intracellular recordings from retinal ganglion cell dendrites (IPSP's were *never* obtained from dendrites). The inhibitory phenomena were only seen as hyperpolarization of the perikaryon and axon membranes, induced by the depolarizing (metabolic) process of the glia (Müller fiber). The intracellular dendritic EPSP's recorded both at "on" and "off" of the stimulus were depolarizing saw-tooth transients, the intracellular ganglion cell spike patterns being synchronous to them. (See Fig. 3, in LAUFER et al., this symposium.) However, the hyperpolarizing inhibitory membrane potential change of the ganglion cell was a steady graded square wave, opposite in sign to, and a mirror image of the depolarizing Müller fiber response.

Electron-microscopy by GLORIA VILLEGAS at this Institute definitely shows that the ganglion cell bodies of the vertebrate retina are embedded in glia (Müller fiber), and that they totally lack synaptic connection, the synapses being found to terminate only on the dendrites (personal communication). Consequently, it is concluded that in the retina the inhibitory process is of glial origin, and not synaptic. This hypothesis, if valid for the whole nervous system, would explain for instance the disagreement concerning the inhibitory mechanisms of the spinal cord (ECCLES-LLOYD, see discussion in Ref. 6).

Thus, the excitability control and inhibition of the neurons depend on opposite metabolic processes, agreeing with the prophesies of EWALD HERING, who attempted to explain the mutual antagonistic interactions of black-white and opponent colors on the basis of opposite metabolic processes depending directly on the cellular responses to stimulation, as has now been found to occur in the glial cells.

It might be suggested that the different velocities of the spreading of the excitability control processes in the glial networks depend on the different diffusion rates of CO_2 and NH_3 in the tissue, these two substances being the critical mediators governing the metabolic processes (glycolysis, proteolysis) which have opposite effects on the electrical glial cell reactions. It is tempting to suggest that the analeptic and ataraxic effects of CO_2 and NH_3 are caused by a direct influence on the glial metabolism. It is also suggested, that the specific and often opposite effects on different parts of the nervous system of many drugs, ultimately depends on whether the enzymatic systems in the different cells favor or inhibit the release of CO_2 or NH_3. In this connection it is of interest to mention that carbonic anhydrase shows an 80 times higher concentration in the glia than in the neuron (E. GIACOBINI, personal communication).

Most likely anesthetics, sedatives and in general neurotropic drugs exert their effects by interfering with the glial metabolism, which controls the excitability and membrane permeability characteristics of the neurons. According to this view the primary effect is on the glial cell which mediates the metabolic influence on the nerve cell membrane. Certain drugs like Tridione (anti-serotonin) produce color vision disturbances, probably by influencing the glial metabolism. Serotonin, pseudo-cholinesterase, etc. are localized in glial cells, and are also involved in the mechanisms of many psycho-tropic drugs. Administration of serotonin or serotonin-like compounds elicits schizophrenic-like symptoms (W. WOOLLEY).

Probably the fundamental cause of epilepsy will be found in disturbances of the glial cell metabolism. Lack of CO_2 (hyperventilation epilepsy) or a rapid lowering of the temperature (shivering) produces a condition of hyperexcitability and uncoordinated nervous activity. We found that the retinal ganglion cells which had been largely disengaged from the glial control showed an uncoordinated, periodic, high frequency firing and hyperexcitability, while simultaneously large glial oscillations were observed.

The wavelength dependences of the retinal S-potentials correlate exactly with the psycho-physical processes for brightness and color vision (HERING, MÜLLER,

ADAMS, SCHRÖDINGER, JUDD, TALBOT, HURVICH), suggesting that the overall activity of the brain is under direct glial "programming-engramming" control. Comparing Fig. 3 with Fig. 4 one finds the agreement very striking indeed.

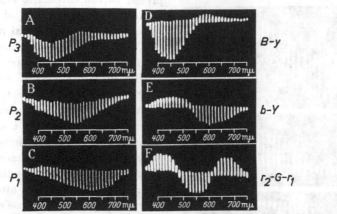

Fig. 3. *A-C* different L-responses obtained from the horizontal cells. *D* the C-response recorded from the Müller fiber; *E* the opposite polarity response of the amacrine glia; *F* the triphasic C-response obtained from tangential glial cells at the level of the proximal dendrites of the ganglion cells. *Mugillidae*

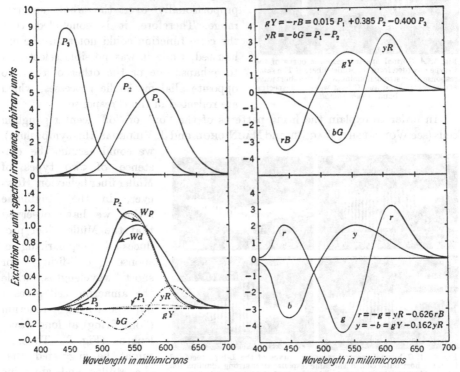

Fig. 4. Diagram illustrating the zone theory of v. KRIES and G. E. MÜLLER (from JUDD, Ref. 3)

The spectral response curves of Fig. 3 were obtained from glial cells in the fish (!) retina, while the zone theory diagram of Fig. 4 is based on psychophysical experiments on man (!).

$P_1 - P_2 - P_3$ corresponds to the tri-chromatic receptor input (Young-Helmholtz), while $b - y$ and $r - g - r$ are the opponent processes (Hering) elaborated by integrative, glial-neuronal interactions. The $B - y$ response might be interpreted as the chromatic mechanism of a deuteranope, and $b - Y$ of a protanope (would explain the neutral point differences), while $r_2 - G - r_1$ would correspond to the mechanism of a tetartanope (Fig. 3).

By illuminating the retina with a very strong light of a spectral band either from the long or from the short wave ends, it was possible to show that the hyperpolarizing or the depolarizing components alternately could be exhausted (Fig. 5). However, it was not possible to achieve a corresponding selective alteration of the L-type of spectral response curve (Fig. 6). After a strong illumination the L-type of spectral response curve was reduced proportionally over the whole spectral range. Therefore, it is concluded that the cone function could not easily be exhausted, while it was possible selectively to exhaust one or the other of the two opposite glial metabolic processes, which are reflected in the C-response.

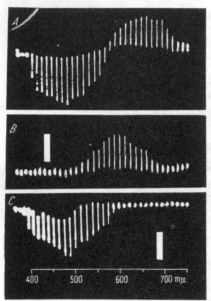

Fig. 5. *A* Normal spectral response curve of the C-type recorded from the Müller fiber. *B* The same response after strong illumination with a short wave end spectral band and *C* long wave end spectral band. *Centropomidae*

In order to explain the firing patterns of the "on" or "off" center ganglion cells (see Wolbarsht, Wagner and MacNichol, and J. Villegas, this symposium), we could assume the existence of two types of Müller fiber behavior. However, in the Mugillidae retina we have observed that the Müller fiber produces a hyperpolarizing response ("on"-firing) for short wavelengths, while the amacrine cell gives a hyperpolarizing reaction ("on"-firing) at long wavelengths (Fig. 3). Thus, it might be suggested that the Müller and amacrine glia are responsible for the

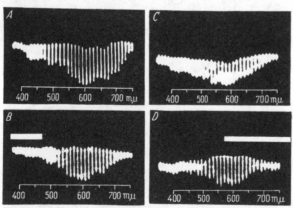

Fig. 6. *A*, *C* Normal spectral response curves of the L-type recorded from the horizontal cell. *B* The same response after strong illumination with a short wave end spectral band and *D* long wave end spectral band. *Centropomidae*

two types of ganglion cell firing pattern. The spike firing at "off" is interpreted as the release of the glial inhibitory control, the dendritic EPSP then being able to produce enough outward current through the initial segment of the axon to initiate the spikes (see SVAETICHIN, *16, 17*). It is further assumed that the spatial interactions of opponent colors and black-white both depend on the control function of the Müller fiber networks and also possibly the amacrine glia. We may suggest that the "on-off" transients seen at the neutral point of the C-response, these transient responses also being produced by white light, are important for black-white and contrast phenomena.

It is suggested that memory and learning depend on permanent changes of the protein-enzyme "programming-engramming" systems of the glial networks. These changes would be based on phenomena similar to the ones occurring in anaphylaxia (genetic memory, drug resistance, immunologic tolerance), in which mast-cells and smooth muscles are involved, the latter being cells which can be considered similar to the glial and pigment cells (also serotonin sensitive). The inborn instinctive behavior would depend on a genetic glial protein memory.

Sleep and alertness would be controlled in the same way as that in which the glial networks regulate dark and light adaptation in the retina (*11*). In the dark adapted state the GMP is low, 10 mV, and so is also the trans-retinal steady potential (SP) which probably corresponds to the trans-cortical steady potential, the glia-neuron system exhibiting pronounced oscillatory phenomena (*4*), the retina functioning at high sensitivity and showing only spatio-temporal summation processes. In the light adapted state the GMP reaches an equilibrium level of 35 mV and the SP increases to 10 mV; the rhythmic activity is reduced, and the retina now performs accurate spatio-temporal and wavelength discriminations and advanced integrative functions. It can be assumed that the state and mode of functioning of the retina is reflected into the cortex influencing its level of sleep and alertness; and that is why we have our eyes closed when asleep.

Would anybody expect a violin, with its frequency source (strings and bow) and resonance chamber, to produce marvellous melodies without a player modulating all the possible sounds and effects according to his own style ? The neuronal circuits appear to be an instrument which the glia is modulating.

Summary

1. A description is given of the localization of the origin of the retinal S-potentials by means of micro-electrodes filled with a lithium carmine solution. The luminosity (L) type of responses were found to be recorded from the large horizontal cells, while the chromatic (C) type of responses were recorded from the Müller fibers, both being glial structures.

2. The structure of the retina is described, on the basis of ultrastructural studies made by GLORIA VILLEGAS in this Institute. The glial networks and barriers and their functional aspects are emphasized.

3. Our new findings of glial-neuronal interaction are discussed; the experimental results show the dependence of the glia-neuron system on glial cell metabolism, this being responsible for setting the membrane potentials and thus the excitability levels of the neurons, as well as being involved in inhibition, the latter being shown in the retina to be glial and not synaptic. These results demonstrate that neurophysiology can only be investigated successfully if the glia-neuron system is considered as a whole.

References

1. Gerschenfeld, H. M., F. Wald, J. A. Zadunaisky and E. De Robertis: Function of astroglia in the water-ion metabolism of the central nervous system. An Electron Microscope Study. Neurology 9, 412 (1959).
2. Glees, P.: Neuroglia, morphology and function. Oxford: Blackwell Scientific Publications 1955.
3. Judd, D. B.: Current views on color blindness. Docum. ophthal. ('s-Grav.) 3, 251—287 (1949).
3a. Körnmüller, A. E.: Die Elemente der nervösen Tätigkeit. Stuttgart: Georg Thieme, 1947.
4. Laufer, M., G. Svaetichin, G. Mitarai, R. Fatehchand, E. Vallecalle and J. Villegas: The effect of temperature, carbon dioxide and ammonia on the neuron-glia unit. This symposium.
5. Lorente de Nó, R.: A study of nerve physiology. Stud. Rockefeller Inst. med. Res. 131, 132 (1947).
6. Lloyd, D. P. C.: On the monosynaptic reflex inter-connections of hind-limb muscles. Proc. of the 2nd. International Meeting of Neurobiologists, Amsterdam. 289—297(1959).
7. MacNichol, E. F., L. MacPherson and G. Svaetichin: Studies on spectral response curves from the fish retina. Symp. on Visual Problems of Color, Teddington, England, National Physical Laboratory (1957).
8. — and G. Svaetichin: Electric responses from the isolated retinas of fishes. Amer. J. Ophthal. 46, p. 2, 26—46 (1958).
9. Mitarai, G.: The origin of the so-called cone potential. Proc. Japan Acad. 34, 299—304 (1958).
10. — Determination of ultra-microelectrode tip position in the retina in relation to S-potential. J. gen. Physiol. 43, p. 2, 94—98 (1960).
11. — G. Svaetichin, E. Vallecalle, R. Fatehchand, J. Villegas and M. Laufer: Glia-neuron interaction and adaptational mechanisms of the retina (1960). This symposium.
11a. Müller, G. E.: Darstellung und Erklärung der verschiedenen Typen der Farbenblindheit nebst Erörterung der Funktion des Stäbchenapparates sowie des Farbensinns der Bienen und Fische, Göttingen 1924.
11b. Über die Farbenempfindungen. Psychophysische Untersuchungen. Z. psychol., Erg.-Bd. 17, 1, 435 (1930)
12. Polyak, S. L.: The retina. Chicago: Chicago University Press 1941.
13. Ramon y Cajal, S.: Histologie du système nerveux de l'homme et des vertebres. Madrid: Instituto Ramon y Cajal 1952.
14. Rochon-Duvigneaud, A.: Les yeux et la vision des vertèbres. Paris: Masson et Cie. (Editeurs) Libraires de l'Académie de médecine (1943).
15. Sjöstrand, F. S.: Electron-microscopy of myelin and of nerve cells and tissue. In: John N. Cumings (Editor) Modern Scientific Aspect of Neurology. 188—231. London: Edward Arnold Publishers, Ltd. 1960.
16. Svaetichin, G.: Analysis of action potentials from single spinal ganglion cells. Acta physiol. Scand. 24, suppl. 86, 23—57 (1951).
17. — Component analysis of action potentials from single neurons. Exp. Cell Res. suppl. 5, 234—261 (1958).
18. Villegas, G. M.: Electron Microscopic Study of the Vertebrate Retina. J. gen. Physiol. 43, p. 2, 15—43 (1960).
19. — Comparative ultrastructure of the retina in fish, monkey, and man. (1960). This Symposium.
20. Walls, G. L.: The vertebrate eye and its adaptive radiations. Michigan 1942.

Discussion pg. 493

The Effect of Temperature, Carbon Dioxide and Ammonia on the Neuron-Glia Unit*

By

Miguel Laufer, Gunnar Svaetichin, Genyo Mitarai, Richard Fatehchand, Edmundo Vallecalle and Jorge Villegas

With 4 Figures

The intra-cellular origins of the luminosity and chromatic S-potentials have been located (8), by means of glass micro-electrodes containing a lithium carmine solution. Since the responses were found to originate in glial structures (horizontal cells and Müller fibers respectively), they were considered to be extra-neuronal correlates of the processes occurring in the nerve cells. This induced our group to examine as far as possible the relations between the glial and the neuronal behavior, and it has now become clear to us that the glial cells are definitely involved in the control of excitability in the nervous system.

Up to now, it has generally been considered that the functions of the glial tissues in the central nervous system are restricted to the support and the nourishment of the neurons, these cells entirely accounting for the generation, regulation, and conduction of all types of nervous activity. It has only very recently been demonstrated (1, 6, 9) that there is no real extra-neuronal space in the central nervous system, and that the neuron and glia cell membranes remain closely packed after the tissue has been maintained in either a hypertonic or a hypotonic medium.

The present paper reports some preliminary results of the behavior of glial and neuronal structures under the influence of temperature, carbon dioxide and ammonia.

Methods

The following preparations were used in the experiments to be described:

a) The isolated retina of a shallow water fish *(Centropomidae)* and of the toad *(Bufo vulgaris)*.

b) The spinal ganglion, sciatic nerve and muscle of the toad.

All the specimens were placed in a moist chamber, in an atmosphere of $O_2 + 5\%$ CO_2 unless otherwise stated. The recordings were made with glass micro-electrode filled with 2.5 Mol. KCL, and having a resistance of maximally 100 megohm. To produce temperature changes in the preparations, water was used to heat or cool the chamber underside, this consisting of a microscope cover glass 0.17 mm in thickness. The temperature was measured by a micro-thermocouple on the surface of the tissue under study. When it was required to study the effect of a particular gas, this was circulated through the chamber. A detailed description of the technique used, and the light stimulation unit, is given elsewhere (4, 7).

Results

a) **Temperature changes.** The effects on the trans-membrane potentials and on the responses to stimuli will be discussed. The temperature of the specimen could be reduced or increased by 10°C in less than five seconds from room

---

* From the Department of Physiology, Instituto Venezolano de Investigaciones Cientificas, Caracas, Venezuela.

temperature (about 24°C). Responses were repetitively evoked by light stimuli (for the retinal structures), or by electrical stimulation (for the spinal ganglion and sciatic nerve).

Cooling. Effect on resting potentials. For the glial structures (horizontal cells and Müller fibers), the GMP (glial membrane potential) could be reduced in one second by up to 60% of the initial value (20—40 mV). An example is shown in Fig. 1, "C" indicating the instant at which cooling commenced. Similar behavior was observed in the trans-retinal and pigment layer steady potentials. However, cooling produced an opposite but less marked effect on the membrane potentials of neuronal structures (cell body, dendrites, and axons), the resting potentials increasing by between 10 and 60% of the initial values.

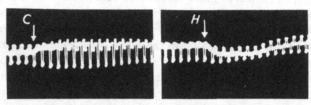

Fig. 1. Effect of temperature change on the GMP and S-potentials of a MÜLLER glial cell in retina. *C* and *H* indicate the starts of cooling and heating respectively. *Centropomidae*

Cooling. Effect on responses. For the glial structures, there was a marked increase in the L-response and the hyperpolarizing part of the C-response, both of these increasing at the same rate, while the depolarizing C-response decreased. These effects are shown in the left hand picture of Fig. 1. The changes in response were reversible unless the low temperature was maintained for several minutes. In the latter case, the GMP remained at its low value, but the S-potentials gradually reduced in amplitude and their rise and decay times increased. The effect of cooling was to reduce the trans-retinal responses (ERG). In the neuronal structures, the spike potentials and the dendritic transient potentials increased by up to 60% of their initial values, while their rise and decay times markedly increased (specially the decay time, which doubled). These effects accompanied the increase in membrane resting potential.

Heating. Effect on resting potentials. As shown in Fig. 1, the GMP of the glial structures increased, "H" indicating the instant at which heat was applied; increases of up to 60% were recorded. Similar behavior was evident in the trans-retinal and pigment layer steady potentials. These changes were somewhat slower than those produced by cooling, and became irreversible if the temperature was maintained above 30°C for longer than one minute. On the other hand, the neuronal structures showed decreased membrane potentials, these changes also being slower than those produced by lowering the temperature.

Heating. Effect on responses. The increase in the GMP of the glial structures was accompanied by a decreasing hyperpolarizing response (to extinction), and by an increase in the depolarizing C-response. These effects are shown in the right hand picture of Fig. 1. The ERG showed a marked increase, while the neuronal spike potentials and the dendritic transient potentials decreased by about 50%.

b) Carbon dioxide. *Effect on resting potentials.* The effect of carbon dioxide on the glial and neuronal structures appeared immediately. For the glial structures, the GMP increased to a new steady value in less than five seconds; this change was reversible unless an excessive amount of gas had been used. In Fig. 2, the arrows indicate the instances of application of carbon dioxide. Here (A) is one experiment and (C) another, (C) comprising the two bottom pictures. Equally fast changes occurred in the trans-retinal and pigment layer steady potentials, although these decreased. On the other hand, the neuronal structures showed decreases in their membrane potentials, these changes being smaller and slower than those in the glial structures.

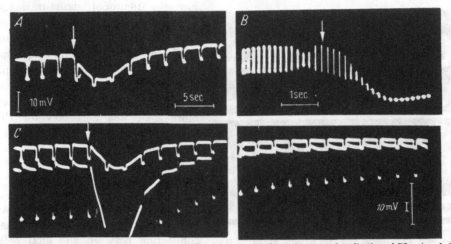

Fig. 2. Effect of carbon dioxide on a horizontal glial cell. Arrows indicate instants of application of CO_2. A and C show effect on GMP and S-potentials; the bottom right hand picture is a continuation of C. The effect of CO_2 on oscillatory phenomena is shown in B; vertical lines indicate oscillation amplitudes. *Centropomidae*

Effect on responses. The hyperpolarizing responses of the horizontal cells and Müller fibers, the trans-retinal responses (ERG), and the neuronal action potentials (spike potentials and dendritic transient potentials) markedly reduced in amplitude, finally disappearing if sufficient carbon dioxide was used. The effects on the hyperpolarizing responses of the glial cells are shown in (A) and (C) of Fig. 2. The depolarizing C-responses at first increased as the GMP increased, but subsequently gradually diminished. When the carbon dioxide supply was cut off, the responses became comparable to those obtained before application of the gas. Similar effects were observed if the retina was initially maintained in a pure oxygen atmosphere, and 5% carbon dioxide then added, or if one breathed on the preparation. In the case of the neuronal structures, the rise and decay times of the action potentials progressively increased to about twice their initial values.

c) **Ammonia.** *Effect on resting potentials.* For the membrane GMP, most marked effects were obtained with the application of only a very small amount of ammonia vapor, the GMP reducing by up to 50% of its initial value. Increases were observed in the membrane potentials of the neuronal structures, and the transretinal and pigment layer steady potentials, but these changes were small. The effect of ammonia occurred immediately, having a maximum influence in less than five seconds. The changes were reversible unless a large amount of the vapor was applied for a long time, in which case the GMP remained low and did not recover when the supply of vapor ways cut off.

Effect on responses. For the glial structures, the decreasing GMP was accompanied by an increase in the L-response and in the hyperpolarizing C-response, and by a decrease in the depolarizing C-response. These changes in amplitude occurred very rapidly, were up to 50% of the initial amplitudes, and could be reversed unless the vapor was applied for more than five seconds or in a large amount. In the latter case, the GMP became very low (a few mV) and the response decreased to vanishing point. A small amount of ammonia changed the ERG to a P III, which we have shown to be the action potential of the photoreceptors.

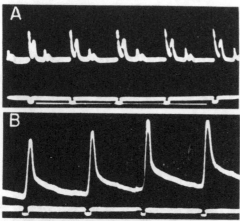

For the neuronal structures, the application of a small amount of ammonia increased the spike and dendritic transient (Fig. 3) potentials by up to 50%, these showing an irreversible decrease if sufficient ammonia had been applied (much more than was necessary for the irreversible changes to occur in the glial structures).

Fig. 3. Intracellular recording from a retinal ganglion cell dendrite. *A* The resting membrane potential was 30—40 mV, and the depolarizing saw-tooth transients appeared at "on" and at "off" of the alternating red (indicated on lower beam) and blue light stimuli. *B* This record was obtained from the same dendrite after exposure to NH₃, the resting level now being increased by about 50% and also the transient responses, which were slower and only seen at "on", the responses to blue light being very small. Due to the long refractory period the duration of the light stimuli was too short (200 msec) for evoking transients at "off". Light adapted fish retina. *Centropomidae*

Comments

Our experimental results indicate that there is an intimate functional connection between the glial cells and the neurons, the glia controlling neuronal excitability. Opposite effects are induced in the glial and neuronal structures by temperature change, and by the application of carbon dioxide or ammonia. These agents produce changes in the glial and neuronal responses which are closely related to changes in the GMP, although the neuronal membrane potentials alter much less than the GMP. For instance, an increased GMP is accompanied by a reduced glial response, a decrease in neuronal membrane potential, and reduced neuronal spike and dendritic transient potentials. Table 1 summarizes the results obtained. However, for muscle, a structure without glial tissue, neither temperature change, carbon dioxide nor ammonia produced any effects comparable to those which we have described. It is also of interest that no changes of the kind we have discussed could be produced by the application in high concentration to our preparations of the following agents: HCl, H_2SO_4, $NaOH$, Na_2CO_3, $(NH_4)_2SO_4$. This was also the case for pure oxygen or nitrogen; the small changes which were observed with these gases were slowly occurring and partly due to the consequent lack of carbon dioxide.

For intact glia-neuronal units in situ, the membrane potential changes due to temperature are in fact much greater than those to be expected from the Nernst equation (8). According to this equation, a 3% alteration in membrane potential is produced by a 10°C temperature change, and this was only found if the glial

Table 1. *Comparative effects of temperature, carbon dioxide and ammonia*

	Glia horizontal L-response Light adapted (fish)	Glia Müller C-response Light adapted (fish)	Perikaryon spinal ganglion (toad)	Dendrite retinal ganglion cell (fish)	Axon myelinated (toad)	Muscle striated (toad)	Pigment layer steady pot. Light adapted (toad)	Transretinal steady pot. and erg Light adapted (toad)
Resting **COLD**	Decrease	Decrease	Increase	Increase	Increase	No	Decrease	Decrease
Response	Increase	+ Decrease — Increase	Increase	Increase	Increase			Decrease
Resting **HEAT**	Increase	Increase	Decrease	Decrease	Decrease	No	Increase	Increase
Response	Decrease	+ Increase — Decrease	Decrease	Decrease	Decrease			Increase
Resting **CO₂**	Increase	Increase	Decrease	Decrease	Decrease	No	Decrease	Decrease
Response	Decrease	+ Increase — Decrease	Decrease	Decrease	Decrease			Decrease
Resting **NH₃**	Decrease	Decrease	Increase	Increase	Increase	No	Increase	Increase
Response	Increase	+ Decrease — Increase	Increase	Increase	Increase			Increase

cells were in a non-functional state. Glial activity can be reduced by using a well dark adapted retina, since in this case the GMP is known to be very low (4). In this condition, the glial cells are relatively unaffected by temperature change, by CO_2, or by ammonia. However, the glial-neuronal system now appears to be unstable, as shown by the appearance of oscillatory phenomena recorded from glial structures during darkness (equivalent to a sleep condition). These oscillations diminished very much in amplitude under dim light (Fig. 4), or if the GMP was increased by means of a small amount of carbon dioxide (Fig. 2B). As shown in Fig. 4, the oscillations mainly consist of two frequency components, a slow one of between 3 and 6 c/s, and a fast one between 30 and 40 c/s. The GMP can also be very much reduced by the application of a large amount of ammonia to the retina. The excitability control exerted by the glial cells is now much reduced, since the ganglion cells exhibit random firing.

There is evidence from other work that neuron behavior is functionally connected with glial activity. Morphological studies show that there is no significant extra-cellular space in the nervous system (1, 6, 9), and this supports our contention that the glial cells are intimately involved in nervous activity. Extra-neuronal compartments have been postulated, the "x" phase (5), to explain large effluxes of sodium and potassium from the squid giant axon. Further, HYDÉN and PIGON (2) conclude, from the concentrations of different substances in nerve and glial cells, that the neurons and glia represent two systems which are linked energetically and apparently constitute a functional unit in the central nervous system. Since we found that there is a close correlation between the GMP and changes in glial and neuronal responses, it is logical to relate the excitability control exerted by the slow L-fraction of the electrotonus in the intact sciatic nerve (3) to glial (Schwann cell) activity. If the glia is in a non-functional state, control of the nerve cells is lost and these behave abnormally.

Up to now, the glial system has been thought of as a blood-brain barrier. But if we consider it as a blood-brain bridge, and keep in mind the fundamental role it has as an extra-neuronal space in the central nervous system (for electrolytes,

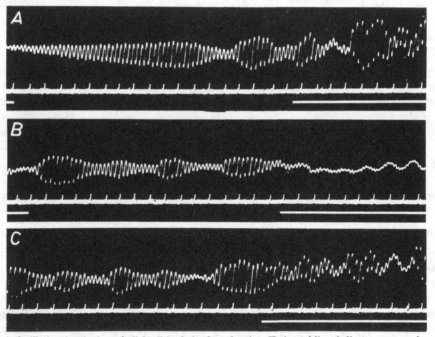

Fig. 4. Oscillations in a horizontal glial cell in dark-adapted retina. Horizontal lines indicate presence of weak light stimulus. Time markers 100 msec. *Centropomidae*

metabolites, hormones and drug pathways), we are more inclined to emphasize its function in regulating and maintaining the excitability levels in the nervous system and in relating this system with the internal medium of the body.

Summary

The effects of temperature, carbon dioxide and ammonia were examined on glial and neuronal structures in a shallow water fish (Centropomidae) and in the toad (Bufo vulgaris). Each of these agents produced opposite effects on the membrane potentials and parallel changes in the responses of the glial and neuronal structures; the changes in the glial and neuronal responses were closely related to changes in the glial membrane potentials. The results show that there is an intimate functional connection between the glial cells and the neurons, the glia controlling neuronal excitability. If glia activity is reduced, the glial-neuronal system becomes unstable, as shown by the appearance of oscillations and by random firing of the neurons.

References

1. Gerschenfeld, H. M., F. Wald, J. A. Zadunaisky and E. de Robertis: Function of astroglia in the water-ion metabolism of the central nervous system. An Electron Microscope Study. Neurology 9, 412 (1959)
2. Hydén, H., and A. Pigon: A cytophysiological study of the functional relationship between oligodendroglial cells and nerve cells of deiters nucleus. J. Neurochem. 6, 57 (1960).
3. Lorente de Nó: A study of nerve physiology. Stud. Rockefeller Inst. med. Res. 131, 132 (1947).
4. Mitarai, G., G. Svaetichin, E. Vallecalle, R. Fatehchand, J. Villegas and M. Laufer: Glia-neuron interaction and adaptational mechanisms of the retina (1960). This symposium.
5. Shanes, A. M., and M. D. Berman: Kinetics of ion movement in the squid grant axon. Gen. J. Physiol. 55, 279—300 (1955).
6. Sjöstrand, F. S.: Electron-microscopy of myelin and of nerve cells and tissue. John N. Cumings (Editor). Modern Scientific Aspect of Neurology. 188—231. London: Edward Arnold Publishers, Ltd. 1960.
7. Svaetichin, G., and R. Jonasson: A technique for oscillographic recording of spectral response curves. Acta physiol. scand. 39, suppl. 134, 3—16 (1956).
8. — M. Laufer, G. Mitarai, Richard Fatehchand, E. Vallecalle and J. Villegas: Glial control of neuronal networks and receptors (1960). This symposium.
9. Villegas, G. M.: Electron microscopic study of the vertebrate retina. J. gen. Physiol. 43, p. 2, 15—43 (1960).

Glia-Neuron Interactions and Adaptational Mechanisms of the Retina*

By

Genyo Mitarai**, Gunnar Svaetichin, Edmundo Vallecalle, Richard Fatehchand, Jorge Villegas and Miguel Laufer

With 13 Figures

The graded electrical response (S-potential) recorded intracellularly from the fish retina (*28, 29*) has been found to originate in two different types of glial cells: (a) the L-type from the horizontal cell; and (b) the C-type from the Müller fiber (*33*). Our theory of neuron-glia interaction leads us to believe that the S-potentials reflect the metabolic processes taking place in the glial cells, the glial function being intimately coupled with the activity of the neurons and receptors, on which components the glial cells exert a metabolic excitability control.

The first part of this paper deals with the question as to whether the glial responses selectively reflect the functioning of the rods and cones in different states of adaption. The results of our present studies show that the S-potential obtained in the strictly scotopic state reflected rod activity only, while in the complete photopic state the effects of the cones were only observed. Mitarai and Yagasaki (*14*) described differences of the latencies and the rise and decay times of the L-response; these changes, which depend on the adaptational conditions of the retina, were confirmed in the present work. Numerous studies have attempted to prove a photochemical theory of retinal adaptation, without however any real success, as has been pointed out by Rushton (*24, 25*). Therefore, it appeared

* Department of Physiology, Instituto Venezolano de Investigaciones Cientificas, Caracas, Venezuela.

** Present address: Institute of Environmental Medicine, Nagoya Univ., Chikusa-Ku, Japan.

worthwhile to look for neurophysiological mechanisms of retinal adaption, based on a glial excitability control of the neurons and receptors. The second part of this paper is a comparative study of well-known phenomena observed in light and dark adaptation in man, and the behavior of the glial cell potentials under corresponding conditions in the fish retina.

Methods

The live fish *(Centropomus)* was dark-adapted for 12 hours before the experiment started, and then, following the original method of manipulation (*28, 29*), the retina was isolated in dim red light, and kept in a moist atmosphere of $O_2+5\%$ CO_2. If the isolated retina was exposed to light shortly before the experiment,

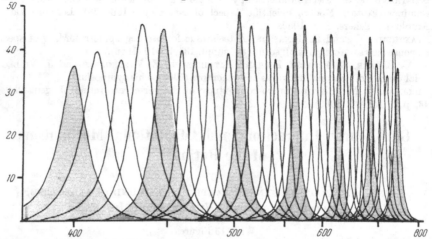

Fig. 1. Transmission curves of the 34 interference filters used in the photostimulator unit, based on data furnished by the manufacturer (BALZER, LICHTENSTEIN). *Abscissae* wavelengths in millimicrons. *Ordinates* transmission in percent

a true scotopic response could not be obtained, even if the retina was kept in darkness for long periods afterwards. In these series of experiments the pigment layer had been removed. For a general description of the experimental procedure see references *13, 15, 28*, and *29*. A micropipette electrode filled with 2.5 mol KCL-solution was used for the recordings. Finely tapered electrodes, having a resistance of about 100 megohms, and a tip diameter of less than 0.1 μ were selected. These electrodes could maintain a constant resting potential and an unchanged response for about 30 minutes, permitting the observation of adaptation processes. At this point, we wish to express our thanks to Professor TSUNEO TOMITA (Keio University, Tokyo) for instructing us on the production of finely tapered electrodes with the pulling machine and the glass capillaries provided by the Takahashi Company (Tokyo, Japan).

The recent work in this laboratory has been carried out with a new photostimulator and it is therefore necessary to provide some information on this equipment, which is similar in most details to the one described in earlier papers (*13, 29* and *32*). In this new stimulator unit, 34 interference filters (BALZER, LICHTENSTEIN) of almost equal wavelength intervals were mounted at equal angular distances close to the periphery of a circular "plexiglas" plate (radius 30 cm). This interference filter wheel was rotated by an electric motor, and a linear potentiometer attached to the wheel provided the voltage for the wavelength sweep of the oscilloscope. The transmission curves of the interference filters used are shown in Fig. 1, the peak wavelength being given by the numbers in Fig. 2. The interference filters were combined with neutral filters in such a way that each one transmitted approximately equal light energy as measured by a black-body thermocouple. An oscillographic recording of the relative energy calibration obtained by means of the thermocouple amplifier system is shown in Fig. 2. The difference in amplitude of the two responses indicated by the bar in the bottom

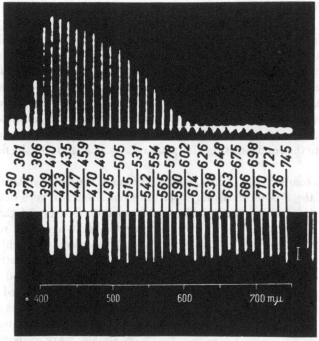

Fig. 2. *Below* Oscillographic relative energy calibration curve showing only peak parts of thermoelectric responses, caused by absorption of radiant energy passing the filters 399 to 745 mμ. *Center* Numbers give the maxima of transmission of the 34 interference filters of the photostimulator. The amplitude difference the two thermoelectric responses below in the right hand corner (indicated by the bar) corresponded to an 8% change of radiant energy. *Above* Recording of spectral response curve of the "General Electric" photocell GL-929

right hand corner of Fig. 2, corresponded to an 8% change of the radiant energy. Hence, the error in matching the relative energies transmitted through the filters from 410—745 mμ was smaller than $\pm 4\%$. Somewhat less energy was available for the filters having a peak wavelength shorter than 410 mμ. A test recording (Fig. 2, top) of the spectral curve of a photocell (General Electric, GL-929) confirmed that the spectral energies were matched with an error of less than $\pm 4\%$. The light source of the photostimulator was a 1000 watt xenon high pressure lamp (Osram, XBO-1001), fed from a stabilized DC supply (Ing. Halstrup, Freiburg i. Br., Germany).

The light used for stimulation in the present studies was projected through the retina from the vitreous side and focussed with a microscope objective to a spot of 40 μ diameter at the receptor level (*32*). The background illumination or adaptation was restricted to a circular area of diameter 500 μ.

The relative intensity of light was varied by a set of neutral density filters, which were mounted on two wheels in such a way that they could easily be combined to produce a range of densities covering $\overline{6.9}$ Log units in density steps of $\overline{0.3}$ *(29)*. In this way a logarithmic scale of relative light intensities was obtained; in the text the intensity of the light stimulus is indicated by the total density of the neutral filters which have been interposed in the light beam of the photostimulator.

1. Trans-retinal potentials

a) The ERG. When the micro-electrode touched the exposed surface of the receptor layer of the isolated fish retina, the indifferent electrode being in contact with the vitreous side, focal illumination (spot diameter 40 μ) evoked a slow response (ERG) having an amplitude of less than 1 mV. This potential change was mainly a receptor side negative going, transient (b-wave) in the dark-adapted state using weak light stimuli, and predominantly a receptor side positive, square wave (a-wave, P. III) after adaptation to light. In the recordings from the fish retina used in these experiments the b-wave was small compared to the large b-wave seen in the ERG recordings from the frog, this difference presumably being related to the concentration of bipolar cells, which is low in the fish and high in the frog.

In order to compare the spectral characteristics of these transretinal potentials with those of the S-potentials, the spectral response curves were determined in the different states of adaptation. The spectral response curve of the transient,

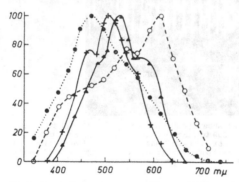

Fig. 3. Spectral response curves of trans-retinal recordings (ERG) obtained from the fish retina *(Centropomidae)*. Scotopic state: dotted line and filled circles. Mesopic state: continuous lines, crosses and triangles. Photopic state: broken lines and open circles

receptor side negative response (b-wave) recorded at night from the strictly dark-adapted retina, showed one maximum situated at about 470 mμ (Fig. 3, dotted line and filled circles), whereas the corresponding curve for the receptor side positive, square wave response (a-wave, PIII) obtained after adaptation to light, had its peak at about 600 mμ (Fig. 3, broken line and open circles). In the transitional "mesopic" state the spectral response curves showed maxima at 505 and 531 mμ with submaxima at 470 and 602 mμ. Such a change of the spectral response maxima with adaptation corresponds to a "Purkinje phenomenon", the submaxima observed in the dark-adapted and mesopic states indicating the presence of three different photopigments in the rods having their maxima at 470, 505 and 531 mμ, which is in agreement with the common finding of several rod pigments in the retina of fish *(4, 5)*.

b) The receptor potentials. Focal stimulation (spot diam. 40 μ) of the light-adapted isolated fish retina deprived of the pigment epithelium, produced a receptor side positive transient response at "on" (a-wave), and a DC change lasting during the period of stimulation (PIII), followed by a negative going transient at "off" (cf. MOTOKAWA et al., *17, 18*). When all interacting electrical responses to light stimuli produced by the retinal neurons and glial cells had been abolished, for instance by exposing the retina to small amounts of NH_3, it was possible to obtain a receptor side positive, square-wave shaped response (without transients) showing an amplitude twice (or more) as large as that of the trans-retinal potential recorded before the exposure to NH_3, this response being strictly localized to the illuminated receptors. Studies in this laboratory (*12, 34*) have definitely shown that this receptor side positive square wave (P III, *10*) is produced by the photo-receptors. The spectral response curve of this receptor potential obtained after exposure to NH_3, had in the dark-adapted state its maxima at about 470 and 531 mμ, while in light-adapted conditions the maximum was at about 554 mμ. This "Purkinje shift" of the receptor potential shows that both the rods and the cones when exposed to light, produced a square-wave shaped graded potential, the apical ends of the photoreceptors going positive. In the light-adapted state the latency of the receptor potentials (cones) was about

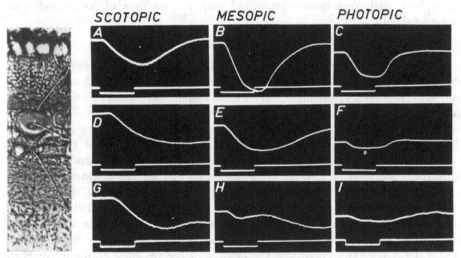

Fig. 4. Left: micrograph showing (radial) section of fish retina. Oscillograms of S-potentials recorded from different glial cells in different states of adaptation. A—C external horizontal cell responses; *D—F* internal horizontal cell responses; *G—I* Müller fiber responses

8 msec., being always shorter than the latency of the S-potentials (15—18 msec) recorded under the same experimental conditions. In the scotopic and mesopic retina, the rise and decay times of the receptor potentials (rods and cones) were much slower than when the retina had been light-adapted. (Compare the corresponding behavior of the S-potentials described below.) The rise time of the receptor potential was shorter than that of the S-potential.

   c) **The steady potential (SP).** The trans-retinal steady potential (SP) reaches values of maximally 10 mV in frog (*22*) and is somewhat lower in the fish, the receptor side being negative. In the dark-adapted state the SP is low, 1—2 mV, and increases with adaptation to light (*20*), this occurring also in the absence of

the pigment epithelium. Hence, the SP must be somehow involved in the processes of adaptation. Studies by the group of this laboratory (34) have shown that
the main part of the SP is produced by two different structures: 1. the photoreceptors, this confirming the earlier observations (22), and 2. by the pigment
epithelium. In the dark-adapted retina the glial membrane potential (GMP) of
the Müller fiber and the internal horizontal cell is low (see below), and so is also
the SP. Under different experimental conditions exposing the retina to temperature
changes, CO_2, NH_3, etc., the SP recorded across the receptor layer, and also
across the isolated pigment layer, always reacted in the same way as the membrane
potential of the glial cells. Hence, it is concluded that the SP reflects the glial
metabolic control of the retinal adaptation (excitability). The SP depends somehow
on the mutual interaction between 1. the receptor and its pigment cell, and 2.
the receptor and the Müller fiber-horizontal cell networks.

Very likely the trans-retinal steady potential (SP) is of the same origin as the
trans-cortical steady potential (21), both of them depending on the metabolic
activity of the glial networks, which controls the excitability level of the neurons.
The spreading depression of Leao which also has been observed in the retina (9) is
probably a glial phenomenon connected with contractions of astro-glial cells
(horizontal cell).

2. The S-potentials

a) The external L-response. When a micro-electrode was advanced into a
strictly scotopic retina to a depth of $80-100$ μ, a DC shift of about 35 mV suddenly
appeared; however, surprisingly, only a small response or none at all was obtained
even when a light stimulus was applied which was strong for the dark-adapted
retina. For examining this kind of response a high amplification was necessary
(Fig. 4, $A-C$). At maximum stimulus intensity, the latency of this type of
L-response was approximately 20 msec, the rise time 150 msec and the decay
time about 300 msec (Fig. 4, A). Once the retina had become adapted to a weak
background light, the response increased in amplitude without showing any
change in the resting potential level (Fig. 4, B). A continuous and stronger light
adaptation caused a small increase of the resting GMP level, while the response
amplitude decreased, the rise and decay times of the response becoming shorter
(Fig. 4, C). Under this condition, the latency of the response gradually reached
15 msec, the rise and decay times being shortened to a mere 50 msec. The threshold of the response was found to be $\overline{3.9}$ on the scale of relative light energy used
in these experiments (see methods), the amplitude increasing proportionally to
the logarithmic change of the stimulus intensity between $\overline{3.6}$ and $\overline{0.9}$ (Fig. 9).

The spectral response curve of this kind of L-response had its maximum at
590 mμ, this peak and the general shape of the curve remaining constant throughout all different states of adaptation (Fig. 5, $A-C$). Histological localization of
the micro-electrode recording site after marking with lithium carmine (33),
showed that this type of S-potential was obtained from an external horizontal cell,
hence it is called "the external L-response". The characteristics are in summary
the following: 1. the resting membrane potential was always high; 2. the threshold
was fairly high and the response comparatively fast; 3. the spectral response curve
did not show any "Purkinje shift," the maximum always corresponding to the

photopic peak value of 590 mμ. From the work of GLORIA VILLEGAS (*36, 37, 38*) we know that the horizontal cells show no connections with the synaptic endings of the receptors, but are in membrane to membrane contacts with the dendritic network of the external plexiform layer and with the cell bodies of the sparsely occurring external type of bipolar. On the basis of these facts two possibilities can be suggested: 1. either the external horizontal cell is selectively connected only to the cone system, or 2. since the metabolic linkages between the external

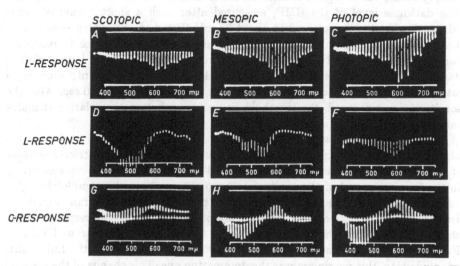

Fig. 5. Spectral response curves recorded from the external horizontal cell (A—C) the internal horizontal cell (D—F) and the Müller fiber (G—I) in different states of adaptation

horizontals and the bipolar cells are structurally restricted, this could be the reason for the high threshold of response observed in the external type of horizontal cell.

b) **The internal L-response.** When in a dark-adapted retina the electrode was additionally advanced by about $10-20\ \mu$, it passed from an external horizontal cell into an internal one. The resting membrane potential (GMP) was now only about 10 mV and remained at this same level when the electrode was advanced further into a second internal horizontal cell (deeper down). The internal type horizontal cell, which forms the two innermost of the three horizontal cell layers, differs structurally from the row of external horizontals; therefore, it was not surprising to find that the external and internal horizontals could also be distinguished from each other on the basis of their functional characteristics. In the dark-adapted state the internal horizontals showed a low GMP of 10 mV or less, while the sensitivity to light stimuli was very high, having a threshold intensity of $\overline{6.3}$ on the relative light intensity scale; which also approximately was the threshold stimulus for our own eyes adapted to the same level of illumination. A stimulus intensity of $\overline{4.8}$ was sufficient to produce a maximal response reaching the saturation level (Figs. 8 and 9). The latency of the response in the dark-adapted state was long and about 50 msec, the response being very slow with a rise time of about 300 msec and a decay of more than 1 sec. Thus, the charcteristics of the internal L-response in the dark-adapted state agree well with the description of the S-potential in the dark-adapted conditions given by MITARAI and YAGA-SAKI (*14*).

When turning on the lights in the room for a moment one could see that the strictly dark-adapted retina had an intense reddish-violet color indicating that the rods possibly contained a mixture of "rhodopsin and porphyropsin". Such an exposure to light, which was too short to produce any observable bleaching of the rod pigments, was enough to change the characteristics of the internal L-response. The darkness level of the GMP, measured after such a short period of light-adaptation, had now increased to about 35 mV (Fig. 4, *E*, *F*), which seems to be a kind of "equilibrium" value for the light-adapted state, since it remained constant at this magnitude even when the retina was kept for a long period in darkness. The response after light-adaptation was also different, showing a latency of about 15 msec, with rise and decay times of about 50 sec. Also the sensitivity was reduced, the threshold being about $\overline{3.9}$ on the relative stimulus intensity scale (Figs. 8 and 9).

Studies on the spectral response curves of the internal type of L-response obtained in dark- and light-adapted conditions showed that in the strictly scotopic state the maximum was situated at about 470 mμ, having very low sensitivity in the long wave end of the spectrum (Fig. 5, *D*), while in the completely light-adapted retina the spectral response curve peaked at about 590 mμ (Fig. 5, *F*). In the transitional (mesopic) state of adaptation the spectral response curve showed in addition to the maximum at about 470 mμ another one around 531 mμ. Further adaptation increased the peak at 590 mμ until finally in the fully light-adapted state, this maximum was the dominating one. This change of the spectral response curve maximum with the state of adaptation apparently corresponds to a "Purkinje phenomenon".

These experiments clearly show that the internal horizontals are interacting with bipolars which carry the information from both rods and cones.

c) **The C-response.** Advancing an electrode from the receptor side of a dark-adapted retina down to the second level of the internal horizontals, the GMP generally was found to be low (10 mV) and in that case the electrode tip was localized in an internal horizontal cell. However, at about every fifth penetration with the electrode into the dark-adapted (*Centropomus*) retina a higher GMP of about 20 mV was observed, the tip of the electrode being at a depth corresponding to the level of the second layer of internal horizontal cells; however, in that case a spectral response curve of the C-type was obtained. Histological localization proved that the electrode tip had entered the expanded part which contains the nucleus of a Müller fiber (*33*). It was at first thought that the C-response was exclusively due to the cone system, as the experiments seemed to prove. However, the present results provide evidence that the rod system also somehow contributes to the C-response (*42*), as the Müller fiber in the scotopic state yields a response strikingly similar to the internal L-response, both being characterized by: 1. a long (50 msec) latency, 2. slow (300 msec) rise and (more than 1 sec) decay times (Fig. 4, *G*), 3. a peak of the spectral response curve at 470 mμ, with a submaximum at 531 mμ, and 4. at low sensitivity to red light (Fig. 5, *G*). It must be emphasized that in the dark-adapted retina the GMP of the Müller fiber always was higher

(20 mV) than that of the internal horizontal cell (10 mV), and that also correspondingly the threshold for the C-response ($\overline{4.8}$) was high compared to that of the internal L-response ($\overline{6.3}$). In connection with the light adaptation process, the GMP level of both the Müller fiber and the internal horizontal cell increased, and finally stabilized at a photopic "equilibrium" level of about 35 mV, the C- and L-response now showing equal thresholds. At a higher intensity of the stimulus light ($\overline{2.4}$) even in the dark-adapted state, the C-response of course displayed the typical reversal of the polarity of the response evoked by spectral lights from the long wave end (Fig. 6). Since the strictly scotopic threshold stimulus as well as the GMP of the C-response differed from those of the internal L-response, it can be suggested that the Müller fiber is less intimately linked to the rod system than is the internal horizontal cell.

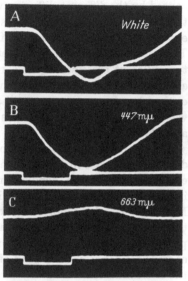

Fig. 6. Scotopic C-responses to white, blue and red stimuli of 150 msec duration

In the course of light-adaptation the rise and decay of the C-response became faster as the resting level and the amplitude of the positive response to red light increased. Simultaneously, the spectral response curve peak of the depolarizing response shifted from 602 to 663 mμ, the neutral point moving from 565 to 590 mμ. The maximum of the hyperpolarizing part remained constant at about 470 mμ throughout the adaptational process.

3. Spreading of the metabolic control of excitability in the glial networks

a) **Spreading velocity of the S-potentials.** It has earlier been pointed out that the L-response "apparently originates in the star-shaped horizontal cell" (31) and "that the ends of their prolongations have close membrane to membrane contacts and form a continuous network perpendicular to the receptor" (36) and further, "that it was observed that the excitations spread to adjacent horizontal cells" (31). When a restricted area of the retina was stimulated with a light spot of high intensity, S-potentials could be recorded up to several millimeters away from the illuminated part. Furthermore, illumination of a restricted area of a dark-adapted retina changed the state of adaptation, as seen from the S-potentials which were recorded from the surrounding retinal regions which had not been exposed to light. It was therefore important to measure the velocity of the spreading of the different S-potentials in the fish retina. This was done by recording the response latencies at different distances from the spot of illumination; the experiments showed that the L-response propagated with a velocity of about 0.35 m/sec, this also being the speed of propagation of the hyperpolarizing process of the C-response, while the velocity of the depolarizing response was only about 0.15 m/sec. Under the same experimental conditions (isolated retina, room temperature 24°C) the

L-response and the hyperpolarizing part of the C-response evoked at the site of illumination, showed a latency of 18 msec, while the focal latency of the depolarizing process of the C-response was 40 msec.

According to the studies described in other papers of this symposium (*12, 33*) the spreading of the excitability control of the glial networks actually seem most likely to correspond to an intra- and inter-glial spreading of a metabolic reaction. We have some indication that this spreading is mediated by the diffusion of CO_2 and NH_3, and that possibly the two different speeds of propagation observed are caused by the different diffusion velocities of CO_2 and NH_3 in the glial cells. Thus the spreading of the S-potentials is not likely to be simply a membrane phenomenon, but rather the spreading of a metabolic reaction involving the whole cell. This view is supported by the fact that in one and the same Müller fiber there are two different processes of the C-response with different spreading velocities, and also by the observation that the hyperpolarizing reaction could be promptly evoked by an exposure to small amounts of CO_2, while the depolarizing process was initiated by minute amounts of NH_3 (large amounts of NH_3 blocked all glial activity irreversibly).

As a general conclusion from our studies we may state that two fundamentally different processes in the glial cells control neuronal excitability: 1. the process corresponding to the depolarizing reaction of the Müller fiber, which causes inhibition of the ganglion cell firing, and 2. the hyperpolarizing processes of the Müller fiber and the horizontal cell which cause a general graded regulation of the excitability level of the neurons and receptors. In the retina the hyperpolarizing process of the glial cells manages in a "plastic" way the adaptational phenomena of wide retinal areas, this kind of control reaction being the only one existing in the horizontal cell.

These studies show that the glial networks and the spreading in them of the processes which control excitability are of basic importance for the understanding of the retinal phenomena of adaptation. Further, these findings offer a new approach to research on the functional mechanisms of the cortex and the nervous system in general.

b) **Spatial amplitude distribution curves of the S-potentials.** In order to study the spatial amplitude distributions of the different S-potentials and also to compare those with the spatial distribution of the trans-retinal responses (ERG), a series of experiments was carried out in which measurements were made of the amplitudes of the potentials evoked by a 40 μ stimulus spot. The spot could be moved along a line which crossed the recording site of the micro-electrode, the response amplitudes being plotted against the distances of the stimulus spot from the recording site. For this purpose a special scanning apparatus was used, the design of which was as follows. The microscope objective used for focussing the light spot on the retina was attached to a micro-manipulator (Leitz), which was moved by a motor-driven linkage so as to constrain the spot to perform a scanning of the retina along consecutive parallel lines, the micro-electrode tip being in the center of the scanned area (rather like TV scanning). The retina was either continuously illuminated by the moving spot, or the light was automatically flashed on after each 350 μ of scanning movement. The two co-ordinates of the scanning motion operated proportionally the X and Y deflections of the oscilloscope, the output signal of the DC amplifier used for the micro-electrode recording being added to the Y-deflection of the oscilloscope. In this way a two co-ordinate scanning area with the superimposed responses could be pictured on the oscilloscope screen.

This same equipment also proved useful for studies on the spatial distributions and spatio-temporal interactions of the ERG and the ganglion cell spikes, the spikes being conveniently presented by brightness modulation of the oscilloscope spot. This kind of arrangement also permits studies of spatial interactions between a spot kept in a fixed position and a second scanning spot of different wavelength. A similar arrangement has been described and successfully used by MOTOKAWA et al. (19, 27).

The oscillographic recordings reproduced in Fig. 7 illustrate results of measurements obtained with this scanning apparatus. However, in this case only the X-axis scanning was operated, the light spot describing a straight line which

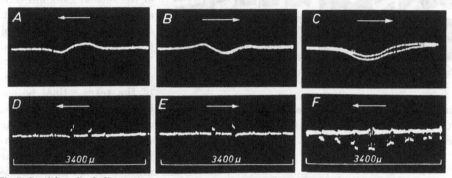

Fig. 7. Spatial amplitude distribution curves of photopic trans-retinal potentials (A, B and D, E) and of L-response (C, F) obtained with the scanning method described in text. A—C obtained with stimulus light continuously on, while in D—F the light was flashed on after each 350 μ of scanning movement. Diameter of light spot 40 μ. Scanning speed 0.3 mm/sec. Duration of flash 200 msec. Recording electrode kept in center of the scanning width of 3400 μ

crossed the recording site of the micro-electrode, this being situated in the center of the scanning width of 3400 μ. Fig. 7, C shows the spatial amplitude distribution curve of the internal type of L-response, recorded when the spot of light continuously illuminated the retina during the scanning cycle. The overlapping of the two superimposed curves, both obtained with the same direction of scanning, was due to a drift of the resting GMP. Corresponding measurements obtained by flashing the spot on for a duration of 200 msec after every 350 μ distance of scanning movement are shown in Fig. 7, F.

In the same way, recordings were obtained of the external type of L-response, and separately for the depolarizing and hyperpolarizing parts of the C-response. The spatial amplitude distribution curves thus obtained for these different S-potentials proved to be very similar for the same conditions of adaptation and intensity of stimulation. The scanning curves were approximately symmetrical on both sides of the center of recording, the shape of the curves being independent of the scanning direction for a scanning speed of 0.3 mm/sec. The scanning curves of the external L-response and the depolarizing part of the C-response were always broader, covering a distance about 25% greater than the equivalent curves for the internal L-response and the hyperpolarizing part of the C-response. The experiments show that the S-potentials could be evoked over a wide area of the retina, in agreement with earlier reports (*31, 41*).

c) **Comparison of S-potentials with trans-retinal responses.** In a number of extensive studies, Motokawa et al. (*17, 18, 19*) (see also Mitarai, *16*) have analyzed the trans-retinal potential evoked by restricted illumination of the fish retina, and have shown that the receptor-side positive response, obtained when the spot was close to the electrode, reversed to a negative on when the stimulating light was moved some 500 μ away from the recording site. These same authors (*19*) also demonstrated a very interesting correlation between the spike patterns of the retinal ganglion cells and the spatial distribution and polarity reversal of the trans-retinal responses. We have confirmed the studies, the scanning curves of the trans-retinal potentials being basically the same as those obtained by the Japanese authors.

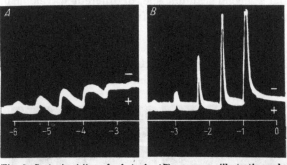

Fig. 8. Scotopic (*A*) and photopic (*B*) responses illustrating relationship between amplitude and logarithmic stimulus intensity

It is of interest to notice the direction dependent assymmetry obtained in the scanning curves of the trans-retinal potentials. This can be seen in Fig. 7, comparing *A* with *B* and *D* with *E*, and is due to the mixture of temporal effects with the spatial interaction phenomena. However, when using the same speed of scanning (0.3 mm/sec) no temporal or directional effects were observed in the recordings of the S-potentials. Thus, it is seen that the scanning curves of these two kinds of potentials are strikingly unlike. Indeed, while the trans-retinal response showed a reversal of polarity when the stimulus spot was advanced towards or moved away from the central region of recording, there was no polarity reversal and only an amplitude change in the corresponding recordings of the S-potential.

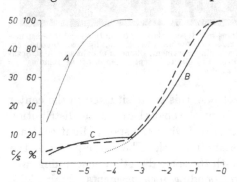

Fig. 9. Amplitude-intensity relation curve in dark-(*A, C*) and light-(*B*) adapted states, and critical fusion frequency curve (broken line) for sun-fish (Ref. *43*)

It turned out to be a difficult task to correlate the spreading velocities of the S-potentials with the propagation velocity of the receptor surface-negative trans-retinal potential, this being the potential which spreads from an illuminated area to the surrouding non-illuminated regions, and which response has been described by Motokawa et al. (*17, 18*) and Mitarai (*16*). In recent studies (*19*), it was demonstrated that the receptor surface-negative spreading response either was associated with (excitatory) "on" discharges or with (post-inhibitory) spike firings at "off", depending on the type of ganglion cell being involved. Thus, the receptor surface-negative potential could be accompanied by excitatory or inhibitory effects as well, whereas only the depolarizing polarity of the S-potential is associated with inhibition. In their measurements of the propagation velocity of this trans-retinal potential (*18, 19*) values were obtained varying between 0.067 and 0.160 m/sec giving a mean value of 0.112 m/sec. Due to the large interactions occurring between the receptor surface-negative and the surface-positive potentials, we were not able to determine the spreading velocity of this trans-retinal potential with an accuracy permitting a comparison with the spreading velocity values obtained for the S-potentials. We are inclined to interpret the trans-retinal recordings as representing complex interactions of potentials produced by different retinal structures (receptors, bipolars, and ganglion cell dendrites), while probably the S-potentials are not directly contributing to the ERG, the glial excitability control of the neurons being only indirectly reflected in the trans-retinal recordings. Thus we have reached the conclusion that at the moment it is difficult to correlate directly the intra-cellular glial responses with the trans-retinal recordings.

4. Amplitude-intensity relation of the S-potentials

The series of S-potential recordings shown in Fig. 8 were obtained from an internal horizontal cell, the different intensities of the light stimuli used being given by the logarithmic scale at the bottom of the figure (*28, 29, 30*). The records

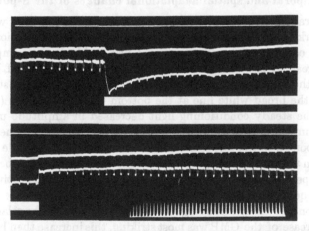

Fig. 10. Change of test response and GMP during and after conditioning light. Top record taken with five times less amplification than lower record. Top horizontal line is zero potential for the low amplification record. Time position of conditioning light shown by broad white line. Time calibration pips are at 1 sec intervals, and their height (10 mV) gives voltage calibration for lower record

in *A* were obtained with an amplification one third of that for *B*, in order to match curve *C* of Fig. 9, whereupon the retina was thoroughly light-adapted and the tracings shown in Fig. 8, B were recorded, these responses matching curve *B* of Fig. 9. The threshold of the response *A* (Fig. 8) was at about $\overline{6.3}$ and it became saturated at about $\overline{3.6}$ of the relative intensity scale. The photopic response *B* (Fig. 8) appeared at about 4.2 and saturated at about 0.6. The corresponding amplitude-intensity relation curves for the scotopic response (*A*) and for the

photopic response (B) have been plotted in Fig. 9. These curves illustrate the
so-called "straight line portion" of the semi-logarithmic relationship, which for
the scotopic state extends from $\overline{6.0}$ to $\overline{4.2}$, and for the photopic from $\overline{3.3}$ to $\overline{0.6}$.
The light intensity used for evoking the maximal, saturated scotopic response
coincided with the threshold intensity of the photopic one; the Purkinje shift
occurring at an intensity level of about $\overline{3.6}$. Thus, the cone system started to
function when the rod system had reached its maximum working level, corresponding to the "rod-cone break" of the adaptation curve. The difference of
25 mV, observed between the GMP levels in the light- and dark-adapted conditions, reflects two metabolic equilibrium levels of the glial excitability control
of the retinal neurons and receptors (adaptation). The continuous curve $B-C$
(Fig. 9) was obtained by replotting curve A in such a way that the maximum
point of C corresponded to the minimum value of B. This overall curve is identical
with the critical flicker fusion curve obtained on the live sun-fish, in which frequencies above 10 c/s corresponded to the cones (30, 43). Sᴠᴀᴇᴛɪᴄʜɪɴ (30) showed
that this flicker fusion curve could be explained by the rates of the rises and
decays of the S-potentials, and this is in good agreement with our present findings
showing that the S-potentials reflect the glial control mechanism of the retinal
excitability. The glial function as pointed out by Vᴀʟʟᴇᴄᴀʟʟᴇ et al. (35) corresponds to the after-potentials of the neurons which determine the maximum
frequency of firing.

5. Temporal and spatial adaptational changes of the S-potential

a) Temporal effect. In these series of experiments S-potentials were obtained
from the dark-adapted retina by repeated test flashes (duration 150 msec),
whereupon a continuous conditioning light was suddenly superimposed on the
stimulated area. As can be seen in Fig. 10, a transient internal -L-response was
produced by the continuous conditioning light, the duration of the stimulus being
indicated by the broad white line at the bottom of the recordings (Fig. 10). The
response to the steady conditioning light decreased in amplitude until finally a
new equilibrium GMP level was reached. As the result of applying the conditioning
light, the responses to the test stimuli were diminished in amplitude in the beginning, and then they increased again as the GMP was reduced. The behavior of the
GMP was depending on previous adaptational conditions. The time necessary
to reach an equilibrium GMP level was long in the scotopic state and short in
the photopic one. If the conditioning light was $\overline{3.6}$ or more on the relative intensity
scale, the increase of the GMP was most striking, this increase then being followed
by a slow decay which lasted for several minutes. During the non-equilibrium mesopic
transition from rod to cone activity the GMP remained at its highest level (Fig. 11,
continuous line). Therefore, the B and C curves of Fig. 9 were obtainable only
at their corresponding equilibrium levels, which were reached some time after the
application of the adapting light. In the photopic state, even abnormally strong
conditioning illumination did not increase the GMP level more than maximally
about 10 mV above the ordinary photopic equilibrium level of 35 mV, which
was found under ordinary room light illumination.

In the mesopic non-equilibrium state where the GMP level, due to the high
sensitivity of the rod system, was brought close to the saturation point of the response,

the responses to the test flashes were small and sometimes indistinguishable (Fig. 12, *F*, *G*). However, as soon as the GMP decreased again, the test responses reappeared. This same behavior was observed also on the hyperpolarizing component of the C-response (Fig. 12, *A—D*), which indicates that the C-response is influenced by the rod activity as well. On the other hand, it was seen that in connection with the high GMP (evel in the transitional state, the sensitivity to red light had increased (Fig. 12*C*), and that it decreased again when the normal photopic equilibrium level of 35 mV was reached (Fig. 12, *D*).These experiments clearly showed that the amplitude of the hyperpolarizing S-potential was inversely proportional to the GMP, whereas the depolarizing component of the C-responses was proportional to the GMP.

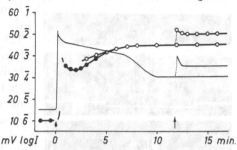

Fig. 11. Process of change of GMP (continuous line) and threshold (filled and open circles) during (between arrows) and after conditioning light. Filled circles illustrate threshold of rod activity and open circles of cone activity. Voltage (mV) scale is for GMP and log scale for threshold

b) **Spatial effects.** In order to study the influence of the photopigment concentration on the adaptational mechanisms, the test light and the conditioning (adapting) light were applied to separate retinal areas 1.5 mm apart from each

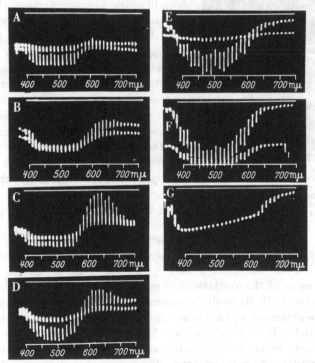

Fig. 12. Recordings *A—D* illustrate changes occurring in GMP and spectral characteristics of C-response when passing from scotopic (*A*) to mesopic (*B*, *C*) and photopic (*D*) states. Recordings *E—G* show changes of scotopic internal L-response (*E*), when adapted to light (*F*, *G*). *B*, *C* and *G* show saturation of hyperpolarizing components. Distance between line of wavelength scale (below) and upper line (zero potential) is calibrated to 100 mV for the low amplification GMP recordings

other. Under these experimental conditions any bleaching by the conditioning light of the photopigment could be excluded in the area where the test flash was supplied. Yet, the results were identical with those obtained in the experiments described above in which the test light was spatially superimposed on the conditioning light, which is in agreement with the observations of FATEHCHAND et al. (6). The results prove that the adaptational changes in the retina are primarily controlled by the glial networks (GMP) and that the state of adaptation is not critically related to the concentration of the photopigments in the receptors.

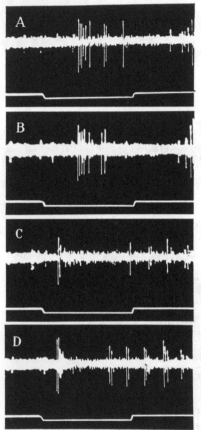

Fig. 13. Effect of change from dark (A) to light-(B) adaptation on ganglion cell spikes. Differences seen in spike amplitudes are due to glial control of ganglion cell membrane potential level (see also SVAETICHIN et al. this symposium)

6. Adaptational changes and the spike firing of the ganglion cells

Fig. 13 shows the retinal ganglion cell spikes obtained in the dark-adapted state (A) and after adaptation to light (B—D). During the non-equilibrium transitional state the spike firing was blocked for a certain period after onset and cessation of a conditioning light, reflecting the behavior of the S-potential as described above. In the dark-adapted state the spikes showed a long "on" and "off" latency and a long duration of the repetitive firings, while in light-adapted conditions the "on" and "off" latencies were shorter and so also the duration of the repetitive discharges. There was a clear relation between the firing patterns of the ganglion cells and the behavior of the S-potentials (39, 40), which is in agreement with our interpretation that the glial networks exert a metabolic controlling action on the neurons and receptors.

Comments

In his pioneering work RAMON y CAJAL maintains that the function of the horizontal cell in the fish retina is that of "a store-house of nervous energy" by which the "tension of the excitation" is reinforced in order to enable it to reach the higher centers (23). Recently, electronmicroscopists and neurochemists (3, 7, 8, 11, 26) have examined a possible morphological and biochemical glial-neuronal relationship, and a high metabolic rate has been postulated for the glial cells.

The non-photochemical "alpha-adaptation" has been assumed to depend on spatial and temporal reorganizations of the neuronal networks in the course of adaptation. However, corresponding experimental evidence has not been available (2). Our present studies show that the adaptational phenomena depend on the function of the glial networks, and that the spatial effects are caused by a spreading of the glial reaction in the retina. These results lead us to the conclusion that the fundamental mechanism for the retinal adaptation is based on the glial metabolic reaction. BARLOW, FITZHUGH and KUFFLER (2) demonstrated that the "lateral inhibition" of the light-adapted retina disappeared in dark-adaptation. Such integrative retinal phenomena of the spatial-temporal interactions (1) can be explained on the basis of the function of the glial cells (35), and our recent experiments (33) show that in the retina the inhibitory effects on the ganglion cell firing are controlled by the Müller fiber glia.

The conclusion is that neuronal events influence the glial cell metabolism, the latter reciprocally controlling the excitability of the neurons (12, 33) just as in feedback systems, and that feedback furnished by the glial system may play an important part in stabilizing retinal behavior (35).

Acknowledgements

We want to express our thanks to the director of IVIC Dr. Marcel Roche for his unfailing interest and trust in our work.

Thanks are due to Mr. W. KRATTENMACHER for the design and construction of the photo-stimulator. We also would like to express our thanks to Messrs. ANTONIO D'YAN and BERNHARD GRAF for the design and construction of the apparatus for light spot scanning of the retina, for assisting in technical matters and for help in producing the pictures.

Summary

1. The electro-physiological analysis of neurons and glial cells which has been presented at this symposium, shows the existence of a close functional interaction between these two types of cells, and further that the excitability of the neuron is controlled metabolically by its glial satellites. It is concluded from the experimental findings described in the present paper that the retinal excitability or level of adaptation is fundamentally controlled by the metabolic activity of the glial networks.

2. By measuring threshold, latency, rise and decay times and the spectral sensitivity during the change from dark- to light-adaptation, it is shown that the external horizontal cells are linked only to the photopic luminosity system, the internal horizontal cells to both the scotopic and the photopic luminosity systems, and the Müller fibers to the chromatic and the scotopic (rod) systems.

3. The adaptational changes of the GMP have been studied in both the transient (mesopic) and the equilibrium (scotopic, photopic) states. In the steady state the sensitivity of the retina (as seen in the glial hyperpolarizing response and ganglion cell firing) was inversely proportional to the GMP. In the course of light-adaptation, the increase of the GMP was accompanied by a Purkinje shift.

4. The alpha-adaptation produced by small spot illumination of the retina was found to be due to a spreading in the glial networks of the metabolic excitability processes.

5. The present results lead us to suppose that the glial networks provide feedback in the retinal functional organization, this feedback controlling and stabilizing the retinal sensivity (see VALLECALLE et al. this symposium).

References

1. BARLOW, H. B.: Summation and inhibition in the frog's retina. J. Physiol. (Lond.) 119, 69—88 (1953).
2. — R. FITZHUGH and S. W. KUFFLER: Change of organization in the receptive fields of the cat's retina during dark adaptation. J. Physiol. (Lond.) 137, 338—354 (1957).
3. Biology of Neuroglia. Springfield, U.S.A.: Windle, F. W. (editor). Charles C. Thomas 1958.
4. CRESCITELLI, F.: The natural history of visual pigments. Ann. N. Y. Acad. Sci. 74, 230 255 (1958).
5. DARTNALL, H. J. A.: The visual pigments. London: Methuen 1957.
6. FATEHCHAND, R., G. SVAETICHIN, G. MITARAI and J. VILLEGAS: Location of the non-linearity in horizontal cell response to retinal illumination. Nature (Lond.) 189, 463—464 (1961).
7. GERSCHENFELD, H. M., F. WALD, J. A. ZADUNAISKY and E. DE ROBERTIS: Function of astroglia in the water-ion metabolism of the central nervous system. An electron microscope study. Neurology (Minneap.) 9, 412 (1959).
8. GLEES, P.: Neuroglia, morphology and function. Oxford: Blackwell Scientific Publications 1955.
9. GOURAS, P.: Spreading depression of activity in amphibian retina. Amer. J. Physiol. 195, 28—32 (1958).
10. GRANIT, R.: Sensory mechanisms of the retina. Oxford: Oxford University Press 1947.
11. HYDÉN, H.: The neuron. Chapter in the cell. Vol. 4, 1, 215—323. J. Brachet & A. Mirsky editors. New York: Academic Press 1960.
12. LAUFER, M., G. SVAETICHIN, G. MITARAI, R. FATEHCHAND, E. VALLECALLE and J. VILLEGAS: The effect of temperature, carbon dioxide and ammonia on the neuron-glia unit. This symposium 457—463 (1961).
13. MACNICHOL., and G. SVAETICHIN: Electric responses from the isolated retinas of fishes. Amer. J. Ophthalm. 46, p. 2, 26—46 (1958).
14. MITARAI, G., and Y. YAGASAKI: Resting and action potentials of single cone. Ann. Rep. Res. Inst. Environm. Med. Nagoya Univ. 2, 54—61 (1955).
15. — The Origin of the so-called cone potential. Proc. Jap. Acad. 34, 299—304 (1938).
16. — Slow potentials of the isolated carp retina. J. Jap. physiol. Soc. (1959).
17. MOTOKAWA, K., T. OIKAWA and T. OGAWA: Slow potentials induced from the illuminated part into the surrounding area of the retina. Jap. J. Physiol. 9, 218—227 (1959).
18. — — K. TASAKI and T. OGAWA: The spatial distribution of electric responses to focal illumination of the carp's retina. Tohoku J. exp. Med. 70, 151—164 (1959).
19. — E. YAMASHITA and T. OGAWA: Slow potentials and spike activity of retina. J. Neurophysiol. 24, 101—110 (1961).
20. MÜLLER-LIMMROTH, H. W.: Der Einfluß der Belichtung auf das Bestandspotential des Froschauges. Z. Biol. 104, 275—283 (1954).
21. O'LEARY, J. L., and S. GOLDRING: Changes associated with forebrain excitation processes: d. c. potentials of the cerebral cortex. Handbook of Physiology, Vol. 1, 315—328. Baltimore: Waverly Press 1959.
22. OTTOSON, D., and G. SVAETICHIN: Electrophysiological investigations of the frog retina. Cold. Spr. Harb. Symp. quant. Biol. 17, 165—173 (1952).
23. POLYAK, S. L.: The retina. Chicago: University Press 1941.
24. RUSHTON, W. A. H., and R. D. COHEN: Visual purple level and the course of dark adaptation. Nature (Lond.) 173, 301—304 (1954).
25. — and F. W. CAMPBELL: Measurement of rhodpsin in the living human eye. Nature (Lond.) 174, 1096—1097 (1954).
26. SJÖSTRAND, F. S.: Electron-microscopy of myelin and of nerve cells and tissue. Modern scientific aspect of neurology. 188—231. London: John N. Cumings (Editor) Edward Arnold Publishers 1960.
27. SUZUKI, H., N. TAIRA and K. MOTOKAWA: Spectral response curves and receptive fields of pre- and post-geniculate fibers of the cat. Tôhoku J. exp. Med. 71, 401—415 (1960).
28. SVAETICHIN, G.: The cone action potential. Acta physiol. scand. 29. suppl. 106, 565—600 (1953).

29. —, and R. Jonasson: A technique for oscillographic recording of spectral response curves. Acta physiol. scand. **39**, suppl. 134, 3—16 (1956).
30. Svaetichin, G.: Receptor mechanisms for flicker and fusion. Acta physiol. scand. **39**, suppl. 134, 47—54 (1956).
31. —, and W. Krattenmacher: Photostimulation of single cones. XXI Internat. Congr. Physiol. Sci. 267 (1959).
32. — — and M. Laufer: Photostimulation of single cones. J. gen. Physiol. **43**, p. 2, 101—114 (1960).
33. —, M. Laufer, G. Mitarai, R. Fatehchand, E. Vallecalle and J. Villegas: Glial control of neurol networks and receptors. This symposium, p. 445—456.
34. —, G. Mitarai, M. Laufer and J. Villegas: Manuscript in preparation (1961).
35. Vallecalle, E., and G. Svaetichin: The retina as model for the functional organization of the nervous system. This symposium, p. 489—492.
36. Villegas, G. M.: Electron microscopy of the fish retina. XXI Internat. Congr. Physiol. Sci. 267 (1959).
37. — Electron microscopic study of the vertebrate Retina. J. gen. Physiol. **43**, p. 2, 15—43 (1960).
38. — Comparative ultrastructure of the retina in fish, monkey and man. This symposium, p. 3—13.
39. Villegas, J.: Studies on the retinal ganglion cells. This symposium, p. 481—489.
40. Wagner, H. G., E. F. MacNichol and M. L. Wolbarsht: The response properties of single ganglion cells in the goldfish retina. J. gen. Physiol. **43**, p. 2, 45—62 (1960).
41. Watanabe, K., and T. Tosaka: Functional organization of the cyprinid fish retina as revealed by discriminative responses to spectral illumination. Jap. J. Physiol. **9**, 84—93 (1959).
42. Willmer, E. N.: Human color vision and the perception of blue. J. Theoret. Biol. **1**, 172—179 (1961).
43. Wolf, E., and G. F. Wolf: Threshold intensity of illumination and flicker frequency for the eye of the sun fish. J. gen. Physiol. **19**, 495—502 (1936).

Studies on the Retinal Ganglion Cells*

By

Jorge Villegas

With 5 Figures

In recent studies (*6, 15*), it has definitively been proved, by histological localization of the recording electrode tip, that the S-potential has an intracellular origin in the tangential and radial glial systems of the retina; the L-response was obtained in the horizontal cells and the C-response in the Müller fibers. Each glial cell, in close contact with several neurons, acts together with them as a functional unit, and provides a metabolic active extraneuronal space. The excitability, and the electrical potentials recorded in the system, are closely related to the metabolic activity of the glial cells.

Since their description in the frog retina (*2*), the response patterns of single ganglion cells have been analyzed by many workers, and several attempts have been made to establish a clear correlation between the ganglion cell response and the slow potentials in the retina (*1, 5, 7*).

In the present work on the isolated fish retina (Centropomidae), it was possible to find some functional relationship between the glial cells response (*S*-potential)

* Department of Physiology, Instituto Venezolano de Investigaciones Cientificas Caracas. Venezuela.

and the ganglion cell activity. The techniques and methods employed in these
studies have been described in prior reports (6, 10, 11).

Glial cell response. Single and simultaneous records of the ganglion and glial
cell responses to different intensities and wavelengths of a 25 μ diameter light
stimulus were obtained. The characteristics of the observed glial response were
similar to those which have been previously described for the same experimental
preparation (4, 6, 12, 14, 15).

Ganglion cell responses. On penetrating from the receptor side of the retinal
surface, the recording site for a maximal amplitude of the spike potential was

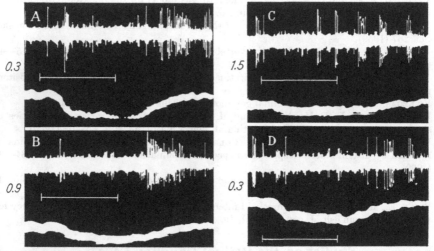

Fig. 1. Relation between ganglion cell spike firing and response amplitude of horizontal cell on changing intensity
of stimulus. Constant duration of 300 msec and wavelength 519 mμ. Log. intensity of stimulus light indicated on
left of each record

always below the level of the last position where glial cell responses could be
obtained. The depth of the recording site could be measured, within about 2 μ
error, by means of a needle gauge attached to the micromanipulator holding the
glass electrode.

Response patterns. The ganglion cells showed the three main types of response
pattern described in the frog retina (2). The "on-off" type was the most frequent
under photopic conditions, but this was not so in the scotopic state.

Two types of "on-off" responses were observed: the first one showed a clear
wavelength dependence, shifting from a pure "on" to a pure "off" discharge as the
stimulus wavelength was changed. The second one depended on the intensity
of the stimulus light, shifting from a pure "on" or a pure "off" to an "on-off"
discharge, when the stimulus intensity was increased above a particular value.
This behavior was independent of the wavelength of the stimulus.

Two different types of pure "off" ganglion cell units were also noticed: the
first one, illustrated in Fig. 2, gave a single burst of impulses at "off" and did not
show any spontaneous activity. The second one, illustrated in Fig. 1, showed
a rhythmical repetitive discharge even in dark periods and under different levels
of background illumination. A stimulus of low intensity produced a short supression of the spontaneous activity at "on" and a slight increment at "off". On

increasing the intensity of the stimulus, the number of spikes and the latency of the "off" firing increased in a similar way to some units described in the cat retina (3).

The "on" type of ganglion cell response pattern also showed the two different characteristics which have been described by several authors: that is, a single burst, or an initial high frequency burst followed by a steady discharge during the total duration of the stimulus. In no case did the "on" cells show any change in pattern with variation of the wavelength.

Wavelength dependence. As previously described, only one type of "on-off" units showed wavelength dependence; when stimulated with light of short wavelength some of these cells fired at "on", while others fired at "off"; in both cases, the response to long wavelength stimuli was opposite to the short wavelength response, being a pure "off" and a pure "on" discharge respectively at threshold intensities. A clear opposition

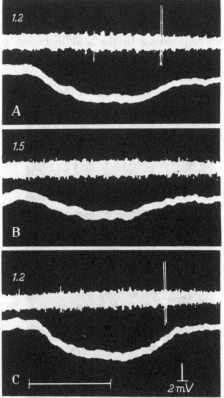

Fig. 2. Relation between ganglion cell spike firing and response amplitude of horizontal cell on changing intensity of stimulus. Constant duration of 300 msec and wavelength 591 mμ. Log. intensity of stimulus light indicated on left of each record

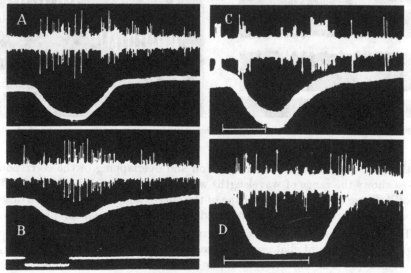

Fig. 3. Relation between ganglion cell and horizontal cell responses. Stimulus intensity lower in B than in A. Stimulus duration doubled from C to D

31*

could be observed between these two groups of units, both groups having a common range of wavelengths in which they fired both at "on" and at "off", corresponding to the middle region of the visible spectrum.

The spectral response curve of both these two types of cell, measured by the constant response method and also by the constant intensity method, exhibited a maximum at 490 mμ for the short wavelengths and another maximum at 640 mμ

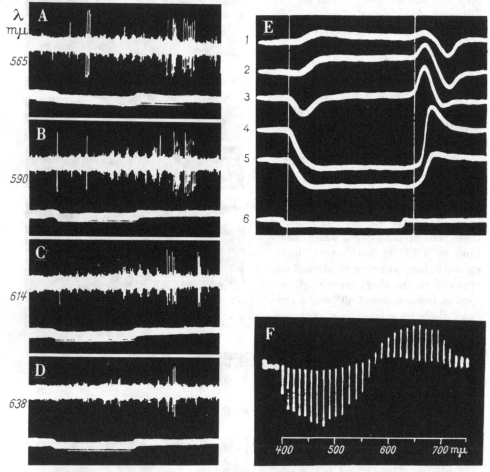

Fig. 4. Relation between ganglion cell and Müller fiber responses on changing the wavelength of stimulus

for the long wavelengths. The intersection and overlapping of the corresponding curves shows the range of wavelengths where these units fired both at "on" and at "off". Some variations in the shape of the curves and in the maximum observed at long wavelengths could be related to different adaptational conditions (6).

The close correlation between the spike pattern and the spectral response curve of the C-type of glial response agrees with earlier descriptions in the gold-fish retina (5). An observed example of this correlation is shown in Fig. 4 where the responses to different wavelengths were recorded with constant stimulus intensity and duration. In A to D of Fig. 4, it is seen that the ganglion cell unit fired at "off" at long wavelengths and both at "on" and "off" at short wavelengths. To the wavelength of 590 mμ, which corresponds to the neutral point of the C-response shown in F of Fig. 4, and to the glial response shown in E_3 of Fig. 4, the response of the ganglion cell was a single spike at "on" and a double discharge at "off". At very short or very long wavelengths the ganglion cell discharge appeared only at "on" and only at "off" respectively. The corresponding responses of the glial cell are shown in E_1 to E_4 of Fig. 4, the wavelengths decreasing from the top to the bottom of the picture. The presence of a double "off" discharge of the

ganglion cell, as well as a negative phase of the positive glial response and a positive phase of the negative going glial response, seems to be due to oscillations caused by the high intensity stimuli used.

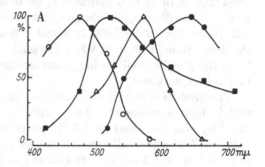

In Fig. 5 are shown some experimental results obtained in the optic tectum (Fig. 5 A) and in the retina in situ (Fig. 5 B) of the same fish (Centropomidae). There is a clear correlation between these results and the ones illustrated in Fig. 4. The neutral point and the maxima of the spectral response curve in F of Fig. 4, correspond respectively in Fig. 5 to the intersection of the "on" and "off" curves and to the maxima of the "on" and "off" responses. The pure "on" and the pure "off" types of cell were found to have identical spectral response curves, as measured by both the constant response and the constant intensity methods, with the maximum at a wavelength of 590 mμ

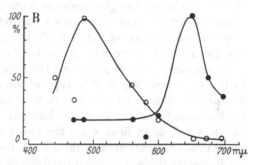

Fig. 5. Spectral response curves recorded in the optic tectum (A) and the retina in situ (B) of Centropomidae. Open circles "on" response, filled circles "off" response, of wavelength dependent "on-off" unit. Triangles pure "on" unit. Squares pure "off" unit. Vertical scales in percent of number of spikes, horizontal scales wavelength in mμ

under photopic conditions. The pure "on" and the pure "off" types of cell had substantially the same thresholds at any particular wavelength. Similar results were obtained in the optic tectum.

When the glass capillary micro-electrode had penetrated about 50 μ below the level of the C-response, intracellular recordings from the ganglion cell body were sometimes obtained. The "on" discharge appeared superimposed on a positive going square wave for long wave-length stimuli, and at short wave-lengths the "off" discharge just followed a negative going square wave (16). It was also possible to obtain, above the level of the cell body recordings (just below the recording site of the C-response or the lowest level L-response), depolarizing saw-tooth transients at "on" and "off", which by their characteristics appeared similar to the slow optic nerve or ventral root potentials (p. 460, Fig. 3).

These intracellular responses likely are recordings from ganglion cell dendrites. They were sometimes wave-length dependent but always depolarizing EPSP's.

Intensity dependence. Using a light stimulus of constant duration and wavelength, the intensity was decreased in steps of 0.6 log. units, starting at 0.3 log. units below the maximum intensity (see methods, in ref. 6). Some results are shown in Fig. 1, where the glial cell response had reached a maximal hyperpolarizing amplitude of 2.4 mV in A, 1.3 mV in B, 0.9 mV in C and 1.8 mV in D. The corresponding responses of the ganglion cell changed from an "on-off" discharge in A to a pure "off" discharge in B, a rhythmical "on" discharge at a frequency of 10 c/s in C and then again to an "on-off" discharge in D. It can be seen that the discharge of the ganglion cell started when the response of the glial cell crossed the 1.2 mV level, in A and D both at the rise and decay times, and at the decay time in B; in C, where the glial cell response did not cross the 1.2 mV level, the ganglion cell discharge was similar to the spontaneous firing shown by this unit in darkness.

The records obtained from another unit are shown in Fig. 2. Starting (A) with a light stimulus of 1.2 log. units on the relative intensity scale (6), the intensity was decreased by 0.3 log. units in B and then increased to its initial value in C. The glial cell response reached a maximum hyperpolarizing amplitude of 3.2 mV in A, 1.2 mV in B and 3.2 mV in C. The ganglion cell fired only during the decay time of the glial response when the latter crossed the 1.2 mV level in A and C. No ganglion cell response was obtained when the amplitude of the glial response was 1.2 mV or less, 1.2 mV being the "threshold" level. This ganglion cell unit showed no spontaneous activity in darkness.

A similar relationship between the ganglion and glial cell responses is evident in the records of Fig. 3. The type of intensity dependent variation previously described is illustrated in A and B. In C and D the intensity of the stimulus was kept constant, but the stimulus duration was doubled for D. In both cases the ganglion cell units fired when the rising and decaying phases of the negative going glial responses crossed the 1.2 mV level.

Receptive fields. The receptive fields of different ganglion cells were measured using a spot of 25 μ diameter, and were found to be homogeneous and oval in shape, the two main diameters being 275 and 200 μ. No difference in response pattern was found between center and periphery under photopic conditions, whether the light stimulation was white or monochromatic. The threshold for each unit was constant over the whole receptive field, and when the stimulus spot was located outside the receptive field, an increment of at least one log. unit of the stimulus light intensity was still only able to produce very erratic responses of the unit being tested.

Comments

From the present experimental results it is deduced that there is a clear correlation between glial responses and the activity of ganglion cells.

It is evident that there exists a critical "threshold" amplitude of the glial response, as observed when a ganglionar response is evoked, this "threshold" being very close to the 2 mV value calculated for a similar experimental preparation on the basis of flicker fusion studies (12).

Since it has been shown that the S-potential reflects the glial excitability control of the neurons and cannot be considered a generator potential for producing spikes in the neurons (6, 15), its "threshold" amplitude should be understood as being the level of the glial reaction elicited by the neuronal events that initiate the firing of the ganglion cells.

The presence in neuronal elements of opposite types of temporal patterns which are or are not dependent on wavelength, having the same spectral response curve for each of the opponents, seems to reflect the mechanisms for spatial contrast (black-white, opponent color). In studies of the glial responses (Centropomidae) which have been carried out so far, we have only found one polarity for the L-type of response and only one pattern for the C-type, the latter being negative going at short wavelengths and positive going at long wavelengths. This suggests that bipolar cell mechanisms are involved in building up systems of particular spectral sensitivities and, in conjunction with the very good agreement which exists between the diameters for homogeneous receptive fields obtained for the ganglion cells in the present work and the magnitude of the plateau of the spatial amplitude distribution curves of the glial responses (6), leads to the conclusion that a glial cell together with all the bipolars with which it is in close contact, form a functional unit connected to one ganglion cell and partially related to other ganglion cell units. We have described in other papers (6, 15) the behavior of the receptor potential, this showing only one polarity and a small receptive field; on the other hand, the ganglion cell distributions and their synaptic connections seem to provide a retinal mosaic means for spatial discrimination. When the fish moves, so that a particular part of the retinal image is moved between receptive fields of opposite temporal characteristics, the stimulus which provokes a given sensation in a certain field produces the opponent one in the next field, making spatial discrimination possible. This simple organization provides a fine grain contrast discrimination mechanism for photopic and a coarser but low threshold one for scotopic vision. For this arrangement two types of bipolar cell are required; the first one would be effective for excitation of the ganglion cells during the negative going phase and the second one during the positive going phase of the glial response. The experimental evidence for this assumption is clear, since two groups of ganglionar response patterns can be built up. One group of elements is the pure "on", and the short wavelengths "on" and long wavelengths "off", these always firing during the relative negative going phase of the glial response. The other group consists of the pure "off", and the short wavelengths "off" and long wavelengths "on" units, these always firing during the relative positive going phase of the glial response. Without this assumption of at least two different excitatory types of bipolar cells it seems impossible to understand how two opposite temporal patterns are obtained at the ganglion cell level from only one type of temporal pattern at the glia-bipolar level. However, another explanation is perhaps possible, since in the retina of another fish (p. 453, Fig. 3) opponent patterns of glial C-response have been recorded. One may therefore expect that in the Centropomidae retina this other type of C-response also exists, but has not yet been observed since the amacrine cells are too small.

As has been suggested (6, 15), the spatio-temporal and wavelength discrimination carried out by the retina is under the direct control and programming by the glial networks, rather than by the neuronal circuits according to the concepts based on the classical neuron theory.

Further studies are necessary in order to establish a more detailed correlation between these glial and ganglion cell responses and the retinal mechanisms of vision.

Summary

The response patterns of single ganglion cells to light stimuli of different intensities and wavelengths are studied and related to the glial cell responses, in the fish retina (Centropomidae).

The glial response (S-potential) is not considered to be a generator potential for the spike discharge of the ganglion cells. However, a "threshold" amplitude (1.2 mV) for the glial response is found, this being the amplitude of the glial reaction elicited by the neuronal events that initiate the firing of the ganglion cells.

The receptive fields of single ganglion cells show no difference in pattern between center and periphery to a 25 μ diameter light stimulus, whether white or monochromatic light is employed. The threshold for each unit is constant over the whole receptive field. There is agreement between the diameters of the receptive fields of the ganglion cells and the magnitude of the plateau in the spatial amplitude distribution curves of the glial responses, this being interpreted as evidence for glial-bipolar functional units connected to one ganglion cell and partially related to other ganglion cells.

Ganglion cell units showing opposite temporal patterns, but having identical spectral response curves for each of the opponents, and whose maxima and inflection points correspond respectively to the maxima and inflection points of the spectral response curves of the glial cells, are described. Two groups of ganglion cell response patterns are built up. One group is the pure "on" and the short wavelengths "on" and long wavelengths "off" units, these always firing during the relative negative going phase of the glial response. The other group consists of the pure "off", and the short wavelengths "off" and long wavelengths "on" units, these always firing during the relative positive going phase of the glial response. Two types of bipolar cell are assumed; the first one would be effective for excitation of the ganglion cells during the negative going phase and the second one during the positive going phase of the glial response. These facts are considered to reflect the retinal mechanisms for spatial contrast (black-white, opponent color) and discrimination.

References

1. Gouras, P.: Graded potentials of bream retina. J. Physiol. (Lond.) 157, 487—505 (1960).
2. Hartline, H. K.: The responses of single optic nerve fibers of the vertebrate eye to illumination of the retina. Amer. J. Physiol. 121, 400 (1938).
3. Kuffler, S. W.: Discharge patterns and functional organization of mammalian retina. J. Neurophysiol. 16, 37—68 (1953).
4. MacNichol jr., E. F., and G. Svaetichin: Electric responses from the isolated retina of fishes. Amer. J. Ophthal. 46, 26—46 (1958).
5. —, M. L. Wolbarsht and H. G. Wagner: Electrophysiological evidence for a mechanism of color vision in the goldfish. In "Light and Life", pp. 795—814. New York: McElroy, W. D., and B. Glass, edit. John Hopk. Press 1961.

6. MITARAI, G., G. SVAETICHIN. E. VALLECALLE, R. FATEHCHAND, J. VILLEGAS and M. LAUFER: Glia-neuron interactions and adaptational mechanisms of the retina. This symposion 463—481 (1961)
7. MOTOKAWA, K., E. YAMASHITA and T. OGAWA: Slow potentials and spike activity of retina. J. Neurophysiol. 24, 101—110 (1961).
8. OTTOSON, D., and G. SVAETICHIN: Electrophysiological investigations of the frog retina. Cold Spr. Harb. Symp. quant. Biol. 17, 165—173 (1952).
9. — — The electrical activity of the retinal receptor layer. Acta physiol. scand. 29, 31—39 (1956).
10. SVAETICHIN, G.: The cone action potential. Acta physiol. scand., supp. 106, 565—600 (1953).
11. —, and R. JONNASON: A technique for oscillographic recording of spectral response curves. Acta physiol. scand. 39, supp. 134, 3—16 (1956).
12. — Spectral response curves from single cones. Acta physiol. scand. 39, supp. 134, 17—46 (1956).
13. — Receptor mechanism for flicker and fusion. Acta physiol. scand. 39, supp. 134, 47—54 (1956).
14. —, and E. F. MACNICHOL jr.: Retinal mechanism for chromatic and achromatic vision. Ann. N. Y. Acad. Sci. 74, 385—404 (1958).
15. —, M. LAUFER, G. MITARAI, R. FATEHCHAND, E. VALLECALLE, and J. VILLEGAS: Glial control of neuronal networks and receptors. This symposion 445—456 (1961).
16. WIESEL, T. N.: Retinal inhibition and excitation in the cats retinal ganglion cells with intracellular electrodes. Nature, (Lond.) 183, 264—265 (1959).

The Retina as Model for the Functional Organization of the Nervous System

By

EDMUNDO VALLECALLE* and GUNNAR SVAETICHIN**

With 2 Figures

The unclassical characteristics of the S-potentials have been puzzling from the very beginning, and the demonstration of their glial origin increased the problems necessitating a revision of the conventional neurophysiological concepts. In the course of the attempts to give an interpretation of our experimental findings concerning the glial cell behavior in correlation to ordinary neurophysiological views, it became evident that for any explanation of a normal organized neuronal activity whatever, it is obligatory to take into account the close and permanent relationship existing between metabolism and the electrical potentials. The present paper represents a preliminary and very short exposition of our working hypothesis which offers a general interpretation of a possible functional organization of the nervous system. This presentation is based on: 1. the experimental data collected since 1953 on the electrophysiology of the glial cells (partly still unpublished), 2. an extensive panoramic review of comparative physiology and related fields and 3. a superficial attempt to apply concepts from the communication theory on the studies of the nervous system. Under these circumstances this analysis does not pretend to be either detailed or conclusive, since more time is

* Department of Physiology, Vargas Medical School, Central University of Venezuela, Caracas, Venezuela.
** Department of Physiology Instituto Venezolano de Investigaciones Cientificas, Caracas, Venezuela.

needed to digest and present the large amount of information which has been gathered concerning the integrative function of neurons, receptors and glial cells.

In the retina the signals seem to be elaborated in the following way. The generator system works by stepwise summation through metabolic compensation and phosphorylative oxydative coupling. Light reaction enables the resynthesis of the photopigment, triggers the oxybiotic process and in the completely light-adapted conditions the receptor photopigment represents an extra power supply. As a feature characteristic of the whole nervous system, the metabolic steps and the coupling processes are obtained through superimposed tangential (planar) compartments coupled by radial conductors. The oxybiotic glycolysis increases from the external plexiform layer towards the internal one. The patterns obtained are related

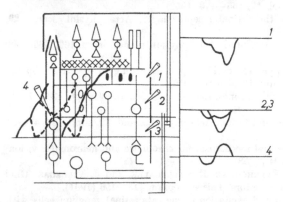

Fig. 1. Schematic drawing showing the different compartsments of the retina and the overall shape of spectral responses in each compartment, (1) — the photopic, (2—3) — the scotopic-photopic, and (4) — the chromatic. The scheme intends to reproduce the tangential and radial organizations and the convergence at a node (ganglion cell)

to many factors; among the important ones there are the physical dimensions of the stimulus and the functional metabolic organization of the retina. Two very general mechanisms seem evident: 1. the tangential one which is quantitatively related to the background illumination, working as a summation process converging the signals to the ganglion cells (Fig. 1), and 2. the straight line system representing the foveal system. In a closer correlation to the classical description of the retina, the tangential system carries scotopic and photopic brightness information (L-response) converging from recruited receptorial areas. The differentiating straight line system (C-response) works through the following patterns: in the recordings from the Müller fiber short wavelength stimuli give a hyperpolarizing response and long wave end stimuli a depolarizing response, the amacrine glial cell showing an inverse spectral dependence. In the dark-adapted state, when the system is unloaded (open loop), the responses to weak stimuli are hyperpolarizing for all wavelengths corresponding to "on" firing of the ganglion cells, while the wavelength dependent, opposite polarity response are obtained, when there is an overload of the system in the light-adapted state (closed loop), the ganglion cells fire only at "off". This type of response has been described as the chromatic C-response and it is also the one involved in black-white contrast, the contrast being more pronounced at minimal intervals between "on" and "off" discharges caused by the scanning image. This represents a fundamental process of the fovea and is considered a kind of "stiffness mechanism" of the neuronal circuits. According to these concepts the glia function as a "relaxation pump", being the slow adapting biochemical storage compartment, which represents the basic mechanism of a mnemonic control of the neuronal circuits. The past events form an important conditioning background for the instantaneous ones in a glial mechanism for facilitation and inhibition.

It is tempting to imagine the formation of the code through the following very general mechanisms: 1. a feed forward input which supplies in part the tangential glial controller making available an added duplicated signal, 2. a negative feedback which is assured through the radial Müller fiber glia which is in parallel with the conductors (this negative feedback is not identical to an output feedback; it is more similar to a feedback in the chemical sense), and 3. a time integral process,

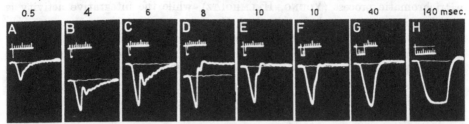

Fig. 2. Illustration of oscillatory phenomena seen in the S-potentials recorded from the light-adapted retina to certain durations of light stimuli (A—H). (Reproduced from SVAETICHIN: Acta Physiol. Scand. 1953, 29, Suppl. 106. Fig. 16)

which implies the existence of a structure for storing the information and which adds the accumulated information to the instantaneous one. In this way a progressive activation is observed as the signals accumulate, and once the balance of the system has been reached, there is a feeding into the input of a signal of opposite sign. One important problem concerning such networks is their stability. Actually, oscillations can occur either due to the "stiffness" or due to the latency delays and differences (phase component latency differences, synaptic delays or Müller fiber feedback delays). Such oscillations were often observed with short flashes (Fig. 2) or when in the experiments the excitability control of the glial networks had been reduced for instance by lack of CO_2 or after application of NH_3, cocain etc. These oscillations are normally avoided through a metabolic damping effect of the glia, which introduces a lag behind the output so as to compensate the initial delay and inhibit the neuron before the error has reached the zero value. Such a system is known as a derivative control by phase advance and retardation and it causes a cutting off of the ganglion cell firing and a differentiation of the signal with respect to time. In practice this means a glial setting of the excitability levels of the neuronal circuits.

The retina appears to be a model for the whole nervous system working as a servo-mechanism with three term controls: 1. set point, 2. additional activation related to the time integral of the signals, and 3. phase mechanism (phase advance for the correction of the delay latencies, and phase retardations identical to the initial input, which looks as a feed forward input). In the retina and generally in the whole nervous system there seems to exist a mechanism to restrain oscillations caused by threshold delays, this system being characterized by fast alternative activation at the neutral points of the opponent processes, this mechanism reminding of the "dithers" of communication systems.

The experimental findings stimulate further generalizations through comparative physiology and phylogenesis. The same organization probably exists as a decoding system of the retinal signals in the cortex, each layer of the retina approximately corresponding to a cortical one. The flow of information from the input system is converging towards nodes. The encoded signals are built up by algebraic summation and dispersion in time of the spatiotemporal patterns of the retinal areas. From the geniculate to the cortex the reverse operation represents the decoding. A highly suggestive support for these interpretations is given by the striking identity existing between the psychophysical processes described by MÜLLER, ADAMS, SCHRÖDINGER, JUDD, TALBOT, HURVICH and the spectral response curves recorded from the retinal glial cells (see Figs. 3 and 4 in SVAETICHIN et al. this conference, p. 453 implying that the receptorial input works through a trichromatic process (YOUNG, HELMHOLTZ), while the integrative activity is based on an opponent color mechanism (HERING).

Gross anatomy reveals that the central receptorial areas have the same general organization, moreover that they are spatially oriented in a three-dimensional system (sagittal, vertical and frontal). The bilateral frontal symmetry and the sagittal and caudo-cephalic assymetry introduce a cross-over of the signals with the final aspects of a doubly crossed control system where the automatic coordination takes place.

Phylogenetic studies support the above statements, since the evolution from the pre-chordal to the vertebrate shows that the nervous system is developed from a radial converging system with tonic responses, into a converging-metameric one which introduces asynchronism in the system. Thus, evolution leads from a tonic non-discriminative response to a tetanic discriminative one. Moreover, the pre-chordal branchial system seems to be closely related to metabolic control, growth, nutrition, instinctive behavoir etc. for the purpose of conservation of the individual and the species. The close connections actually observed between the branchial input and the rhinencephalic-hypothalamic centers implies the presence of important vegetative emotional and affective components in visual, auditive and olfactory sensations influencing the instinctive behavior. This is the evolutional background for the vegetative and visceral neurotic disorders (psychosomatic medicine). The primitive metabolic importance of the branchial input can be considered the base for the subjective character of sensation.

In a general view the neuronal and glial networks appear as mutual analyzers of their metabolic activities, inducing by local interactions and recruitments progressively the harmonious function of the whole collectivity of cells. Each experience appears like a stress which through the glial-neuronal networks can be compensated and so represents a gain or learning — or unfortunately not. Thus, even for the psychological processes the old physiological postulate is valid: "life is a permanent fight against death".

Summary

The S-potentials recorded from the fish retina since 1953 (SVAETICHIN) are obtained from glial satellite cells of the neurons. The characteristics of these potentials make them similar to metabolic potentials which accompany the chemical events known as sodium and potassium pumps.

On the basis of the experimental results gathered since 1953, it appears that the retinal mechanism is a model for the whole nervous system functioning as a servo mechanism with set point, phase mechanism, additional activation related to the time integral of the signal and dither mechanism for the neutral points of the opponent processes. The glial satellite cells set the excitability of the neurons, and the line of power of the servo system is represented by the glia.

Discussion

to Svaetichin, Laufer, Mitarai, J. Villegas and Vallecalle

With 1 Figure

H. Barlow: Svaetichin, Villegas and Vallecalle have been suggesting that the ionic movements of functional importance in the c.n.s. are those which occur between nerve cells and glia cells, rather than those between nerve cells and extracellular fluid. The main evidence is that under the electron microscope glia cells appear to surround the nerve cells completely, and I want to point out that such appearances can be very deceptive as far as function is concerned. In the periphery, where we know more about how the nerve cell works. The Schwann cell surrounds the axon almost everywhere: but, in myelinated axons at least, it is through that very small fraction of the total axon surface which is not surrounded by Schwann cells that the all-import inward Na^+ ion current passes during the action potential.

It looks as though the function of the Schwann cell is to prevent unnecessary ionic exchange between nerve cell and extra-cellular fluid. Perhaps this is also the function of glial cells in the c.n.s.

G. Svaetichin: Electronmicroscopy shows that no extracellular space exists in the central nervous system (Sjöstrand, De Robertis, Gloria Villegas and others). Also the myelinated axon is normaly completely covered by the Schwann cells which are analogue to glia. A free axon surface at the node of Ranvier exists only under abnormal conditions when the Schwann cells have been pulled apart in connection with the dissection etc. (Antonio Gallego, personal communication and own observations).

Recent experiments in our laboratory show (Laufer et al. and Svaetichin et al., this symposium), that the sciatic nerve kept in air or oxygen in the absence of 5% CO_2 does not function normally, and further, that isolated axons or a sciatic nerve 5—10 minutes after the opening of the peri-neuronal sheath change their behaviour. These findings agree with earlier observations of Lorente de Nó.

It is concluded that the difference in behavior depends on the functional state of the Schwann cell, and that the absence of CO_2 and also the opening of the peri-neurium brings the Schwann glia out of its normal state of function. The metabolic systems of the glial cells are apparently very sensitive to the experimental conditions, such as presence of CO_2, NH_3, temperature changes etc.

It is concluded that the Schwann glia controls metabolically the excitability of the axon; the L-Fraction of the membrane of Lorente de Nó most likely corresponds to the Schwann cell function.

When the Schwann cell does not operate, the axon behaves in agreement with the classical studies on isolated axons. The movement of ions across the axonal membrane may be different when the permeability is controlled by the metabolism of a normally functioning glial or Schwann cell.

A. Arduini: It is asked whether the volume ratio of horizontal cells is always so large as to permit the ion concentration to remain constant.

G. Svaetichin: Our preliminary interpretation (Fatehchand et al.,[1]) based on ion concentration differences might be difficult to defend. We are now inclined to explain our results on the basis of metabolic processes occurring in the glial cells.

R. Jung: Svaetichins und Vallecalles interessante Gliazellhypothese ist nicht nur für die langsamen Potentiale der Retina zu diskutieren, sondern auch von allgemeiner Bedeutung für die Hirnpotentiale des EEGs. Wenn die retinale Glia im Parallelschluß mit Neuronen und Synapsen langsame Potentiale erzeugt — und das wäre eine Revolution unseres elektrophysiologischen Denkens — so wird die Glia auch im Gehirn etwas mit den langsamen Wellen zu tun haben. Kornmüllers Postulat einer sekretorischen Funktion der Gliazellen als Ursache der Hirnpotentiale war elektrophysiologisch schwer zu verstehen, und Svaetichins

---

[1] Nature (Lond.) 189, 463 (1961).

Vorstellung erscheint einleuchtender, ist mir aber noch nicht klar genug. Die Hirnpotentiale sind nur durch geometrisch ausgedehnte, senkrecht zur Kortexoberfläche gerichtete Generatoren mit Dipolcharakter zu erklären, wie die präsynaptischen Fasern und Dendriten. Wenn die Glia langsame Potentiale erzeugen soll, die wie Retinogramm und EEG Dipol- und Vektorcharakter haben und in weiter Entfernung nachweisbar sind, so müßten ausgedehnte, parallel orientierte Gliastrukturen, ähnlich den Spitzendendriten, vorhanden sein. Anatomisch findet sich aber im Cortex ein Gestrüpp von Gliazellen und dies wäre für die Produktion gerichteter Potentiale wenig geeignet, da die größten Gliazellen, die Astrocyten, eine allseits radiäre Struktur haben. Den retinalen Müllerzellen ähnliche gleichgerichtete Glia-Elemente finden sich ähnlich den Schwann-Zellen nur um die Nervenfasern, und diese sind mehr in der weißen Substanz als im Cortex parallel orientiert. Die größten langsamen Potentiale kommen aber gerade nicht aus der weißen Substanz, sondern aus dem Cortex. Zur Erklärung der langsamen Cortexpotentiale müßte man dann einen parallelgeschalteten Gliaapparat um die Dendriten und präsynaptischen Nervenendigungen annehmen.

Wenn die Rolle der Glia in der Retina sichergestellt ist und Parallelschaltung mit den neuronalen, Elementen Transmembranpotentiale und Elektrolytverhältnisse geklärt sind, müssen wir uns auch ernstlich mit diesen Fragen im ZNS befassen. Über Einzelheiten der retinalen Receptorpotentiale werden GRÜSSER und SVAETICHIN heute abend diskutieren (vgl. S. 56 ff).

P. GLEES: I have 2 comments: 1. Although the individual Müller neuroglia cell reaches through the whole length of the retina no similar expanded glia cell reaches from the ventricular wall or from the white matter to the surface of the brain. In the cortex we have a multiple arrangement of smaller glia cells which however seal the surface of the brain in a continous limiting membrane. Therefore the conditions in the retina cannot be analogue to the glial arrangement in the cortex.

2. Dr. VILLEGAS' and SVAETICHIN's pictures show the virtual absence of extracellular spaces in the retina, confirming the electronmicroscopical studies of the cerebral cortex. His news that neuroglial elements in the retina such as Müller's fibres can be attributed with the fact of electrolyte movements deserve special and general attention as this would mean that neuroglia represent the extracellular "spaces" for neurones. This would demand special metabolic requirements of neuroglia as electrolytes have to be pumped in or out of neuroglial membranes and electrolytes are not freely available extracellularly.

G. SVAETICHIN (to JUNG and GLEES): ACHUCARRO described in the nervous system syncytial glial networks which he considered of functional importance. Electronmicroscopy shows membrane to membrane connected gliacells, which form continuous radial and tangential nets in the retina. Our experiments demonstrate a spreading of the S-potential in these glial networks. The findings may possibly explain the large extension of the cortical electrical dipoles if we assume that the glial networks are working together with the neurons; these structures may also be the sources of the brain waves.

It has to be pointed out that dehydration after histological fixation causes a tremendous shrinkage of the gliacells. Our experience is that freezing sectioning of fixated material without subsequent dehydration is most favorable for studying of the glial structures in the light microscope.

(to GLEES): For Dr. GLEERS second question I refer to the discussion of VILLEGAS and SJÖSTRAND. Apparently the glianeuron double membrane can be considered functionally as one asymetrical membrane without apparent extracellular space. The demonstrated electronmicrographs are all from the work of Dr. GLORIA VILLEGAS, and it is of course not surprising to find that the ultrastructure of the retina and cortex is practically identical.

Further, we do agree with the general statements of Prof. GLEES.

K. O. DONNER: Comparing SVAETICHIN's results with those on neuronal discharges and antagonistic on-off-curves there seems to be a difference in Svaetichin's C-response in different states of adaptation and no direct relation between the potentials recorded by SVAETICHIN and the impulse frequencies, recorded by WOLBARSHT, DE VALOIS and others. I don't know, if rod activity has been well controlled in all these cases and some of the results may be explained by rod-cone antagonism, which may have nothing to do with colour vision.

G. SVAETICHIN: For the relations of C-responses to the generation of impulses in different adaptational states and also interaction of rods and cones the paper by MITARAI et al. in this symposion gives most of the answers which are possible at our present stage of knowledge.

D. HURVICH-JAMESON: In Dr. SVAETICHIN's remarks he suggests that in the retina the large cells carry brightness information and the small cells carry color information and visual acuity. I do not understand the assumed separation between brightness information and acuity, since acuity for achromatic patterns depends on the gradient of brightness information in the image. The cells assumed to respond to brightness must therefore be involved in visual acuity in terms of the difference in brightness information from one image area to the rest.

G. SVAETICHIN: This is a speculation, but it is reasonable to assume that the spatial interaction in the retina (black-white, wavelength, visual acuity) is taken care of by the small ganglion cells in cooperation with the Müller fibers and glial amacrine cells, while the brightness information involves the large ganglion cells with widely spread dendritic arborisations. At low level illumination the dark adapted retina mainly shows summation in space and time and poor discriminative function.

The spatial interaction of the glia-neuron system develops and sharpens with the log intensity increase of illumination, while the spike frequency of the large ganglion cells which carry the brightness information also is proportional to the log intensity of light.

O.-J. GRÜSSER: Die von Dr. SVAETICHIN beschriebenen *Submaxima* in der spektralen Empfindlichkeit der intraretinalen Potentiale sind überraschend, wenn man berücksichtigt, daß der Zerfall eines oder mehrerer Photopigmente die spektrale Empfindlichkeit dieser Potentiale bestimmt. Die bisher bekannten Photopigmente haben „glatte" Absorptionskurven. Könnten die Submaxima nicht auch durch die Konstruktion des Spektralfilterrades bedingt sein, bei dem die Abstände relativ zu den max-Werten der Filter angebracht sind? Aus technischen Gründen sind daher die zeitlichen Abstände der verschiedenen Farbreize nicht gleich. Da die Potentialhöhe der intraretinalen langsamen Potentiale jedoch vom vorausgehenden Dunkelintervall abhängig ist, könnte so das Auftreten von Submaxima in der Konstruktion der Reizanordnung begründet sein.

G. SVAETICHIN (zu GRÜSSER): Die Submaxima unserer spektralen Antwortkurven können aus folgenden Gründen keine Artefakte unseres Lichtreizgerätes sein: Wir haben einen neuen sorgfältig getesteten Photostimulator benutzt (vgl. S. 464) bei dem die Abstände zwischen den Interferenzfiltern konstant waren, und wir haben diese Submaxima damit noch exakter bestimmt. Folgende Spektralregionen zeigen solche Maxima: 420, 440, 470, 540, 590, 650 und 690 mμ.

Bei den spectral response curves der C- und L-Typen verschiedener Tierarten finden sich die Submaxima in den gleichen Spektralregionen. Diese Spitzen korrelieren erstaunlich gut mit den Submaxima des menschlichen Sehens (SPERLINGs psychophysische Messungen, COPENHAVER und ARMINGTONs ERG-Registrierungen, RUSHTONs und WHEALEs Photopigmentmessungen). Wir glauben, daß diese Photopigmente wichtige Komponenten des cellulären Atmungssystems sind (Carotine, Hämocroteine). Dies stimmt überein mit früheren Hinweisen von ARVANITAKI-CHALAZONITIS und SIR RAMAN. Unsere Experimente zeigen, daß die elektrische Aktivität der Zapfen (entsprechend P_3 des ERG) sofort durch sehr kleine Mengen von Cyanid aufgehoben wird.

Schließlich ist noch zu sagen, daß die Organisation der Gegenfarbenpotentiale auch durch verschiedene Gliasysteme kompliziert wird. Die Zapfenpotentiale selbst zeigen zwar im Gegensatz zu unseren früheren Vorstellungen keine Umkehr bei Komplementärfarben, sondern gleiche Polarität mit verschiedenen Maxima bei Lichteinwirkung verschiedener Spektralfarben (vgl. Abb. S. 453). Erst nach der Glia-Neuronverarbeitung dieser photochemischen Eingangsprozesse entstehen die beiden Polaritäten der Gegenfarben, wobei wiederum Blau-gelb (B-y) und Gelb-blau (Y-b)-Typen zu unterscheiden sind, wie die Abb. 3D, E, S. 453 zeigt; wahrscheinlich gibt es auch Verschiebungen im Rot-grün-Bereich bei anderen Species.

Abb. 1 zeigt einen solchen verschobenen Neutralpunkt von einer anderen Zentropomiden-Fischart in verschiedener Gliazellen. Die Bedeutung dieser umgekehrten Potentiale „Rg" und „Gr" ist noch nicht völlig geklärt. Sicher ist nur, daß sie in verschiedenen Tiefen der Retina vorkommen. Abb. 3 und 4 auf S. 453 geben die beste Übersicht über die verblüffenden Korrelationen, die sich zwischen Gliazellregistrierungen der Fisch-Retina (Abb. 3) und den psychophysischen Messungen beim Menschen (Abb. 4) gefunden haben. Sie entsprechen etwa den Voraussagen von G. E. MÜLLERs Theorie von 1924, der nach psychophysischen Ergebnissen diese Struktur des Farbsystems in verschiedenen Schichten der Retina vorausgesagt hat.

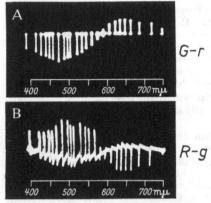

Fig. 1. Spectral response curves showing opposite polarities recorded from 2 different glia cells in the isolated fish retina. Depolarizing responses are upwards in both records. A: short wave hyperpolarization (in green), G-r long wave hyperpolarization (in red). R-g Hyperpolarization corresponds to on-firing in the correlated ganglion cells

Dies ist wiederum ein Beispiel dafür, daß die subjektive Sinnesphysiologie der Neurophysiologie wichtige Anregungen geben kann.

G. SVAETICHIN u. E. VALLECALLE (Schlußwort): Es ist sehr verlockend, die Konzeption der Glia-Neuron-Wechselwirkung, die wir nach Beobachtungen in Retina, Spinalganglien und myelinisierten Nerven entwickelt haben, zu verallgemeinern. Eine Anwendung auf die Hirnpotentiale und die Funktionsmechanismen des ZNS bietet sich als Erstes an, wie wir in unserem letzten Vortrag und in der Diskussion mit JUNG und GLEES ausgeführt haben. Jedoch hat die Erklärung der durch die Glia regulierten elektrobiologischen Phänomene noch große Interpretationsschwierigkeiten, weil man sie noch nicht mit den heute gültigen Ionen-Theorien widerspruchslos vereinigen kann.

Die verspätete Einsendung unserer Mitteilungen auf diesem Symposion war hierdurch mitbegründet. Wir mußten unsere Ansichten erst durch neue Experimente bestätigen, modifizieren und klären.

Unsere ersten Erklärungsversuche der Gliazellpotentiale gingen davon aus, die Glia einfach als extraneuronales Ionencompartement anzusehen [FATEHCHAND et al.: Nature 189, 463—464 (1961)]. Diese auf dem Symposion mehrfach diskutierte Erklärung mußte nun durch eine andere Interpretation ersetzt werden, die durch eine große Zahl experimenteller Ergebnisse gestützt ist: Danach haben die Gliazellen eine Stoffwechselkontrolle über die Erregbarkeit der Neurone (metabolic excitability control of the neurons). Wir haben in unseren obigen Arbeiten gezeigt, wie in der Retina die glialen Reaktionen von einer Zelle zur nächsten, innerhalb des retinalen Glia-Netzwerks sich ausbreiten und dadurch die Erregbarkeit der Neurone beeinflussen. Der Dipolcharakter der corticalen Potentiale, den Prof. JUNG erwähnt hat, könnte erklärt werden, wenn man eine enge Wechselwirkung zwischen Neuronen und Glia-Netzwerk annimmt. Ferner zeigt sich, daß die glialen Membranpotentiale Oscillationen zeigen, die den sog. Hirnwellen ähneln. Diese oscillierende Aktivität, die sich im Gliazell-Netzwerk ausbreitet, erzeugt wiederum rhythmische synchronisierte Erregbarkeitsänderungen im corticalen Neuronensystem. Nach unseren Untersuchungen haben wir den Eindruck, daß die Neurone und ihre Synapsen, ebenso wie die Receptoren ausschließlich Erregungsträger sind und daß ihre Erregbarkeit, einschließlich aller Hemmungen metabolisch durch die Glia-Netze kontrolliert werden. Die Gliazellen bilden wahrscheinlich die „Programm-Engramm-Einheit" des Nervensystems, wenn wir dieses als eine große Rechenmaschine ansehen. KORNMÜLLERs Vorstellungen über die Erregungs- und Hemmungskontrolle der Glia-Satelliten auf die Nervenzelle zeigen somit gewisse Ähnlichkeiten mit den Deutungen, zu denen wir auf Grund unserer Retina-Experimente gelangt sind. Es bedarf aber noch vieler Arbeit, bis man diese Deutungen auch im ZNS experimentell nachweisen kann.

Namenverzeichnis

Die **fett** gedruckten Seitenzahlen bezeichnen den Beginn der Hauptreferate, die durch (Disk.) ergänzten Seitenzahlen den Beginn der Diskussionsbemerkungen

Die normal gedruckten Seitenzahlen weisen auf Zitate innerhalb des Textes, die *kursiv* gedruckten Seitenzahlen auf Literaturzitate hin

Sachverzeichnis

Printed in the United States
by Baker & Taylor Publisher Services

Printed in the United States
by Baker & Taylor Publisher Services